Stroke

Stroke

A Clinical Approach
Second Edition

Louis R. Caplan, M.D.

Professor and Chairman, Department of Neurology, Tufts University School of Medicine; Neurologist-in-Chief and Chairman, Department of Neurology, New England Medical Center, Boston, Massachusetts
Former Professor of Neurology, University of Chicago Pritzker School of Medicine, Chicago, Illinois

With a Foreword by *C. Miller Fisher*, *M.D.*, Professor of Neurology Emeritus, Harvard Medical School, Boston, Massachusetts

Illustrations by *Juan Sanchez-Ramos*, *M.D.*, *Ph.D.*, Assistant Professor of Neurology, University of Miami School of Medicine, Miami, Florida

Butterworth–Heinemann
Boston   London   Oxford   Singapore   Sydney   Toronto   Wellington

Every effort has been made to ensure that the drug dosage
schedules within this text are accurate and conform to standards
accepted at time of publication. However, as treatment recommendations vary in the light of continuing research and clinical
experience, the reader is advised to verify drug dosage schedules
herein with information found on product information sheets.
This is especially true in cases of new or infrequently used drugs.

 Recognizing the importance of preserving what has been written,
it is the policy of Butterworth–Heinemann to have the books it
publishes printed on acid-free paper, and we exert our best efforts
to that end.

Library of Congress Cataloging-in-Publication Data

Caplan, Louis R.
 Stroke : a clinical approach / Louis R. Caplan , with a
foreword by C. Miller Fisher ; illustrations by Juan Sanchez-
Ramos. — 2nd ed.
  p. cm.
 Includes bibliographical references and index.
 ISBN 0–7506–9181–6 (alk. paper)
 1. Cerebrovascular disease. I. Title.
 [DNLM: 1. Cerebrovascular Disorders—diagnosis.
2. Cerebrovascular Disorders—therapy. WL 355 C244s]
RC388.5.C33 1993
616.8'1—dc20
DNLM/DLC
for Library of Congress   92–49251

British Library Cataloguing-in-Publication Data

A catalogue record for this book is available from the British
Library.

Butterworth–Heinemann
80 Montvale Avenue
Stoneham, MA 02180

10 9 8 7 6 5 4 3 2 1

Printed in the United States of America

Contents

Foreword

Advances in the understanding, diagnosis, and treatment of cerebrovascular disease continue to flow from clinics in North America, Europe, and Japan. This highly complex field has become a demanding specialty within the domain of neurology. Unfortunately, no two stroke cases are the same, and we are reminded of the observation of a London cockney that "there ain't more than one average Englishman in a hundred." To know one's way in this intricate endeavor requires very special knowledge and experience. A fine appreciation of the practical nuances calls for a Stradivarian clinical skill. Simplified discourse is precluded.

In this volume, Dr. Caplan addresses these needs as he presents an unusually complete and admirably balanced account of the clinical and pathological aspects of the many different types of cerebrovascular disorder. The stamp of the master clinician, the in-depth expert, is evident in its pages. Moreover, the appropriate use of the most modern investigative technologies is discussed in detail. Each subject is covered in a clear, uncomplicated way. Retaining the essential while excluding the irrelevant, this unique textbook reflects the author's special interest and long involvement in cerebrovascular disease. Current relevant facts are offered in such abundance that the reader is afforded the genuine prospect of becoming an instant mini-expert.

The ultimate goal, of course, is the prevention of strokes, and the promised land is increasingly discernible. At medical rounds I recently expressed to internists the admonition that if a patient of theirs has a stroke, the physician should be regarded as at fault. The statement, although exaggerated, phrased the challenge in the correct perspective; it did not fall on deaf ears. Control of hypertension, anticoagulation of atrial fibrillators, auscultation for carotid bruits, proscription of tobacco, institution of antiatherosclerosis measures, heeding of TIAs, treatment of early symptoms as an emergency, and other measures give promise of conquering stroke. The crucial front-line anti-stroke thrust is in the hands of the patient's personal physician. It is the neurologist's task to instruct and advise. Front-line physicians will find that in his treatise Dr. Caplan has spelled out the rationale for their essential contribution.

C. MILLER FISHER

Preface

Now here you see, it takes all the running you can do just to keep in the same place.

Queen of Chess, in *Through the Looking Glass*, by Lewis Carroll

To present medicine in terms that will make the reader work—to present puzzles like those which confront us at the bedside, and then to offer at the end of each case my own solution of these puzzles—is the plan pursued. We learn by that which makes us work, not by any attempt to present truth as a free gift.

Richard C. Cabot, *Case Histories in Medicine*, third edition, Wm Leonard, Boston, 1928

Six years have passed since the first edition of *Stroke: A Clinical Approach* was published. The time is ripe for a second edition. There are three major motives for a rewrite. First, much has changed since 1985, when the first edition was written. Stroke has become an increasingly fertile field for basic and clinical research. There are now more neurologists and other clinicians specializing in the care of stroke patients. More data, more reports, more publications, more meetings, and more stroke-related research have been issued in the past 5 years than during any comparable past period of time. Technology has also advanced dramatically. Magnetic resonance imaging (MRI), magnetic resonance angiography (MRA), transcranial Doppler (TCD), and single photon emission computed tomography (SPECT) were unknown or in their infancy at the time of the first edition. Ultrasound technologies have improved greatly and are now commonplace in most hospitals in North America and much of Europe. Echocardiography and other technologies for diagnosing cardiac lesions and rhythm abnormalities have also advanced dramatically. Other technologies—such as digital venous subtraction angiography (DVSA), oculoplethysmography (OPG), and measurements of cerebral blood flow by inhalation of radioactive xenon, to mention only a few—have disappeared or have become greatly deemphasized. New, potentially powerful, treatment modalities, such as recombinant tissue plasminogen activator (rTPA) and percutaneous intravascular angioplasty, have surfaced and are being tested. The changes are so vast that, like the Queen of Chess in the preceding quotation, most of us must run hard simply to keep pace with progress in the field. If it is difficult for stroke experts and researchers to keep up, imagine how impossible it must be for those not specializing in stroke. I therefore wanted to bring the material more up to date with present knowledge and clinical practice.

A second reason for a rewrite is that seldom does anyone get things just right the first time. My own clinical rereading of the text, as well as critiques and reviews by others, clearly uncovered inadequacies and flaws in the first edition. I felt that a second try would make the book better. Many readers criticized the diagrammatic artist's representations of imaging tests and radiographs in the first edition. Also, the first writing did not include discussions of stroke in the young, stroke and cerebrovascular disease in surgical patients, or spinal-cord strokes. These omissions have been corrected. Other areas have been expanded and modified to make the coverage more complete.

Third, the authorship of this book has changed. The first edition was written with the great help of Dr. Robert Stein, who was then first a stroke fellow and later a junior faculty member at the Michael Reese Hospital, University of Chicago, with me. Since then, he has left academia for the attractions of clinical practice in an idyllic spot on the coast of Maine. Continuing to write the book in collaboration would have been difficult and would have greatly lengthened the production time. His contributions have been sorely missed. The idea for the first edition was his, and his absence has increased my work considerably. Single authorship, however, has made the style, writing, and philosophy more uniform and even.

The second edition, like the first, has as its major aim to convey an approach to the patient with cerebrovascular disease. Data sharing and didactic writing do not always translate into better care. I have kept and even expanded in this edition the use of cases as a teaching method. As Cabot (the founder of the Cabot cases—the clinicopathological conferences in the *New England Journal of Medicine*) said (in a statement preceding the quotation cited at the beginning of this preface), having the reader puzzle over the patient sets the wheels of thinking and learning in motion, and it increases the yield to the reader. For more than a decade, I and my colleagues have used real stroke cases as the major means of teaching at annual courses of the American Academy of Neurology. Actively thinking about the case definitely augments learning and is preferred over pure didactic exposition.

The general organization of the first edition has been retained. In Part I, on general principles, I have added an introductory chapter that emphasizes the importance of stroke and that attempts to place our present knowledge and approach into historical perspective. Readers cannot grasp fully where the present state of knowledge is and where it is going unless they have a general idea of where it has been. I have rearranged the order of the next chapters in this section. Now, basic pathology, anatomy, and patho-physiology are considered first. These basic foundation topics rightfully should precede a discussion of diagnosis. In the first edition, the diagnosis chapter appeared first, to catch the readers' interest. However, putting the cart before the horse only made the discussion more difficult to write and harder for the reader to follow. The section on pathophysiology has been greatly expanded. This prepares the reader better for discussions on the rationale for diagnostic testing strategies and treatment, and it clarifies the questions to be asked and answered. The chapters on laboratory diagnosis and on treatment have been nearly completely rewritten, using a problem-oriented approach and bringing the material up to date.

In Part II, the major meat of the book, which covers the various stroke mechanisms, syndromes, and problems, I have added new chapters on stroke in children and young adults, spinal-cord strokes, and strokes and cerebro-vascular disease in patients who have had surgery or in whom surgery is con-templated or already planned. I also have expanded all of the other chapters in this section, adding more detailed and newer information. Part III, on stroke prevention, complications, and rehabilitation, has not been greatly modified. These topics, although very important, are not the major focus of this book. The main theme is the approach to the patient with acute stroke. I could not omit entirely discussions of prevention and rehabilitation, so these chapters are brief and attempt to emphasize succinctly the key salient points. A fuller discussion of complications would venture into the entire field of internal medicine.

In addition to those individuals who helped make the first edition possible, I want to acknowledge and thank others that have directly or in-directly influenced this writing. Especially important have been my stroke fellows at Tufts—Drs. Dana DeWitt, Ken Ho, Nicolle Danault, Ed Feldmann, Conrad Estol, Barbara Tettenborn, Frank LaFranchise, Phil Teal, and Axel Rosengart. My colleagues on the New England Medical Center Stroke Service—Drs. Michael Pessin and Dana DeWitt—have been indis-pensable. Drs. Sam Wolpert, Eddie Kwan, and Mary Anderson helped select and interpret radiographic material. Other individuals at Tufts—Drs. Allen Ropper, Bruce Ehrenberg, Ed Bromfield, John Kelly, Paul Rosman (neu-rology), Tom O'Donnell, Bill Mackey, Mike Belkin (vascular surgery), Deeb Salem, Herb Levine, Nat Pandyan (cardiology), Bruce Furie (coagulation hematology)—have been very helpful. Colleagues elsewhere in North America and Europe have helped me to develop ideas and philosophies and deserve my recognition and gratitude. These individuals include Drs. C. Mil-ler Fisher, H. J. Barnett, J. P. Mohr, Tony Furlan, Carlos Kase, Mark Fisher, Harold Adams, Jose Biller, Mark Dyken, Don Easton, Steve Levine, Bob Ackerman, Phil Kistler, Mac Reinmuth, Michael Hennerici, Julian Bogousslavsky, Werner Hacke, J. C. Gautier, M-G Boussel, Pierre Amarenco, Jan van Gijn, and many others. Most of all, thanks are due to the stroke patients who have taught me so much and to whom I am eternally indebted. I hope and pray that this book in some small measure helps in the care of future stroke patients.

LOUIS R. CAPLAN, M.D.
Boston, Massachusetts

Preface to the First Edition

Stroke is a very common, yet complex, entity. The third leading cause of death in the United States, it is also an important cause of prolonged morbidity. The past decade has witnessed an explosion of new diagnostic technologies capable of unraveling abnormal cerebral anatomy and function, as well as the structure and function of the brain's vascular supply. New treatment strategies and techniques have proliferated.

Unfortunately, this revolution in technology and neuroscience has left a communication gap between the physician–scientists at academic centers, where the new data are being generated, and the practitioners who care for stroke patients. Most advances have been published in specialty scientific journals. When information is gathered into book form, the result has often been multiauthored compendia that emphasize the complexities, uncertainties, and controversies in stroke diagnosis and treatment. These larger volumes present diverse material from many authors with different views, sometimes without a guiding hand to organize the huge mass of data and lead the clinician through the labyrinth. No wonder many physicians, especially nonneurologists, feel lost in this maze of technology and controversy!

This is a book by clinicians, aimed primarily at physicians who care for patients with stroke. It has three important features that we hope distinguish it from other stroke compendia and legitimize its existence: (1) It is written entirely by two authors and describes a single approach to the stroke patient. (2) It is a "how-to" manual that describes a practical approach to the evaluation, diagnosis, and treatment of the stroke patient. (3) It incorporates, wherever possible, data and strategies gained from our experience with the Harvard and Michael Reese stroke registries and the National Stroke Data Bank. Our goal has been to interpret and organize the newer advances into practical terms referable to the daily care of stroke patients. The book is intended as a manual for the general practitioner, internist, or surgeon confronted with stroke patients and for the medical student and house officer in training. We hope it may prove useful as a general framework or modus operandi for the neurologist, neurosurgeon, or vascular surgeon who does not specialize in stroke.

Part I presents general information and considerations, including bedside and laboratory diagnosis; a brief review of cerebral anatomy, pathology, and pathophysiology; and principles of treatment. Part II, the core of the book, discusses specific stroke subtypes. The essentials of clinical presentation, diagnosis, and treatment are discussed for the various types of occlusive disease, cerebral embolism, hypoxic–ischemic encephalopathy, and hemorrhagic disorders. Part III briefly considers prevention, complications, and rehabilitation.

The book is pragmatic and details a unified, rational approach to diagnosis and treatment. It is not meant to be a repository of definitive and balanced knowledge, hypotheses, and concepts. Basic science and laboratory data are included only when they contribute to the understanding and practical management of the stroke patient. We briefly introduce the physician to computer logic in an attempt to make the approach to stroke more systematic and measurable. Whenever possible, we include quantitative data from our own stroke registry experience, most of it previously unpublished, to allow estimation of probabilities. Of course, certainty in stroke is the exception and not the rule. Where no solid scientific data exist to guide management in a particular situation, we explain what we do and why. In the chapters on specific stroke syndromes, we use the case analysis method, which closely mimics the usual clinical situation and is easier to digest than didactic exposition. We also translate applications of the newer technologies into simple, pragmatic, utilitarian advice for the clinician. All figures, including illustrations of radiological findings, are presented as drawings rather than photographs, in order to highlight the appearance of the various lesions that occur in stroke patients. References are limited to essential work and are not meant to be exhaustive. At times, original classic sources have been chosen, rather than the most recent work, in an effort to acquaint the reader with the richness of the stroke literature.

We wish to thank the teachers, colleagues, and students who made this book possible. Distinction between student and teacher is always artificial, even transparent, since the best teachers are eternal students who ably share their zest and style of learning, and our students teach us more than we know. Drs. Derek Denny-Brown, Walle Nauta, C. Miller Fisher, Raymond D. Adams, Flaviau Romanul, and H. Richard Tyler are probably most responsible for kindling and nurturing the senior author's interest in the nervous system and stroke. Many colleagues merit our special thanks: those at Boston's Beth Israel Hospital, especially Drs. Chaim Mayman, Nicholas Zervas, and Arthur Rosenbaum; coworkers in the Harvard Stroke Registry, especially Drs. J. P. Mohr and Howard Bleich; colleagues at the Michael Reese Hospital, especially Drs. Daniel Hier, Allan Burke, James Goodwin, Morris Fisher, Lonnie Amico, Larry Ferguson, Gerry Luken, Gerry Moss, Steve Gould, Dushyant Patel, and Masoud Hemmati; colleagues at the New

England Medical Center, especially Drs. Michael Pessin, L. Dana DeWitt, R. Michael Scott, William Shucart, and Samuel Wolpert; former Stroke Fellows Drs. Elizabeth Zaraspe-Yoo, Phil Gorelick, Cathy Helgason, and Michael Kelly, and all the resident physicians who worked with us at the Harvard Medical School, the University of Chicago, and Tufts University.

LOUIS R. CAPLAN
ROBERT W. STEIN
Boston, Massachusetts

Stroke

PART I

General Principles

CHAPTER 1

Introduction and Perspective

It was then that it happened. To my shock and incredulity, I could not speak. That is, I could utter nothing intelligible. All that would come from my lips was the sound *ab* which I repeated again and again. . . . Then as I watched it, the telephone handpiece slid slowly from my grasp, and I, in turn, slid slowly from my chair and landed on the floor behind the desk. . . . At 5:15 in that January dusk I had been a person; now at 6:45 I was a case. But I found it easy to accept my altered condition. I felt like a case.

Eric Hodgins[1]

Cheshire puss. . . . Would you tell me please which way I ought to go from here? That depends a great deal on where you want to get to, said the cat. I don't much care where, said Alice. Then it doesn't matter which way you go, said the cat. So long as I get somewhere, Alice added. Oh, you're sure to do that, said the cat, if you only walk long enough.

Lewis Carroll[2]

The past is always with us, never to be escaped; it alone is enduring; but amidst the changes and chances which succeed one another so rapidly in life, we are apt to live too much for the present and too much in the future.

William Osler[3]

Numbers

In the United States, about 500,000 individuals have a stroke and 150,000 die from stroke each year, and about 2 million stroke survivors are living in the United States at any one time.[4] For a very long time, stroke has been the third leading cause of death in the United States and in many other countries, surpassed as a killer only by heart disease and cancer. Strokes are an even more important cause of both short-term and prolonged disability. Survivors of a stroke are often unable to return to work or to assume their former effectiveness as citizens, spouses, friends, and parents. The economic cost of stroke is enormous. The American Heart Association estimated that in 1989 alone, the cost of stroke was approximately $13.5 billion.[4] This figure included the cost of physician and nursing care, hospital and nursing-home services, the cost of medications and other treatments, and lost productivity because of disability.

Important Medical and Historical Figures Who Had a Stroke

The history of the world has undoubtedly been altered by stroke. Many important innovators in science, medicine, and politics have had their productivity cut prematurely short by stroke. Marcello Malpighi, one of the early microscopists, discoverer of capillaries and the microscopic anatomy of the lungs, kidneys, and spleen, died of an apoplectic right hemiplegia.[5] Louis Pasteur, at age 46, had a left hemiparesis, although he continued to make important advances until additional strokes impaired his function at age 65.[5]

Three important figures in twentieth-century neurology—Russell Dejong,[6] the first editor of the journal *Neurology;* Raymond Escourolle, the great French neuropathologist; and Houston Merritt, longtime Columbia professor and writer of Merritt's *Neurology*—were badly disabled by multiple strokes in their later years. Two of the most important political figures of the early twentieth century, Vladimir Lenin and Woodrow Wilson, had intellectual impairment due to stroke while they were at the helms of their countries in critical times in history. Lenin, at age 52, had the sudden onset of dysarthria and right hemiparesis. An observer noted that "often as he spoke, the words were slurred, and he paused several times like a man who has lost the thread of his argument."[5] Wilson, the architect of the League of Nations, had a series of small strokes that left him pseudobulbar and with a left hemiparesis at a time that he was ardently working for world peace and cooperation. The heads of state who met at Yalta and elsewhere to divide up the spheres of influence after World War II—Franklin Roosevelt, Winston Churchill, and Josef Stalin—were, at the time, suffering from severe cerebrovascular disease.[7] Roosevelt subsequently died of a fatal stroke after years of very severe hypertension.[8] Who knows how history might have been different if the brains of our leaders had not been addled by stroke.

The Personal Tragedy of Stroke

The mortality, morbidity, and economic toll of stroke is very impressive. Knowledge that our leaders and heroes may have brains damaged and even riddled with brain infarcts and hemorrhages is undoubtedly very sobering. Yet even more important, in my own opinion, is the effect of stroke on the individual victim. What could be worse than to suddenly become unable to speak, move a limb, stand, walk, see, read, feel, write, or think? The loss of function is often instantaneous and totally unanticipated; impairments may be transient or permanent, slight or devastating. The first common term for stroke, *apoplexy*, literally meant, in Greek, "struck suddenly with violence."[9] Stroke patients tell us graphically about the personal tragedy of their illness. Eric Hodgins, the popular author of *Mr. Blandings Builds His Dream House*, wrote an autobiographical account of his stroke, which he titled *Episode*, from which I quoted at the beginning of this chapter.[1] He changed from a functioning human in one moment to a helpless, dumb invalid, "a case," in the next. Imagine an articulate author dependent for his livelihood on his use of language being totally unable to speak. Surely, the brain is wholly responsible for intelligence, capability, character, wit, humor, personality, and most of the characteristics that make us recognizable as individuals and as humans. Losing brain function can be dehumanizing and often places individuals in very dependent situations. For these reasons, most individuals fear stroke more than any other disease, with the possible exception of cancer. All of us would like to exit this life with our capabilities and minds intact, despite the inevitable aging of our bodies.

When I conjure in my own mind the personal tragedy of stroke, I picture one of my own patients, Herman Blumgart, an extremely gifted physician, teacher, and investigator. He was, for many years, physician-in-chief at the Beth Israel Hospital in Boston.[10] His early investigations in coronary artery disease were landmark advances in our understanding of vascular disease of the heart.[11,12] Yearly, he gave the introductory lecture to incoming Harvard Medical School students about the joys and responsibilities of being a physician. I recall his vivid, very articulate lectures and bedside demonstrations. He was, in many ways, the model physician. He was also a very vocal advocate on behalf of patients. His lecture "Caring for the Patient," presented in 1963 and reported in the *New England Journal of Medicine*, remains a model exposition on doctoring, as valid today as when it was originally delivered.[13] Tragically, this master of communication was rendered, in an instant, severely aphasic. His Wernicke-type aphasia was so severe that he could barely communicate verbally his basic needs and could hardly understand the queries and spoken and written statements of others. He could no longer read, eliminating one of his lifelong joys. As a junior staff neurologist, I was one of his physicians. The angst and frustration of his plight was written clearly on his face each time I saw him. This personal disaster was more palpable and dramatic for me than even the Shakespearean depictions of the tragic figures of Hamlet and Lear. There, but for the grace of God, go I, and of course, go all of us.

A Brief History of Stroke

In any human endeavor, the future is influenced and colored by the past. As the Wonderland dialogue between Alice and the Cheshire Cat (cited at the beginning of this chapter) teaches, where you are going depends a great deal on where you have been and where you want to go.[2] Osler, and most other important medical innovators, were very aware of their debt to history and of their inevitable entanglement with the past as well as the present and future.[3] Herein is only a very sketchy review of some important people and milestones, to convey a sense of the historical context of the present state of knowledge and ignorance in the field of stroke. Of course, the following view of history is eclectic, biased, and very personal and should be clearly recognized as such.

Hippocrates (circa 400 B.C.) was probably the first to write about the medical aspects of stroke.[5,9] He and his followers were mostly interested in *prognosis*, predicting for the patient and family the outcome of an illness.[14] Hippocrates was a keen observer, and he urged careful observation and recording of phenomenology. Hippocrates wrote in his aphorisms on apoplexy, "persons are most subject to apoplexy between the ages of forty and sixty,"[15] and attacks of numbness might reflect "impending apoplexy."[9] He astutely noted, "when persons in good health are suddenly seized with pains in the head and straightaway are laid down speechless and breathe with stertor, they die in seven days when fever comes on."[5,16] This description of subarachnoid hemorrhage shows the Hippocratic emphasis on observation and prognosis. Hippocrates also observed that there were many blood vessels connected to the brain most of which were "thin," but two (the carotid arteries) were stout. The Greeks recognized that interruption of these blood vessels to the brain could cause loss of consciousness, and so they named the arteries *carotid*, from the Greek word *Karos*, meaning "deep sleep."

A few hundred years after Hippocrates, *Galen* (131–201 A.D.) described the anatomy of the brain and its blood vessels from dissections of animals. Although his early writings emphasized observation and experimentation, much of his later works combined mostly theorizing and speculation, in which he attributed disease to a disequilibrium between putative body humors and secretions, such as water, blood, phlegm, bile, and so forth.[14] Galen and his voluminous writings dominated the 1300 years following his death. Thus, during the ensuing Dark and Middle Ages, persons who called themselves physicians gained their knowledge solely from studying the Galenic texts, considered at the time to be the epitome of all medical wisdom. Dissection, experimentation, and personal observations were discouraged and not considered scholarly.

Andreas Vesalius (1514–1564) challenged the Galenic tradition by dissecting humans and relying on his own personal observations instead of Galen's writings. Vesalius could not find the rete mirabile of blood vessels that Galen had described (presumably in a lower animal). Vesalius's dissections were published in a volume entitled *De Humani Corpis Fabrica* (usually referred to as the *Fabrica*), which contained the detailed drawings his young artist and collaborator Jan Kalkar reproduced as woodcuts and copper plates.[5,17] The seventh book of the *Fabrica* contains 15 diagrams of a brain.

These were the most detailed neuroanatomical studies up to that time.[5] By all accounts, Vesalius had a great flair for lecturing and teaching, and his works and personage stimulated much interest in anatomy.[14]

During the last half of the seventeenth century, two important physicians, *Johann Jakob Wepfer* (1620–1695) and *Thomas Willis* (1621–1675), made further anatomical and clinical observations. Wepfer wrote a popular treatise on apoplexy, which was originally published in 1658 and had five subsequent editions.[5,18] Wepfer performed meticulous examinations of the brains of patients dying of apoplexy. He described the appearance of the carotid siphon and the course of the middle cerebral artery in the sylvian fissure. Obstruction of the carotid and vertebral arteries was recognized as a cause of apoplexy, the blockage preventing sufficient blood from reaching the brain.[19] He also was the first to show clearly that bleeding into the brain was an important cause of apoplexy. Willis, a neuroanatomist, best known for his *Cerebri Anatome*, which contained a description of a circle of anastamotic vessels at the base of the brain, was also a well-known clinician and an astute observer. Willis recognized transient ischemic attacks and the phenomenology of embolism, as well as the existence of occlusion of the carotid artery.[19,20]

During the eighteenth century, one of the true giants in medical history *Giovanni Battista Morgagni* (1682–1771) was able to focus attention on *pathology* and the cause of disease. Up to that time, anatomy and prognostic formulas had prevailed. Morgagni, a distinguished professor of anatomy at the University of Padua, had a vision that the secret to understanding disease was to carefully perform necropsies on humans with illnesses and then to correlate the pathological findings with their symptoms during life. Although the clinicopathological method is now taken for granted, this was a new approach for physicians in the eighteenth century. Morgagni labored his entire career to meticulously collect material for his epic work, *De Sedibus et Causis Morborum per Anatomen Indagatis*, which was published when he was 79 years old.[14,21] *De Sedibus* is a five-volume work organized in the form of 70 letters to a young man, describing the cases collected. The first volume was titled *Disease of the Head*. Morgagni's clinical descriptions of patients were detailed but contained no formal physical or neurological examinations because these were not performed in his time.

One of Morgagni's descriptions illustrates the style and content of the book. "A certain man, who was a native of Genoa, blind of one eye, and liv'd by begging, being drunk, and quarreling with other drunken beggars, receiv'd two blows by their sticks; one on his hand which was slight, and another violent one at the left temple so that blood came out of the left ear. Yet soon after, the quarrel being made up, he sat down at the fire with them . . . and again fill'd himself with a great quantity of wine, by way of pledge of friendship being renewed; and not long after, on the same night, he died."[14] Necropsy showed a large epidural hematoma. Morgagni also described cases of intracerebral hemorrhage and recognized that paralysis was on the side of the body opposite to the brain lesion. Morgagni's work shifted the emphasis from anatomy alone to inquiry about diseases and their pathology, causes, and clinical manifestations during life.

During the early years of the nineteenth century, a very influential treatise on apoplexy was written by prominent Irish physician John Cheyne (1777–1836). Cheyne's book, which appeared in 1812, was titled *Cases of Apoplexy and Lethargy with Observations upon the Comatose Diseases.*[22] In it, he sought to separate the phenomenology of lethargy and coma from apoplexy. Cheyne's description of the neurological abnormalities was more detailed than those of his predecessors, and the "morbid appearances" of the patients' brains were emphasized, following the example of Morgagni. One illustrative patient was a woman of 32, who was near the end of her pregnancy. After a headache, she became less responsive. Cheyne found that "she preserved the power of voluntary motion of the left side, but the right was completely paralytic. She seemed perfectly conscious when raised, attempted to speak, but could not articulate; she signified by pointing with her left hand that she desired to drink."[22] After a historical review of her case, Cheyne discussed the available treatments (blood-letting, emetics, purges, external applications) and then described 23 other cases. The pathological findings included clear descriptions of brain softenings and intracerebral and subarachnoid hemorrhages.[22] From the time of Cheyne, developments were made concurrently in the clinical, anatomical, and pathological aspects of stroke.

John Abercrombie contributed a more detailed clinical classification of apoplexy in his general text published in 1828.[23] Abercrombie used the presence of headache, stupor, paralysis, and outcome to separate apoplectics into three clinical groups. In the first group, which he termed *primary apoplexy*, the onset was sudden, unilateral paralysis; rigidity and stupor were present; and the outcome was poor. These patients probably had large intracerebral hemorrhages or large brain infarcts. In the second group, patients had sudden headache, vomiting, and either faintness or falling but no paralysis. Undoubtedly, these patients had subarachnoid hemorrhages. In the third group, there was unilateral paralysis, often with abnormal speech, but neither stupor nor headache was present. This group must have had small infarcts or parenchymatous hemorrhages. Abercrombie also speculated on etiological mechanisms, mentioning spasm of vessels, interruption of the circulation, and rupture of diseased vessels causing hemorrhage.[9,23]

In the middle of the nineteenth century, dissemination of knowledge about the pathology of stroke came with the publication of four atlases, each containing plates of brain and vascular lesions. Hooper's atlas, published in 1828, clearly illustrated pontine and putaminal hemorrhages and a subdural hematoma.[24] Cruveilher (1835–1842),[25] Carswell (1838),[26] and Bright[27] also published atlases containing lithographs of systemic and neuropathological lesions. Bright, better known for his work on nephritis, collected more than 200 neuropathological cases and specimens[9] and included illustrations of 25 nervous-system specimens, including cerebrovascular cases, in his volume on nervous-system disorders.[27]

During the later portion of the nineteenth and the early years of the twentieth centuries, the anatomical details of the cerebral vessels and their supply were studied carefully. Detailed observations of the distribution of the arteries and veins in the cranium were made by Düret, a French neurosurgeon, first working in Charcot's laboratory;[28,29] by Stopford in Britain;[30] and later, by Foix, who dissected pathological specimens at the Salpetriere in France.[31-34] Foix (Figure 1.1) made many key anatomical and clinical observations. Also during this same period, clinicians gathered more information on the phenomenology in patients with stroke. The bulk of these data involved clinical descriptions, with little insight into pathogenesis, laboratory confirmation, or treatment. The general medical and neurological texts of Osler,[35] Gowers,[36] and Wilson[37] contained very detailed descriptions of the clinical findings and prognosis of many stroke syndromes. The clinicopathological method culminated in descriptions by Foix and his colleagues of the syndromes of infarctions in the regions of the middle cerebral artery,[33,34] posterior cerebral artery,[34,38] anterior cerebral artery,[34,39] and vertebrobasilar artery.[32,34]

Later reports by Fisher (Figure 1.2), who analyzed the findings in patients with internal carotid artery occlusions[40] and cerebellar[41] and basal ganglionic[42] hemorrhages and lacunar infarcts,[43] and by Kubik and Adams, who described the findings in patients with basilar artery occlusions,[44] carried on the example set by Foix. All of these reports contained meticulous descriptions of the signs and symptoms found in patients with infarcts and hemorrhages in various vascular and brain distributions. Elegant and thorough as these descriptions were, their limitations included reliance on only the fatal cases because precise diagnosis was not possible during life; predominance of anecdotal cases, with few data on the incidence and frequency of findings in large series of patients with the specific described conditions; insufficient availability of technology to allow ready diagnosis or clarification of the pathogenesis or pathophysiology of the vascular lesions and their effects on the brain; and little knowledge about the effectiveness of treatment.

During the twentieth century, especially the 1970s and 1980s, there has been an explosive growth of interest in and knowledge about stroke for several reasons: *Technology* has allowed better visualization of the anatomy and functional aspects of the brain and of vascular lesions during life. New *surgical and medical treatments* are now possible. *Therapeutic trials* have begun to evaluate systematically the efficacy and safety of some of these treatments. *Databases and registries* of large numbers of well-studied stroke

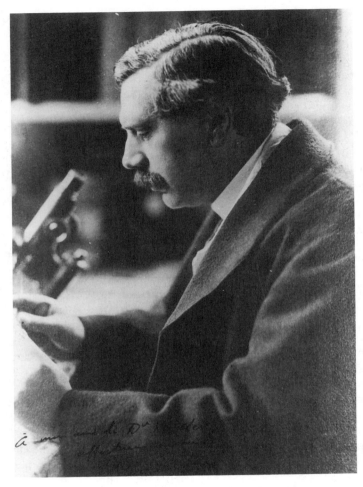

FIGURE 1.1   Charles Foix in his laboratory at the Salpetriere.

patients have helped in the identification and quantification of the most common clinical and laboratory findings in the various stroke syndromes. *Epidemiological studies* have pinpointed more accurately the risk factors for stroke-prevention strategies.

The technological revolution probably began with the work of the Portugese neurosurgeon Moniz (1874–1955). Moniz surgically exposed and temporarily ligated the internal carotid artery in the neck and then rapidly injected by hand a 30 percent solution of sodium iodide, taking skull films later at regular time intervals.[45] He first used the technique for studying patients suspected of having brain tumors, but he later studied stroke patients. By the time of his monograph on angiography in 1931,[46] Moniz had studied

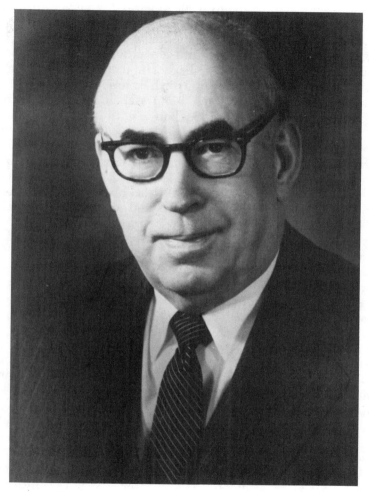

FIGURE 1.2   C. Miller Fisher.

180 patients; had switched to another opaque-contrast agent, Thorotrast, because of convulsions that had occurred following the injection of sodium iodide; and had demonstrated the occurrence of occlusion of the internal carotid artery during life.[46,47] Modern angiography began with the work of Seldinger, in Sweden, who devised a technique by which a small catheter could be inserted into an artery over a flexible guidewire after withdrawing the needle.[48] Catheter angiography of selected vessels in the carotid and vertebral circulations was then possible without surgical incisions. Newer dyes and filming techniques have since made angiography safer and more definitive.

Hounsfield of the research laboratories of EMI in Britain originated the concept of computed tomography (CT). The instrument was first tried at the Atkinson-Morley hospital in London.[5] CT scanners were first introduced to North America in 1973. Films from first-generation scanners were very primitive, but by the late 1970s, third-generation scanners had made CT a very useful, almost indispensable, diagnostic technique. By the mid-1980s, CT was readily available throughout North America and most of Europe. CT allowed clear distinction between brain ischemia and hemorrhage and allowed definition of the size and location of most brain infarcts and hemorrhages. The advent of nuclear magnetic resonance into clinical brain imaging in the mid-1980s was a further major advance. Magnetic resonance imaging (MRI) proved superior to CT in showing old hemosiderin-containing hemorrhages and in imaging vascular malformations, lesions abutting on bony surfaces, and posterior fossa structures. MRI also made it easier to visualize lesions in different planes by providing sagittal, coronal, and horizontal sections. More recently, improved filming techniques have begun to make it possible to image the brain vasculature through the technique of magnetic resonance angiography (MRA).[49]

Ultrasound was introduced to medicine in 1961 by Franklin and colleagues, who used Doppler shifts of ultrasound to study blood flow in canine blood vessels.[5,50] B-mode ultrasound was soon used to provide images of the extracranial carotid arteries noninvasively. By the early 1980s, B-mode, continuous-wave, and pulsed-Doppler technology was readily available, which could reliably detect severe extracranial vascular occlusive disease in the carotid and vertebral arteries in the neck. Sequential ultrasound studies allowed physicians to study the natural history of the development and progression of these occlusive lesions and to correlate the occurrence and severity of disease with stroke risk factors, symptoms, and treatment. In 1982, Aaslid and colleagues introduced a high-energy bidirectional pulsed-Doppler system that used low frequencies to study intracranial arteries, termed *transcranial Doppler ultrasound* (TCD).[51] TCD has made possible noninvasive detection of severe occlusive disease in the major intracranial arteries during life, as well as sequential study of these lesions.[52] Introduction of echocardiography and ambulatory cardiac rhythm monitoring in the 1970s and 1980s greatly improved cardiac diagnoses and detection of cardiogenic sources of embolism. By the early 1990s, clinicians could safely define the nature, extent, and localization of most important brain, cardiac, and vascular lesions in stroke patients. Accurate diagnosis using modern technology facilitated clinical-imaging correlations in patients with nonfatal strokes, and this paved the way for monitoring the effects of various treatments.

During the middle years of the twentieth century, clinicians had advanced knowledge of clinical phenomenology by personally studying and describing small groups of patients. In 1935, Aring and Meritt studied a group of patients coming to necropsy at the Boston City Hospital, in order to clarify the differential diagnosis between brain hemorrhages and infarcts.[53] Subsequently, Fisher and his colleagues and students studied and described the clinical findings in small numbers of patients with various cerebrovascular syndromes. During the 1970s and 1980s, the technological advances described made it possible to define the clinical and laboratory features of nonfatal, even minor, strokes and prestroke vascular lesions. With better knowledge of clinical and morphological features, clinicians naturally sought more quantitative data. How often did intracerebral hemorrhages or lacunar infarcts occur? How often did each of the clinical symptoms and signs occur in each subtype of stroke? Clinicians recognized that valid statistically meaningful data could not be collected unless large numbers of patients with a wide spectrum of representative cases were studied and analyzed. The advent of computers in medicine in the 1970s greatly facilitated the storage and analysis of large quantities of complex data. Collection of data on large numbers of stroke patients began with the series of Dalsgaard-Nielsen in Scandinavia,[54] and with a series of patients seen by clinicians at the Mayo Clinic in Rochester, Minnesota.[55,56] The Harvard Cooperative Stroke Registry in the early 1970s was the first computer-based registry of prospectively studied stroke patients.[57] During the 1970s and 1980s, a number of other stroke registries and databases provided more quantitative information about clinical and laboratory phenomena and diagnoses.[58–62] Community-based studies in South Alabama;[63] Framingham, Massachusetts;[64] Oxfordshire in Great Britain;[65] the Lehigh Valley in Pennsylvania;[66] and various regions in North Carolina, Oregon, and New York[67] have generated important epidemiological data. Computer-based registries and data banks have undoubtedly assisted collection and analysis of a wide variety of clinical, radiological, pathological, and epidemiological information.[68,69] The present text has relied heavily on data from these studies, especially those in which I was personally involved.[57,59,61]

During the second half of the twentieth century, there were major advances in therapeutic capabilities, especially in cerebrovascular surgery. In 1951, Fisher had suggested the possibility of surgery on stenotic lesions of the extracranial carotid artery: "It is conceivable that some day vascular surgery will find a way to by-pass the occluded portions of the internal carotid artery during the period of ominous fleeting symptoms."[5,40] Carrea, Molins, and Murphy, in Buenos Aires, performed an anastomosis from the external carotid to the internal carotid artery in a patient with severe internal carotid artery stenosis in October 1951, but their report did not appear until 1955.[5,47,70] Eastcott, Pickering, and Rob also performed an anastomosis, this time from the common carotid artery to a segment of the internal carotid artery above an occlusion, in London in May 1953, and their report appeared before that of the Argentine authors.[5,71] DeBakey said that he had performed the first carotid artery thromboendarterectomy in August 1953, but the case was not reported until many years later.[72] Advances in surgical technique, angiography, and anesthesia led to great improvements in the techniques of endarterectomy during the 1950s and 1960s. By the mid-1960s, carotid endarterectomy became a very common routine surgical procedure. Vascular surgeons also began to operate with technical skill on the extracranial subclavian, vertebral, and innominate arteries for posterior circulation occlusive disease.[5,47,73,74]

The advent of the dissecting microscope and other instrumentation advances led to new capabilities for intracranial surgery. Microsurgery on small- and medium-sized arteries facilitated surgical treatment of aneurysms and vascular malformations and made possible anastomoses and even embolectomy involving small basal and surface arteries of the brain.[75,76] In the 1970s, bypass procedures using the dissecting microscope created anastomoses between extracranial arteries such as from the superficial temporal and occipital artery branches of the external carotid artery to the middle cerebral and posterior inferior cerebellar arteries.[75-78] These procedures became very popular until a randomized controlled study proved that the anterior circulation bypasses, as then performed, were no better—and were sometimes worse—than medical therapy. Subsequent improvements in neuroanesthesia and intensive care helped reduce the morbidity and mortality of cerebrovascular surgery on the brain and its vasculature.[79]

Medical treatment also changed dramatically during the middle and later portions of the twentieth century. The lack of remedial treatments in the preceding eras was, at least partially, responsible for disinterest in defining the cause of stroke because little could be done in any case. The appearance of effective antihypertensive medicines in the middle years of the twentieth century clearly reduced the incidence of brain parenchymal hemorrhages and also reduced the frequency of ischemic stroke and occlusive vascular disease. Anticoagulant therapy with heparin and dicumarol were introduced as treatments for patients with occlusive cerebrovascular disease in the 1950s. Wright and colleagues at Cornell,[80-82] and Millikan, Siekert, and Whisnant at the Mayo Clinic[83] pioneered the use of dicumarol for cerebrovascular indications. The presence of a potentially useful therapy further stimulated interest in stroke and was a factor in generating a meeting of individuals interested in cerebrovascular disease at Princeton, New Jersey, in 1954.[84] This was to be the first of the biennial Princeton conferences that bring together stroke experts and investigators from around the world to discuss problems, advances, and research in stroke. The emergence of stroke as a potentially treatable disease also helped promote the creation in 1967 of a Stroke Council as part of the activities of the American Heart Association.[85] This council convened its first international stroke conference in Dallas, Texas, in 1976. The journal *Stroke*, also an outgrowth of the American Heart Association, began publication in 1970 with Millikan as its first editor.

If anticoagulants or other treatments were to be effective, therapy should be started in early or premonitory phases of stroke. Fisher had emphasized the presence of temporary short-lived episodes of neurological symptoms, which he termed *transient ischemic attacks (TIAs)* in his patients with occlusion of the internal carotid artery.[40] Although others, including Hippocrates, Willis, and Gowers,[36] had mentioned the occurrence of these attacks, in the era before Fisher, they were generally not well known in the broader medical community. In 1953, Fisher and Cameron reported a patient with multiple TIAs and basilar artery disease, in whom the attacks ceased after introduction of heparin and the anticoagulant phenylindandione.[5,86] The authors commented, "Transient phenomena preceding the onset of a stroke are much more frequent than is commonly believed, for the patient often neglects them, while his physician does not inquire about their occurrence once paralysis has occurred."[86] Analysis of the usual time-sequence features of stroke by physicians at the Mayo Clinic and elsewhere led to the introduction and popularization of terms that attempted to capture the tempo of the symptoms and signs. These designations included progressing stroke, reversible ischemic neurological deficits, completed strokes, and so forth. It was hoped that these designations would be simple and easy to distinguish by physicians not sophisticated in neurology and that the designations would predict prognosis and response to various treatments. Unfortunately, these terms proved difficult to define. Furthermore, experience showed that they did not predict whether the patient would show a brain infarct on neuroimaging studies; nor did they predict the prognosis, the nature of the vascular process causing the ischemia, or the response to various treatments.[87,88] Their utility now is solely for descriptive purposes. These terms *do not* represent diagnoses or the basis for treatment selection.

In 1950, Craven commented on the use of aspirin as an agent that might prevent thrombosis. Craven had observed that dental patients who took aspirin often bled after tooth extractions, and he reasoned that aspirin might be interfering with the normal clotting process.[5,89] Only later was aspirin shown to affect platelet adhesion and aggregability. Aspirin was not used for the treatment of cerebrovascular symptoms until the early 1970s.[90] However, by the mid-1970s, aspirin use was so widespread that therapeutic trials of its effectiveness were designed and reported.[91,92] Thrombolytic therapy to lyse clots in stroke patients had been tried briefly in the early 1960s but had been abandoned and discredited because of an unacceptable high complication rate.[93] During the 1980s, streptokinase and recombinant tissue plasminogen activator were shown to be effective in the treatment of acute coronary artery thrombosis, and these drugs were introduced as investigational agents to treat patients with cerebrovascular thrombi.[94,95] Other potentially effective pharmacological agents became available after 1950 and included corticosteroids and mannitol and other osmotically active agents, to treat brain edema; beta-adrenergic blocking agents and angiotensin-converting enzyme inhibitors, to better control arterial hypertension; and calcium-channel blocking agents, to control blood pressure, diminish cerebrovascular vasoconstriction, and inhibit Ca^{++} entry into ischemic cells.

Physicians' armamentaria of surgical and medical treatments had grown impressively, but there were few objective data on the effectiveness, safety, and utility of the various treatments. Reliance on anecdotal reports of treatment responses in very selected, small samples of patients clearly was not very satisfactory. During the 1970s and 1980s, methodology was developed and improved for more systematic, planned, scientific, statistically based study and analysis of large series of representative patients prospectively entered in multicenter randomized, controlled therapeutic trials.[96] Therapeutic trials of the effect of aspirin and other agents that alter platelet functions were helpful in suggesting the utility of these drugs in some patients.[91,92] More recently, trials have also shown the effectiveness of anticoagulation in preventing brain embolism in patients with atrial fibrillation.[97–99] Trials have been and are being used to evaluate the effectiveness of various surgical procedures, such as carotid endarterectomy[100–103] and extracranial to intracranial bypass procedures.[104] At the time of this writing, trial methodology, design, and statistical analysis is still being improved and modified. Well-conceived trials offer great promise for the study of the treatment of common cerebrovascular conditions in the future. Barnett, Fields, and Toole have been pioneers in the introduction and performance of stroke treatment trials. Unfortunately, however, the expense, requirements for very large numbers of patients, need for clearly verifiable commonly occurring end points, and other practical considerations make these multicenter trials unsatisfactory for studying the treatment of many cerebrovascular conditions.[105]

Stroke as a Model Example of Brain and Vascular Disease

Stroke is the prototype of a focal, well-circumscribed brain lesion. Fisher is fond of saying that neurology is learned "stroke by stroke." Knowledge of the symptoms and signs in patients with focal brain infarcts and hemorrhages has been instrumental in developing an understanding of the functioning of various brain structures and regions. Awareness of the clinical findings in patients with frontal-lobe hemorrhages has undoubtedly helped clinicians to recognize tumors, focal infections, atrophies, and other disease processes located in the frontal lobes. The ability to localize infarcts and hemorrhages precisely with CT and MRI has greatly facilitated study of anatomical–physiological correlations. Study of stroke patients and stroke animal models has improved understanding of brain electrophysiology, chemistry, pharmacology, and overall physiology.

Stroke also provides a model for the study of vascular diseases. Atherosclerosis, embolism, and thrombosis are all usually systemic disorders that affect many critical organs in addition to the brain. Information about the morphology, development, and etiology of lesions in the cerebrovascular bed has undoubtedly influenced knowledge of vascular conditions that affect the coronary, renal, and limb arteries. Of course, the corollary is also true; stroke clinicians clearly can and should gain from clinicians and researchers who study vascular diseases affecting these other body regions. Similarly, study of patients with cardioembolic strokes has advanced knowledge about the heart and its diseases. Stroke patients often have abnormalities of blood coagulation. Elucidation of clotting and bleeding dysfunction underlying stroke has advanced general knowledge about the formed and serological elements of the blood and the vascular endothelium and about their functions in coagulation.

Stroke Care

It is not possible to overemphasize that the care of strokes is not the same as the care of stroke patients. Most strokes result from systemic illnesses, such as hypertension, atherosclerosis, cardiac diseases, and coagulopathies. These conditions profoundly affect other body organs and general health, as well as the brain and central nervous system. Unfortunately, specialists sometimes only see and treat one portion of the body and limited aspects of the general problem, similar to the proverbial blind men feeling isolated parts of the elephant. As physicians, we must be sure that the general systemic disorders, such as hypertension and atherosclerosis, receive deserved detailed and long-term attention. As entry portals into the health-care system, clinicians seeing stroke patients can and should become key figures in preventing disease and in correcting unhealthy practices.

Strokes create other health problems. These include not only the acute complications that are discussed in Chapter 18, but also problems such as increased wear and tear on the joint structures of the hip, knee, and ankle because of altered gait; aspiration and recurrent bronchopulmonary infections; and poor bladder emptying, with an increased frequency of urinary-tract infections. Strokes also have profound social, psychological, and economic effects on stroke sufferers and their families and friends. Physicians caring for stroke patients must consider all of the multiple facets of the condition and must liberally employ other medical and ancillary health personnel. The family often needs nearly as much attention, education, and compassion as the patient. In another book, I have devoted considerable attention to the general approach toward and care of patients, especially those with neurological illnesses.[106]

The other organs exist to keep the brain functioning normally. Any change in the brain's function and activity profoundly affects living. There is no medical task that is more complex, more multifaceted, more important, and potentially more rewarding than caring for a stroke patient.

References

1. Hodgins E. Episode: report on the accident inside my skull. New York: Atheneum, 1964:7–14.
2. Carroll L. Alice's adventures in wonderland. New York: Dutton, 1929:93–94.
3. Osler W. Aequanimitas. In: Aequanimitas with other addresses to medical students, nurses and practitioners medicine. Philadelphia: Blakiston, 1932:8–9.
4. American Heart Association. 1989 stroke facts. Dallas, 1989.
5. Fields WS, Lemak NA. A history of stroke: its recognition and treatment. New York: Oxford University Press, 1989.
6. Gilman S, Russell N. DeJong, 1907–1990. Ann Neurol 1991;29:108–109.
7. Friedlander, WJ. About three old men: an inquiry into how cerebral atherosclerosis has altered world politics. Stroke 1972;3:467–473.
8. Bruenn HG. Clinical notes on the illness and death of president Franklin D. Roosevelt. Ann Int Med 1970;72:579–591.
9. McHenry LC, Jr. Garrison's history of neurology. Springfield, Ill.: Charles C. Thomas, 1969.
10. Linenthal AJ. First a dream. The history of Boston's Jewish hospitals, 1896 to 1928. Boston: Beth Israel Hospital, 1990:276–294.
11. Blumgart HL, Schlesinger MJ, Davis D. Studies on the relation of the clinical manifestations of angina pectoris, coronary thrombosis, and myocardial infarction to the pathological findings. Am Heart J 1940;19:1–9.
12. Blumgart HL, Schlesinger MJ, Zoll PM. Angina pectoris, coronary failure, and acute myocardial infarction. JAMA 1941;116:91–97.
13. Blumgart HL. Caring for the patient. N Engl J Med 1964;270:449–456.
14. Nuland S. Doctors, bibliography of medicine. Birmingham, Ala.: Libraries of Gryphon Editions, 1988.
15. Adams F. The genuine works of Hippocrates: translated from the Greek. Baltimore: Williams and Wilkins, 1939.
16. Clark E. Apoplexy in the Hippocratic writings. Bull Hist Med 1963; 37:301–314.
17. Vesalius A. De Humani Corporis Fabrica. Basileae, Italy: J Oporini, 1543.
18. Wepfler JJ. Observationes Anatomicae, ex Cadaveribus Eorum, quos Sustulit Apoplexia, cum Exercitatione de Ejus Loco Affecto. Schaffhausen, Germany: Joh. Caspari Suteri, 1658.
19. Gurdjian ES, Gurdjian ES. History of occlusive cerebrovascular disease: I. From Wepfer to Moniz. Arch Neurol 1979;36:340–343.
20. Toole JF. The Willis lecture: transient ischemic attacks, scientific method, and new realities. Stroke 1991;22:99–104.
21. Morgagni GB. The seats and causes of disease investigated by anatomy. Translated by B Alexander. London: Millar and Cadell; 1769. Birmingham: Classics of Medicine Library.
22. Cheyne J. Cases of apoplexy and lethargy with observations upon the comatose diseases. London: J Moyes Printer, 1812.
23. Abercrombie J. Pathological and practical researches on diseases of the brain and spinal cord. Edinburgh: Waugh and Innes, 1828.
24. Hooper R. The morbid anatomy of the human brain illustrated by coloured engravings of the most frequent and important organic diseases to which that viscus is subject. London: Rees, Orme, Brown and Green, 1831.

25. Cruveilhier J. Anatomie pathologique du corps humain: descriptions avec figures lithographiées et coloriées des diverses alterations morbides dont le corps humain est susceptible. Paris: J.B. Bailliere, 1835–1842.
26. Carswell R. Pathological anatomy: illustrations of the elementary forms of disease. London: Longman, 1838.
27. Bright R. Reports of medical cases, selected with a view of illustrating the symptoms and cures of diseases by a reference to morbid anatomy: vol II. diseases of the brain and nervous system. London: Longman, Rees, Orme, Brown, and Green, 1831.
28. Duret H. Sur la distribution des arteres nouricieres du bulbe rachidien. Arch Physiol Norm Pathol 1873;2:97–113.
29. Duret H. Recherches anatomiques sur la circulation de l'encephale. Arch Physiol Norm Pathol 1874;3:60–91,316–353.
30. Stopford JS. The anatomy of the pons and medulla oblongata. J Anat Physiol 1928;50:225–280.
31. Foix C, Hillemand P. Irrigation de la protuberance. C R Soc Biol [Paris] 1925;92:35–36.
32. Foix C, Hillemand P. Les arteres de l'axe encephalique jusqu'au diencephale inclusivement. Rev Neurol [Paris] 1925;41:705–739.
33. Foix C, Levy M. Les ramollissements sylviens. Rev Neurol [Paris] 1927;43:1–51.
34. Caplan LR. Charles Foix—the first modern stroke neurologist. Stroke 1990;21:348–356.
35. Osler W. The principles and practice of medicine. 5th ed. New York: D Appleton, 1903.
36. Gowers WR. A manual of disease of the nervous system. London: J and A Churchill, 1893.
37. Wilson SAK, Bruce AN. Neurology. 2nd ed. London: Butterworth, 1955.
38. Foix C, Masson A. Le syndrome de l'artere cerebrale posterieure. Presse Med 1923;31:361–365.
39. Foix C. Hillemand P. Les syndromes de l'artere cerebrale anterieure. Encephale 1925;20:209–232.
40. Fisher CM. Occlusion of the internal carotid artery. Arch Neurol 1951;65:346–377.
41. Fisher CM, Picard E, Polak A, et al. Acute hypertensive cerebellar hemorrhage: diagnosis and surgical treatment. J Nerv Ment Dis 1965;140:38–57.
42. Fisher CM. Clinical syndromes in cerebral hemorrhage. In: Fields W, ed. Pathogenesis and treatment of cerebrovascular disease. Springfield, Ill.: Charles C Thomas, 1961:318–342.
43. Fisher CM. Lacunes: small, deep cerebral infarcts. Neurology 1965;15:774–784.
44. Kubik CS, Adams RD. Occlusion of the basilar artery: a clinical and pathological study. Brain 1946;69:73–121.
45. Moniz E. L'encephalographie artérielle, son importance dans la localisation des tumeurs cérébrales. Rev Neurol [Paris] 1927;2:72–90.
46. Moniz E. L'angiographie Cerebrale. Paris: Masson, 1931.
47. Gurdjian ES, Gurdjian ES. History of occlusive cerebrovascular disease: II. after Moniz with special reference to surgical treatment. Arch Neurol 1979;36:427–432.
48. Seldinger SI. Catheter replacement of the needle in percutaneous arteriography. Acta Radiol 1953;39:368–376.

49. Edelman RC, Mattle HP, O'Reilly GV, et al. Magnetic resonance imaging of flow dynamics in the circle of Willis. Stroke 1990;21:56–65.

50. Franklin DL, Schlegel WA, Rushner RF. Blood flow measured by Doppler frequency shift of back-scattered ultrasound. Science 1961;134:564–565.

51. Aaslid R, Markwalder TM, Nornes H. Non-invasive transcranial Doppler ultrasound recording of flow velocity in basal cerebral arteries. J Neurosurg 1982; 57:769–774.

52. Caplan LR, Brass LM, DeWitt LD, et al. Transcranial Doppler ultrasound: present status. Neurology 1990;40:696–700.

53. Aring CD, Meritt HH. Differential diagnosis between cerebral hemorrhage and cerebral thrombosis. Arch Int Med 1935;56:435–456.

54. Dalsgaard-Nielsen T. Survey of 1000 cases of apoplexia cerebri. Acta Psychiatr Neurol Scand 1955;30:169–185.

55. Whisnant JP, Fitzgibbons JP, Kurland LT, et al. Natural history of stroke in Rochester, Minnesota 1945 through 1954. Stroke 1971;2:11–22.

56. Matsumoto N, Whisnant JP, Kurland LT, et al. Natural history of stroke in Rochester, Minnesota 1955 through 1969: an extension of a previous study 1945 through 1954. Stroke 1973;4:20–29.

57. Mohr JP, Caplan LR, Melski JW, et al. The Harvard Cooperative Stroke Registry: a prospective registry. Neurology 1978;28:754–762.

58. Kunitz S, Gross CR, Heyman A, et al. The Pilot Stroke Data Bank: definition, design, and data. Stroke 1984;15:740–746.

59. Caplan LR, Hier DB, D'Cruz I. Cerebral embolism in the Michael Reese Stroke Registry. Stroke 1983;14:530–536.

60. Chambers BR, Donnan GA, Bladin PF. Patterns of stroke: an analysis of the first 700 consecutive admissions to the Austin Hospital Stroke Unit. Aust N Z J Med 1983;13:57–64.

61. Foulkes MA, Wolf PA, Price TR, et al. The Stroke Data Bank: design, methods, and baseline characteristics. Stroke 1988;19:547–554.

62. Bogousslavsky J, Mille GV, Regli F. The Lausanne Stroke Registry: an analysis of 1000 consecutive patients with first stroke. Stroke 1988;19:1083–1092.

63. Gross CR, Kase CS, Mohr JP, et al. Stroke in south Alabama: incidence and diagnostic features—a population based study. Stroke 1984;15:249–255.

64. Wolf PA, Kannel WB, Dauber TR. Prospective investigations: the Framingham study and the epidemiology of stroke. Adv in Neurol 1978;19:107–120.

65. Oxfordshire Community Stroke Project. Incidence of stroke in Oxfordshire: first year's experience of a community stroke registry. Br Med J 1983;287: 713–717.

66. Alter M, Sobel E, McCoy RC, et al. Stroke in the Lehigh Valley: incidence based on a community-wide hospital registry. Neuroepidemiology 1985;4: 1–15.

67. Yatsu FM, Becker C, McLeroy K, et al. Community hospital-based stroke programs: North Carolina, Oregon, and New York: I. goals, objectives, and data collection procedures. Stroke 1986;17:276–284.

68. Mohr JP. Stroke data banks [editorial]. Stroke 1986;17:171–172.

69. Caplan LR. Stroke data banks, then and now. In: Courbier R, ed. Basis for a classification of cerebrovascular disease. Amsterdam: Excerpta Medica, 1985:152–162.

70. Carrea R, Molins M, Murphy G. Surgical treatment of spontaneous thrombosis of the internal carotid artery in the neck. Carotid–carotideal anastomosis. Acta Neurol Latinoamer 1955;1:71–78.
71. Eastcott HHG, Pickering GW, Rob CG. Reconstruction of internal carotid artery in a patient with intermittent attacks of hemiplegia. Lancet 1954;2:994–996.
72. DeBakey ME. Successful carotid endarterectomy for cerebrovascular insufficiency: nineteen year follow-up. JAMA 1975;233:1083–1085.
73. Crawford ES, DeBakey ME, Fields WS. Roentgenographic diagnosis and surgical treatment of basilar artery insufficiency. JAMA 1958;168:509–514.
74. DeBakey ME, Crawford ES, Cooley DA, et al. Cerebral arterial insufficiency: one to 11 year results following arterial reconstructive operation. Ann Surg 1965;161:921–945.
75. Jaccobson JH, Wallman LJ, Schumacher GA, et al. Microsurgery as an aid to middle cerebral artery endarterectomy. J Neurosurg 1962;19:108–115.
76. Yasargil MG. Microsurgery applied to neurosurgery. Stuttgart, Germany: Georg Thieme Verlag, 1969:108–109.
77. Yasargil MG, Krayenbuhl HA, Jacobson JH. Microneurosurgical arterial reconstruction. Surgery 1970;67:221–233.
78. Maroon JK, Donaghy RMP. Experimental cerebral revascularization with autogenous grafts. J Neurosurg 1973;38:172–179.
79. Ropper AH, Kennedy SF, eds. Neurological and neurosurgical intensive care. Rockville, Md: Aspen, 1988.
80. Wright IS, McDevitt, E. Cerebral vascular disease: significance, diagnosis, and present treatment, including selective use of anticoagulant substances. Ann Int Med 1954;41:682–698.
81. McDevitt E, Carter SA, Gatje BW, et al. Use of anticoagulants in treatment of cerebral vascular disease. JAMA 1958;166:592–596.
82. Groch SN, McDevitt E, Wright IS. A long-term study of cerebral vascular disease. Ann Int Med 1961;55:358–367.
83. Millikan CH, Siekert RG, Whisnant JP. Anticoagulant therapy in cerebral vascular disease—current status. JAMA 1958;166:587–592.
84. Millikan CH (ed.). Cerebral vascular diseases. Transactions of the Second Conference Held under the Auspices of the American Heart Association. Princeton NJ, Jan 16–18, 1957. New York: Grune & Stratton, 1958.
85. Caplan LR. The stroke council and the young investigator award. Mayo Clin Proc 1989;64:125–128.
86. Fisher CM, Cameron DG. Concerning cerebral vasospasm. Neurology 1953;3:468–473.
87. Caplan LR. Are terms such as *completed stroke* or *RIND* of continued usefulness? Stroke 1983;14:431–433.
88. Caplan LR. TIAs—we need to return to the question, what is wrong with Mr. Jones? Neurology 1988;38:791–793.
89. Craven LL. Experiences with aspirin [acetylsalicylic acid] in the nonspecific prophylaxis of coronary thrombosis. Mississippi Valley MJ 1953;75:38–44.
90. Harrison MJG, Marshall J, Meadows JC, et al. Effect of aspirin in amaurosis fugax. Lancet 1971;2:743–744.

91. Fields WS, Lemak NA, Frankowski RF, et al. Controlled trial of aspirin in cerebral ischemia. Stroke 1977;8:301–316.
92. Canadian Cooperative Study Group. A randomized trial of aspirin and sulfinpyrazone in threatened stroke. N Engl J Med 1978;299:53–59.
93. Meyer JS, Gilroy J, Barnhart ME, et al. Therapeutic thrombolysis in cerebral thromboembolism: randomized evaluation of intravenous streptokinase. In: Millikan CH, Siekert R, Whisnant JP, eds. Cerebrovascular diseases. New York: Grune & Stratton, 1964:200–213.
94. Del Zoppo GJ, Zeumer H, Harker LA. Thrombolytic therapy in stroke: possibilities and hazards. Stroke 1986;17:595–607.
95. Sloan MA. Thrombolysis and stroke: past and future. Arch Neurol 1987;44: 748–768.
96. Beaudry MA, Hachinski VC. Cerebrovascular disease. In: Porter RJ, Schoenberg BS, eds. Controlled clinical trials in neurological disease. Boston: Kluwer Academic, 1990:113–129.
97. Peterson P, Godtfredsen J, Boysen G, et al. Placebo-controlled randomized trial of warfarin and aspirin for prevention of thromboembolic complications of chronic atrial fibrillation: the Copenhagen AFASAK Study. Lancet 1989;1: 175–179.
98. The Boston area anticoagulation trial for atrial fibrillation investigators: the effect of low dose warfarin on risk of stroke in patients with nonrheumatic atrial fibrillation. N Engl J Med 1990;323:1505–1511.
99. Stroke prevention in atrial fibrillation study group investigators: preliminary report of the stroke prevention in atrial fibrillation study. N Engl J Med 1990;322:863–868.
100. Fields WS, North RR, Hass WK, et al. Joint study of extracranial arterial occlusion as a cause of stroke: organization of study and survey of patient population. JAMA 1968;203:955–960.
101. Veterans Administration Cooperative Study. Role of carotid endarterectomy in asymptomatic carotid stenosis. Stroke 1986;17:534–539.
102. North American Symptomatic Carotid Endarterectomy Study Group. Carotid endarterectomy: three critical evaluations. Stroke 1987;18:987–989.
103. Asymptomatic Carotid Atherosclerosis Study Group. Study design for randomized prospective trial of carotid endarterectomy for asymptomatic atherosclerosis. Stroke 1989;20:844–849.
104. EC/IC Bypass Study Group. Failure of extracranial–intracranial bypass to reduce the risk of ischemic stroke. N Engl J Med 1985;313:1191–1200.
105. Caplan LR. Clinical trials in neurology especially stroke: the clinician's role. In: Hachinski V, ed. Controversies and challenges in neurology. Philadelphia: FA Davis, 1991.
106. Caplan LR. The effective clinical neurologist. Boston: Blackwell, 1990.

CHAPTER 2

Basic Pathology, Anatomy, and Pathophysiology of Stroke

Stroke is anything but a homogeneous entity. Disorders as different as rupture of a large blood vessel, with flooding of the brain with blood, and occlusion of a tiny artery, with softening in a small but strategic brain site, both qualify as strokes. These two pathological caricatures of stroke subtypes are as divergent as grapes and watermelons, two obviously very dissimilar substances that are included together under the large category of *fruit.* *Stroke* refers to any damage to brain or central nervous system structures caused by abnormalities of the blood supply. The term *stroke* is usually used when the symptoms begin acutely, while *cerebrovascular disease* is a more general term that carries no connotation as to the tempo of brain injury. Of course, many patients with badly diseased vessels have had no injury to brain tissue. Almost by definition, the blood-vessel disorder precedes and subsequently leads to the brain injury. Recognition of the vascular problem before the brain becomes damaged may offer the clinician a window of opportunity during which brain damage can be prevented. At times, even when brain injury has occurred, the individual is unaware of any symptoms, and neurologists may not be able to detect any abnormalities on neurological examination. Sophisticated neuroimaging techniques have recently taught clinicians that such "silent strokes" are quite common.

Diagnosis and treatment of stroke patients requires a basic understanding of the anatomy, physiology, and pathology of the two major structures involved—the brain and spinal cord—and of the blood vessels that supply blood to these structures. To be effective, clinicians caring for stroke patients must have an intimate familiarity with (1) the appearance of the normal brain and its various lobes and regions; (2) the appearance of brain tissue damaged by various vascular disorders; (3) the usual locations and course of arteries supplying the brain and spinal cord; and (4) the frequency, location, and appearance of diseases of the cerebrovascular system. Note that this discussion includes a number of words related to vision. Many of the diagnostic tests used, especially imaging of the brain and blood vessels, produce pictures. *Clinicians must be able to visualize what the structures and diseases look like.* For this reason, this chapter relies heavily on illustrations.

This chapter offers succinct and simple coverage of the topics just mentioned. It begins by introducing the different mechanisms of brain damage in stroke. These stroke mechanisms are the major players, the key actors in the drama of stroke. Their characterization, recognition, and treatment form the meat of this book. Normal vascular anatomy and distribution are then described and illustrated. Next, the usual distribution and frequency in the blood vessels and in the brain of these different mechanisms are discussed and diagrammed. The chapter closes with a discussion of stroke pathophysiology, the dynamics of the functional response of the vascular system and brain to the primary injuries.

Pathology: Mechanisms of Cerebrovascular Damage to Brain Tissue

When confronted by a stroke patient, the clinician should ask, "What is the mechanism of the brain dysfunction? What pathological process is active in this patient?" There are two major categories of brain damage in stroke patients: (1) *ischemia*, a lack of blood flow, depriving brain tissue of needed fuel and oxygen; and (2) *hemorrhage*, the release of blood into the extravascular space within the cranium. Bleeding damages the brain by cutting off connecting pathways and by causing localized or generalized pressure injury to brain tissue; biochemical substances released during and after hemorrhage also may adversely affect nearby vascular or brain tissues.[1,2]

Ischemia

Ischemia can be further subdivided into three different mechanisms: thrombosis, embolism, and decreased systemic perfusion.

Thrombosis

By convention, *thrombosis* refers to an obstruction of blood flow due to a localized occlusive process within one or more blood vessels. The lumen of the vessel is narrowed or occluded by an alteration in the vessel wall or by superimposed clot formation (e.g., see sequence in Figure 2.1). The commonest type of vascular pathology is *atherosclerosis*, in which fibrous and muscular tissues overgrow in the subintima, and fatty materials form plaques that can encroach on the lumen. Next, platelets adhere to the plaque crevices and form clumps that serve as nidi for the deposition of fibrin,

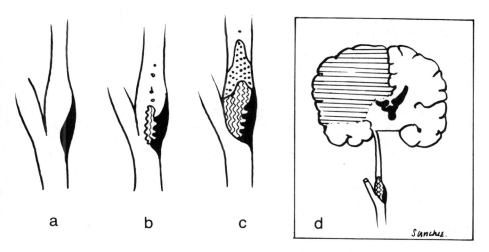

FIGURE 2.1   Internal carotid artery atherosclerotic lesions: (a) plaque; (b) plaque with platelet-fibrin emboli; (c) plaque with occlusive thrombus; (d) recent ischemic cerebral infarct due to internal carotid artery occlusion.

thrombin, and clot.[3,4] Atherosclerosis affects chiefly the larger extracranial and intracranial vessels.[5,6] Occasionally, clot forms within the lumen because of a primary hematological problem, such as polycythemia, thrombocytosis, or a systemic hypercoagulable state. However, the smaller penetrating intracranial vessels are more often damaged by hypertension than by atherosclerotic processes.[7,8] In such cases, increased arterial tension leads to hypertrophy of the media and deposition of fibrinoid material into the vessel wall, a process that gradually encroaches on the already small lumen.

Less common vascular pathologies leading to obstruction include *fibromuscular dysplasia*,[9] an overgrowth of medial and intimal elements that compromises vessel contractility and luminal size; *arteritis*, especially of the Takayasu[10] or giant-cell type;[11] *dissection of the vessel wall*,[12] often with luminal or extraluminal clot temporarily obstructing the vessel; and *hemorrhage into a plaque*,[13] leading to acute or chronic luminal compromise. At times, the focal vascular abnormality is a functional change in the contractility of blood vessels. Intense focal vasoconstriction can lead to decreased blood flow and thrombosis. Dilation of blood vessels also alters local blood flow, and clots can form in dilated segments.

Embolism

In *embolism*, material formed elsewhere within the vascular system lodges in a vessel and blocks the blood flow. In contrast to thrombosis, embolic luminal blockage is not due to a localized process originating within the blocked vessel. The material arises proximally, most commonly from the heart; from major arteries such as the aorta, carotid, and vertebral arteries; and from systemic veins (Figure 2.2). *Cardiac* sources of embolism include the heart valves, endocardium, and either clot or tumor within the atrial or ventricular cavities.[14] *Artery-to-artery* emboli are composed of clot, platelet clumps, or fragments of plaques that break off from the proximal vessels.[15] Clots originating in *systemic veins* travel to the brain through cardiac defects such as an atrial septal defect or a patent foramen ovale, a process termed *paradoxical embolism.*[16] Also, occasionally, air, fat,[17] plaque material,[18] particulate matter from injected drugs,[19] bacteria,[20] and tumor cells enter the vascular system and appear to embolize to cerebral vessels.

Decreased systemic perfusion

In this circumstance, diminished flow to brain tissue is due to low systemic perfusion pressure. The most common causes are cardiac pump failure (most often due to myocardial infarction or arrhythmia) and systemic hypotension (due to blood loss or hypovolemia). In such cases, the lack of perfusion is more generalized than in localized thrombosis or embolism and affects the brain diffusely and bilaterally. Poor perfusion is most critical in border zone or so-called watershed regions at the periphery of the major vascular-supply territories (e.g., on Figure 2.3, compare b with both a and c).[21,22] Asymmetrical effects can result from preexisting vascular lesions, causing an uneven underperfusion.

Damage caused by ischemia

All three mechanisms of ischemic injury lead to temporary or permanent injury to tissue. Permanent injury is termed *infarction.* Capillaries or other vessels within the ischemic tissue may also be injured, so that reperfusion can lead to leakage of blood into the ischemic tissue, a hemorrhagic infarct. The extent of brain damage depends on the location and duration of the poor perfusion and the ability of collateral vessels to perfuse the tissues at risk. Brain and vascular injuries may cause swelling during the acute phase, producing local edema. In the chronic phase, glial scars form, and macrophages gradually ingest the necrotic tissue debris, within the infarct leading to shrinkage of the volume of the infarcted tissue or a frank cavity.

Hemorrhage

Hemorrhage can be further subdivided into two subtypes: subarachnoid and intracerebral.

Subarachnoid hemorrhage

In *subarachnoid hemorrhage,* blood leaks out of the vascular bed onto the brain's surface and is disseminated quickly via the spinal fluid pathways into

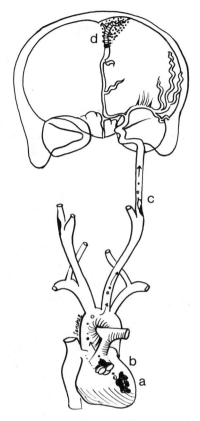

FIGURE 2.2 Examples of potential sources of embolism: (a) cardiac mural thrombus; (b) vegetations on heart valve; (c) emboli from carotid plaque. Also shown: (d) infarcted cortex in area supplied by terminal anterior cerebral artery due to embolism.

the spaces around the brain (Figure 2.4).[23] Bleeding most often originates from aneurysms or arteriovenous malformations, but bleeding diatheses or trauma can also cause subarachnoid bleeding. A ruptured aneurysm releases blood rapidly at systemic blood pressure, suddenly increasing intracranial pressure, whereas bleeding from other causes is usually slower and at lower pressures.

Intracerebral hemorrhages

The terms *intracerebral* and *intraparenchymal hemorrhage* describe bleeding directly into the brain substance. The cause is most often hypertension, with leakage of blood from small intracerebral arterioles damaged by the elevated blood pressure.[24-28] Bleeding diatheses, especially from the

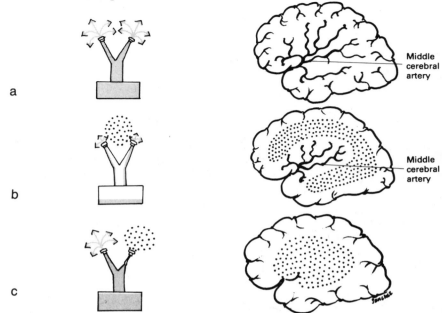

FIGURE 2.3   In heart (pump) failure and watershed infarction, (a) normal pump and arterial circulation do not occur; instead, due to (b) low pump pressure and border-zone ischemia, water goes to the center of hoses (arteries), and stippled areas show poor flow. In contrast, with (c) "blocked hose" and middle cerebral-artery infarction, water flow is deficient in the center of supply (stippled area).

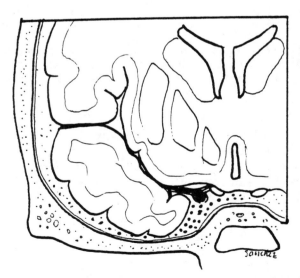

FIGURE 2.4   Subarachnoid hemorrhage: Blood is seen spreading from a ruptured aneurysm into the subarachnoid space.

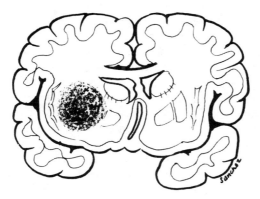

FIGURE 2.5 Intracerebral or intraparenchymal (putaminal) hemorrhage: Note mass effect and shift of cerebral midline.

iatrogenic prescription of anticoagulants or from trauma, vascular malformations, and vasculopathies (such as amyloid degeneration) can also cause bleeding into the brain. Parenchymatous hemorrhages occur in a localized region of the brain (Figure 2.5). The degree of damage will depend on the location, rapidity, volume, and pressure of the bleeding.

Intracerebral hemorrhages are at first soft and dissect along white-matter fiber tracts. When bleeding dissects into the ventricles or onto the surface of the brain, blood is introduced into the cerebrospinal fluid. The blood clots and solidifies, causing swelling of adjacent brain tissues. Later, blood is absorbed, and, after macrophage clearing of the debris, a cavity or slit forms that may disconnect brain pathways. The intracranial cavity is a closed system. The bony skull, vertebral column, and dura mater act as a fortress protecting the brain from outside injury. In adverse situations, such as swelling or hemorrhage arising inside the fortress, these structures may constitute a prison, restricting and strangulating their enclosed contents and forcing herniation of tissue from one compartment to another.[29–31]

The Stroke Mechanism Guides Treatment

The problems in these five major subtypes of stroke—thrombosis, embolism, decreased systemic perfusion, subarachnoid hemorrhage, and intracerebral hemorrhage—are quite distinct and require different treatment strategies. Some therapies suitable for ischemia would be disastrous if the problem were hemorrhage; for example, using anticoagulants or opening a blood vessel to diminish supposed ischemia would augment hemorrhage. Even within the various subcategories of ischemia, treatment depends on the subtype. Other major subtypes also require differing treatments; for example, operating on a blood vessel for supposed local thrombosis might be unnecessary if the problem were embolism and would certainly be ineffective in preventing subsequent emboli from arising proximally. The origin of the embolism also affects treatment: Embolism arising from the heart requires different therapeutic strategies than embolism arising from localized vessel plaques. In regard to systemic hypoperfusion, pump failure or hypovolemia due to intestinal bleeding needs urgent attention, which would be needlessly delayed by inappropriate angiography or a futile search for a localized extracranial vascular lesion. In subarachnoid hemorrhage, the major aim of treatment is to prevent the next aneurysmal leak, whereas in intracerebral hemorrhage, rebleeding is rare, and treatment is aimed at controlling local bleeding and pressure.

In order to treat the stroke patient optimally, the physician must identify the correct mechanism of stroke. Because it is not always possible to be absolutely certain of the single true mechanism, the clinician often must consider the possibility of more than one mechanism, such as thrombosis or embolism, and must evaluate for each. At times, more than one mechanism is operant; for example, in subarachnoid hemorrhage, the blood may cause spasm of blood vessels and thus induce local ischemia. A thrombus obstructing a carotid artery can also fragment and lead to distal artery-to-artery embolism.

Anatomy: Common Anatomical Sites of Vascular and Brain Lesions

Clinical neurology differs from most medical specialties in its emphasis on and even obsession with anatomy. In order to localize and repair damage to water pipes, the effective plumber must be aware of exactly where the pipes are, what they supply, and where they are most likely to be damaged by various hazards. Abnormal neurological signs and symptoms depend more on the localization of the brain injury than on its mechanism. Although all portions of the lung or liver look and function identically, the brain certainly does not. The nervous system is a world of uncountable individual nerve cells and networks, each with quite different and unique characteristics but working together. Each of the various mechanisms of stroke just reviewed has its own preferences for anatomical brain loci. Identification of the location of the stroke depends on analysis of the abnormal neurological symptoms and signs, and on interpretation of brain imaging and electroencephalography. This section of this chapter reviews the important anatomical facts about the extracranial and intracranial arteries,[32] their normal regions of supply, and the most common loci for various vascular pathologies. Next, the anatomical predilections of the major stroke mechanisms within the brain are outlined. This subject is discussed more extensively in the second part of this book, where specific stroke syndromes are addressed.

Normal Vascular Anatomy

The common carotid artery (CCA) bifurcates in the neck, usually opposite the upper border of the thyroid cartilage, into the *internal carotid artery* (ICA), which runs posteriorly as a direct extension of the CCA, and the *external carotid artery* (ECA), which courses more anteriorly and laterally. The ICA travels behind the pharynx and gives off no neck branches. The ICA then enters the skull through the carotid canal within the petrous bone and forms an S-shaped curve, first coursing within the petrous temporal bone and then within the cavernous sinus. This intracavernous portion of the ICA is usually termed the *carotid siphon* because of its shape. The siphon portion of the ICA gives off an ophthalmic artery branch that exits anteriorly; the ICA then penetrates the dura and from its supraclinoid portion gives off anterior choroidal and posterior communicating arteries before bifurcating into the *anterior cerebral artery* (ACA), which courses medially, and the *middle cerebral artery* (MCA), which courses laterally (Figure 2.6).

The ECA has two major vascular channels that ordinarily supply the face, which can act as collateral circulation if the ICA occludes: the *facial artery*, which courses along the cheek toward the nasal bridge, where it is termed the *angular artery*, and the *preauricular artery*, which terminates as the superficial temporal artery. The other important arterial supply of the face involves the frontal and supratrochlear branches from the ophthalmic artery (ICA system), which supply the medial forehead above the brow. When the ICA occludes, these ECA branches can be an important source of collateral blood supply. The patterns of collateral circulation from ECA to ICA are illustrated subsequently in Figure 3.2.

The ACA courses medially until it reaches the longitudinal fissure and then runs posteriorly over the corpus callosum. It supplies the anterior medial portion of the cerebral hemisphere and gives off deep branches to the caudate nucleus and the basal frontal lobe. At times, the first portion of the ACA is hypoplastic on one side, in which case the ACA from the other side supplies both medial frontal lobes. The anterior communicating artery connects the right and left ACAs and provides a means of collateral circulation from the anterior circulation of the opposite side when one ACA is hypoplastic or occludes.

The main stem of the MCA courses laterally, giving off lenticulostriate artery branches to the basal ganglia. As it nears the sylvian fissure, the MCA trifurcates into a small anterior temporal branch and large superior and inferior trunks. The superior trunk supplies the lateral hemisphere above the sylvian fissure, and the inferior trunk supplies the temporal and inferior parietal lobes below the sylvian fissure. The regions of brain supplied by the ACA, MCA, and posterior cerebral artery (PCA) are outlined in Figures 2.7 through 2.9.

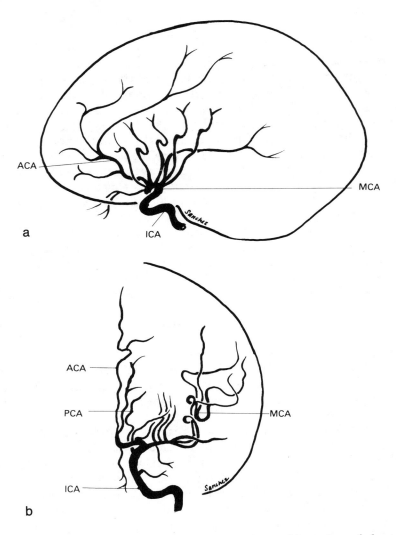

FIGURE 2.6 (a) Lateral and (b) anteroposterior views of branches of the internal carotid artery (ICA). ACA = anterior cerebral artery; MCA = middle cerebral artery; PCA = posterior cerebral artery.

Traditionally, by convention, the carotid artery territories just described are referred to as the *anterior circulation* (front of the brain), while the vertebral and basilar arteries and their branches are termed the *posterior circulation* (because they supply the back of the brain). Each ICA supplies roughly two fifths of the brain by volume, while the posterior circulation accounts for about one fifth of the total. Despite its much smaller size, the posterior circulation contains the *brainstem*, a midline strategically critical

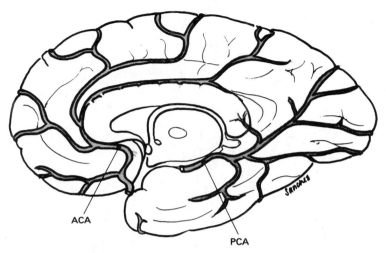

FIGURE 2.7   Anterior (ACA) and posterior (PCA) cerebral arteries: medial view of sagittal section.

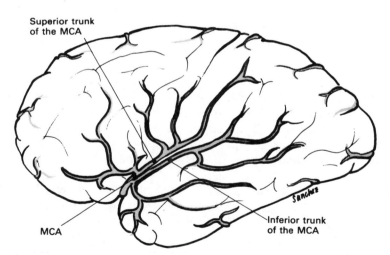

FIGURE 2.8   Middle cerebral artery (MCA): lateral view, with superior and inferior trunk branches.

structure without which consciousness, movement, and sensations could not be preserved. The posterior circulation is constructed quite differently from the anterior and consists of vessels from each side (the vertebral and anterior spinal artery branches), which unite to form midline arteries that supply the brainstem and spinal cord. Within the posterior circulation, there

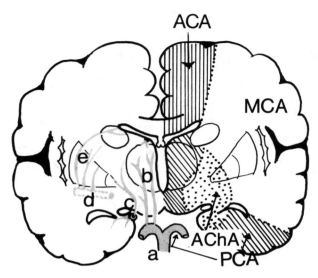

FIGURE 2.9   Coronal view: The right side depicts territories supplied by the anterior cerebral artery (ACA), middle cerebral artery (MCA), posterior cerebral artery (PCA), and anterior choroidal artery (AChA). The left side depicts individual vessels: (a) basilar artery; (b) thalamoperforators, which originate in the PCA; (c) Ach; (d) MCA; (e) lenticulostriate arteries.

is a much higher incidence of asymmetric, hypoplastic arteries, of variability of supply, and of retention of fetal circulatory patterns.[33,34] The proximal portions of the posterior circulation on the two sides differ. On the right, the subclavian artery arises from the innominate artery, a common channel supplying both the anterior and posterior circulations. On the left side, the subclavian artery usually arises directly from the aortic arch after the left CCA.

The first branch of each subclavian artery is the vertebral artery (VA) (Figure 2.10). The VA courses upward and backward until it enters the transverse foramen of C6 or C5 (sixth or fifth cervical vertebra) and runs within the intravertebral foramina, exiting to course behind the atlas before piercing the dura mater to enter the foramen magnum. Its intracranial portion ends at the medullopontine junction, where it joins the contralateral VA to form the basilar artery. In the neck, the VAs have many small muscular and spinal branches. The intracranial portion of the VA gives off major posterior and anterior spinal artery branches, penetrating vessels to the medulla, and the large posterior inferior cerebellar arteries (PICAs).

The basilar artery runs in the midline along the clivus, giving off bilateral anterior inferior cerebellar artery (AICA) and superior cerebellar artery (SCA) branches before bifurcating at the pontomesencephalic junction

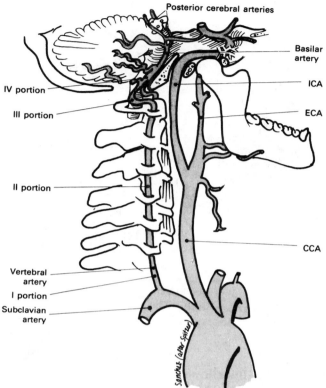

FIGURE 2.10 Lateral view depicting the vertebral and carotid arteries in the neck, the brainstem, and the cerebellum.

into its terminal PCA branches (Figure 2.10). The vascular supply of the brainstem has been worked out by Foix,[35–37] Stopford,[38] and Gillilan[39] and is illustrated in Figure 2.11. The PCAs give off penetrating vessels to the midbrain and thalamus, course around the cerebral peduncles, and then supply the occipital lobes and inferior surface of the temporal lobes (Figures 2.7 and 2.9).

The circle of Willis allows for connections between the anterior circulations of each side, through the anterior communicating artery, and between the posterior and anterior circulations of each side, through the posterior communicating artery (Figure 2.12).

Distribution of Vascular Pathology

Thrombosis

Atherosclerotic narrowing most commonly occurs at the origin of the ICA in the neck. The remainder of the nuchal ICA is seldom affected, but the

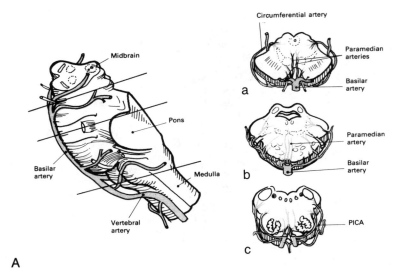

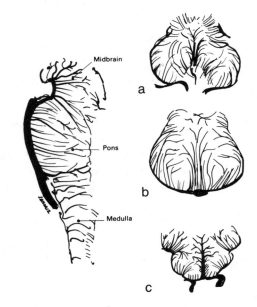

FIGURE 2.11   The vascular supply of the brainstem. (A) Penetrating brainstem arteries. (B) Drawing based on angiographic postmortem opacification of arteries: (a) midbrain; (b) pons; (c) medulla. (After Carpenter MB, *Core Text of Neuroanatomy*. Baltimore, MD: Williams and Wilkins, 1978, p. 333.)

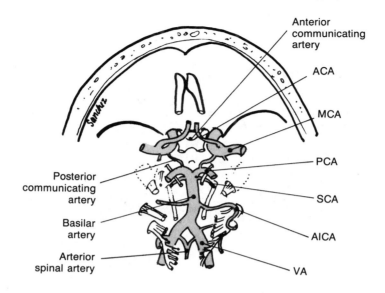

FIGURE 2.12 Internal surface of the skull, showing exit of the cranial nerves and their relationship to the arteries of the circle of Willis.

carotid siphon is also a frequent site for atheroma. The supraclinoid carotid artery and the main-stem MCA and ACA are affected less often in the general population,[40-42] although in black, Chinese, and Japanese patients, MCA disease is more common than is disease of the ICA.[42-46]

Sites of predilection for atheroma in the posterior circulation include the proximal origin of the VA and the subclavian artery, the proximal and distal ends of the intracranial vertebral artery, the basilar artery, and the origins of the PCAs.[34,42,47] Figure 2.13 depicts the most frequent loci of atherosclerosis, which rarely affects the distal superficial branches of the cerebral (ACA, MCA, PCA) or cerebellar (PICA, AICA, SCA) arteries.

Lipohyalinosis and medial hypertrophy secondary to *hypertension* affect primarily the penetrating lenticulostriate branches of the MCA, the anterior perforating vessels of the ACA, the thalamogeniculate penetrators from the PCA, and the paramedian perforating vessels to the pons, midbrain, and thalamus from the basilar artery[48] (Figure 2.14). At times, atheromatous plaques within parent arteries or microatheromas within the orifices of branches cause blockage of penetrating vessels.[49] The distribution of atheromatous branch disease is the same as that of lipohyalinosis.

Dissection—traumatic or spontaneous tearing of a vessel wall with intramural bleeding—usually involves the distal extracranial carotid and vertebral arteries.[12,50] Less common are dissections of the intracranial ICA, MCA, VA, and basilar arteries.[12,50-52] *Temporal arteritis* characteristically affects the ICA and VAs just before they pierce the dura to enter the cranial

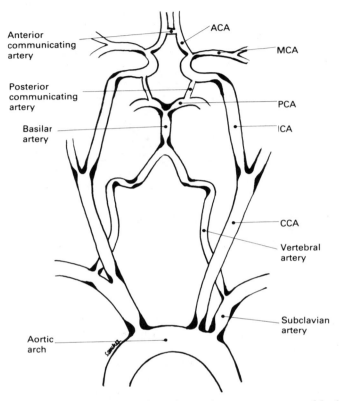

FIGURE 2.13   Sites of predilection for atherosclerotic narrowing; black areas represent plaques.

cavity, as well as the branches of the ophthalmic arteries before they pierce the globe.[11,53]

Embolism

Emboli can block any artery, depending on the size and nature of the embolic material. Large emboli, often clots formed within the heart, can block even large extracranial arteries, such as the innominate, subclavian, carotid, and vertebral arteries in the neck. More often, smaller thrombi formed in the heart or the proximal arteries embolize to block intracranial arteries, such as the ICA, ACA, VA, basilar artery, PCAs, and both the MCA and its superior and inferior trunks. Within the anterior circulation, there is a strong predilection for emboli to go to the MCA and its branches. Small balloons released into the ICAs in experimental animals follow flow patterns to travel to MCA branches.[54] Within the posterior circulation, thrombi preferentially

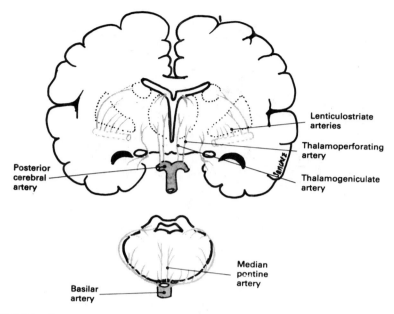

FIGURE 2.14 Penetrating arteries prone to lipohyalinosis and microaneurysms: the thalamogeniculate and lenticulostriate vessels and arteries to the pons.

block the intracranial VA, the distal basilar artery, and the PCAs. Smaller fragments—such as tiny or fragmented thrombi, platelet or platelet–fibrin clumps, cholesterol crystals or other fragments from atheromatous plaques, and calcified fragments from valve and vessel surfaces—tend to embolize to superficial small branches of the cerebral and cerebellar arteries and the ophthalmic and retinal arteries.

Intracerebral hemorrhage

Intracerebral hemorrhage is often due to hypertensive damage to small penetrating vessels and has the same vascular distribution as lipohyalinosis (Figures 2.14, 2.15).[55] Charcot and Bouchard originally described in 1872 microaneurysms, which they believed ruptured, causing intracerebral hemorrhage.[25,26] More-recent studies indicate that sudden increases in blood pressure and blood flow can also cause these same penetrating arteries to break, even in the absence of any chronic hypertensive changes.[27,28]

Subarachnoid hemorrhage

Cerebral aneurysms most often affect junctional regions of the larger vessels of the circle of Willis. The ICA–posterior-communicating-artery junction,

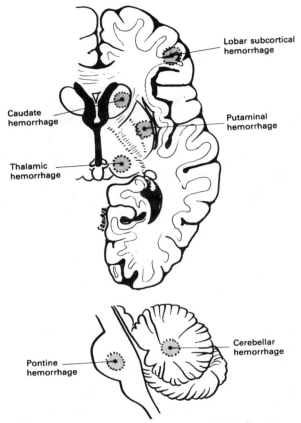

FIGURE 2.15   Horizontal cerebral section and sagittal brainstem section, showing commonest sites of intracerebral hemorrhage.

anterior communicating artery, and MCA trifurcation are the commonest sites. The supraclinoid ICA, pericallosal artery, vertebral–PICA junctions, and apex of the basilar artery are also frequent sites (Figure 2.16).[56,57] Arteriovenous malformations that cause the syndrome of subarachnoid hemorrhage are either located in the brain, abutting on pial or ventricular surfaces, or situated within the ventricular system or the subarachnoid space. Some large malformations are located entirely within the subarachnoid cerebrospinal fluid compartment.

Distribution of Brain Pathology

Ischemia

It is difficult to separate the distribution of brain lesions due to thrombosis from those due to embolism because in many patients, thrombosis of a

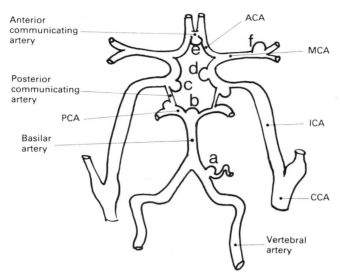

FIGURE 2.16 Commonest sites of intracerebral aneurysms; (a) PICA, (b) basilar artery, (c) posterior communicating artery, (d) ICA, (e) anterior communicating artery, and (f) bifurcation of the MCA.

vessel can lead to distal artery-to-artery embolism. Usually, the region of ischemia tends to be in the center of the supply of the occluded vessel. The extent and size of the infarct will depend on the rate of occlusion, adequacy of collateral circulation, and resistance of brain structures to ischemia. In patients with angiographically documented occlusion of the ICA in the neck, Ringelstein and colleagues distinguished those patients with an intra-arterial embolus to the MCA and its branches ("occlusio supra occlusionem") from those with cortical and subcortical infarcts that were thought to be related to diminished blood flow secondary to the carotid occlusion.[58] Figure 2.17 depicts diagrammatically some of the patterns of infarction in patients with ICA occlusions. In a separate study, Ringelstein and his colleagues studied the distribution of lesions in the brain in patients with cardiogenic cerebral embolism.[59] Figure 2.18, derived from their report, illustrates their findings.

In systemic hypoperfusion, in contrast, the regions most vulnerable to ischemia are in the border zones between major vessel supply zones (Figure 2.17). The situation has been likened to a watering system for a field.[60] If a hose is blocked and the pressure of water in the pump is kept constant, the portion of the field least well supplied will be at the center of the blocked hose (refer back to Figure 2.3b). More water will flow through the open hoses to supply the edges of supply of the blocked hose. However, if pump pressure is reduced, water will trickle out each hose, and only the center of each hose

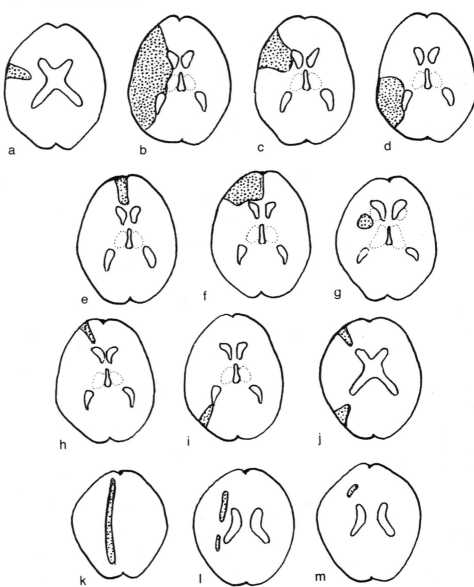

FIGURE 2.17   Most common CT locations of infarcts in the anterior circulation—infarcts are shown by hatched gray: (a) wedge-shaped MCA infarct, (b) entire MCA territory, (c) superior-division MCA, (d) inferior division MCA, (e) ACA, (f) ACA and MCA, (g) striatocapsular infarct, (h) wedge-shaped anterior watershed infarct, (i) wedge-shaped posterior watershed infarct, (j) anterior and posterior watershed infarcts, (k) linear watershed infarct, (l) ovular deep watershed infarct, (m) small white-matter watershed infarct. (From Caplan LR. Cerebrovascular disease: larger artery occlusive disease. In: Appel S, ed., Current Neurology, Vol 8, Chicago: Year-book Medical 1988, 179–226; reprinted with permission.)

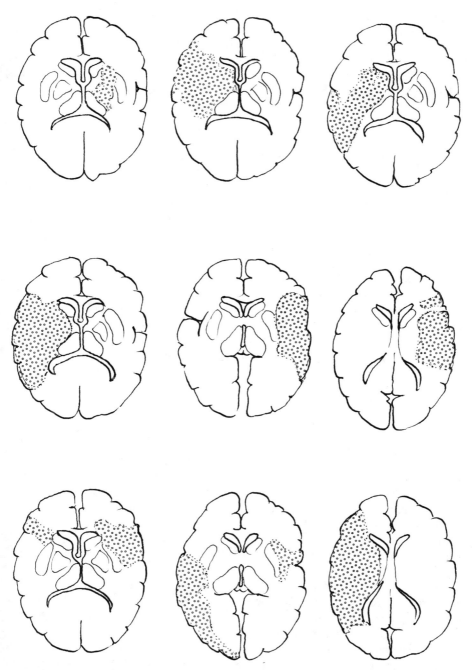

FIGURE 2.18   Infarctions in patients with embolic strokes (reprinted with permission from E.B. Ringelstein et al., "Computed tomographic pattern of proven embolic infarctions," *Annals of Neurology* 1989;26:759–765).

will get water (see Figure 2.3c). Low pressure will reduce flow to the border regions or watersheds between hoses. Another way to look at the distribution of damage in patients with low flow is the concept of the distal fields.[21] The region receiving less blood is the farthest from the center of the longest vessels. These are especially at the edges of the major vessel distributions and most often are more posterior in the hemispheres.

Intracerebral hemorrhage

The commonest brain locations for hypertensive intracerebral hemorrhages are the putamen (lateral ganglionic region) (40%), thalamus (12%), lobar white matter (15–20%), caudate nucleus (8%), pons (8%), and cerebellum (8%) (Figure 2.15). Hemorrhages due to arteriovenous malformations have no special predilection but are most often either subcortical or near the brain surface. Hemorrhages due to amyloid angiopathy also are usually lobar and do not seem to affect the basal ganglia or posterior fossa structures.

Hemorrhages due to illicit drugs, especially cocaine and amphetamines, have the same general distribution as hypertensive hemorrhages, probably because the mechanism of bleeding is probably an acute increase in blood pressure. Hemorrhages in patients on anticoagulants seem to preferentially involve the cerebral white matter and the cerebellum.[61]

Physiology and Pathophysiology of Brain Ischemia and Hemorrhage

Ischemia

Normal metabolism and blood flow

The brain is a very metabolically active organ. Unlike other body organs, the brain uses glucose as its sole substrate for energy metabolism. Glucose is oxidized to CO_2 (carbon dioxide) and H_2O (water). Glucose metabolism leads to conversion of adenosine diphosphate (ADP) into adenosine triphosphate (ATP). A constant supply of ATP is needed to maintain neuronal integrity and to keep the major extracellular cations Ca^{++} (calcium ions) and Na^+ (sodium ions) outside the cells, and the intracellular cation K^+ (potassium ions) within the cells. Production of ATP is much more efficient in the presence of oxygen. Although in the absence of oxygen, anaerobic glycolysis leads to formation of ATP and lactate, the energy yield is relatively small, and lactic acid accumulates within and outside of cells.[62] The brain requires and uses approximately 500 ml of oxygen and 75 to 100 mg of glucose each minute, a total of 125 gm of glucose each day.[63]

These requirements for oxygen and glucose translate into a need for lots of oxygenated blood containing adequate sugar. Even though the brain is a relatively small organ, accounting for only 2% of adult body weight, the brain uses about 20% of the cardiac output when the body is resting.[63]

Cerebral blood flow (CBF) is normally about 50 ml for each 100 gm of brain tissue per minute, and cerebral oxygen consumption—usually measured as the cerebral metabolic rate for oxygen ($CMRO^2$)—is normally about 3.5 ml/100 gm/minute.[62] By increasing oxygen extraction from the bloodstream, compensations can be made to maintain $CMRO^2$ until CBF is reduced down to a level of 20 to 25 ml/100 gm/minute.[62] Positron emission tomography (PET) now allows for measurements of CBF, $CMRO^2$, and oxygen extraction fraction (OEF), as well as the cerebral metabolic rate for glucose (CMRgl) in various brain regions of interest.[64]

Brain energy use and blood flow depend on the degree of neuronal activity. In 1890, Roy and Sherrington first demonstrated the ability of the brain to augment local blood flow in response to regional changes in neuronal activity.[65,66] PET now shows that using the right hand increases metabolism and CBF in the left motor cortex. Clearly, it is critical for survival of brain tissue that there be systems to maintain CBF despite changes in systemic blood pressure. The capacity of the cerebral circulation to maintain relatively constant levels of CBF despite changing pressure has traditionally been termed *autoregulation*. CBF remains relatively constant when mean arterial blood pressures are between 50 and 150 torr.[62] When blood pressure has been chronically raised, both the upper and lower levels of autoregulation are raised, indicating a higher tolerance to hypertension but also increased sensitivity to hypotension.[67]

Blood-flow velocities within the intracranial arteries vary from 40 to 70 cm/second.[63] When CBF increases or an artery narrows, the velocity in that segment of artery increases. At first glance, increased velocity in response to a reduction in luminal diameter seems paradoxical. One must try, however, to visualize a simple everyday example of velocity of liquid flow, an ordinary garden hose. When using the hose to wash off a pavement or a patio, in order to generate a high-pressure jet of water, the nozzle is turned to reduce the luminal diameter. The narrower the nozzle lumen, the more pressure in the stream until the lumen is nearly effaced, at which time water dribbles out, and velocity becomes greatly reduced. This analogy may be useful to recall in Chapter 4, when considering *transcranial Doppler*, an ultrasound device that has the capability of measuring blood-flow velocities in segments of the major basal arteries.

Local brain effects of ischemia

When blood flow to a brain region is reduced, survival of the at-risk tissue depends on the intensity and duration of the ischemia and the availability of collateral blood flow. Animal experiments have allowed for estimates of thresholds of ischemia in the brain (Figure 2.19).[62] At blood-flow levels around 20 ml/100 gm/minute, electroencephalographic (EEG) activity is affected. $CMRO^2$ also begins to fall when CBF is diminished below 20 ml/100 gm/minute. At levels below 10 ml/100 gm/minute, cell membranes and func-

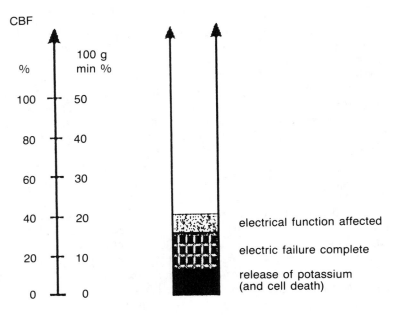

FIGURE 2.19   Thresholds of ischemia.

tions are severely affected. Neurons cannot survive for very long at blood flows below 5 ml/100 gm/minute.

When neurons are rendered ischemic, a number of biochemical changes occur, which potentiate and enhance cell death: K^+ *moves across the cell membrane into the extracellular space, and* Ca^{++} *moves into the cell,* where it both greatly compromises the ability of intracellular membranes to control subsequent ion fluxes and causes mitochondrial failure;[64] normally, there is a tenfold gradient difference between extracellular and intracellular (cytosolic) Ca^{++}. Decreased oxygen availability leads to production of oxygen molecules with unpaired electrons, termed *oxygen free radicals*. These free radicals cause peroxidation of fatty acids in both cell organelles and plasma membranes, severely damaging the cell functions.[68] With decreased oxygen availability, anaerobic glycolysis leads to an *accumulation of lactic acid* and a decrease in pH. The resulting *acidosis* also greatly impairs cell metabolic functions.

Recently, interest has mounted in the activity of local neurotransmitters, often referred to as *excitatory neurotransmitters*.[68–70] In regions of ischemia, concentrations of these neurotransmitters, glutamate, aspartate, and kainic acid, are significantly increased.[68,69] Hypoxia, hypoglycemia, and ischemia cause energy depletion and an increase in glutamate release but a decrease in glutamate uptake. This increased availability of glutamate causes vulnerable neurons to receive toxic exposure to glutamate, thereby increasing the likelihood of cell death. Glutamate entry opens membranes and increases Na^+ and Ca^{++} influx into cells. Large influxes of Na^+ are followed by entry of chloride ions and water, causing cell swelling and edema. Glutamate is an agonist at both N-methyl-D-aspartate (NMDA) and non-NMDA (kainate and quisqualate) receptor types, but only NMDA receptors are linked to membrane channels with high calcium permeability.[70,71] Antagonism of NMDA receptors might limit the damage caused by excitatory neurotransmitters. Knowledge of these changes in the neuronal and extracellular spaces is important in a subsequent (Chapter 5) discussion of treatment strategies to limit ischemia.

These aforementioned local metabolic changes cause a self-perpetuating cycle of changes that lead to increasing neuronal damage and cell death. Changes in ionic concentrations of Na^+, K^+, and Ca^{++}, release of oxygen free radicals, acidosis, and release of excitatory neurotransmitters further damage cells, leading to more local biochemical changes, which in turn cause more neuronal damage. At some time, the process of ischemia becomes irreversible, despite reperfusion of tissues with adequate oxygen and glucose-rich blood. In fact, once this process has become irreversible, reperfusion can lead to delivery to the local ischemic site of more Ca^{++}, oxygen free radicals, neurotransmitters, and other metabolites.

The degree of ischemia caused by blockage of an artery varies in different zones supplied by that artery. In the center of the zone, blood flow is lowest, and ischemic damage is most severe. On the periphery of blood supply, collateral blood flow allows delivery of blood, although at a rate lower than normal. Referring to Figure 2.19, metabolism at the center of supply may be reduced sufficiently to cause cell necrosis (0–10 ml/100 gm/minute), while at the periphery, supplies of 10 to 20 ml/100 gm/minute, might stun the brain, causing electrical failure but not permanent cell damage. The zone of dysfunctional, but not dead, brain surrounding the center of infarction has traditionally been referred to as the *ischemic penumbra*. Garcia and Anderson eloquently describe this region as follows: "Penumbral neurons are thought to be paralyzed in a shadowy state between life and death, merely awaiting the restoration of either adequate blood flow or other as yet unknown conditions before resuming full life."[68] Some neurons are thought to be more vulnerable to hypoxia and decreased fuel supply than other neurons, termed *selective vulnerability.*

Arterial occlusion and reaction to the occlusive process

Cerebral ischemia cannot be viewed as a static anatomicopathological process. It is a dynamic, often unstable, condition. Brain tissue, in imminent danger of irreversible death, nevertheless often recovers remarkably well, leaving no trace of its previous precarious situation. In order to treat the patient optimally, the physician must understand the various factors affecting the outcome. The discussion of pathophysiology so far has centered on the function and metabolism of local regions of brain tissue. To understand the variety of factors affecting outcome, I now turn to a more macroscopic view of both the process of arterial occlusion and the way in which occlusive changes are handled by the body.

Vascular occlusion most often begins with formation of atherosclerotic plaques within extracranial and large intracranial arteries. Atherosclerotic plaques cause cerebral ischemia in a variety of ways. Progressive intimal thickening leads to stenosis or occlusion of the vessel, with reduced distal flow. The plaque often interrupts the endothelium and then ulcerates. A breach of the vascular endothelium disrupts the smooth vascular lining and initiates a process of platelet adherence to the vessel wall. The tiny hemostatic plug then enlarges by aggregation of platelets to each other.[72] ADP, epinephrine, and collagen can all increase platelet aggregation. Activated platelets release ADP and arachidonic acid. In the presence of the enzyme cyclo-oxygenase, arachidonic acid is metabolized to prostaglandin endoperoxides, which can be converted by thromboxane synthetase to *thromboxane* A_2, a very potent vasoconstrictor and inducer of further platelet aggregation and secretion.[3] At the same time, the vessel wall may secrete *prostacyclin*, a potent vasodilator and inhibitor of platelet aggregation.[73] Both vascular patency and the formation of platelet fibrin clots may be determined by the balance between thromboxane A_2 and prostacyclin and other factors.

Atherosclerotic plaques thus interact with blood platelets to form nidi of loosely adherent platelets and fibrin that can break off and embolize distally. The platelet nidus can initiate the coagulation cascade, leading to formation of an occlusive thrombus. Plaque hemorrhage also can lead to rapid reduction in the vascular lumen and may predispose to thrombus formation with subsequent embolization. When a critical plaque size and reduction in luminal area are reached, the occlusive process seems to accelerate. Reduced luminal size and plaque bulk change the physical mechanical properties of blood flow and local turbulence.[74,75] Cracking, ulceration, and clot formation are promoted and accelerated by these changes in flow dynamics.[74–76]

In many cases, the occlusive lesion is an embolus formed more proximally, in which case vascular occlusion is quite sudden. Thrombi can also form in situ when the body's coagulation system has been activated and the blood is hypercoagulable. In some patients with hypercoagulability, thrombi form simultaneously or sequentially in multiple systemic, extracranial and intracranial arteries and veins. In others, with arterial lesions (e.g., arterial atherosclerotic plaques or dissections), the process of occlusive thrombosis is accelerated at sites of vascular disease. Hypercoagulability can be a lifelong hereditary problem. Systemic diseases such as regional enteritis and thrombocytosis can cause increased clotting. The process of atherothrombosis (e.g., in the coronary or cerebrovascular systems) can also activate serological coagulation factors that promote further thrombosis.[77–79]

Much of the treatment of patients with thromboembolic stroke concerns attempts to affect or reverse the coagulation process or to facilitate clot lysis or removal. Clinicians treating patients with ischemia should be familiar with the general features of blood coagulation in order to effectively choose and monitor antithrombotic and thrombolytic therapies.

The final step in the coagulation cascade is the conversion of the soluble protein *fibrinogen* into insoluble polymers termed *fibrin*. These strands of fibrin form a network of fibers that entangle the formed blood elements (platelets, erythrocytes, and leukocytes) into a clot. Fibrin is quite adhesive and has the capability of contracting. The fibrinogen → fibrin reaction occurs when Factor II, *prothrombin*, is converted to *thrombin*. Clearly, the amounts of circulating fibrinogen and prothrombin are important factors in these reactions.

Prothrombin can be activated in two different ways: In the so-called extrinsic system of coagulation, a tissue or endothelial injury releases thromboplastic substances, which in turn cause both platelet activation and activation of some of the blood serine protease coagulation factors, especially Factors V, VII, and X. Activation of Factor X (usually termed *Stuart Factor*) catalyzes the reaction of prothrombin to thrombin. Activation of platelets causes them to agglutinate, to adhere to the injured vessel wall, and to release various intracellular substances, which in turn activate the coagulation system.[80–83]

The complementary intrinsic coagulation system refers to blood-coagulation factors that circulate in inactive forms (Factors V, VIII [antihemophilic globulin], IX, X, XI, XII) and are intrinsic to the blood. Activation of Factor XII (Hageman factor) from an inert precursor form to an activated form trips off a series of reactions, often described as the "coagulation cascade," in which the various blood-clotting factors are sequentially converted to their active enzymatic forms. Ultimately, these reactions lead to activation of Factor X, which catalyzes the prothrombin → thrombin reaction.[80–83] Thrombin, in turn, in addition to converting fibrinogen to fibrin, has a profound influence on blood platelets, causing them to swell, aggregate, and release substances that affect vascular tone and blood coagulability.[82]

Also important are various natural inhibitors of coagulation: antithrombin III, protein C, and protein S. Deficiencies in any of these serum proteins can cause increased coagulability. There are also naturally occurring factors that act to lyse clots once they are formed. Tissue plasminogen activator and other substances activate another serum protein, plasminogen, to form *plasmin*, a potent fibrinolytic enzyme. Plasminogen is also activated by various coagulation factors, such as Factor XII, so that the process of coagulation itself activates the thrombolytic system. Various plasmin inhibitors ("antiplasmins") are also present.[84]

Pathologists recognize and describe three different types of thrombi:[81]

(1) *Red thrombi* are composed mostly of red blood cells and fibrin, and they form in areas of slowed blood flow. Their formation does not require an abnormal vessel wall or tissue thromboplastin (Figure 2.20). (2) *White thrombi*, in contrast, are composed of platelets and fibrin and are poor in red blood cells (Figure 2.21). White clots form almost exclusively in areas in which the vessel wall or endothelial surface is abnormal, characteristically in fast-moving bloodstreams. (3) *Disseminated fibrin deposition* in small vessels. These types of thrombi are distinct and are affected by different therapeutic agents. In many cases, the thrombus begins as a white platelet fibrin clot and then a red thrombus is laid down as a cap over the initial platelet mass.[81,82]

When a major artery occludes, a crisis is created. Pressure drops distal to the occlusion, and the brain region supplied by that vessel is acutely deprived of blood. Diminished blood flow in turn activates protective mechanisms that serve to restore needed blood flow to the ischemic region. Low pressure helps to draw blood from higher-pressure regions. Collateral circulation increases. Ischemic cell damage causes release of lactic acid and other metabolites. The resulting local tissue acidosis leads to vasodilation, augmenting regional CBF.[85] If brain tissue is deprived of blood and needed nourishment for too long, it dies. At times, there are varying grades of ischemia, ranging from irreversible cell death in the most deprived zone to a reversible situation of diminished electrical activity but normal or only slightly elevated extracellular potassium concentration in the threatened ischemic penumbral zone.[68,69,86] The severity of the ischemic crisis depends on the rate of vascular occlusion. A vessel that has gradually occluded may already have evoked abundant collateral circulation, so that final occlusion produces less stress on the system.

Factors affecting tissue survival

The survival of the brain regions at risk depends on a number of factors: (1) the adequacy of collateral circulation, (2) the state of the systemic circulation, (3) serological factors, (4) changes within the obstructing vascular lesion, and (5) resistance within the microcirculatory bed.

The Adequacy of Collateral Circulation. Congenital deficiencies in the circle of Willis and prior occlusion of potential collateral vessels decrease the available collateral supply. Hypertension or diabetes diminishes blood flow in smaller arteries and arterioles and thus reduces the potential of the vascular system to supply blood flow to the needy region.

The State of the Systemic Circulation. Cardiac pump failure, hypovolemia, and increased blood viscosity all reduce CBF.[87–89] The two major determinants of blood viscosity are the hematocrit and the fibrinogen level. In patients with hematocrits in the range of 47 to 53, lowering of the hematocrit by phlebotomy to below 40 causes flow to increase by a mean of 50 percent.[87] Blood pressure is also very important. Elevation of blood pressure

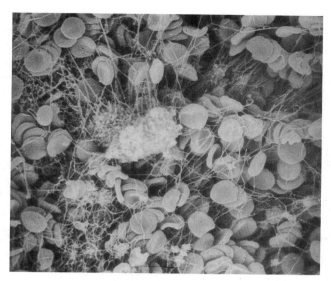

FIGURE 2.20   Phase microscope image of a *red thrombus*, composed of fibrin and erythrocytes, formed in a thrombogenic system, in a vessel with a low flow rate (courtesy of S.H. Hanson and Ch. Kessler, Emory University, Division of Hematology).

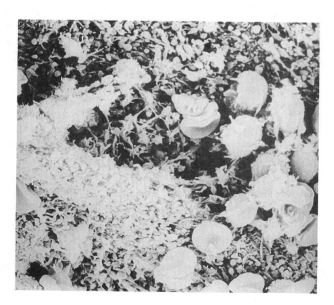

FIGURE 2.21   Phase microscope image of a white fibrin–platelet thrombus formed in a high-flow system (courtesy of S.H. Hanson and Ch. Kessler, Emory University, Division of Hematology).

except at malignant ranges increases CBF. Surgeons take advantage of this fact by injecting catecholamines to raise blood pressure and flow artificially during the clamping phase of carotid endarterectomy. Low blood pressure significantly reduces flow. In some patients, the balance is so tenuous that simply sitting in bed or standing lowers collateral pressure enough to induce symptoms.[90,91]

Serological Factors.   The blood functions as a carrier of needed oxygen and other nutrients to the tissues. Hypoxia is clearly detrimental because each milliliter of blood delivers a less-than-normal oxygen supply to the tissues. Low blood sugar similarly increases the risk of cell death. Evidence is now accumulating that higher-than-normal blood sugar also can be detrimental to the ischemic brain.[92,93] Elevated serum calcium levels[94,95] and high blood-alcohol content[96] may also be important detrimental variables.

Changes within the Obstructing Vascular Lesion.   Embolic occlusive clots do not adhere to the vessel wall of the recipient artery and frequently move on. The moving embolus can block a more distal intracranial artery, causing added or new ischemia, or it may fragment and pass through the vascular bed. Clot formation activates an endogenous thrombolytic system that includes tissue plasminogen activator (tPA).[84] Inhibitors of tPA are also present in variable concentrations. Sudden obstruction to a vascular lumen can cause reactive vasoconstriction (spasm), which in turn causes further luminal compromise. Thrombolysis, passage of clots, and reversal of vasoconstriction all promote reperfusion of the ischemic zone. If reperfusion occurs quickly enough, the stunned, reversibly ischemic brain may recover quickly. The occlusive clot may propagate further proximally or distally along the vessel, blocking potential collateral channels. The distal end of the thrombus can also break loose and embolize to an intracranial receptive site. Hypercoagulable states promote such extension of thrombi.

Resistance within the Microcirculatory Bed.   The vast majority of CBF does not occur in the large macroscopic arteries at the base of the brain or along the surface. Most flow occurs through microscopic-sized vessels: the arterioles, capillaries, and venules. The resistance to flow in the vessels is affected by prior diseases, such as hypertension and diabetes, which often cause thickening of vessel walls. Experimental animals and human subjects that have been hypertensive prior to a vascular occlusion fare worse than individuals previously normotensive, presumably because of these changes in the microcirculatory bed. Both hyperviscosity and diffuse thromboses within the capillaries and microvessel bed greatly reduce flow through the microcirculation. Ischemic insults may produce biochemical changes that lead to platelet activation, clumping of erythrocytes, and plugging of the microcirculation. Ames referred to these changes as causing a "no reflow" state in the microvascular bed, even when large arteries are reperfused.[97] In general, studies of CBF are very sensitive to changes in resistance in the microcirculatory bed. Remember that flow is inversely proportional to resistance in the vascular bed, the majority of which is microcirculatory.

Edema and pressure changes within the brain and cranial cavity may also influence survival of brain tissue and patient recovery after a vascular occlusion. There are two types of brain edema: (1) water accumulation inside cells, termed *cytotoxic edema;* and (2) fluid within the extracellular space, often termed *vasogenic edema.*[98] Extracellular edema is also often referred to as "wet edema" because in such cases, the cut surface of the brain oozes edema fluid, whereas intracellular (cytotoxic) edema is termed dry edema.[98] Cytotoxic edema is caused by energy failure, with movement of ions and water across the cell membranes into cells. Extracellular edema is caused by hydrostatic pressure factors, especially increased blood pressure and blood flow, and by osmotic factors. When proteins and other macromolecules enter the brain extracellular space because of breakdown of the blood–brain barrier, they exert an osmotic gradient pulling water into the extracellular space. This vasogenic edema accumulates more in the cerebral and cerebellar white matter because of the difference in compliance between gray and white matter.[98]

Brain swelling due to cytotoxic edema means a large volume of dead or dying brain cells, which implies a very bad outcome. On the other hand, edema within the extracellular space does not necessarily require severe neuronal injury, and fluid in the extracellular compartment can potentially be mobilized and removed. In any case, severe edema may cause gross swelling of the brain; shifts in position of brain tissue, with potential pressure damage; and herniation of brain contents from one compartment to another.

Intracranial pressure may also be increased, leading to increased morbidity and decreased CBF. When intracranial pressure is increased, the pressure in the venous sinuses and draining veins must also increase if blood is to be drained from the cranium. There must be a gradient between venous pressure and intracranial pressure for drainage to occur. Also, in order for tissue perfusion to occur, arterial pressure must be considerably higher than venous pressure. Blood flow is already compromised in the presence of vascular occlusion. Increased intracranial pressure places an additional stress on the system, forcing even higher the flow values required for tissue survival. Brain edema and increased intracranial pressure also cause headache, decreased levels of consciousness, and vomiting.[99] Pressure shifts and herniation cause pressure-related damage to adjacent tissues and signs of dysfunction of the compressed structures.[31,100] Because pressure shifts and herniations are more common after intracerebral hemorrhage, because of the additional factor of the presence in the brain of an extra mass of tissue (hematoma), I discuss herniations further subsequently, in regard to intracerebral hemorrhage.

Events during the first three weeks after vascular occlusion

Considerable clinical experience indicates that the tenuous balance created by occlusion of a major artery is temporary and usually resolves in 2 to 3 weeks at most. During this period, any systemic changes, such as decrease in fluid volume or positional or pharmacologically mediated drops in blood pressure, can be associated with worsening of symptoms. By 3 weeks, either the brain tissue has died, causing a brain infarct, or collateral sources of blood flow develop, which adequately supply the region at risk. By 2 to 3 weeks, collateral circulation stabilizes, and the patient is less vulnerable to positional or circulatory changes. In addition to causing ischemia through low perfusion, the occlusive thrombus, which at first loosely adheres to the vessel wall, can propagate distally or can fragment and embolize to a distal artery. By 2 to 3 weeks, the clot has become more adherent and has much less tendency to embolize. Most studies of anterior[101,102] and posterior circulation ischemia[103,104] document a very low incidence of progression of acute ischemic deficits after 2 weeks.

During the hours, days, and early weeks after an occlusion, the question of death or survival of at-risk brain tissue can be viewed as a clash between factors acting to worsen ischemia and natural body responses that act to prevent or limit ischemia. Table 2.1 summarizes these "good guys" versus "bad guys" responses, which are useful to keep in mind when treatment is discussed. Obviously, the clinician hopes to build on the body's natural defenses and counteract the factors that promote ischemia.

This process of shifting vulnerability translates clinically into fluctuating variable symptoms and signs during the early period after a vascular occlusion. Acute blockage of an artery often translates into the sudden onset of symptoms. After occlusion, a weighing of the balance of positive and adverse factors toward the adverse side causes transient deficits or causes fluctuating, stepwise, or gradual worsening of neurological symptoms and signs. Sudden worsening is often related to distal embolization.

Intracerebral Hemorrhage

Hemorrhage into the brain parenchyma is often preceded by hypertensive damage to small cerebral penetrating arteries and arterioles. Small aneurysmal dilations, first hypothesized by Charcot and Bouchard in the 1870s, pepper the penetrating vascular territories of hypertensive patients[25,26,28] and in some patients represent weak points that rupture under increased arterial tension. In the majority of patients, abrupt elevation in blood pressure causes rupture of small penetrating arteries that had no prior vascular damage.[27,28] Leakage from these small vessels produces a sudden but local pressure effect on surrounding capillaries and arterioles, causing them in turn to break.[104] An avalanche-type effect ensues, in which vessels at the circumference break, adding volume to the gradually enlarging hemorrhage (Figure 2.22). The accumulation of hematoma at the periphery can be likened to a snowball rolling down hill, gathering volume along its circumference as it descends. High blood pressure and this avalanche effect enlarge the hemorrhage, while mounting local pressure acts as a tamponade to the bleeding.

TABLE 2.1
The Balancing of Factors after Vascular Occlusion

Factors Promoting Ischemia	versus	Body Responses Acting to Limit Ischemia
1. Decreased blood flow 2° to occlusion		1. Opening of collateral vascular flow
2. Embolization of clot		2. Passing and fragmentation of emboli
3. Propagation of clot and activation of coagulation factors and inhibitors of thrombolysis		3. Activation of thrombolytic factors
4. Diminished flow due to hypotension, hypovolemia, poor cardiac output		4. Improvement in general conditions

Trauma, bleeding disorders, and degenerative changes in congenitally abnormal blood vessels within arteriovenous malformations also may initiate intracerebral bleeding, which then progresses in a manner similar to hypertensive intracerebral hemorrhage. The gradual increase in size of the hematoma translates clinically into gradual worsening of symptoms and signs during the period until the hematoma attains its final size. Hematomas can stop enlarging and may drain themselves by emptying into the ventricular system or the cerebrospinal fluid (CSF) at the pial surface.

If the hemorrhage becomes sizable, the increase in intracranial volume must increase intracranial pressure. When intracranial pressure rises, the venous pressure in the draining dural sinuses increases pari passu. In order to perfuse the brain, the arterial pressure must rise to produce an effective arteriovenous difference. Thus, the patient with intracerebral hemorrhage may have a markedly elevated blood pressure merely secondary to the hemorrhage, not necessarily reflecting the true level of the premorbid pressure. While lowering this pressure does help to stop bleeding, caution must be exercised because the elevated pressure also helps to perfuse the areas of brain not damaged by the hemorrhage.

Patients with intracerebral hemorrhage often worsen during the first 24 to 48 hours after their initial symptoms. This worsening can be due to continued bleeding but most often is related to the development of edema around the lesion,[105,106] to the effects of the lesion on blood flow and metabolism, and—in large hemorrhages—to shifts in brain contents and herniations. Effects caused by masses in patients with hematomas are more common than in patients with ischemia because an extra volume of substance has been added (blood in the hematoma), in addition to the surrounding edema. Most often, pressure effects in hemispheral hematomas result in a shift of the midline without herniation of brain contents (Figure 2.23). The brain is compartmentalized by bony fortresses (anterior, middle, and posterior fossas) and by dural structures (falx cerebri and tentorium cerebelli), which, under normal circumstances, contain fully their usual

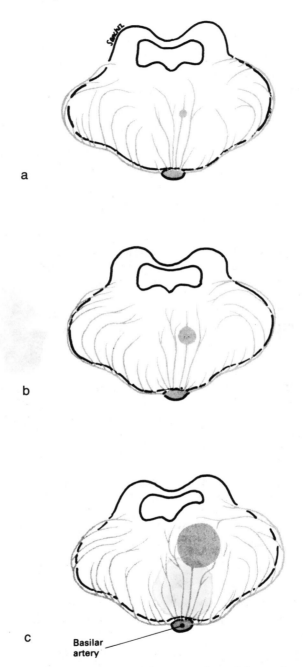

a

b

c

Basilar
artery

FIGURE 2.22   Avalanche-type effect in pontine hemorrhage, showing gradual development of hemorrhage due to rupture of small vessels on the periphery of the hemorrhage.

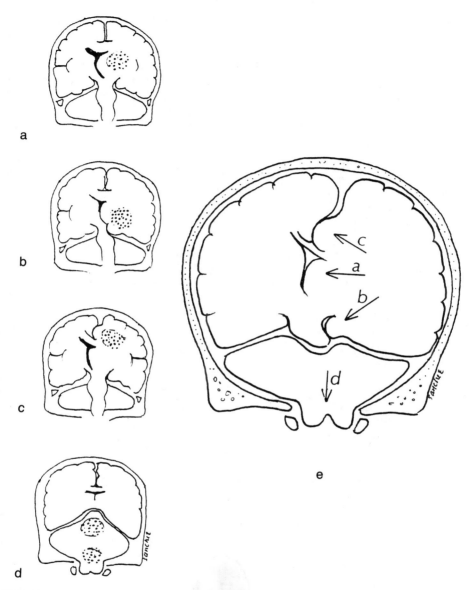

FIGURE 2.23   Shifts and herniations: Displacement of brain tissues due to mass-producing strokes are illustrated by patients with hematomas. (a) Basal ganglionic hematoma causes compression of the ipsilateral ventricle and shift of the midline to the opposite side. (b) Deep hematoma causes uncal herniation. The medial temporal lobe exerts pressure on the upper brainstem. (c) Frontal hematoma causes herniations of the cingulum under the falx cerebri. (d) Cerebellum hematoma causes increased posterior fossa pressure with herniation of the cerebellum (e) through the foramen magnum. These patterns are also illustrated on the larger figure to the right.

contents. When mass effects are severe, brain tissue bulges or spills out of its usual abode into a different compartment—a process called "herniation."[28,31,100]

Brain shifts and herniations and their effects are depicted in Figure 2.23. The commonest are (1) herniation of the temporal lobe through the tentorial notch, to compress the midbrain (Figure 2.23a); (2) symmetrical, downward pressure by the swollen hemispheres on the rostral brainstem, causing elongation (Figure 2.23b); (3) herniation of the anterior medial frontal lobe, usually of the cingulate gyrus, under the falx cerebri (Figure 2.23c); (4) herniation of the cerebellum upward through the tentorial notch, to compress the brainstem (Figure 2.23d); (5) downward herniation of the cerebellar tonsils through the foramen magnum, compressing the medulla and upper cervical spinal cord (Figure 2.23d).

Shifts in brain contents can also lead to compression or stretch of arteries and infarction in areas of supply and secondary hemorrhages. The most common loci of secondary vascular changes leading to infarction involve the PCA, where it passes between the tentorium and the medial temporal lobe and the ACA adjacent to the falx (Figure 2.24). Distortion of the

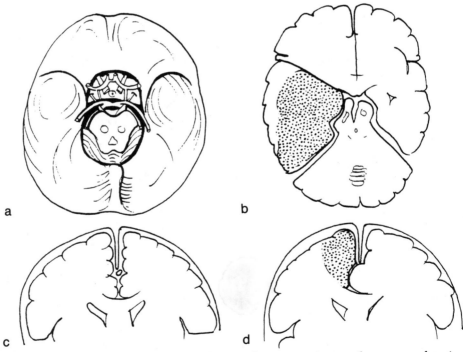

FIGURE 2.24   Infarcts due to compression of arteries: (a) normal anatomy showing PCA crossing up and over the edge of the tentorium; (b) infarction of medial temporal lobe due to compression of PCA between herniated uncus and tentorium; (c) anatomy showing ACA in relation to falx; (d) infarction of medial frontal lobe, due to compression of ACA against falx.

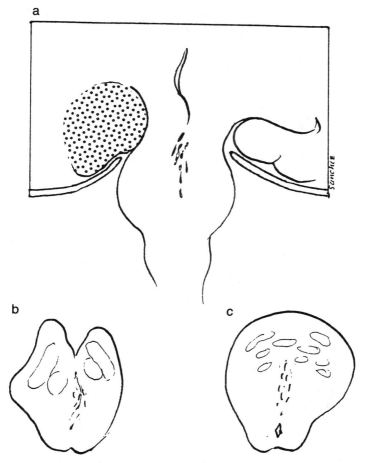

FIGURE 2.25 Düret hemorrhages: (a) herniation with compression of midbrain (longitudinal view); (b) midbrain cross-section; (c) pons cross-section.

upper brainstem at the tentorial opening often leads to secondary hemorrhages in the brainstem. These usually involve the midline and paramedian vessels and are called "Düret hemorrhages," after the French clinician and researcher who first described them.[28,107] Düret hemorrhages are illustrated in Figure 2.25.

The ventricular system may also be compressed at variable sites. Hematomas in the putamen or cerebral lobes may distort the foramen of Monro, causing dilation of the contralateral lateral ventricle. Thalamic hematomas often obstruct and compress the third ventricle, leading to hydrocephalus of both lateral ventricles. Cerebellar hemorrhages can compress the forth ventricle or cerebral aqueduct, leading to obstructive hydrocephalus of the third and lateral ventricles. These examples of hydrocephalus are depicted in Figure 2.26.

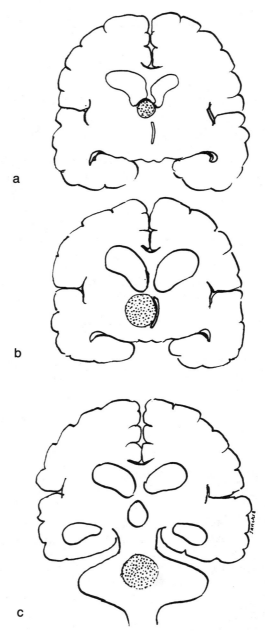

FIGURE 2.26 Strokes causing hydrocephalus: (a) hematoma blocking foramen of Monro, causing dilation of the ventricle on the left; (b) thalamic hematoma compressing the ventricle, causing dilation of the lateral ventricles; (c) cerebellar hematoma compressing the fourth ventricle, causing dilation of the third ventricle and lateral ventricles.

Shifts in brain contents, herniations, and secondary infarctions, as well as Duret hemorrhages and hydrocephalus, all cause clinical worsening of signs and symptoms.

Subarachnoid Hemorrhage

Subarachnoid bleeding nearly always abruptly increases intracranial pressure (ICP). Systemic blood pressure and volume must be maintained or augmented to preserve brain perfusion in the face of the increased ICP. After the initial bleeding, three major risks affect subsequent events: rebleeding, vasoconstriction, and hydrocephalus. Once the outer wall of abnormal blood vessels, most often aneurysms and arteriovenous malformations, has been breached, the vessels are vulnerable to *rebleeding*. Clearly, a second or third bleed poses substantial threats for survival because each bleed increases ICP and the amount of blood in the CSF. Arteries bathed in bloody CSF often become constricted. *Vasoconstriction*, often termed *vasospasm*, can be local or more diffuse, and it frequently leads to ischemia, brain edema, and infarction.[108,109] Blood within the CSF can clog the absorptive membranes, leading to communicating *hydrocephalus*, dilation of all of the ventricular system. At times, the initial bleed or subsequent bleeds are into the brain, as well as on its surface. In these patients, the discussion of intracerebral hemorrhage also applies because they have both intracerebral and subarachnoid hemorrhages.

Having laid the basic building blocks for understanding the mechanisms of stroke, I proceed directly to clinical diagnosis at the bedside, and then laboratory diagnosis.

References

1. Kapp J, Mahaley M, Odom G. Cerebral arterial spasm: III. partial purification and characterization of spasmogenic substances in feline platelets. J Neurosurg 1968;29:350–356.
2. Ropper A, Zervas N. Cerebral blood flow after experimental basal ganglia hemorrhage. Ann Neurol 1982;11:266–271.
3. Weiss H. Platelet physiology and abnormalities of platelet function. N Engl J Med 1975;293:531–540,580–588.
4. Moncada S, Vane J. Arachidonic acid metabolites and the interactions between platelets and blood-vessel walls. N Engl J Med 1979;300:1142–1147.
5. Baker A, Iannone A. Cerebrovascular disease: I. the large arteries of the circle of Willis. Neurology 1959;9:321–332.
6. Fisher CM, Gore I, Okabe N, et al. Atherosclerosis of the carotid and vertebral arteries—extracranial and intracranial. J Neuropathol Exp Neurol 1965;24:455–476.
7. Fisher CM. Lacunes: small deep cerebral infarcts. Neurology 1965;15:774–784.
8. Fisher CM. The arterial lesions underlying lacunes. Acta Neuropathol 1969;12:1–15.

9. Houser O, Baker H, Sandok B, et al. Cephalic arterial fibromuscular dysplasia. Radiology 1971;101:605–611.
10. Vinijchalkul L. Primary arteritis of the aorta and its main branches (Takayasu's arteriopathy). Am J Med 1967;43:15–27.
11. Goodwin J. Temporal arteritis. In: Vinken P, Bruyn G, eds. Handbook of clinical neurology: vol 39, pt 2. neurological manifestations of systemic diseases. Amsterdam: North Holland, 1980:13–342.
12. Fisher CM, Ojemann R, Roberson G. Spontaneous dissection of cervico-cerebral arteries. Can J Neurol Sci 1978;5:9–19.
13. Imparato A, Riles T, Mintzer R, et al. The importance of hemorrhage in the relationship between gross morphologic characteristics and cerebral symptoms in 376 carotid artery plaques. Ann Surg 1983;197:195–203.
14. Caplan LR, Hier DB, D'Cruz I. Cerebral embolism in the Michael Reese Stroke Registry. Stroke 1983;14:530–536.
15. Fisher CM. Observations of the fundus oculi in transient monocular blindness. Neurology 1959;9:333–347.
16. Jones H, Caplan LR, Come P, et al. Paradoxical cerebral emboli: an occult cause of stroke. Ann Neurol 1983;13:314–319.
17. Dines D, Linscheid R, Didier E. Fat embolism syndrome. Proc Mayo Clin 1972;47:237–241.
18. Beal M, Williams R, Richardson E, et al. Cholesterol embolism as a cause of transient ischemic attacks and cerebral infarction. Neurology 1981;31:860–865.
19. Atlee W. Talc and cornstarch emboli in eyes of drug users. JAMA 1972;219:49–51.
20. Hart RG, Foster JW, Luther MF, et al. Stroke in infective endocarditis. Stroke 1990;21:695–700.
21. Mohr J. Neurological complications of cardiac valvular disease and cardiac surgery including systemic hypotension. In: Vinken P, Bruyn G, eds. Handbook of clinical neurology: vol 38, pt 1. neurological manifestations of systemic diseases. Amsterdam: North Holland, 1979:143–171.
22. Romanul F, Abramowicz A. Changes in brain and pial vessels in arterial boundary zones. Arch Neurol 1964;11:40–65.
23. Symonds C. Spontaneous subarachnoid hemorrhage. Q J Med 1924;18:93.
24. Caplan LR. Intracerebral hemorrhage. In: Tyler H, Dawson D, eds. Current neurology: vol. 2. Boston: Houghton Mifflin, 1979:185–205.
25. Cole F, Yates P. Intracerebral microaneurysms and small cerebrovascular lesions. Brain 1967;90:759–768.
26. Rosenblum W. Miliary aneurysms and "fibrinoid" degeneration of cerebral blood vessels. Hum Path 1977;8:133–139.
27. Caplan LR. Intracerebral hemorrhage revisited. Neurology 1988;38:624–627.
28. Caplan LR, Kase C. Intracerebral hemorrhage. Boston: Butterworth, 1993.
29. Finney L, Walker A. Transtentorial herniation. Springfield, Ill.: Thomas, 1962.
30. Fisher CM. Observations concerning brain herniation. Ann Neurol 1983;14:110.
31. Ropper AH. Lateral displacement of brain and level of consciousness in patients with acute hemispheral mass. N Engl J Med 1986;314:953–958.
32. Stephens R, Stilwell D. Arteries and veins of the human brain. Springfield, Ill.: Thomas, 1969.

33. Lie T. Congenital malformations of the carotid and vertebral arterial systems, including the persistent anastomoses. In: Vinken P, Bruyn G, eds. Handbook of clinical neurology: vol 12, pt 2. vascular diseases of the nervous system. Amsterdam: North Holland, 1972:289–339.

34. Caplan LR. Vertebrobasilar occlusive disease. In: Barnett HJM, Mohr J, Stein B, Yatsu F, eds. Stroke: pathophysiology, diagnosis and management. New York: Churchill Livingstone, 1986:549–619.

35. Foix C, Hillemand P. Contributions a l'etude des ramolissements protuberentiels. Rev Med 1926;43:287–305.

36. Foix C, Hillemand P. Les arteres de l'axe encephalique jusqu'a diencephale inclusivement. Rev Neurol 1925;32:705–739.

37. Caplan LR. Charles Foix—the first modern stroke neurologist. Stroke 1990;21:348–356.

38. Stopford J. The arteries of the pons and medulla oblongata. J Anat Physiol 1915,1916;50:131–164,255-280.

39. Gillilan L. Anatomy and embryology of the arterial system of the brainstem and cerebellum. In: Vinken P, Bruyn G, eds. Handbook of clinical neurology: vol 11, pt 1. vascular diseases of the nervous system. Amsterdam: North Holland, 1972:24–44.

40. Fisher CM. Clinical syndromes in cerebral arterial occlusion. In: Fields W, ed. Pathogenesis and treatment of cerebrovascular disease. Springfield, Ill.: Thomas, 1961:151–181.

41. Castaigne P, Lhermitte F, Gautier JC, et al. Internal carotid artery occlusion: a study of 61 instances in 50 patients with postmortem data. Brain 1970; 93:231–258.

42. Caplan LR. Cerebrovascular disease: large artery occlusive disease. In: Appel S, ed. Current neurology: vol 8. Chicago: Yearbook Medical, 1988:179–226.

43. Gorelick PB, Caplan LR, Hier DB, et al. Racial differences in the distribution of anterior circulation occlusive cerebrovascular disease. Neurology 1984; 34:54–59.

44. Caplan LR, Gorelick PB, Hier DB. Race, sex, and occlusive cerebrovascular disease: a review. Stroke 1986;17:648–655.

45. Kieffer S, Takeya Y, Resch J, et al. Racial differences in cerebrovascular disease: angiographic evaluation of Japanese and American populations. AJR 1967; 101:94–99.

46. Feldmann E, Daneault N, Kwan E, et al. Chinese–white differences in the distribution of occlusive cerebrovascular disease. Neurology 1990;40:1541–1545.

47. Moossy J. Morphology, sites, and epidemiology of cerebral atherosclerosis. Res Publ Assoc Res Nerv Ment Dis 1966;51:1–22.

48. Mohr JP. Lacunes. Stroke 1982;13:3–11.

49. Caplan LR. Intracranial branch atheromatous disease. Neurology 1989;39: 1246–1250.

50. Caplan LR, Zarins C, Hemmatti M. Spontaneous dissection of the extracranial vertebral artery. Stroke 1985;16:1030–1038.

51. O'Connell BF, Towfighi J, Brennan RW, et al. Dissecting aneurysms of head and neck. Neurology 1985;35:993–997.

52. Caplan LR, Baquis GD, Pessin MS, et al. Dissection of the intracranial vertebral artery. Neurology 1988;38:868–877.

53. Wilkinson I, Russell R. Arteries of the head and neck in giant cell arteritis. Arch Neurol 1972;27:378–391.
54. Gacs G, Merei FT, Bodosi M. Balloon catheter as a model of cerebral emboli in humans. Stroke 1982;13:39–42.
55. Fisher CM. Clinical syndromes in cerebral hemorrhage. In: Fields WS, ed. Pathogenesis and treatment of cerebrovascular disease. Springfield, Ill.: Thomas, 1961:318–342.
56. Bull J. Contribution of radiology to the study of intracranial aneurysms. Br Med J 1922;2:1701–1708.
57. Alpers B. Aneurysms of the circle of Willis. In: Fields WS, ed. Intracranial aneurysms and subarachnoid hemorrhage. Springfield, Ill.: Thomas, 1965:5–24.
58. Ringelstein E, Zeumer H, Angelou D. The pathogenesis of strokes from internal carotid artery occlusion. Stroke 1983;14:867–875.
59. Ringelstein EB, Koschorke S, Holling A, et al. Computed tomographic pattern of proven embolic brain infarctions. Ann Neurol 1989;26:759–765.
60. Zulch K, Behrends R. The pathogenesis and topography of anoxia, hypoxia, and ischemia of the brain in man. In: Meyer J, Gastant H, eds. Cerebral anoxia and the EEG. Springfield, Ill.: Thomas, 1961:144–163.
61. Kase C, Robinson K, Stein R, et al. Anticoagulant-related intracerebral hemorrhage. Neurology 1985;35:943–948.
62. Jafar JJ, Crowell RM. Focal ischemic thresholds. In: Wood JH, ed. Cerebral blood flow. New York: McGraw-Hill, 1987:449–457.
63. Toole JF. Cerebrovascular disorders. 4th ed. New York: Raven Press, 1990.
64. Frackowiak R, Lenzi G, Jones T, et al. Quantitative measurements of regional cerebral blood flow and oxygen metabolism in man using ^{15}oxygen and positron emission tomography: therapy, procedure, and normal values. J Comput Assist Tomogr 1980;4:722–736.
65. Roy CS, Sherrington CS. On the regulation of the blood-supply of the brain. J Physiol (London) 1890;11:85–108.
66. Friedland RP, Iadecola C. Roy and Sherrington (1890): a centennial reexamination of "On the regulation of the blood-supply of the brain." Neurology 1991;41:10–14.
67. Symon L. Pathological regulation in cerebral ischemia. In: Wood JH, ed. Cerebral blood flow. New York: McGraw-Hill, 1987:413–424.
68. Garcia JH, Anderson ML. Pathophysiology of cerebral ischemia. CRC—Critical Reviews in Neurobiology 1989;4:303–324.
69. Collins RC, Dobkin BH, Choi DW. Selective vulnerability of the brain: new insights into the pathophysiology of stroke. Ann Intern Med 1989;110:992–1000.
70. Olney JW. Neurotoxicity of excitatory amino acids. In: McGeer P, Olney JW, eds. Kainic acid as a tool in neurobiology. New York: Raven Press, 1978:95–121.
71. MacDermott AB, Mayer ML, Westbrook GL, et al. NMDA-receptor activation increases cytoplasmic calcium concentration in cultured spinal cord neurons. Nature 1986;321:519–522.
72. Shaltil S, Bennett J. Platelets and their membranes in hemostasis: physiology and pathophysiology. Ann Intern Med 1980;94:108–118.
73. Moncada S, Higgs E, Vane J. Human arterial and venous tissues generate prostacyclin (prostaglandin 4) a potent inhibitor of platelet aggregation. Lancet 1977;1:18–20.

74. Hennerici M, Sitzer G, Weger H-D. Carotid artery plaques. Basel: Karger, 1987.
75. Caplan LR, Pessin MS. Symptomatic carotid artery disease and carotid endarterectomy. Ann Rev Med 1988;39:273–299.
76. Fisher CM, Ojemann RG. A clinico-pathologic study of carotid endarterectomy plaques. Rev Neurol (Paris) 1986;142:573–589.
77. Fisher M, Francis R. Altered coagulation in cerebral ischemia. Arch Neurol 1990;47:1075–1079.
78. Tohgi H, Kawashima M, Tamura K, et al. Coagulation–fibrinolysis abnormalities in acute and chronic phases of cerebral thrombosis and embolism. Stroke 1990;21:1663–1667.
79. Coull B, Goodnight S. Antiphospholipid antibodies, prethrombotic states, and strokes. Stroke 1990;21:1370–1374.
80. Gorelian M. A guide to disorders of hemostasis. Ann Intern Med 1966; 65: 782–795.
81. Deykin D. Thrombogenesis. N Engl J Med 1967;276:622–628.
82. Mustard JF, Murphy EA, Rowsell HC, et al. Factors influencing thrombus formations in vivo. Am J Med 1962;33:621–647.
83. Rybak ME. Disorders of hemostasis. In: Noble J, ed. Textbook of general medicine and primary care. Boston: Little Brown, 1987:535–552.
84. Sloan M. Thrombolysis and stroke. Arch Neurol 1987;44:748–768.
85. Raichle M. The pathophysiology of brain ischemia. Ann Neurol 1983;13:2–10.
86. Astrup J, Siesjo B, Simon L. Thresholds in cerebral ischemia: the ischemic penumbra. Stroke 1981;12:723–725.
87. Thomas D, du Boulay G, Marshall J, et al. Effect of hematocrit on cerebral blood flow in man. Lancet 1977;2:941–943.
88. Thomas D, Marshall J, Russell RW, et al. Cerebral blood flow in polycythemia. Lancet 1977;2:161–163.
89. Tohgi H, Yasmanouchi H, Murakami M, et al. Importance of the hematocrit as a risk factor in cerebral infarction. Stroke 1978;9:369–374.
90. Caplan LR, Sergay S. Positional cerebral ischemia. J Neurol Neurosurg Psychiatry 1976;39:385–391.
91. Toole J. Effects of change of head, limb, and body position on cephalic circulation. N Engl J Med 1968;279:307–311.
92. Ginsberg M, Welsh F, Budd W. Deleterious effect of glucose pretreatment on recovery from diffuse cerebral ischemia in the cat. Stroke 1980;11:347–354.
93. Plum F. What causes infarction in ischemic brain? Neurology 1983;33: 222–233.
94. Hass W. Beyond cerebral blood flow, metabolism, and ischemic thresholds: an examination of the role of calcium in the initiation of cerebral infarction. In: Meyer J, Lechner H, Reivich M, et al., eds. Cerebral vascular disease: vol 3. Proceedings of the 10th International Salzburg Conference. Amsterdam: Excerpta Medica, 1981:3–17.
95. Gorelick PB, Caplan LR. Calcium, hypercalcemia and stroke. Current Concepts of Cerebrovascular Disease (Stroke) 1985;20:13–17.
96. Hillbom M, Kaste M. Ethanol intoxication: a risk factor for ischemic brain infarction in adolescents and young adults. Stroke 1981;12:422–425.
97. Ames A III, Wright RL, Kouada M, et al. Cerebral ischemia: II. the no-reflow phenomenon. Am J Pathol 1968;52:437–453.
98. O'Brien MD. Ischemic cerebral edema: a review. Stroke 1979;10:623–628.

99. Ropper AH. Brain edema after stroke, clinical syndrome and intracranial pressure. Arch Neurol 1984;41:26–29.
100. Ropper AH. A preliminary MRI study of the geometry of brain displacement and level of consciousness with acute intracranial masses. Neurology 1989;39:622–627.
101. Barnett H. Delayed cerebral ischemic episodes distal to occlusion of major cerebral arteries. Neurology 1978;28:769–774.
102. Fisher CM. Occlusion of the internal carotid artery. Arch Neurol Psychiatry 1951;65:346–377.
103. Caplan LR. Occlusion of the vertebral or basilar artery. Stroke 1979;10: 277–282.
104. Jones H, Millikan C, Sandok B. Temporal profile of acute vertebrobasilar system infarction. Stroke 1980;11:173–177.
105. Fisher CM. Pathological observations in hypertensive cerebral hemorrhage. J Neuropathol Exp Neurol 1971;30:536–550.
106. Herbstein D, Schaumberg H. Hypertensive intracerebral hematoma: an investigation of the initial hemorrhage and rebleeding using Cr 51 labeled erythrocytes. Arch Neurol 1974;30:412–414.
107. Duret H. Traumatismes cranio-cerebaux. Paris: Librarie Felix Alcan, 1919.
108. Heros RC, Zervas NT, Varsos V. Cerebral vasospasm after subarachnoid hemorrhage: an update. Ann Neurol 1983;14:599–608.
109. Hijdra A, van Gijn J, Nagelkerke NJD, et al. Prediction of delayed cerebral ischemia, rebleeding, and outcome after aneurysmal subarachnoid hemorrhage. Stroke 1988;19:1250–1256.

CHAPTER 3

Diagnosis and the Clinical Encounter

A 36-year-old man, JH, becomes confused at work and is brought to the hospital. Upon arrival, it is obvious that his left limbs are weak. He is very sleepy and at times barely arousable. The nurse in the emergency ward at the hospital calls you, his physician, and relates that your patient is having a stroke.

Information Used for Stroke Diagnosis

The patient vignette describes a severely ill man; the clinician's first task is to decide what is the matter with him. This chapter follows the process of diagnosis by a stepwise consideration of the facts in his case. Before proceeding with the specific case example, however, the general process of stroke diagnosis is reviewed. Clinical diagnosis is often difficult, but the process becomes simple and more logical if approached systematically. I routinely follow several steps and rules and urge each individual clinician to become familiar with the diagnostic methods that he or she uses. Routines and thoroughness prevent errors made by snap guesses or impulsive diagnoses. I have elaborated elsewhere in much more detail on the subject of clinical neurological diagnoses[1,2] and only summarize very briefly the main points here.

First, the clinician must decide on the key questions to be asked. Answers are difficult unless the questions are clearly framed. The most general questions should be asked first, followed by the more specific ones. In neurology, two diagnostic questions always require an answer: (1) What is the disease mechanism—the pathology and pathophysiology? and (2) where is the lesion(s)—the anatomy of the disorder? In regard to the stroke patient, the *what* question concerns which of the five stroke mechanisms (hemorrhage—subarachnoid or intracerebral; ischemia—thrombotic, embolic, or decreased global perfusion) is present. Of course, before distinguishing among stroke mechanisms, clinicians should first ask whether the findings could be caused by a nonvascular process, such as a brain tumor, intoxication, or traumatic injury that mimics stroke. The *where* question concerns the anatomical location of the disorder, both in the brain and in the vascular system.

Usually, different data are used to answer these two quite different questions. In determining stroke mechanism, the following clinical bedside data are helpful:

1. ecology—the past and present personal and family illnesses of the patient
2. the presence and nature of past strokes or transient ischemic attacks (TIAs)
3. the time of the onset of the symptoms
4. activity at the onset of the stroke
5. the temporal course and progression of the findings (Did the stroke come very suddenly, with the deficit maximal at onset; did it progress in a stepwise, remitting or progressive fashion; or were there fluctuations between normal and abnormal?)
6. accompanying symptoms such as headache, vomiting, and decreased level of consciousness

The responses to these items can all be gleaned from a careful history from the patient, a review of physicians' and medical records, and data collected from observers, family members, and friends. These data are primarily *historical* and require little sophisticated knowledge of neurology. The general physical examination, which uncovers disorders not known from the history, adds to the data used for diagnosing the stroke mechanism. Elevated blood pressure, cardiac enlargement or murmurs, and vascular bruits are examples of physical findings that influence the identification of the stroke mechanism.

Diagnosis of stroke location is made using different data:

1. analysis of the neurological symptoms and their distribution
2. the findings on neurological examination

The history and knowledge of general systemic diseases tells the clinician *what* is wrong; the neurological examination tells more *where* the disease process is located.

Mechanism and anatomical diagnoses are not absolute. *More realistic are estimates of probability.* In one patient, intracerebral hemorrhage may be the most likely diagnosis, by far, but embolism and thrombosis are also possible and should not be eliminated from consideration. In another patient, there might be an apparent toss-up between thrombosis and embolism.

The process of diagnosis involves two basic techniques: (1) *hypothesis generation and testing,* and (2) *pattern matching.* As the patient relates the history, the clinician should be thinking of a possible diagnosis and testing that hypothesis by asking additional questions that will help confirm or refute the hypothesis. For example, an elderly patient with known coronary and peripheral-limb atherosclerosis has a left hemiparesis noted on awakening. In such a case, I think of thrombosis because that would be a common stroke mechanism, considering the ecology, so I then ask whether there had been prior transient episodes of left-limb symptoms. Their presence would strongly favor thrombosis.

Anatomical hypotheses are also generated. A left hemiparesis raises the possibility of a right cerebral or brainstem lesion, so I ask about accompanying visual, sensory, or brainstem symptoms that would help generate a more specific anatomical localization. The process of anatomical diagnosis is much like locating a missing person. First, the clinician must determine whether the person is in the United States before limiting the whereabouts to Massachusetts, then the Boston vicinity, then to a specific street in the Brookline neighborhood. Similarly, regarding the diagnosis of mechanism, the physician must decide on ischemia versus hemorrhage before hypothesizing about subtypes of ischemia. The physician must identify thrombosis versus embolism versus global hypoperfusion before distinguishing subtypes of thrombosis, such as lacunar or large artery, anterior or posterior circulation. Thus, the clinician proceeds systematically from the more general to the more specific. Clearly, the amount of available data may limit reasonable hypotheses to the most general inferences. In some patients, few historical data are available.

The other technique used by most clinicians is *pattern matching.* For example, I recognize the person I call "Jim" by comparing the individual in front of me with a mental image of Jim that I conjure up in my mind's eye. I do not ordinarily list individual features (e.g., height, glasses, hair style). Similarly, clinicians try to identify a constellation of findings that match their mental images of patterns of stroke mechanisms and pathology and anatomy.

Though the preceding description indicates a sequence of analysis, *diagnosis of* what *and* where *should proceed concurrently as well as sequentially.* While obtaining the patient's history, have the patient elucidate information that will allow prediction of the probability of various stroke mechanisms and locations. At the end of the history, be prepared to list these and to assign rough probability estimates. Next, think about and plan the examination. In this patient, what additional findings are important and will help to confirm or refute the preliminary diagnoses. What data will allow more specificity? In the patient with left hemiparesis, the presence of a left visual field deficit or left visual neglect would localize the lesion to the right cerebral hemisphere. Nystagmus or a gaze palsy to the right would favor a brainstem site. A right carotid bruit or a cholesterol crystal in the right ocular fundus would favor a right carotid artery site. After the general and neurological examinations, reexamine the original hypotheses and their probabilities. New or unexpected findings from the examinations might stimulate new hypotheses or might confirm or refute prior hypotheses. A blood pressure of 260/140 torr would clearly increase the likelihood of hemorrhage. The absence of a pulse or presence of papilledema on examination would change prior estimated probabilities.

Next, proceed to ask what laboratory tests might help refine the hypotheses in place at the end of the history and the examinations. Also, initial laboratory test results will help determine the need for other tests. Laboratory tests should also be planned, reviewed, and ordered sequentially (this topic will be elaborated in Chapter 4). Overall, the process of diagnosis should be logical, systematic, and sequential.

Procedure for Diagnosis of Stroke Mechanism and Brain Localization

Mimicking a Computer

Computers have taught clinicians to be more aware of the process and mechanics of diagnosis. In an individual patient, how would a computer estimate the most likely stroke mechanism diagnosis? Physicians may not always have ready access to a computer and the necessary software to take advantage of computer diagnosis. They can, however, emulate the logic and methodology of the computer process for a more systematic diagnostic strategy. One technique of computer diagnosis is the use of Bayes's theorem.[3,4] Needed for this methodology are knowledge of (1) the incidence of each illness (in this case, stroke mechanism) in the population studied, and (2) the incidence of a given finding in each illness (stroke mechanism). Armed with this information and the findings in the individual patient, the computer calculates the probability of a given stroke mechanism. The use of probabilities mimics the way clinicians usually approach a diagnostic problem. Seldom is a single diagnosis absolutely certain (100%). More often, a given diagnosis—for example, cerebral embolism—is considered most likely (perhaps 70% probable); but thrombotic occlusion also should be considered (perhaps 20%); and intracerebral hemorrhage, although unlikely (10%), is still considered in the differential diagnosis.

Knowing the incidence of the various stroke mechanisms provides what is usually called *a priori odds*. An analysis of data from large stroke studies and registries[5–18] (Table 3.1) shows that approximately 80 percent of all strokes are ischemic and 20 percent are hemorrhagic. Therefore, if no other specific information were available about a stroke patient, the diagnosis of ischemic stroke would be correct four out of five times, but subarachnoid hemorrhage would be correct for fewer than 1 patient in 10. The remainder of the computer prediction uses individual factors (e.g., headache preceding stroke, activity at onset, prior evidence of atheroscle-

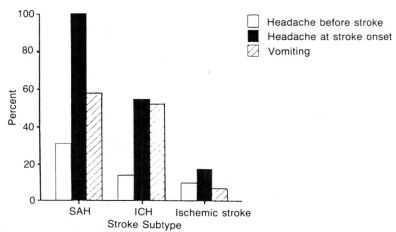

FIGURE 3.1 Graph showing frequency of headache patterns and vomiting in patients with ischemic strokes and hemorrhages in the Michael Reese and University of Illinois stroke registries. From Gorelick PB, Hier DB, Caplan LR, et al. Headache in acute cerebrovascular disease. Neurology 1986;36:1445–1450 with permission.

rosis) to predict the mechanism. For example, Table 3.2 presents the relative incidence of headache during the days or weeks preceding stroke. Relatively few patients had headaches preceding stroke, but the finding was slightly more common in patients with thrombotic stroke and intracerebral hemorrhage and less common in patients with either subarachnoid hemorrhage or cerebral embolism. In this example, the difference in incidence is small. By contrast, headache at or near the onset of stroke (Table 3.3) invariably occurred in patients with subarachnoid hemorrhage but was clearly less often present in patients with other mechanisms of stroke.

These data can also be presented in graphic form: Figure 3.1, from a study of patients seen on the stroke service at the Michael Reese Hospital and the University of Illinois,[19] depicts the frequency—by stroke subtype—of headache preceding stroke (often called "sentinel headache") and headache at onset. The computer and the alert physician sum the individual data items, factor in the a priori odds, and arrive at a total probability for a given stroke mechanism in each stroke patient. During the discussion of individual data items in the remainder of this chapter, I include important data results from my own stroke-registry experience.

Ecology

Included within this broad heading are prior medical diseases and demographic data that might predispose the patient to have one or more of the stroke mechanisms. When called to see a patient with stroke, the physician usually has available some background information from the family, another physician, or the clinician's own past knowledge. For example, a call

TABLE 3.1
Incidence of Type of Stroke in Various Studies

Study	Reported	N	Thrombosis	LA	Lacune	ICU	Embolism	ICH	SAH	Total Ischemia	Total Hemorrhage
							Percentage				
Aring and Merritt[5]	1935	407	81	—	—	—	3	—	—	84	15
Whisnant et al.[6]	1971	548	75	—	—	—	3	10	5	78	15
Matsumoto et al.[7]	1973	993	71	—	—	—	8	10	6	79	16
Kannell et al.[8]	1965	90	63	—	—	—	15	4	18	78	22
Harvard Stroke Registry[9]	1978	694	—	34	19	—	31	10	6	84	16
Michael Reese Stroke Registry[10]	1983	472	—	18	13	30	17	14	8	78	22
Austin Hospital[11]	1983	700	—	45	23	18	8	6	excluded	94	6
South Alabama[12]	1984	160	—	6	13	40	26	8	6	85	14

Study	Year	No. of Patients									
Pilot Stroke Data Bank[13]	1984	928	—	19	11	25	22	11	13	77	24
Lausanne Stroke Registry[14]	1988	1000	—	43	13	8	20	11	excluded	89	11
Stroke Data Bank[15]	1988	1805	—	6	19	32	14	13	13	71	26
Lehigh Valley Stroke Registry[16]	1989	2639	60	—	9	—	20	9	excluded	91	9
Oxfordshire Community Stroke Project[17]	1990	675	—	—	—	—	—	10	5	81	15
Community Hospital-Based Stroke Program[18]	1990	4129	32	—	—	—	11	5	2	60	10

Note: Thrombosis = unspecified nonembolic ischemic infarct; LA = large artery occlusive disease; ICU = infarct cause unknown; ICH = intracerebral hemorrhage; SAH = subarachnoid hemorrhage. — = Not labeled as such by the study. Because of missing data, the percentages do not add up to 100%.

TABLE 3.2
Headache Preceding Stroke (from Harvard Stroke Registry)[9]

	Thrombosis	Embolus	ICH	SAH
Yes	27 (8.2%)	8 (4%)	6 (8%)	1 (3%)
No	291 (89%)	177 (87%)	61 (77%)	27 (87%)
Other	9 (2%)	18 (9%)	12 (15%)	3 (10%)
	327	203	79	31

Note: "Other" usually means no data (patient aphasic, stuporous, or information not available). ICH = intracerebral hemorrhage; SAH = subarachnoid hemorrhage. Percentages do not always add up to 100, due to rounding.

TABLE 3.3
Headache at Onset of Stroke

	Thrombosis	Lacune	Embolus	SAH	ICH	INF
HSR	12%	3%	9%	78%	33%	—
MRSR	29%	16%	17%	98%	80%	13%

Note: SAH = subarachnoid hemorrhage; ICH = intracerebral hemorrhage; INF = cause unknown; HSR = Harvard Stroke Registry;[9] MRSR = Michael Reese Stroke Registry.[10]

from the hospital emergency room might describe a "65-year-old man with angina pectoris, two prior 'heart attacks,' diabetes, and hypertension who arrived here today with . . ." This information leads the physician to consider the particular stroke mechanisms in the patient who is about to be seen. In the preceding example, the presence of diabetes and coronary artery disease strongly favors a diagnosis of associated atherosclerosis of the extracranial cervical vessels and a thrombotic (or artery-to-artery embolus) mechanism of stroke. The presence of prior heart disease raises the possibility of arrhythmia, mural thrombosis, ventricular aneurysm, and valvular heart disease—all potential sources of cerebral embolism. The presence of hypertension increases the probability of intracerebral hemorrhage (ICH), especially if the hypertension is severe, a determination that can be made quickly. An alert physician would also be sure to inquire whether the patient was being treated with anticoagulants for the cardiac disease, a factor that would greatly increase the chance of ICH.

The clinician uses the presence of individual risk factors to alter the likelihood that an individual patient has a particular stroke mechanism. Perhaps another example will help clarify this statement. I have said that, on average, 60 percent of strokes are considered thrombotic, 20 percent are embolic, 12 percent are due to ICH, and 8 percent are due to subarachnoid hemorrhage (SAH). The presence of severe hypertension—for example, 220/130 torr—would certainly make hemorrhage, especially ICH, much more likely. This factor would significantly shift the odds toward ICH and slightly to SAH. If another factor, such as age, is then added—for example, if the severely hypertensive patient were a 23-year-old woman—this would make the major alternative diagnosis, thrombotic stroke, much less likely and would further increase the likelihood of a hemorrhagic mechanism. This shift of probabilities can be described as "loading on" or "detracting from" a specific diagnosis: For example, severe hypertension loads heavily on ICH (+ + + +); youthfulness detracts from thrombosis (− − −). Data from prior experience, such as those found in registries, can help determine quantitatively the relative shift of odds.

Table 3.4 lists the incidence of diabetes, hypertension, and coronary artery disease in the various subtypes of stroke in the Harvard Stroke Registry (HSR) and the incidence of other similar variables in the Michael Reese Stroke Registry (MRSR). Note that hypertension was more common in all groups in the MRSR and atherosclerosis more prominent in the HSR. The populations in these two registries were quite different: the HSR included a predominantly white, middle- and upper-class population with a high incidence of atherosclerosis, whereas the MRSR had more young black hypertensive individuals with a lower prevalence of atherosclerosis. Black, Chinese, and Japanese populations have a higher incidence of ICH and intracranial occlusive disease than white populations.[20-27] Table 3.5 lists estimated loading weights that could be assigned to the various risk factors. At times, the effect of a condition is indirect; for example, the presence of diabetes increases the chance of myocardial infarction, which in turn increases the likelihood of a cardiac-origin embolism.

I now return to the patient JH discussed at the very outset of this chapter. I continue to discuss his case and its analysis during the remainder of the discussion of clinical diagnosis.

After the call from the emergency room, before leaving for the hospital, the secretary is asked to pull JH's office chart. He had last been seen 1 year ago, at age 35, because of bronchitis. Notes indicate that he smoked 3 packs of cigarettes a day, had always had normal blood pressures, and had no history of cardiac or neurological symptoms. He had described, however, a very high incidence of heart attacks in his family. He had been overweight, and his blood cholesterol level last year was 295. He was advised to pursue a weight-reduction program, to reduce his intake of fats and cholesterol-containing foods, to stop smoking, and to return for a recheck. He had not returned.

When leaving for the hospital, think about the information known, based on the emergency room nurse's call and on JH's records. The illness was said to have begun rather suddenly, and the brain lesion must be focal because he has an obvious left limb paralysis. Abrupt-onset focal brain lesions are most often strokes, but his youth serves as a reminder to be certain to consider focal brain lesions other than stroke. Brain tumors, abscesses, trauma, and encephalitis can cause focal findings, and without other information, it is not yet certain how abruptly the symptoms began and progressed. If the process is a stroke, as would be statistically most likely, review the background information regarding risks for the different stroke mechanisms. His past smoking, family history of cardiac disease, and high

TABLE 3.4
Incidence of Findings in Each Type of Stroke

	Thrombosis	Lacune	Embolus	ICH	SAH
HSR					
Atherosclerosis[a]	56%	37%	34%	11%	5%
Diabetes	26%	28%	13%	15%	2%
Past hypertension	55%	75%	40%	72%	19%
MRSR					
Angina pectoris	13%	8%	20%	5%	0%
Past MI	23%	16%	40%	12%	0%
Recent MI	7%	12%	12%	3%	0%
Past hypertension	75%	55%	55%	68%	44%

Note: ICH = intracerebral hemorrhage; SAH = subarachnoid hemorrhage; HSR = Harvard Stroke Registry;[9] MRSR = Michael Reese Stroke Registry;[10] MI = myocardial infarction.

[a]Includes peripheral vascular disease, coronary disease, and bruits.

TABLE 3.5
Weighting of Ecological Factors

	Thrombosis	Lacune	Embolus	ICH	SAH
Hypertension	+ +	+ + +		+ +	+
Severe hypertension		+		+ + + +	+ +
Coronary disease	+ + +		+ +		
Claudication	+ + +		+		
Atrial fibrillation			+ + + +		
Sick sinus syndrome			+ +		
Valvular heart disease	+		+ + +		
Diabetes	+ + +	+	+		
Bleeding diathesis				+ + + +	+
Cigarette smoking	+ + +		+		+
Cancer			+ +	+	+
Old age	+ + +	+			−
Black or Japanese origin	+	+		+ +	

Note: ICH = intracerebral hemorrhage; SAH = subarachnoid hemorrhage.

blood cholesterol level suggest to you the possibility of premature atherosclerosis, with large-artery occlusive disease as the mechanism of the stroke. An unusual type of cardiac disease with cerebral embolism is another mechanism that is suggested by the family history of cardiac disease. ICH could also cause left-sided paralysis and sleepiness, but the absence of past hypertension makes this less likely. Make a mental note to quickly check his blood pressure and seek signs of organ damage due to hypertension on examination. The first hypothesis regarding preliminary stroke mechanism is large-artery atherosclerosis with embolism, and ICH also to be seriously considered. Systemic hypoperfusion and SAH seldom cause severe hemiplegia at outset.

So far, few neurological data could help localize the lesion. The patient has a left-sided paralysis, and so the right cerebral hemisphere and right pons are the most likely sites of pathology. The report of confusion at work favors a hemispherical lesion. Plan to ask questions that will promote more precise localization.

Having used the ecological data to shift the usual stroke-mechanism probabilities, carry these probabilities into an investigation of the next data items, such as prior cerebrovascular symptoms, course of illness, accompanying symptoms, and so on, each of which will then further modify the probabilities.

> When you arrive at the emergency room, the nurse says that the patient's pulse and blood pressure are normal. The patient is awake but cannot give any account of his illness. He seems unaware that his left limbs are paralyzed. The coworker who was with him when he became ill says that he suddenly seemed dazed and quickly became hemiplegic, falling to the ground. His wife says that he did not follow previous dietary advise and was still smoking heavily. She said he had not been ill, but a week before he told her that for 10 minutes one morning, his left arm and face had temporarily felt numb, symptoms he attributed to a draft from an air conditioner in the office.

Prior Cerebrovascular Symptoms

Though not especially common, prior cerebrovascular events so heavily load probabilities that they should be given considerable importance. TIAs in the same vascular territory are frequent precursors of thrombotic stroke, so their presence, especially when multiple, is virtually diagnostic of that stroke mechanism. If a patient presenting to the hospital with aphasia and right-limb weakness had had an attack of transient right-handed weakness 3 weeks earlier and an attack of right-face and right-hand numbness and weakness 1 week earlier, the clinician could be relatively certain that the stroke was a result of thrombotic occlusive disease within the left anterior circulation. If, in addition, that same individual had also had a black shade descending over the left eye, causing temporary blindness, the location could be further refined, and it would seem certain that the occlusive lesion involved the carotid artery before its ophthalmic artery branch. The presence, nature, and duration of TIAs are very important. Information about the presence of TIAs must be vigorously and repeatedly sought.

Patients are exceedingly naive about the functions of the body, especially the nervous system. Most stroke patients attribute their weakness, lack of feeling, and visual deficits to the local limbs or to the eyes; they often do not understand that the central nervous system (CNS) control of these functions has been damaged. They often wonder why the head is being studied and imaged rather than the arm or leg, where surely the trouble resides. Patients will usually not volunteer information they feel is unrelated to their present trouble. A woman with visual difficulty will not tell her eye doctor about a vaginal discharge, considering the latter problem in the province of her gynecologist. Similarly, a patient with hand weakness might not tell the physician about prior leg weakness, not realizing that the conditions are related. The same individual will surely not tell the doctor about temporary visual dysfunction, considering the eye problem to belong to the ophthalmologist. Patients often attribute their temporary symptoms to banal causes in the environment—for example, an air conditioner draft, as in the case of JH. Symptoms of TIA must be elicited specifically: "Have you ever had temporary weakness of your right hand, your right leg, your face? Have you had difficulty speaking, seeing, and so forth?" On entry to the hospital, or during the first physician encounter, patients are often not at their optimum performance levels. They may be sick, frightened, or worried and therefore suboptimal observers and witnesses. Many patients have told me on the third or even seventh day of stroke about prior TIAs, having denied their presence when queried on admission.

Some patients cannot provide information about a TIA because of aphasia, altered level of consciousness, amnesia, and so on. Other observers, such as family, hospital visitors, and friends, should be queried because the patient may have told them about prior symptoms, or these individuals may have observed altered function in the patient. Caution must be exercised in exploring symptoms at the patient's work site, because knowledge about a patient's neurological problem might adversely affect job status. Clearly, permission should be sought before approaching employers or coworkers for health information. In this case, the coworker and wife were present and could provide useful data when the patient could not.

In patients with small-vessel disease (lacunar infarction), TIAs are generally less common. In the HSR, TIAs occurred in 23 percent of patients with lacunar disease, compared with 50 percent of patients with large-vessel arteriosclerosis.[9] When present, TIAs are more likely to be stereotyped (e.g., weakness of face, arm, and leg in each attack) and are usually limited to a period of days. In contrast, patients with occlusion of larger blood vessels, such as the ICA in the neck, may have TIAs over a period of weeks or months. It takes longer for a large vessel (8–15 mm in diameter) to occlude than for a small vessel (several hundred microns in diameter) to do so. In large-vessel disease, the TIAs may be less stereotyped, with weakness of a hand in one attack and aphasia and facial numbness in another. The larger the vascular territory, the more opportunity there is for variety. Note, in Table 3.6, that in carotid artery occlusion, the initial TIA most often occurred months before the stroke, whereas the last TIA often preceded the stroke by less than a week. As a vessel occludes, TIAs can become more frequent. Thus, a TIA occurring yesterday is much more ominous than a single TIA that occurred 3 months ago, and the recent TIA would demand more urgent evaluation and treatment.

The term *TIA* designates ischemia, but it does not differentiate between an embolic and a thrombotic mechanism, or between a small-vessel

TABLE 3.6
Transient Ischemic Attacks (TIAs) in Patients with Severe Carotid Artery
Occlusive Disease (from Harvard Stroke Registry)[9]

Time	First TIA		Last TIA	
<1 day	2	(11)	16	(41)
1 day–1 week	9		25	
1 week–1 month	14	(48)	7	(15)
>1 month	34		8	
	59		56	(3 unknown)

and a large-vessel site. Cerebral embolism can produce a transient disorder that would qualify as a TIA. Some evidence supports the notion that embolism is more likely to produce less frequent but longer attacks, whereas low-flow states produce briefer but more frequent attacks. In our experience, shotgunlike repeated episodes of ischemia in the same vascular territory virtually always indicate a critical degree of vessel narrowing. Single but longer attacks are more often associated with an ulcerated plaque or other embolic source.

Occasionally, a patient will present with a history of transient deficits in different vascular territories.

Such a patient was DB, who awakened one night with numbness of his left arm and leg, symptoms that were gone by morning, when he told his wife. Two nights later, while on his way to the bathroom, he noted weakness and numbness of his right limbs. In the morning, his physician could still document slight weakness of the right hand but noted no other abnormalities on examination.

Had this patient confused his left and right sides and mislocalized the initial symptoms? A week later, the same patient suddenly developed a cold, painful right leg, and investigations confirmed bacterial endocarditis as the source of his multiple embolizations.

In our patient, JH, the single TIA provided an important clue in predicting the most probable stroke mechanism. The symptoms involved the left arm and face, making it very unlikely that the cause was a local disturbance in these parts of the body. This must have been a transient brain event and one localized to the same side of the brain, probably the same vascular territory as the stroke. A thrombotic event seems the likely mechanism. TIAs do not usually precede ICH. If the mechanism were cardiac-origin embolism, emboli would have hit the same general target twice in a row. It would help if he were alert enough to tell whether there had been more transient attacks because many attacks in the same territory will make cardiac-origin embolism quite unlikely.

TABLE 3.7
Activity at Onset in Subtypes of Stroke (from Michael Reese Stroke Registry)[10]

Activity at Onset	Thrombosis	Lacune	Infarct (U)	Embolus	ICH	SAH
On arising	40%	50%	31%	17%	13%	15%
Stress	1%	1%	5%	5%	10%	15%
ADL	54%	47%	50%	68%	64%	64%
Unknown	5%	2%	14%	10%	13%	6%

Note: Infarct (U) = cause of infarct undetermined; ICH = intracerebral hemorrhage; SAH = subarachnoid hemorrhage; stress = increased activity—exertion, coition, cough, sneeze, etc.; ADL = ordinary daily activity.

In addition to TIA, past strokes may also help the alert clinician pinpoint a stroke mechanism. A patient with three prior strokes during the past year involving the vertebrobasilar, left carotid, and right carotid systems has a high probability of cerebral embolism. A normotensive patient with several prior ICHs in different loci has a high probability of having a bleeding diathesis or amyloid angiopathy as the cause of a propensity for ICH. JH had no history of a prior stroke.

Activity at Onset

Traditional teaching states that the most thrombotic strokes occur when the circulation is least active and most sluggish—for example, during the night or during a nap, with the deficit usually noticed on arising. Embolism and hemorrhage, in contrast, would be more likely to occur when the circulation is more active or when blood pressure rises. More recent data show that most ischemic[28] and hemorrhagic strokes[29] actually occur during the morning hours especially between 10 A.M. and noon, after the patient has awakened and begun daily activities. Table 3.7 contains data from the MRSR on the incidence of the various stroke mechanisms in relationship to activity at onset. A significant number of hemorrhages do occur at night, and thrombotic deficits can occur during activity. It is, however, very unusual for a thrombotic stroke or a lacune to develop during vigorous physical activity or coition. A particularly common time for embolism to occur is on arising at night to urinate, the so-called *matudinal* (morning) embolus. Coughing or a vigorous sneeze can also shake something loose, resulting in cerebral embolism. The onset in JH was during relatively sedentary activities at work.

Early Course of Development of the Deficit

Table 3.8 contains data from the HSR, MRSR, and Lausanne Stroke Registry, concerning the temporal course of the neurological deficit. Often, the early course gives critical information about the stroke mechanism. A few examples may serve to illustrate.

WC, a previously hypertensive man, suddenly became aphasic and hemiplegic while eating lunch with his family. When initially examined in the emergency room, he was mute and had a severe right hemiplegia. Two hours later, he was much improved and could lift his right leg and say a few words.

The improvement shortly after onset of the deficit argues strongly against an ICH. The deficit, which was maximal at onset and was unassociated with headache, is most compatible with an embolic mechanism. The next case illustrates a different scenario.

RP was admitted to the hospital, and the intern called to say that she had developed a gradually progressive hemiplegia throughout the day. On closer questioning, RP related the following account: At 9:30 A.M., while eating breakfast, her left hand became clumsy, and she dropped a piece of bread. When she climbed the stairs to go to her room, she noticed a slight limp in her left foot. Worried about her problem, she rested for an hour and was comforted when, on rising, she could walk down the stairs without any difficulty and clear the table without a trace of left-hand awkwardness. At midday, while sitting on the couch, her left limbs became weak and she could lift neither her arm nor her leg.

RP's account was typical of a stuttering onset, with improvement in the deficit, followed by worsening. Again, this course would be difficult to understand if the initial deficit had been caused by ICH; the tempo was most compatible with a thrombotic process.

I have called the process of eliciting the historical details from RP "walking through" the course with the patient. Most patients have difficulty quantifying their deficits and estimating the course of their illness. When patients are asked to describe their activities, an alert observer can often better gauge the course of development of the deficit. I encourage clinicians to construct a "course of illness" graph, which depicts the temporal pattern of the findings.[1,30] Inspection of this graph helps to predict stroke mechanism.[30] Such a graph would aid diagnosis in the following case.

BK was admitted to the hospital with a note that stated she had a sudden onset of left hemiplegia while shopping. While the patient was trying on a hat in a store, the shopkeeper had noted a droop of the face and had called for an ambulance, against the patient's wishes. The shopkeeper recalled the patient walking to the next room and gesturing with both hands. When the ambulance arrived ten minutes later, the patient could walk to the ambulance but had a limp and less swing of the left arm. Upon arrival at the hospital, she had a severe left hemiplegia, eyes and head were deviated to the right, and she was vomiting and complained of headache.

The gradual development of a progressive focal deficit, accompanied by gradually developing symptoms of increased ICP suggested ICH, a diagnosis confirmed by computed tomography (CT). In this case, a call to the shop clarified the early course of illness and helped suggest the correct diagnosis.

In patient JH, the onset was very abrupt and presumably maximal at onset because he fell with a hemiplegia. Among the two stroke mechanisms with the highest probability so far—embolism and atherosclerosis with thrombosis—each often has a tendency to begin abruptly and to have maximal deficit at or near onset. Recall from the discussion in Chapter 2 that when atherosclerotic large-artery lesions critically reduce the size of the residual lumen, occlusive thrombosis often develops. Because the thrombus is initially not adherent, portions may break loose and embolize. Sudden, maximal-at-onset deficits in patients with large-artery occlusions are presumed to be caused by artery-to-artery embolism from the site of thrombosis to an intracranial artery. Thus, the onset and course to date do not help choose between the two mechanisms being considered most strongly.

Accompanying Symptoms

Headache is an invariable symptom of SAH. Sudden release of blood into the subarachnoid space increases ICP and usually leads to severe headache, vomiting, and a decrease in the level of consciousness. In ICH, the focal deficit usually develops progressively, and only later, when there has been enlargement of the hematoma, do headache, vomiting, and decreased consciousness develop. Loss of consciousness is common in SAH and is rare in ischemic stroke unless the ischemia involves the brainstem bilaterally. Seizures are not common in the early period of stroke; their presence argues for embolic stroke or ICH. Table 3.9 lists the incidence of accompanying features, by stroke mechanism.

Combining two pieces of information often adds greatly to the accuracy of the probabilities. An example of this is seen in Table 3.10, which analyzes the presence of vomiting for each stroke mechanism, in relation to the stroke's location in the anterior or posterior circulation. Vomiting is common in posterior circulation strokes, presumably because of involvement of the so-called vomiting center in the floor of the fourth ventricle. However, vomiting is rare in ischemic strokes in the anterior circulation, whether thrombotic or embolic. In the anterior circulation, ICH was accompanied by vomiting, presumably because of the associated increase in ICP. Thus, vomiting and anterior circulation location equals ICH. A patient with a right hemiparesis and aphasia who vomits early during the stroke has a high likelihood of harboring an ICH.

Patient JH denied headache but did have lethargy, qualifying as some decrease in level of consciousness. Decrease in level of consciousness is very unusual in lacunar infarction, one subtype of thrombotic stroke. He had not vomited. These features do not, in his case, help differentiate between thrombosis and embolism.

Localization and Detection of the Vascular Lesion

Having pursued the historical features as thoroughly as possible, the clinician should now be ready to perform a general and neurological examination.

TABLE 3.8
Early Course of Deficit

	Thrombosis			Lacune			Embolus			ICH			SAH	
	HSR	MRSR	LSR	HSR	MRSR	LSR	HSR	MRSR	LSR	HSR	MRSR	LSR	HSR	MRSR
Maximal at onset	40%	45%	66%	38%	40%	54%	79%	89%	82%	34%	38%	44%	80%	64%
Stuttering or stepwise	34%	30%	27%	32%	28%	40%	11%	10%	13%	3%	9%	52%	3%	14%
Gradual smooth	13%	14%		20%	24%		5%	1%		63%	51%		14%	18%
Fluctuant	13%	11%	7%	10%	8%	5%	5%	0%	5%	0%	2%	4%	3%	4%

Note: ICH = intracerebral hemorrhage; SAH = subarachnoid hemorrhage; HSR = Harvard Stroke Registry;[9] MRSR = Michael Reese Stroke Registry;[10] LSR = Lausanne Stroke Registry.[14] In LSR, both gradual smooth and stuttering or stepwise were combined as progressive course.

TABLE 3.9
Incidence of Accompanying Symptoms at or near Onset, by Stroke Subtype

	Thrombosis			Embolism			Lacune			ICH			SAH	
	HSR	LSR	SDB	HSR	LSR	SDB	HSR	LSR	SDB	HSR	LSR	SDB	HSR	SDB
Decreased consciousness	15%	13%	14%	20%	12%	29%	3%	3%	2%	39%	50%	57%	68%	48%
Vomiting	11%	—	8%	6%	—	5%	3%	—	1%	46%	—	29%	48%	45%
Seizures	.3%	1%	3%	4%	0%	3%	0%	0%	.1%	7%	7%	9%	7%	7%
Headache	12%	17%	11%	9%	18%	10%	3%	7%	5%	33%	40%	41%	78%	87%

Note: HSR = Harvard Stroke Registry;[9] LSR = Lausanne Stroke Registry;[14] SDB = Stroke Data Bank.[15]

TABLE 3.10
Vomiting and Location and Type of Stroke (from Harvard Stroke Registry)[9]

ICH		
Anterior circulation	19/29	48.5%
Posterior circulation	8/12	67.0%
Thrombosis		
Anterior circulation	3/141	2.0%
Posterior circulation	24/83	29.0%
Embolus		
Anterior circulation	4/198	2.0%
Posterior circulation	6/21	29.0%

While proceeding, the principal aims should be kept in mind. They are (1) to detect vascular and cardiac abnormalities that will aid in determining stroke mechanism and localization of vascular lesions and (2) to localize the process within the CNS. Once the clinician knows where the lesion is in the brain, a knowledge about the anatomy of the vascular supply, about the risk factors in the patient, and about the results of the vascular examination will help the clinician predict the most likely vascular location and process in the patient.

Findings from Examination of the Heart,
Vascular System, and Eyes

Heart

The diagnosis of cardiogenic embolism is important because its evaluation and treatment differ from intrinsic disease of the extracranial and cranial vessels. A careful detailed history of possible cardiac symptoms, angina, myocardial infarction, palpitations or arrhythmia, congestive heart failure, and rheumatic heart disease is as important as the neurological history. The heart should be examined thoroughly, taking time to estimate size, character, and quality of heart sounds and gallops; listening for murmurs is not enough.

Vascular system

Examination of the available systemic and extracranial arteries may give clues to the presence of atherosclerosis or diminished flow not detectable by history. Note the pulse for at least a minute, seeking any irregularities. Feel the radial pulses simultaneously, looking for a significant difference in the strength of the pulse or a delay on one side. In all reported examples of subclavian steal, the diminished blood flow to the arm produced a definite pulse alteration.[31,32] If the pulses are equal and synchronous, it is probably not necessary to check blood pressure in each arm. Feel the femoral and foot pulses and listen to the femoral region for an arterial bruit. Remember that some patients with hyperdynamic circulation—for example, fever, anemia, or hyperthyroidism—have bruits over many peripheral vessels. When a femoral bruit is present, listen over the antecubital and supraclavicular fossas to determine whether bruits are a generalized phenomenon and not necessarily indicative of focal disease.

Next, gently palpate the carotid artery in the neck. Recall that you are feeling the CCA until you reach the bifurcation high in the neck. The ICA then proceeds posteriorly and usually cannot be felt; the ECA projects slightly forward and laterally and can be traced. The left carotid artery is positioned more posteriorly and deeper, so that the carotid pulses rarely feel equal. Feeling a carotid pulse in the neck tells the examiner that the CCA is patent; it gives absolutely no information about the ICA. Even if the proximal ICA is occluded, a pulse can often be seen and felt along the ICA because of propagation of the pulse wave from the CCA. All too often, a bounding carotid pulse is falsely considered evidence against an ICA occlusion. Listening to the carotid artery beginning low in the neck and progressing cranially is important.

Recall that many nonstenosing processes can cause carotid bruits. The commonest of these are transmitted cardiac murmurs, especially aortic stenosis, tortuous vessels, and hyperdynamic circulatory states. Transmitted heart murmurs and hyperdynamic states produce bruits usually heard over the entire vessel, often loudest at the base of the neck. These bruits are usually low-pitched, relatively short, and are invariably heard best over the supraclavicular fossa, perhaps because of the presence of lung tissue just beneath this region, which better transmits the sound. The auscultatory features of a focal vascular constriction can be compared with that of mitral stenosis because each impedes flow and creates a pressure differential beyond the area of blockage. The bruit caused by local constriction of a carotid or vertebral artery is usually

1. *Focal* in location, often loudest at the bifurcation high in the neck and not audible at the base—Osler said that the murmur of mitral stenosis is often limited to the region of a dime; the same explanation is valid for the focality of a focal carotid stenosis.
2. *Long*—It takes longer for blood to course across a constricted vessel; the diastolic murmur of tight mitral stenosis is also long.
3. *High-pitched*—The pressure proximal to a stenosis is higher than that distally. Blood traveling from a high- to a low-pressure area often produces a high-pitched sound.

After listening to the carotid vessels, in a similar way, auscultate over the supraclavicular fossa and then follow the course of each VA, first within the posterior cervical triangle and then up the sternomastoid muscle to the mastoid region. Sometimes, a unilateral vertebral bruit is a reflection of augmented flow, to compensate for a contralateral VA occlusion; the bruit is then on the "wrong side" for the symptoms. The bell of an old-fashioned stethoscope is usually superior to the diaphragm or flat bell of the newer stethoscopes for bruit detection and analysis.

Clues to the patency of the carotid system arteries can also be obtained by careful palpation of the ECA branches on the face. The most readily palpable arteries in normal individuals are the facial artery along the edge of the lower jaw; the preauricular artery just anterior to the ear; and the superficial temporal artery in the temple region. It is important to feel both sides simultaneously to detect a delay or asymmetry of the pulses. When the ECA or CCA on one side is occluded or severely stenosed, the facial, preauricular, and superficial temporal pulses will be diminished on that side, and the regions of supply may feel cool to the touch. When the ICA is occluded before its ophthalmic artery branch, the ECA may supply critical collateral vessels, usually about the orbit.

The augmented flow can often be felt as brisk increased pulsation at the cheek, brow, or inner angle of the eye. Fisher has designated these pulses *ABC* (angular, brow, cheek) for easy recall (Figure 3.2).[33] At times, the superficial temporal artery provides collateral supply to the supraorbital and supratrochlear branches of the ophthalmic artery feeding the low-pressure ophthalmic-carotid system.[34] In the normal situation, blood flows from the ICA to the ophthalmic artery to the supraorbital (frontal artery) and supratrochlear branches cephalad up the brow. In the normal situation, obliteration of these arteries at the brow blocks the distal pulse above it. When there is low pressure in the ophthalmic system, flow goes down these vessels from superficial temporal artery collaterals into the orbit. In that circumstance, obliteration of the brow pulse does not block the forehead pulses, but a finger on the forehead pulses stops the pulsation in the brow,

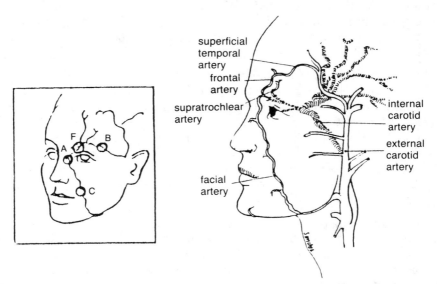

FIGURE 3.2 Lateral view showing internal (ICA) and external (ECA) carotid arteries. ECA branches supply collateral circulation after ICA occlusion. Inset shows palpation points for angular (A), brow (B), cheek (C), and frontal pulses (F).

a reversal of the usual normal pattern of flow. This finding, called the "frontal artery sign,"[34] is the basis for directional Doppler testing of flow into the orbit.

Remember that there is alternative rich collateral circulation at the circle of Willis, especially through the anterior communicating and posterior communicating arteries, which brings collaterals from the opposite cerebral hemisphere and posterior circulation, respectively. Thus, the absence of augmented facial collateral vessels does not mean that the ICA system is not obstructed. On the other hand, the presence of collateral flow through the orbit is diagnostic of a low-pressure ophthalmic–carotid system and thus is important clinically. The technique for detecting this is easy to master at the bedside.

Also feel for the occipital artery behind the mastoid process. This branch of the ECA often provides collateral circulation to the distal extracranial VA in the neck when the VA is occluded at its origin. A bounding occipital artery pulse on one side provides some evidence of VA occlusive disease. In temporal arteritis, the superficial temporal and occipital arteries are often tender, nodular, and pulseless. Compression of these arteries in temporal arteritis often reveals firm arterial walls in contrast to the normal situation.

At times, stenosis of the origin of the ECA produces a bruit that could be confused with an ICA-origin lesion. When the lesion is in the ECA, the bruit can sometimes be traced forward toward the area of the facial artery. Also, blockage of the major ECAs will reduce or obliterate an ECA bruit but will not alter a bruit of ICA origin.[35]

Be sure to feel the femoral and pedal pulses and to inspect the fingers and toes. Claudication and peripheral vascular occlusive disease highly correlate with atherostenosis of the carotid and vertebral arteries in the neck.[9] Cyanosis, coldness, or frank gangrene of digits usually means either embolism from the heart or the aorto-iliac region blocking the distal digital arteries, or in situ thrombosis of digital arteries due to a coagulopathy or severe occlusive peripheral vascular disease. Endocarditis is often associated with tender small nodules in the pulp of the fingers and toes.

JH had a normal-sized heart and rhythm. There were no cardiac murmurs. Blood pressure was 130/70 torr. All pulses were palpable, and there were no vascular bruits. The facial pulses were normal and symmetrical.

The results of the cardiac and vascular examinations provided no new clues in JH. The absence of abnormalities of carotid palpation and auscultation and of palpation of the facial vessels does not exclude severe carotid artery disease in the neck but offers no positive evidence for its occurrence.

Eyes

The eye provides a window into the body's vascular system and can yield clues as to stroke mechanism. *Subhyaloid hemorrhages,* large round hemor-

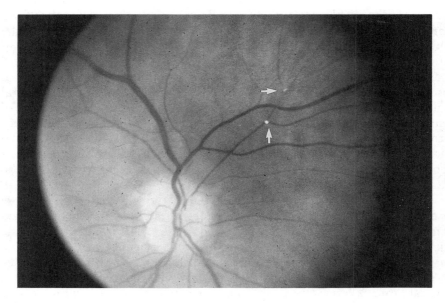

FIGURE 3.3   Cholesterol crystal (white vertical arrow) impacted in branch point of a retinal artery. Above it (horizontal white arrow) is smaller crystal possibly derived from more proximal one.

rhages with a fluid level, represent sudden bleeding below the retina and almost always reflect a very sudden change in ICP. They are frequently seen in patients with SAH and can also occur in suddenly developing large ICHs. The degree of hypertensive retinopathy and arteriosclerotic changes is important to note. In long-standing stenosis of the ICA, the reduced pressure in the ophthalmic artery tributaries may minimize the hypertensive changes ipsilateral to the stenosis. The same phenomenon is well known as the Goldblatt phenomenon in experimental renal artery stenosis. The kidney arteries on the side of the ligature are spared the systemic hypertensive effects, whereas the opposite renal vessels and systemic vessels show advanced hypertension. Cholesterol emboli (Figure 3.3), small fluffy retinal infarcts, white platelet plugs,[36] and venous stasis retinopathy[37,38] all provide clues to a stenosing lesion in the ophthalmic-ICA system and are discussed in more detail in the section on ICA disease in Chapter 6. The iris is also supplied by tributaries of the ophthalmic artery and can reveal ischemic damage in patients with ICA disease.[39]

Stroke Localization

Findings from the Neurological Examination

Clinical localization of the brain lesion is primarily from the findings on neurological examination. It would be impossible and probably unprofitable to review here the full details of the neurological examination. In fact, many nonneurologists feel uncomfortable when confronted with a stroke patient because they feel ill-equipped to detect the neurological findings and to explain them in anatomical detail. Actually, the neurological findings do not have a heavy impact on the diagnosis of stroke mechanism, though the findings do help with the anatomical location of the lesion. The useful anatomical data for practical diagnosis can, in fact, be summarized rather briefly. Rather than systematically reviewing the examination, I comment here only on important, practical, useful features.

I have been impressed that the most important and most frequently missed signs of brain dysfunction involve abnormalities of (1) higher cortical function, (2) level of alertness, (3) the visual and oculomotor systems, and (4) gait.[1] Repeatedly and consistently, these are parts of the examination most frequently overlooked by the nonneurologist, which provide key clues to anatomical localization.

Tests of high-level cortical function

Higher-cortical-function testing should always include examination of language function, especially if the patient has symptoms or signs referable to the right limbs or the right visual field. A good screening test is the writing of a brief paragraph describing the stroke or TIA. Reading a paragraph from a newspaper or a magazine is also helpful. Ask the patient to name objects in the environment and to repeat spoken language. Remember that there is a large difference between *dysarthria* (an abnormality of speech articulation and pronunciation) and *aphasia* (altered content, expression, and understanding of language). If patients are mute and do not write, it is often difficult to be sure whether they are aphasic unless they follow commands or select objects or words from choices in a clearly erroneous manner.

When there are symptoms or signs of dysfunction in the left limbs or visual field, it is especially important to test *visuospatial functions* and to look for *neglect of the left side of space.*[40] Ask the patient to draw a clock or a house, and to copy a single two-dimensional figure. Patients with right hemispheral cortical lesions will often omit the left side of their figures and will display abnormal angles and proportions. Ask the patient to read a brief paragraph or headline or to look at a picture with the examiner. Left neglect is manifested by omitting words, phrases, or people on the left side of the page. Also notice how the patient heeds environmental stimuli to the right and left sides.

Memory can also be affected by a focal CNS lesion, usually involving the PCA territories. The clinician can test memory by asking patients to recall the material contained in the paragraph they read, a picture they were shown, or what they wrote in their own paragraph description. Alternatively, patients may be asked to recall three items that they were shown or were told about. Examination of higher cortical function and the remainder of the neurological examination are discussed in more detail elsewhere.[1]

Level of alertness

Decreased level of consciousness is an important sign of increased ICP or lesions of the brainstem reticular activating system or bilateral cerebral hemispheres.[2,41-43] Nonetheless, often, there is no comment in the record regarding whether the patient was bright and alert or drowsy or delirious. Does the patient require frequent prodding to stay alert? Often, the nurses on the floor or the family who are with the patient for much of the day can better answer this question. They should always be interrogated about the patient's alertness and the appropriateness of mental performance or deviations from premorbid behavior.

Visual and oculomotor function

Much of the mammalian brain is concerned with visual interpretation and exploration, looking and seeing. Large lesions of the posterior hemispheres may produce only visual dysfunction and may leave speech, movement, and other sensations unscathed. Not to *test the visual fields in a stroke patient* is a cardinal sin, similar to failing to palpate the abdomen in a patient with unexplained shock. Test the visual fields by presenting a visual stimulus, usually a finger or pin in the peripheral portion of each visual field in each eye, and determine on confrontation when the patient sees it. Also ask the patient to look at something—a picture, a paragraph, or the scene outside the window. Is there consistent omission of objects on one side?

Probably the most common eye-movement abnormality in patients with stroke is a conjugate-gaze paralysis. The eyes may be deviated to one side, usually the side of the hemispheral lesion, and both eyes fail to look toward the opposite side. This abnormality usually means a frontal or deep hemispheral lesion in the hemisphere opposite to the gaze palsy[44,45] or a lesion in the pons on the same side as the gaze palsy. *Nystagmus,* a rhythmic oscillation of the eyes on horizontal or vertical gaze, is usually diagnostic of a vertebrobasilar location of the stroke, as are dysconjugate palsies or paralysis of movement of one eye or one eye muscle.

Gait

Some patients with cerebellar lesions have a normal examination when recumbent or seated but cannot walk. These patients are all too often discharged from the emergency room only to return later, desperately ill from cerebellar hemorrhage or infarction. Observation of gait also gives a great deal of information about motor function and its symmetry. Is there dragging of one foot, delay in hip flexion on one side, or less arm swing on one side? Are adventitious tremors or odd posturing of a limb seen as the patient walks?

Aspects of motor function

Having covered the usual omissions, I now turn to an evaluation of the motor system. Be sure to test each limb proximally and distally. In central lesions, the most important weakness is usually in the shoulder abductors, arm extensors, finger extensors and abductors, thigh flexors, leg flexors, and foot and toe dorsiflexors and everters. Check for drift of the outstretched hands. Try to estimate the relative motor strength in face, arms, hands, and legs. In hemiparetic patients, are any of these regions disproportionately affected or preserved? Test coordination of each limb by the finger–nose, toe–object maneuvers. Deep tendon reflexes are of little importance in central lesions during the acute stroke, but it is informative to elicit the Babinski response.

Somatosensory functions

In cerebral lesions, higher sensory functions—such as position sense, object recognition, and extinction—are more often affected than elementary pin or touch perception. A useful single screening test is (1) have the patient close the eyes; (2) touch a specific spot on the patient's fingers, hand, or foot; and then (3) direct the patient to touch precisely the same spot with the opposite hand. This test requires no equipment and is an excellent measure of point-position localization, a good reflection of higher sensory tactile function. Of course, at the same time, you are also testing fine touch because if patients cannot feel the touch, they will fail the test. Also, with the patient's eyes still closed, touch both arms, both hands, and then both legs simultaneously, to see whether the patient will apparently extinguish the touch consistently on one side of the body. Again, try to assess the relative sensory involvement in face, arms, hands, and legs for disproportionately severe involvement or sparing.

When you have tabulated in your mind the neurological findings, step back from the bedside and *think*. Where is the lesion likely to be? If there is more than one possible or probable location, you may think of further bedside testing that could distinguish among these possibilities. *Do not leave the bedside before you feel confident in your localization.*

Common Localization Patterns

The neuroanatomic findings can usually be placed in one of seven general categories. The process is simply one of pattern recognition—that is, matching the patient's clinical deficit with that of patients with known lesions in one of the following regions. Also, are there expected findings that are absent or unexpected added findings beyond those described among these patterns?

1. *left hemisphere lesion* (in the anterior hemisphere in the territory of the ICA and its MCA and ACA tributaries)—aphasia, right-limb weakness, right-limb sensory loss, right visual field defect, poor right conjugate gaze, difficulty reading, writing, and calculating
2. *right hemisphere lesion* (in ICA–ACA–MCA distribution)—neglect of the left visual space, difficulty drawing and copying, left visual-field defect, left-limb motor weakness, left-limb sensory loss, poor left conjugate gaze, extinction of the left stimulus of two simultaneously given visual or tactile stimuli
3. *left PCA lesion*—right visual-field defect, difficulty reading with retained writing ability, difficulty naming colors and objects presented visually, good repetition of spoken language, occasional numbness of the right limbs
4. *right PCA lesion*—left visual-field defect, often with neglect, occasionally accompanying left-limb sensory loss
5. *vertebrobasilar territory infarction*—spinning dizziness; diplopia; weakness or numbness of all four limbs or bilateral regions; crossed motor or sensory findings (e.g., numbness or weakness of one side of the face and the opposite side of the body); ataxia; vomiting; headache in the occiput, mastoid, or neck; bilateral blindness or dim vision; on examination, nystagmus or dysconjugate gaze, gait or limb ataxia out of proportion to weakness, bilateral recently acquired weakness or numbness (i.e., one side not due to an old stroke or other defect), crossed signs, bilateral visual-field defects, amnesia
6. *pure motor stroke* (internal capsule or basis pontis)—weakness of face, arm, and leg on one side of the body, without abnormalities of higher cortical function, sensory or visual dysfunction, or reduced alertness
7. *pure sensory stroke* (thalamus)—numbness or decreased sensibility of face, arm, and leg on one side of the body, without weakness, incoordination, visual or higher cortical function abnormalities

In some patients, the findings will be quite limited and will not represent the full clinical syndrome. For example, the abnormality may be limited to aphasia, yet this will be sufficient to place the patient in the category of left-hemisphere anterior circulation disease because no other pattern includes aphasia. Similarly, nystagmus and ataxia are diagnostic of a brainstem or cerebellar process in the category of vertebrobasilar disease. In other patients, the findings are not sufficient to allow definite localization but suggest a number of possibilities. Sudden abnormalities of behavior are found in patients with caudate nucleus,[46,47] thalamic,[48,49] and frontal-lobe infarction. Weakness limited to a single limb could fit into a number of these categories (1, 2, 3, 4, 5, or 6).

The neurological findings also may help predict the stroke mechanism. An example would be a hypertensive patient with pure motor stroke on the right. This lesion is invariably due to a small lacunar infarct in the internal capsule or pons or a small hemorrhage in these areas. A patient with sudden onset of Wernicke-type fluent aphasia without accompanying weakness or motor signs has a left temporal embolus or a small posterior putaminal hemorrhage undercutting the left temporal lobe. We now return to the patient JH who had a very different presentation.

> JH was very sleepy. He could not cooperate for tests of drawing or copying. He was not aware of his left-limb paralysis. He did not notice visual stimuli to his left. His eyes were completely deviated to the right but moved fully to the left with passive head rotation. There was severe paralysis of the left face, arm, and leg, with virtually no movement to pinch or other stimulation. He did not feel touch on his left limbs and could not reliably tell which way his fingers and toes were moved. Pin or pinch was felt as a general discomfort, which he could not localize. Deep tendon reflexes were reduced on the left, and the left plantar response was extensor.

The neurological findings in JH clearly localize the process to the right cerebral hemisphere. The severe motor, somatosensory, and visual loss and lack of awareness of the deficit point to a large lesion involving the frontal and paracentral regions. The decreased level of alertness and the involvement of multiple systems (motor, somatosensory, visual) suggests a large zone of brain abnormality or a deep lesion involving subcortical structures and the internal capsule. Conjugate eye deviation is especially common in deep lesions.

I now review my hypotheses about stroke mechanisms and localization in JH. The site of brain dysfunction is surely the frontal and central portions of the right cerebral hemisphere. The vascular pathway supplying this region involves blood coming from the heart to the aorta to the right innominate, internal carotid, and middle cerebral arteries. Vascular examination has offered no evidence for disease at any of these locations. The ecology suggests the possibility of large-artery occlusive disease, which would be statistically most commonly located at the origin of the ICA in the neck. Atherostenosis at the ICA within the siphon and within the proximal MCA are less likely but possible sites of disease.

Probable stroke mechanisms can be listed, in order of likelihood, as (1) premature atherosclerotic occlusive disease with thrombosis and distal intra-arterial embolization of clot, (2) cardiogenic embolism, and (3) ICH. The clinical findings on neurological examination exclude the possibility of lacunar infarction. The focality of findings and absence of headache exclude SAH. ICH is possible, given the reduction in alertness and the likelihood of a large deep hemispheral lesion, but the absence of risk factors (hypertension, bleeding abnormality, anticoagulation, drug use, etc.) and the presence of a preceding TIA argue very strongly against ICH. The absence of any history of cardiac disease and the normal cardiac findings place cardiogenic embolism below thrombosis as a probable stroke mechanism. I am now ready to test and refine these hypotheses by laboratory and imaging investigations, which are discussed in the next chapter.

Using Information from a Stroke Registry or Data Bank

Early in the discussion of clinical diagnosis, I introduced the computer so that the clinician could attempt to emulate computer logic. I now return to the computer. Suppose that data were available from detailed analyses of patients with stroke. The registry could be the clinician's own data, collected from patients seen at a single institution, or it could be data gleaned by others or pooled from many registries. I have cited information from such registries throughout this chapter.[5-18] Ideally, these registries should include information from each of the categories discussed so far (i.e., demography, risk factors, past TIAs and strokes, onset and course of the deficit, accompanying symptoms, cardiac and vascular abnormalities on examination, and localization from the clinical and imaging tests). The clinicians could then search the registry for patients with characteristics matching their cases. The final diagnosis in these matching cases would help the clinician to estimate more accurately the probability of particular stroke mechanisms and causative vascular lesions in their own patients.

In this chapter, I now go through such a registry search to illustrate the utility. First is a patient who is agitated and has Wernicke's aphasia as the only abnormality on neurological examination. Tables 3.11 to 3.13 document a search on a patient with Wernicke's aphasia, using data from the HSR.[9] From among all testable patients with information about aphasia (469 patients), 54 had Wernicke's aphasia. The distribution of diagnoses in patients with and without Wernicke's aphasia is tabulated in Table 3.11. The Wernicke's aphasia group differs from patients without Wernicke's aphasia because they include more patients with emboli and ICH and fewer examples of thrombosis. However, there are significant numbers of patients showing all stroke mechanisms, so that these data only suggest probabilities. Next, I think of a way to make the groups more specifically like our patient: This patient had no motor weakness. I search again the group with Wernicke's aphasia but now stipulate the absence of motor weakness, so the findings might be more useful. I then look at patients with Wernicke's aphasia with no motor weakness, comparing patients who have Wernicke's aphasia but no weakness with patients who have no Wernicke's aphasia and no weakness (Table 3.12). Now the figures are more impressive because the registry does not contain a single example of thrombosis with Wernicke's aphasia and no weakness. There are, however, a significant number of examples of ICH. From these data, the major differential diagnosis using the past experience of the HSR would be embolus versus ICH.

TABLE 3.11

Diagnosis in Patients with and without Wernicke's Aphasia (from Harvard Stroke Registry)[9]

	Thrombosis	Embolus	ICH	SAH	Total
With Wernicke's aphasia	8 (15%)	35 (65%)	8 (15%)	3 (6%)	54
Without Wernicke's aphasia	222 (53%)	124 (30%)	39 (9%)	30 (7%)	415

Note: ICH = intracerebral hemorrhage; SAH = subarachnoid hemorrhage. Percentages do not always add up to 100 due to rounding.

TABLE 3.12

Diagnosis: Wernicke's Aphasia and No Motor Weakness (from Harvard Stroke Registry)[9]

	Thrombosis	Embolus	ICH	SAH	Total
With Wernicke's aphasia	0 (0%)	12 (75%)	3 (19%)	1 (6%)	16
Without Wernicke's aphasia	56 (58%)	24 (25%)	2 (2%)	14 (15%)	96

TABLE 3.13

Diagnosis: Wernicke's Aphasia and No Motor Weakness or Hypertension (from Harvard Stroke Registry)[9]

	Thrombosis	Embolus	ICH	SAH	Total
With Wernicke's aphasia	0 (0%)	5 (100%)	0 (0%)	0 (0%)	5
Without Wernicke's aphasia	16 (41%)	15 (38%)	1 (3%)	7 (18%)	39

I now think harder and ask whether there is any other parameter that could be added that would differentiate these two conditions: This patient had no history of hypertension and was not hypertensive in the hospital. Hypertension is, of course, common in ICH. If *no hypertension* is added to the list of search criteria (Table 3.13), only five patients remain who have Wernicke's aphasia, no weakness, and no hypertension, and all had cerebral embolism. Using the past experience of the HSR, this patient probably has a cerebral embolus. Of course, the odds would be much higher if the number of patients with Wernicke's aphasia, no weakness, and no hypertension were 100 rather than 5, but the computer has allowed quick and precise comparison of this patient with the experience of the registry.

References

1. Caplan LR. The effective clinical neurologist. Boston: Blackwell, 1990.
2. Caplan LR, Kelly JJ. Consultations in neurology. Toronto: BC Decker, 1988.
3. Bayes T. An essay towards solving a problem in the doctrine of chances. Philos Trans R Soc Lond 1763;53:270–418. Reprinted in Biometrika 1935;45:296–315.
4. Winkler RL. Introduction to Bayesian inference and decision. New York: Holt, Rinehart and Winston, 1972.
5. Aring C, Merritt H. Differential diagnosis between cerebral hemorrhage and cerebral thrombosis. Arch Intern Med 1935;56:435–456.
6. Whisnant J, Fitzgibbons J, Kurland L, et al. Natural history of stroke in Rochester, Minnesota, 1945–1954. Stroke 1971;2:11–22.
7. Matsumoto N, Whisnant J, Kurland L, et al. Natural history of stroke in Rochester, Minnesota, 1955–1969. Stroke 1973;4:20–29.
8. Kannel W, Dawber T, Cohen M, et al. Vascular disease of the brain—epidemiologic aspects. Am J Public Health 1965;55:1355–1356.
9. Mohr J, Caplan LR, Melski J, et al. The Harvard Cooperative Stroke Registry: a prospective registry. Neurology 1978;28:754–762.
10. Caplan LR, Hier D, D'Cruz I. Cerebral embolism in the Michael Reese Stroke Registry. Stroke 1983;14:530–536.
11. Chambers B, Donnan G, Bladin P. Patterns of stroke: an analysis of the first 700 consecutive admissions to the Austin Hospital stroke unit. Aust N Z J Med 1983;13:57–64.
12. Gross C, Kase C, Mohr J, et al. Stroke in south Alabama: incidence and diagnostic features—population-based study. Stroke 1984;15:249–255.
13. Kunitz S, Gross C, Heymann A, et al. The Pilot Stroke Data Bank: definition, design, and data. Stroke 1984;15:740–746.
14. Bogousslausky J, Van Melle G, Regli F. The Lausanne Stroke Registry: analysis of 1000 consecutive patients with first stroke. Stroke 1988;19:1083–1092.
15. Foulkes MA, Wolf PA, Price TR, et al. The Stroke Data Bank: design, methods, and baseline characteristics. Stroke 1988;19:547–554.
16. Friday G, Lai SM, Alter M, et al. Stroke in the Lehigh Valley: racial/ethnic difference. Neurology 1989;39:1165–1168
17. Bamford J, Sandercock P, Dennis M, et al. A prospective study of acute cerebrovascular disease in the community: the Oxfordshire Community Stroke Project—1981–1986. J Neurol Neurosurg Psych 1990;53:16–22.
18. Coull BM, Brockschmidt JK, Howard G, et al. Community hospital-based stroke programs in North Carolina, Oregon and New York: IV. stroke diagnosis and its relation to demographics, risk factors, and clinical status after stroke. Stroke 1990;21:867–873.
19. Gorelick PB, Hier DB, Caplan LR, et al. Headache in acute cerebrovascular disease. Neurology 1986;36:1445–1450.
20. Gorelick PB, Caplan LR, Hier DB, et al. Racial differences in the distribution of anterior circulation occlusive disease. Neurology 1984;34:54–59.
21. Kieffer S, Takeya Y, Resch J, et al. Racial differences in cerebrovascular disease: angiographic evaluation of Japanese and American populations. AJR 1967; 101:94–99.
22. Heyman A, Fields WS, Keating RD. Joint study of extracranial arterial occlusion:

VI. racial differences in hospitalized patients with ischemic stroke. JAMA 1972;222:285–289.
23. Russo LS. Carotid system transient ischemic attacks, clinical, racial, and angiographic correlations. Stroke 1981;12:470–473.
24. Heyden S, Heyman A, Goree J. Nonembolic occlusion of the middle cerebral and carotid arteries: a comparison of predisposing factors. Stroke 1970;1:363–369.
25. Barnett HJM. The international collaborative study of superficial temporal artery–middle cerebral artery anastomosis. In: Rose FC, ed. Advances in stroke therapy. New York: Raven Press, 1982:179–182.
26. Huang CY, Chan FL, Yu YL, et al. Cerebrovascular disease in Hong Kong Chinese. Stroke 1990;21:230–235.
27. Feldmann E, Daneault N, Kwan E, et al. Chinese–white differences in the distribution of occlusive cerebrovascular disease. Neurology 1990;40:1541–1545.
28. Marler J, Price TR, Clark GL, et al. Morning increase in onset of ischemic stroke. Stroke 1989;20:473–476.
29. Sloan M, Price TR, Foukes MA, et al. Circadian rhythmicity of stroke onset: intracerebral and subarachnoid hemorrhage. Ann Neurol 1990;28:226–227
30. Caplan, LR. Course-of-illness graphs. Hospital Practice 1985;20:125–136.
31. Baker R, Rosenbaum A, Caplan LR. Subclavian steal syndrome. Contemp Surg 1974;4:96–104.
32. Caplan LR. Vertebrobasilar occlusive disease. In: Barnett HJM, Mohr JP, Stein B, Yatsu F, eds. Stroke: pathophysiology, diagnosis and management. New York: Churchill Livingstone, 1986:549–619.
33. Fisher CM. Facial pulses in internal carotid artery occlusion. Neurology 1970;20:476–478.
34. Caplan LR. The frontal artery sign: a bedside indicator of internal carotid occlusive disease. N Engl J Med 1973;288:1008–1009.
35. Reed C, Toole J. Clinical technique for identification of external carotid bruits. Neurology 1981;31:744–746.
36. Fisher CM. Observations of the fundus oculi in transient monocular blindness. Neurology 1959;9:333–347.
37. Kearns T, Hollenhorst R. Venous stasis retinopathy of occlusive disease of the carotid artery. Mayo Clin Proc 1963;38:304–312.
38. Carter JE. Chronic ocular ischemia and carotid vascular disease. In: Bernstein EF, ed. Amaurosis fugax. New York: Springer-Verlag, 1988:118–134.
39. Fisher CM. Dilated pupil in carotid occlusion. Trans Am Neurol Assoc 1966;91:230–231.
40. Heir D, Mondlock J, Caplan L. Behavioral deficits after right hemisphere stroke. Neurology 1983;33:337–344.
41. Caplan LR. The patient with reduced consciousness or coma. In: Skillman J, ed. Intensive care. Boston: Little, Brown, 1975:559–567.
42. Plum F, Posner J. Diagnosis of stupor and coma. 3rd ed. Philadelphia: Davis, 1980.
43. Fisher CM. The neurologic examination of the comatose patient. Acta Neurol Scand 1969;45(suppl 36).
44. Mohr J, Rubinstein L, Kase C, et al. Gaze palsy in hemispheral stroke: the NINCDS Stroke Data Bank. Neurology 1984;34(1):199.
45. Tuhrin S, Dambrosia JM, Price TR, et al. Prediction of intracerebral hemorrhage survival. Ann Neurol 1988;24:258–263.

46. Caplan LR, Schmahmann JD, Kase CS, et al. Caudate infarcts. Arch Neur 1990;47:133–143.
47. Mendez MF, Adams NL, Skoog-Lewandowski K. Neurobehavioral changes associated with caudate lesions. Neurology 1989;39:349–354.
48. Graff-Radford NR, Eslinger PJ, Damasio AR, et al. Nonhemorrhage infarction of the thalamus: behavioral, anatomic and physiologic correlates. Neurology 1984;34:14–23.
49. Bogousslavsky J, Regli F, Uske A. Thalamic infarcts: clinical syndrome, etiology, and prognosis. Neurology 1988;38:837–848.

CHAPTER 4

Laboratory Diagnosis

Having reviewed the basic elements on which diagnosis is based and the preliminary diagnostic impressions from the clinical encounter, I now turn to the laboratory. Laboratory investigations should be planned to test, confirm, and elaborate on the hypotheses of stroke mechanism and anatomical localization generated from the clinical encounter. A shotgun approach to laboratory tests should be discouraged. Instead, an individualized and eclectic program of tests should be tailored to the individual patient's problem. Tests should be selected and interpreted sequentially. Results of the initial investigations should help determine the next step in testing.

In this chapter, I consider various tests in relation to the following series of questions, which clinicians should ask sequentially:

1. Is the brain lesion caused by ischemia or hemorrhage, or is it due to a nonvascular stroke mimic?
2. What is the location and morphology of the lesion(s)?
3. What is the nature, site, and severity of the vascular lesion(s)?
4. Are abnormalities of blood constituents causing or contributing to brain ischemia or hemorrhage?
5. Are there abnormalities of brain function and metabolism in regions not shown to be damaged by CT or MRI? Are there abnormalities of blood flow not detected by the macrolevel tests of large artery vascular imaging?

With these questions in mind, I continue to follow JH, the 36-year-old patient with left hemiparesis, as he is put through the diagnostic laboratory tests.

Question 1: *Is the Brain Lesion Caused by Ischemia or Hemorrhage, or Is It Due to a Nonvascular Stroke Mimic?*

Computed Tomography

In 36-year-old JH, the most likely stroke mechanism diagnoses after the clinical encounter are large-artery occlusive disease and cardiogenic em-

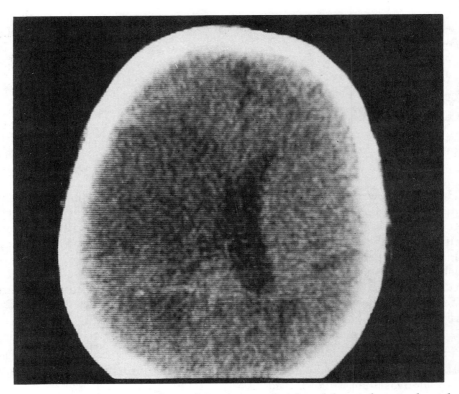

FIGURE 4.1   CT scan, nonenhanced: Large, superficial, and deep infarct in the right MCA territory (on left of figure). The right lateral ventricle is compressed by the swollen brain.

bolism, with infarction of the right frontal and central regions. Hemorrhage from an unusual cause and even nonstroke etiologies are much less likely but possible causes. The next step is a brain-imaging procedure that allows the clinician to distinguish among these possibilities. A CT scan in this patient (Figure 4.1) shows a large, hypodense lesion in the right cerebral hemisphere. This clearly identifies the process as ischemic. A nonvascular lesion large enough to cause a hemiplegia should be readily visible on CT. This lesion conforms very well to the MCA territory and involves the surface and depth in a triangular configuration quite typical for infarction.

CT is readily available in most hospitals and can reliably show ICH. When the mechanism is ischemic, CT may show infarction as a low-density lesion or may initially remain normal.[1] SAH is not as reliably diagnosed by CT, especially if the bleeding is minor or has occurred days previously. Increased density is in the CSF adjacent to bone. Visualization depends more on the hematocrit in the CSF than on the iron content.[2] Because contrast infusions make this meningeal area bright on CT, SAH is particularly difficult to diagnose if there has not been an unenhanced scan. In those circumstances when SAH is suspected from the clinical findings of headache and restlessness, lumbar puncture will be required to confirm or exclude SAH.[3]

Magnetic Resonance Imaging

MRI is probably more sensitive than CT in detecting very early ischemic changes but less securely differentiates ICH from ischemia in acute lesions. MRI shows tomographic sections in multiple planes of proton distribution modified by spin–lattice (T1) and spin–spin (T2) relaxation times.[4,5] Inversion recovery (IR) pulse sequences exploit tissue T1 variations to provide contrast, while T2 information is obtained from spin–echo (SE) sequences. Infarction prolongs the T1 and T2 relaxation constants and appears as a dark, hypointense image on T1-weighted sequences and as a bright hyperintense lesion on T2-weighted films.[4–6] Ischemia alters water content in the cells, changing their response to a magnetic field.

The appearances of ICH are quite different from ischemia but are complex and depend on the duration of time since the bleed and the choice of MRI imaging technique. Hemoglobin derivatives have paramagnetic effects. Imaging appearance depends on the nature of the compound, oxyhemoglobin, methemoglobin, hemosiderin, or ferritin, and whether the substances are present inside cells or in the interstitial extracellular spaces. During the first 12 hours after intracerebral bleeding, hematomas contain mostly oxyhemoglobin, which is not paramagnetic. The hematoma appearance during that time reflects mostly protein and water content. On T1-weighted images the acute hematoma appears as isointense or slightly hypointense (dark), with a surrounding hypointense darker rim. T2-weighted images are often hyperintense (bright) very acutely, reflecting water content. Between 12 and 48 hours after hemorrhage starts, deoxyhemoglobin is formed within extravascular red blood cells (RBCs), especially within the depth of the hematoma. During the next week, oxidation to methemoglobin occurs, beginning at the periphery of the lesion. By day 5 or 6, T1-weighted images show a central area of bright signal due to short T1, and a darker signal around the hematoma due to edema. On T2-weighted images, the center often becomes dark and is surrounded by bright images. Chronic bleeds contain hemosiderin within macrophages and tissues and show as bright, intense areas on T2-weighted images.[4,5,7] In summary, MRI shows hemorrhage less dramatically than CT and requires careful scrutiny of serial images using different acquisition techniques by experienced observers. The presence of mass effects and the location and shape of the lesion can help in the differentiation of hemorrhage from ischemia on MRI. A study comparing CT and MRI found that MRI was more sensitive in detecting infarction within 72 hours of stroke onset but that MRI differentiation between hemorrhage and ischemia during the acute phase was less secure.[7]

Patients with SAH are not easy to study by MRI. Restless, ill patients often have difficulty holding still for the time required to produce high-quality images. The relaxation times of blood admixed with CSF approximate the signal from normal brain parenchyma, especially in T1-weighted images.[5] T2 images often do show a bright signal.

Computed Tomography versus Magnetic Resonance Imaging

In my opinion, brain imaging has become an absolutely integral part of the evaluation of all patients with cerebrovascular disease. Stroke is such a potentially devastating process that clinicians need all of the objective data available to prognosticate, diagnose, and treat individual stroke patients. CT and MRI are noninvasive and safe, and new-generation scanners produce an enormous amount of clinically useful information. I am not convinced at all by the economists who want to save some pennies—not at the expense of the brains of patients.

With improvement in magnetic resonance (MR) imaging, MR has, for the most part, replaced CT in most instances. There are, however, still some advantages of CT. I believe that either a CT or an MRI scan should be performed at least once during the course of stroke in each patient.

In regard to imaging of brain lesions, CT has the following advantages:

1. At present, CT is more readily available. It is generally easier to obtain an acute CT scan in most hospitals than an urgent MRI.
2. CT is now less expensive than MRI.
3. CT imaging and its interpretation is much less dependent than is MRI on selection of technique and filming planes. More experience with CT interpretation makes them easier to read by most clinicians who are not neuroradiologists.
4. CT scans of ICH are easier to interpret than are MRI scans and, in most circumstances, yield adequate data for clinical decision making without the need for MRI scanning.
5. CT images subarachnoid blood as well as MRI does, and the shorter scanning time of CT is important in restless patients whom you do not want to sedate heavily.

Nonetheless, CT has the following disadvantages:

1. CT is not as sensitive as MRI in detecting and imaging acute infarcts.
2. CT is not accurate in delineating lesions adjacent to bony surfaces (e.g., in the orbital, frontal, and temporal lobes). CT is quite inferior to MRI in imaging brainstem and cerebellar infarcts and hemorrhages.
3. CT is mostly a one-plane technique for routine examinations; multiple planes require longer imaging time for reconstruction. MR, by using multiple planes (horizontal, transaxial, coronal, sagittal) shows the

three-dimensional (3D) location of lesions far better than do CT reconstructions.

4.   CT is not as useful in detecting and delineating spinal-cord strokes.

CT and MRI results do depend on the time of the scan in relation to the clinical event. In patients with ischemia, early CT scans are often normal or otherwise not diagnostic. In one study of 29 brain infarcts, 15 were visible on the initial CT taken within 12 hours of stroke onset, and 3 were seen after only 3 hours.[1,8] Contrast enhancement, in my experience, has not been very helpful. In this same study cited, 5 of 15 patients given contrast at the time of the initial scan had enhancement, but in 3 patients, the contrast made lesions isodense and more difficult to visualize than on plain noncontrast films.[9] In only 1 patient, who had multiple infarcts, a single infarct was visible only after contrast and was not seen on the noncontrast scan. During the first days, infarcts are usually round or oval and have poorly defined margins. Later infarcts become more hypodense and darker and are more wedgelike and more circumscribed. Some infarcts that had been hypodense become isodense during the second and third weeks after onset.[10] This so-called fogging effect may obscure the lesion for some time.[1,10] Later, infarcts become hypodense again.[11] Edema also begins to develop within the first days in patients with large infarcts and is manifested by low density surrounding the lesion and mass effect with displacement of adjacent structures.

MRI on the first day of an infarct shows loss of gray–white contrast and decreased intensity (darkness) on T1-weighted images as early as a few hours after stroke onset. Even earlier T2-weighted sequences show hyperintensive bright foci of ischemia.[5,7] During the next days, lesions become darker on T1-weighted and brighter on T2-weighted images. Increased signal on T2-weighted images may be evident years after the stroke.

Despite the fact that a patient clinically has had a TIA and has no residual symptoms or signs at the time of scanning, imaging may show a brain infarct. Nicolaides and colleagues studied 149 patients with hemispheral TIAs and found that 48 percent had an infarct on CT, most often in the symptomatic hemisphere.[12,13] MRI is clearly more sensitive in detecting infarcts in patients with TIAs.[5,12] Kinkle found that 13 of 60 TIA patients (22%) had focal abnormalities visible on CT, while 40 (72%) had lesions visible on MRI.[5] In another study, 50 percent of infarcts shown on CT in TIA patients correlated with symptoms, but 81 percent of the lesions visible on MRI were in regions appropriate to the symptoms.[9,12]

Immediately after the onset of bleeding, intracerebral hematomas are seen on CT as well-circumscribed areas of high density with smooth borders. Sequential scans in some patients have documented continued bleeding with enlargement of the hematomas in later scans.[14,15] Occasionally, a blood-fluid level is seen within acute hematomas. Edema develops within the first days and is seen as a dark rim around the white hematoma. As absorption of blood proceeds, the white image becomes more irregular and hypodense, and edema subsides. Ring enhancement of the outer dark zone may occur and may remain evident for weeks after the bleeding. In patients with low hematocrits, or those scanned initially weeks after stroke onset, hematomas can appear as solely hypodense lesions. I have already discussed the evolution of hematomas on MRI in the section on differentiation of hemorrhage from infarction.

In JH, the CT had shown the lesion quite well and had indicated without a doubt that the lesion was ischemic. I saw no reason to order MRI, with its added expense.

Lumbar Puncture

Lumbar puncture (LP), introduced in clinical medicine by Quincke in 1891, is still an important diagnostic test. LP is especially important in the diagnosis and management of patients with SAH. As has been emphasized, CT and MRI are not very sensitive tests for the detection of SAH, especially if bleeding is minor in degree and occurred days before scanning. The accuracy of CT in documenting subarachnoid blood diminishes after 24 hours.[16] Large SAHs are often preceded by small, warning leaks that are easily overlooked by CT but readily diagnosed by LP. By definition, subarachnoid blood rapidly disseminates and is present in the lumbar theca within minutes. *The absence of blood on LP excludes the diagnosis of SAH.* When blood is present, the quantity of blood and the pressure of CSF can also be measured and followed by later taps. Counting of the number of erythrocytes in the first and third or fourth tubes of CSF and measurement of the CSF hematocrit and spectrophotometric analysis of the CSF give an accurate quantitative database. When RBCs lyse, oxyhemoglobin is released into the CSF, reaches a maximum level in about 36 hours, and gradually disappears between days 7 and 10.[3,17] Bilirubin is first detectable about 10 hours after SAH, reaches a maximum at 48 hours, and persists for about 2 to 4 weeks after large hemorrhages.[3,17] Oxyhemoglobin and methemoglobin are detected at maximal light-absorption peaks at 415 mu on spectrophotometry, and the bilirubin peak is at about 460 mu.[3,18] Sequential LPs with measurement of CSF pressure, quantity of blood, and relative quantities of oxyhemoglobin and bilirubin help to determine the time since the last bleeding and can show evidence of fresh bleeding.

The CSF findings can also help differentiate ICH from ischemia. LPs in most patients with ICH show blood-tinged or xanthochromatic fluid under increased pressure with an increased number of polymorphonuclear leukocytes and an increased protein content.[3,17–20] Using spectrophotometric analysis, oxyhemoglobin and bilirubin can also be detected in higher-than-normal amounts.[11,13] However, some deep hemorrhages do not communicate with the CSF, and LP in these patients can remain normal. CT is a much better diagnostic test than LP in separating brain infarction from hemorrhage.

Question 2: *What Is the Nature, Location, and Morphology of the Lesion?*

In determining the lesion's morphology, the clinician must ask, Exactly where is the lesion? How large is it? What is its extent? What is the effect of the lesion on intracranial structures?

Having separated ischemia from hemorrhage, the clinician needs to know more about the lesion in order to predict the most likely stroke mechanism, localize the underlying vessels involved, prognosticate the probable future course, and select optimal treatment. The laboratory answers to the delineation of the morphology of the brain process usually come from neuroimaging with CT and/or MRI. When these studies are normal or equivocal, tests of brain function, metabolism, and blood flow such as PET, single photon emission CT (SPECT), xenon-enhanced CT (XeCT), EEG, and quantitative neurophysiology can be helpful in localization of the fundamental abnormality in the brain. Clinicians are fortunate to have available clinical data from the neurological examination prior to neuroimaging. Having already made hypotheses about lesion localization, clinicians can match these hypotheses with the imaging results. Does the location of the lesion(s) on CT or MRI explain the clinical signs? Could the lesion(s) be asymptomatic, incidental findings not related to the recent event? Are the clinical signs more severe than would be expected from the imaging studies? A discrepancy might dictate that some tissue, although not morphologically damaged enough to show on scans, is not functioning normally.

What If the Lesion Is an Infarct?

In 80 percent of stroke patients, when CT, MRI, or LP have been indicated, these studies have not shown hemorrhage; an ischemic lesion is present. Analysis of the neuroimaging findings should allow useful information about the lesion location and morphology.

What vascular territory is involved?

Identification of the vessels supplying an area of symptomatic infarction is the first step toward identifying the causative vascular lesion. Ultrasound and vascular-imaging tests can then be aimed at the vessels involved. Once a plumber has pinpointed a blocked sink, the plumber can examine the water tank, the pump, and the pipes that lead to that blocked region, knowing that mischief must be located within that water delivery system. In 36-year-old JH with left hemiparesis, CT has identified an infarct that involves the deep and superficial territory of the right MCA. Infarction is present above and below the sylvian fissure. The responsible vascular lesion must involve the vascular tree proximal to the origin of the lenticulostriate arteries, which supply the deep territory that is infarcted. These vessels branch from the main stem of the MCA. The vascular process probably involves the proximal right MCA. Possibilities from viewing only the imaging data include in situ occlusive disease of the MCA; cardiogenic embolism to the MCA; an intra-arterial embolus from the aorta, right CCA, or ICA; propagation of clot or embolism from the ICA in the siphon.

Suppose that the infarct had involved the paramedian frontal cortex in the supply region of the ACA, in addition to the MCA territory. Clearly, then, the vascular process would have had to originate proximal to the ICA intracranial bifurcation into the ACA and MCA. Similarly, within the posterior circulation, the location of infarction can yield important clues to the location of the vascular process. In a patient with quadriparesis, MRI shows an infarct in the paramedian basis pontis bilaterally. Careful scrutiny of the films also shows a small infarct in the right cerebellum in the territory of the AICA, which originates from the lower to midportion of the basilar artery. The lesion must involve the basilar artery proximal to the AICA branches. The vascular process could be an in situ occlusive lesion within the basilar artery or an embolus to this region arising from the heart, the aorta, the innominate or subclavian arteries, or the vertebral arteries in the neck or intracranially. If the cerebellar lesion had involved the PICA territory, the clinician would know that the vascular lesion must have affected the intracranial VA from which the PICA branches. A knowledge of vascular distribution and supply is essential to localizing the vascular abnormality. Chapter 2 includes diagrams and descriptions of the vascular territories and examples of anterior circulation infarct distributions (Figures 2.6–2.9 and 2.17–2.18).

How large is the infarct?

The size of the lesion is somewhat helpful in prognosis. Although the severity of the clinical deficit is not directly proportional to infarct size, bigger lesions in the same anatomical area cause more severe deficits than small lesions in the same location. The infarct size, as shown on CT or MRI, should be matched in the clinician's mind with the size of the vascular territory involved. The noninfarcted tissue (entire vascular territory minus the infarct) represents the tissue at risk for further ischemia. In order to determine the at-risk tissue, the vascular lesion must be known. For example, a small infarct in the territorial supply of a lenticulostriate branch might represent the entire supply of that small penetrating branch, but if the vascular lesion were in the MCA proximal to that lenticulostriate branch, a large area of cortex would still be at risk for spread of the ischemic damage. Large lesions are also more commonly associated with mass effect and with displacement of intracranial contents, especially if edema develops. Large lesions are also more often accompanied by reduction in the level of alertness. Mass effect and stupor often dictate treatment strategies aimed at these problems.

Are other ischemic lesions present?

So-called silent infarcts are very common;[21] in these patients, clinical manifestations were absent, minor, or forgotten. The presence of silent and symptomatic infarcts can yield clues as to the mechanism of the present symptomatic infarction. Guilt by association—identification by the company it keeps—is an important but by no means an infallible strategy. For example, suppose that a patient is admitted with a pure motor hemiparesis involving his left limbs. CT and MRI do not show a lesion involving the right descending corticospinal system, but five small lacunes in other regions are noted. The likelihood is high that the symptomatic vascular process is lacunar infarction. If CT shows multiple scattered cortical infarcts in different vascular territories, then either cardiogenic embolism or multiple large-artery occlusive disease is the likeliest stroke mechanism.

Are edema or mass effect present?

Edema can develop around infarcts and may even be potentiated by reperfusion of a blocked artery.[22] Sometimes the zone of actual infarction is quite small, but the surrounding edema zone is large. In younger patients, edema may be more threatening than in geriatric patients in whom brain atrophy might allow room for brain expansion. Displacement of midline structures,[23,24] effacement of gyri, encroachment on cisternal spaces, and brainstem displacement can often be judged well on diagnostic-quality CT and MRI scans.

What is the age of the infarct?

There are some general rules for identifying the duration of an ischemic lesion. In the beginning of this chapter, I outlined some sequential changes in brain infarcts, and those have been discussed in more detail elsewhere.[1,4–6,8–10] On CT, well-defined borders, severe hypodensity, and shrinkage of the infarcted brain region all suggest a chronic infarct that is months old. Poor definition from the surrounding brain, edema, mass effect, and contrast enhancement all suggest an acute process. In practice, however, these rules are not often as helpful as clinicians would like them to be. Usually, the history gives the clinician a relatively accurate time of reference. Surprisingly, some very acute lesions quickly become well-delineated and -defined and appear to be older than they actually are. Also, lesions that are months old are not appreciably different by imaging than those that are years old.

What If the Imaging Lesion Represents an Intracerebral Hemorrhage (ICH)?

The presence of a brain hematoma prompts different queries.

Does the location provide a clue as to etiology of the hemorrhage?

Chapter 2 indicated the usual loci of hypertensive brain hemorrhages. These are usually deep and are located in the lateral ganglionic region, subcortex, thalamus, caudate nucleus, pons, and cerebellum. In a hypertensive patient with a hematoma confined to one of these regions, the likelihood of an etiology other than hypertension is quite low. Angiography in patients with hypertension and deep hematomas has had a very low yield for showing aneurysms, arteriovenous malformations (AVMs), or other vascular lesions.[25] Hematomas resulting from aneurysms, so-called meningocerebral bleeds, are invariably contiguous to the aneurysms at the brain base or surface. In amyloid angiopathy, hemorrhages are lobar and are often multiple and can be accompanied by small infarcts.[26,27] Anticoagulant-related ICHs are most often lobar or cerebellar, evolve gradually, and enlarge.[28] AVMs may be located anywhere in the brain, especially in subependymal locations. Calcifications and heterogeneity within the hematoma raise suspicion of an underlying AVM.

How large is the hematoma?

Is there mass effect? By definition, a hematoma represents an extra volume of material in the cranium. Mass effect is more common and more serious in hematomas than in brain infarction. Large size correlates with poor outcome in hematomas at any location. Both mass effect and displacement of adjacent structures are readily analyzed on CT and MRI images.[23,24]

Does the hematoma drain into CSF pathways?

Is it causing hydrocephalus? Hematomas decompress themselves by draining into the CSF on the surface of the brain and into the ventricular system. In the past, ventricular drainage was considered an ominous sign, but now it is recognized that ventricular drainage is not always bad. The alternative to drainage is an increase in the mass of blood within the brain parenchyma. Nature might have already accomplished what the surgeon hopes to gain by drainage. Blockage of the ventricular system is most common at the foramen of Munro (putaminal bleeds) and at the level of the third (thalamic hemorrhage) and fourth ventricle (cerebellar hemorrhage). Dilation of the ventricular system, hydrocephalus, augments the mass effect of the hematoma and is often amenable to surgical decompression with temporary drainage or permanent shunting of CSF fluid.

What If Imaging Studies Show SAH?

Location of blood

What is the location of the blood? Blood may accumulate around a bleeding aneurysm or in the adjacent subarachnoid spaces and cisterns, thus yielding a clue as to the site of bleeding. Blood in the suprasellar cisterns and frontal interhemispheric fissure predicts an anterior communicating artery aneurysm.[1,29,30] Blood localized predominantly in one sylvian fissure suggests an

MCA bifurcation aneurysm on that side.[1,29,30] Thick blood in the pontine and cerebellopontine angle cisterns predicts a posterior fossa aneurysm. Since the early 1980s, Van Gijn and colleagues have identified a pattern of perimesencephalic hemorrhage that seems not to reflect aneurysmal rupture and that has a benign prognosis.[31-33]

How much bleeding has occurred generally or locally? The thickness of blood on CT or MRI correlates roughly with the degree of bleeding. Large subarachnoid bleeds are more often complicated by hydrocephalus and delayed cerebral infarction due to vasoconstriction than are smaller leaks. Vertical layers of blood clot more than 1 mm thick, or local clots larger than 5 × 3 mm in size are often associated with angiographically documented vasoconstriction.[34,35] Repeated LPs, washing away of the blood at the time of aneurysm surgery, and installation of thrombolytic agents such as recombinant tissue plasminogen activator (rtPA) are strategies that have been used to deal with large subarachnoid bleeds.

Are there regions of infarction?

SAH is often complicated by vasoconstriction and delayed ischemic damage. Infarction is most often localized to the territory supplied by the artery harboring the aneurysm but can be located elsewhere. The presence of acute ischemia clearly suggests that vasoconstriction is present. Vasoconstriction can also produce a pattern of generalized brain ischemia without focal infarction.

Is hydrocephalus present?

Blood within the subarachnoid space can diminish the absorptive capability of the arachnoid granulations. Communicating hydrocephalus develops because CSF production exceeds absorption. This complication can be managed by repeated LPs to remove CSF or by temporary or permanent CSF drainage or shunting.

What If CT and MRI Are Negative?

Normal neuroimaging is common in patients with transient ischemia and early after ischemia develops. In these patients, the clinical symptoms and signs provide some clues as to localization. EEG, quantitative EEG mapping, PET, SPECT, and XeCT also help generally to localize the lesion but give information about function and blood flow rather than about morphology.

Question 3: *What Is the Nature, Site, and Severity of the Vascular Lesion(s)?*

Having localized and quantified the process in the brain, the clinician is now ready to turn to the identification of the vascular lesion. It is hoped that the clinical picture and neuroimaging results have narrowed down the vascular region of interest in the individual stroke patient. In patient JH, it is known that the vascular process must be within the right carotid artery system or more proximally (heart, aorta, innominate artery).

What If the Mechanism Is Ischemia?

Ultrasound

Since the early 1980s, major advances in computer technology and electronics have made ultrasound the most important tool in identifying occlusive vascular lesions within the neck and basal cerebral arteries. Ultrasound energy is used to detect interfaces among structures of different densities and to detect moving targets such as RBCs. The ultrasonic information is received through a probe or transducer held over the artery being studied, and the information is converted into electrical energy, either for developing an image or for generating Doppler curves of blood-flow velocity. The technology is so far advanced and so entirely noninvasive that I believe the evaluation of all patients with brain ischemia should include, and indeed begin with, ultrasound testing directly after a CT or MRI scan has been performed and reviewed.

B-mode imaging

High-resolution B-mode ultrasound scanning of the neck provides images in several planes of the neck arteries. Figure 4.2 shows a B-mode image of the carotid bifurcation in the neck, showing a plaque. Advances in technology can show these lesions in different planes (Figures 4.3 and 4.4) and allow 3D reconstruction of the arterial lesions (Figure 4.5). B-mode scanning is quite accurate at the carotid bifurcation in the neck and at the origin of the VA from the subclavian artery. Lesions higher in the neck and more proximally located are technically harder to image well.

B-mode is quite accurate for assessment of the degree of luminal narrowing, in the identification of ulcerations and intraplaque hemorrhages, and for delineating the gross surface-wall characteristics of the carotid arteries.[36] When studied in comparison with angiography and pathological study of the arteries at endarterectomy, B-mode generally has very good sensitivity and specificity (>80%) for detection of significant occlusive lesions).[36,37] B-mode performed by itself does have limitations.[38] The large size of the ultrasound probe and sharp angulation of the vessels sometimes prevents adequate display of the vessels, especially at the VA origin. Calcifications and clots are not imaged. B-mode does not accurately distinguish complete occlusion from severe degrees of stenosis.[38] Analysis of B-mode images also requires experience and familiarity with the vascular anatomy. Arteries can be misidentified, especially from analyzing only one view. Experience has shown that B-mode imaging is enhanced by the addi-

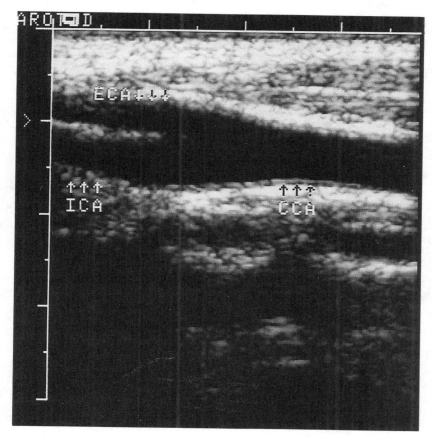

FIGURE 4.2   B-mode ultrasound of carotid artery bifurcation region. On the left is a small plaque near the origin of the ICA (marked by three arrows).

tion of multigated pulsed-Doppler (PD) apparatus. The combined B-mode and Doppler diagnostic systems are called *duplex systems*. The PD in this duplex system helps with identification of the arteries and orientation of B-mode images. The analysis of flow-velocity patterns by Doppler, recorded from different positions within the arterial lumen, provides qualitative and quantitative information about hemodynamic changes. The B-mode images help show the location of the velocity changes. The duplex system offers advantages over either B-mode scanning or Doppler analysis alone.[38,39]

Doppler sonography systems

Continuous-Wave- or Pulsed-Doppler Systems.   There are two main Doppler systems: *Continuous wave (CW) Doppler* measures an average velocity for blood moving through an artery or vein beneath the probe; *PD* is range

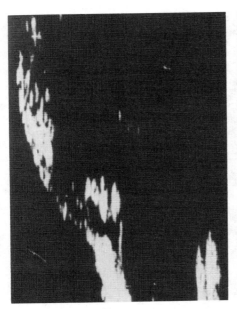 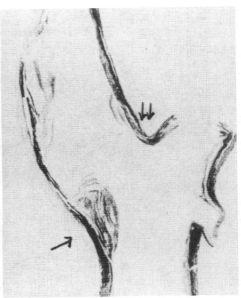

a   b

FIGURE 4.3 (a) B-mode view of the carotid artery. (b) Picture of the stained carotid artery specimen: The two arrows point to the flow divider between the ICA on the left and the ECA on the right. The single arrow points to a plaque in the characteristic location along the posterior wall of the ICA opposite the flow divider. (From Hennerici M, Steinke W. Durchblutungsstorungen des Gehirns—neue diagnostische Moglichkeiten. Verlag Bertelsmann Stiftung, 1987; reprinted with permission.)

gated to measure the velocity of blood in small volumes at specific selected sites within the vessel lumen. The CW Doppler device can readily determine mean flow velocities of the periorbital arteries, the carotid arteries in the neck, and the VAs at their origins and at the cervical region near the skull base (C_1–C_2). Moving the Doppler probe along the course of the carotid and vertebral arteries allows identification of the bifurcation of the carotid arteries and major changes in audible blood-flow signals. Doppler curves can be analyzed using fast Fourier transform (FFT) spectral analysis to detect peak frequencies and broadening of the spectrum.[38,39]

Figures 4.6 and 4.7 show various Doppler curves. The severity of stenosis is estimated by the increase in peak systolic frequency, the presence and severity of poststenotic turbulence, and an increase in diastolic blood-flow velocity.[39,40] Most readers are familiar with the task of washing off a pavement by using a hose. Turning the adjustable end of the hose changes the diameter of the lumen of the nozzle. When the nozzle is tightened, the jet stream of the water is under higher velocity and is more effective in

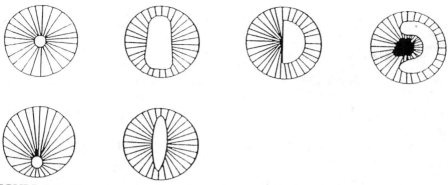

FIGURE 4.4 Transverse sections through various types of plaques. The plaque on the upper right has had an intramural hemorrhage. (From Hennerici M, Steinke W. Durchblutungsstorungen des Gehirns—neue diagnostische Moglichkeiten. Verlag Bertelsmann Stiftung, 1987; reprinted with permission.)

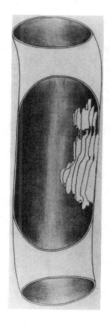

FIGURE 4.5 Three-dimensional reconstruction of a plaque. (From Hennerici M, Steinke W. Durchblutungsstorungen des Gehirns—neue diagnostische Moglich-keiten. Verlag Bertelsmann Stiftung, 1987; reprinted with permission.)

washing the surface. However, if the nozzle is tightened too much, the stream dribbles out or stops altogether. Similarly, in regions of luminal narrowing, blood velocity increases in an inverse proportion to the size of the lumen until a critical reduction in lumen size severely limits flow.

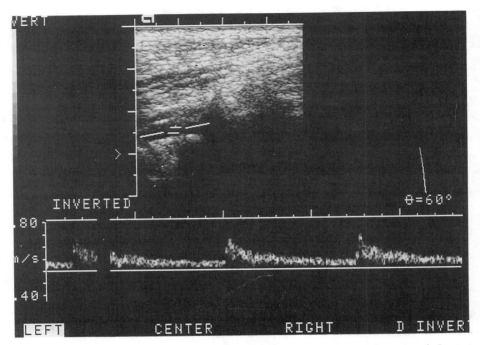

FIGURE 4.6   Duplex scan of a normal VA: Top panel shows a B-mode of the VA (white lines mark the lumen). Bottom panel shows the Doppler spectrum from this artery.

In patients with suspected occlusive disease of the subclavian and innominate arteries, a variety of noninvasive tests can measure blood flow in the arm. The relative velocity of pulsed-wave propagation in the two arms then can be compared. Forearm blood flow can also be studied by oscillography and venous occlusive plethysmography.

Color Doppler Flow Imaging.   Color Doppler flow imaging (CDFI) represents a recent advance in technology. In this technique, the spatial and temporal distribution of color-coded Doppler signals are visualized in real time and displayed as color images superimposed on gray-scale images of the surrounding tissues. This technique is especially good for showing changes in blood-flow patterns near small plaques. This technique has an extremely high sensitivity and accuracy for detecting minor, moderate, and severe degrees of carotid stenosis.[41–43] CDFI improves evaluation of the extent of carotid artery plaques by the simultaneous two-dimensional (2D) display of tissue structure and flow-velocity profile. Real-time images are easier to see and interpret than are curves of velocity. The technology also helps differentiate smooth from irregular surfaces and from ulcerative niches.[41] Unfortunately, severe stenosis cannot always be differentiated from complete

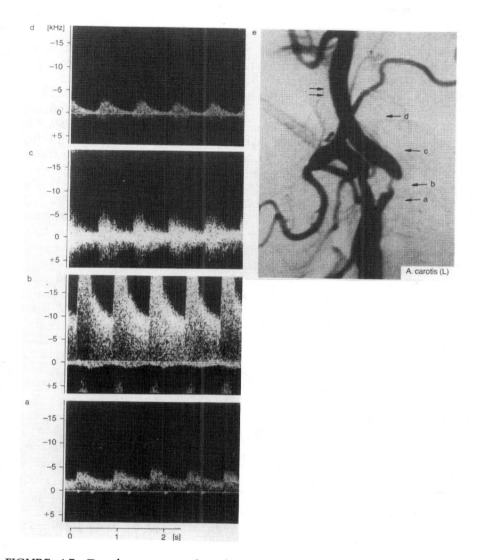

FIGURE 4.7 Doppler spectra taken from various sites from patient with the arteriogram shown on the right. At *a,* the maximal systolic frequency is reduced to 5 kHz; at *b,* there is increased velocity at the region of stenosis to a maximum of 20 kHz, with an endiastolic velocity of 10 kHz; *c* and *d* show velocities within the distal artery. The spectra are broadened and show decreased antegrade velocities. (From von Reutern G, Budingen HJ. Ultraschalldiagnostik der hirnversorgenden Arterien. Georg Thieme Verlag. Stuttgart 1989; reprinted with permission.)

occlusion by CDFI.[41] Nonetheless, the technique shows great promise for showing VA lesions in the neck.

Transcranial Doppler Ultrasound.   One of the major recent advances in the field of analysis of vascular lesions has been the introduction of the transcranial Doppler (TCD) system, which permits study of the intracranial arteries. Extracranial ultrasound examinations use pulse frequencies ranging from 3 to 10 MHz. These ultrasound frequencies cannot penetrate bone sufficiently to reflect signals from the intracranial arteries.[42] Aaslid and colleagues showed that signals could be obtained from the MCA and ACA, using a 2-MHz probe directed intracranially from the temporal bone just above the zygomatic arch. Now, three separate windows are used for probe placement, taking advantage of natural skull foramina or soft-tissue regions.[39,44,45] The temporal window is used for insonating the MCA and its major branches, the proximal ACA, the ICA bifurcation as well as the posterior cerebral arteries. A transorbital probe is placed near the eye and is used for studying blood velocities in the ICA siphon and ophthalmic arteries. A suboccipital window through the foramen magnum allows recording of frequencies from the intracranial VAs and the proximal portion of the basilar artery.[44] Figure 4.8 shows these ultrasonic windows.

Early studies using TCD confirmed normal values and techniques and showed that the technique was very useful in detecting severe stenosis or occlusion of basal cerebral arteries.[39,43–48] The TCD technique is also helpful in showing the hemodynamic effects of extracranial occlusive lesions on velocities in the intracranial branches:[39,45] A microprocessor-controlled directional pulsed-wave adjustable probe is placed at one of the windows and moved until maximal signals are obtained; velocities are then recorded at different depths along the arteries. The recent introduction of 3D display vascular maps helps orient the insonation to the location of the artery being studied. Vascular narrowing due to intracranial occlusive disease, vasospasm, and augmented flow through collateral channels and through AVMs all increase blood velocity. Interpretation of the results depends on integrating information from extracranial and intracranial ultrasound and from study of all of the major intracranial arteries at various depths. (Figures 4.9 and 4.10 show TCD velocity curves in patients with an intracranial and an extracranial lesion, respectively.)

Reserve capacity for augmenting blood flow can be studied using TCD and various vasodilator stimuli.[49] Emboli of all kinds can be detected as sudden alterations in flow, with characteristic sound signals. TCD can also be used to detect paradoxical emboli.[50] Bubbles are injected into an arm vein while the TCD probe is held over the temporal window. In patients without cardiac shunts, no change is noted over the probe. In the presence of cardiac defects with shunting, air emboli are heard and can be recorded.[50]

In patient JH, duplex scanning of the ICAs in the neck suggested an occlusion of the right ICA at its origin (Figure 4.11). The left ICA had only minor disease. TCD showed an inability to detect blood flow in the right MCA. Collateral flow was detected through the right ACA and PCA. There

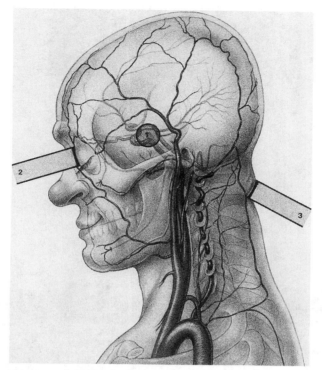

FIGURE 4.8   Diagram showing locations for TCD probes: (1) temporal window, (2) orbital window, (3) suboccipital foramen magnum window. (From von Reutern G, Budingen HJ. Ultraschalldiagnostik der hirnversorgenden Arterien. Georg Thieme Verlag. Stuttgart 1989; reprinted with permission.)

was also some damping of flow in the ICA siphon, presumably due to the proximal ICA obstruction in the neck. The left MCA showed normal velocities.

Magnetic resonance angiography

Although MRA is a very new technique at the time of this writing, it offers many advantages over other noninvasive methods of vascular imaging. Clearly, in the future, clinicians should explore effective noninvasive techniques before catheter angiography with dye installation, provided these noninvasive techniques are readily available and can be performed quickly and urgently. High-quality MRAs of the extracranial and intracranial arteries can be achieved by using gradient-echo techniques and short echo times.[51-55] Not all of the vessels can be imaged at the same time. The arch and extracranial arteries require a different technique and different views than does the circle of Willis. Knowledge of the likely seat of vascular pathology helps the examiner focus on a particular region, thus improving

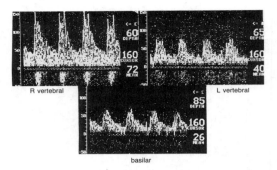

FIGURE 4.9 TCD spectra: The velocities in the right intracranial VA are much higher than in the left VA and the basilar artery. Arteriography showed a region of severe stenosis in the intracranial right VA.

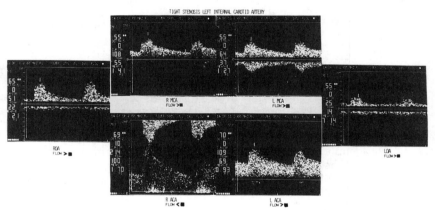

FIGURE 4.10 TCD spectra from a patient with severe stenosis of the left ICA in the neck, showing decreased left MCA velocity and a delta flow velocity > 25 cm/second (delta refers to difference between MCA peak systolic flow velocities on the two sides at 55 mm depth); reversal of flow with slightly increased velocities in the left ACA; increased velocity in the right ACA; and decreased left ophthalmic-artery-flow velocities, compared to the right side.

the yield of the examination. MRI of the brain uses a different technique and is performed separately from MRA. In MRA, veins can be imaged, as well as arteries. Figure 4.12 shows an MRA examination of the neck arteries, and Figure 4.13 is an MRA intracranial examination of a patient with bilateral MCA stenosis.

There are some limitations of the technique.[55] Patients must be cooperative and be able to hold still during the examinations. Patient positioning is critical. At times, the jugular vein can lie over the carotid bifurcation. Overlapping arteries sometimes make images difficult to interpret, a problem most older clinicians are aware of in interpreting arch-contrast

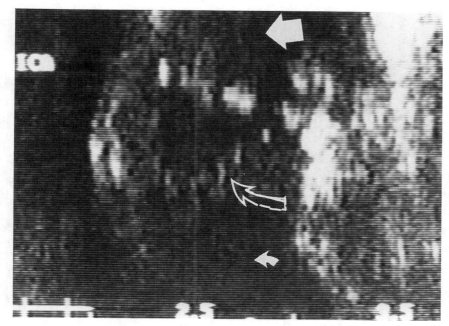

FIGURE 4.11 B-mode scan of the left ICA: The CCA is on top (closed large white arrow); a clot (curved open arrow) occludes the orifice of the ICA; below is the ICA distal to the occlusion (closed small arrow).

angiography and intravenous digital subtraction angiography (DVSA). At present, MRA is expensive and takes time. There have been insufficient correlation studies of MRA with angiographic and pathological findings to define the sensitivity and specificity of the method. Major advantages of MRA are its noninvasive character and the ability it has to display longitudinal images of the cerebrovascular bed. The technology is still in its infancy, and technological advances should lead to further improvement in the technology.

In contrast, ultrasound is mostly able to study arteries at various specific sites and does not provide the same type of visual images as MRA and catheter angiography. At present, until more data are available, MRA should be considered as a screening technique for occlusive disease. Standard angiography may still be needed in many patients, to better delineate the vascular lesions.[55] In patient JH, MRA confirmed a right ICA occlusion in the neck. Intracranial views also showed occlusion of the proximal MCA.

Standard cerebral angiography

Cerebral angiography[55,56] by arterial catheterization remains the standard and tested manner of defining the nature of vascular lesions in the extra-

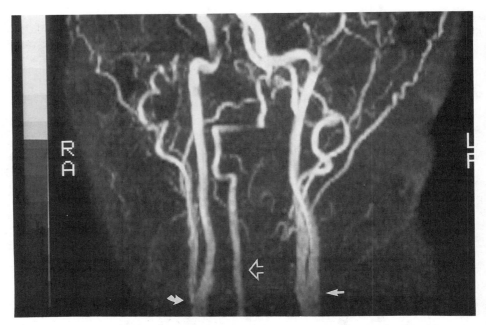

FIGURE 4.12   MRA image of the neck. Right solid arrow shows the left carotid artery; left curved arrow points to the right carotid artery; the outlined arrowhead points to the right VA.

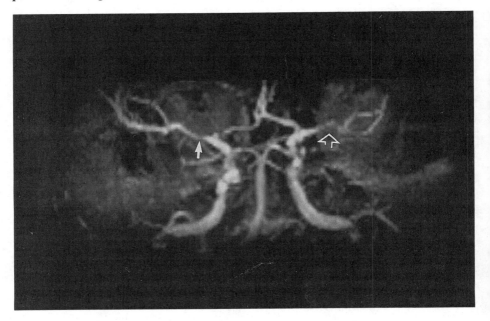

FIGURE 4.13   MRA: The outlined arrowhead points to a severe stenosis of the left MCA; the right MCA has a less severe stenosis (white solid arrow).

cranial and intracranial vessels. The preferred method uses the technique described by Seldinger to selectively catheterize and opacify individual arterial circulations. In experienced hands, angiography reveals very valuable information and has a relatively low incidence of serious complications. Complications depend on the equipment, dye, and catheters used; the amount of dye; the number of injections; the experience of the angiographer; and whether a large arch injection is performed. The general medical and psychological state of the patient, adequacy of hydration, renal function, and nature and severity of vascular disease are also important factors that affect the complication rate.

Angiography should not be limited to patients who are considered surgical candidates. Treatment is most rationally chosen when the stroke mechanism and vascular pathology are well delineated. In general, angiography should be performed on patients in whom some treatments would be feasible and preliminary testing has not revealed sufficient data to arrive at a firm therapeutic decision. Angiography is especially useful in clarifying and defining the nature of occlusive lesions in the anterior and posterior circulations.

Once the decision to perform angiography has been made, the clinician should discuss with the radiologist how the procedure will be performed to maximize clinically useful data and minimize complications. I do *not* advocate arch injections as a routine procedure. Only when it is not possible to catheterize key vessels should a full arch injection be made. When arch injections are performed, they usually precede selective catheterization of vessels. With arch injections, the force of injection and large amount of dye used increase the risk of angiography. Details of the extracranial vessels are usually suboptimal without further selective catheterization, and the intracranial vessels are poorly defined with arch injections. Also, after the use of a large amount of dye, further studies are limited by the need to restrict the total quantity of dye.

Angiography should be tailored to the clinical question and therapeutic alternatives. When possible, neuroimaging (CT or MRI) and ultrasonography should precede angiography. These tests will help the angiographer focus on the particular regions of interest. Screening of other arterial regions may allow the angiographer to limit the angiographic procedure, thus helping to reduce morbidity and, of course, time and expense. The clinician and the angiographer should decide together on the first important data required, considering the clinical context of the study. For example, in a patient with transient aphasia and right hemiparesis, the lesion is within the left ICA territory. CT shows an MCA-territory infarct. In that circumstance, the first angiographic procedure should be to selectively catheterize the left CCA and gain fluoroscopic information about the carotid bifurcation. If the region is widely patent, a selective ICA injection with biplane (anteroposterior and lateral) images of the nuchal and intracranial carotid artery can be performed. If obvious and severe disease at the carotid bifurcation is seen at fluoroscopy, a small amount of dye can be carefully introduced and selective films taken, using several different angles of the carotid bifurcation, before proceeding further. Later, intracranial opacification can and should be done—but carefully. Fluoroscopy or films of the common carotid origin can be made on the way out of or into this vessel. If there is no surgical lesion and the films contain sufficient data to allow a therapeutic decision, angiography can be terminated. If insufficient data are available from the initial study, then proceed to obtain the next important data.

Analysis of possible results of the ICA study may help to illustrate. If the study defines severe stenosis of the main-stem MCA and if, in the responsible clinician's opinion, anticoagulation is indicated, additional studies would not be needed. If, however, a surgical lesion were found at the ICA bifurcation, visualization of the right carotid system would be important for the surgeon. If the ICA is completely occluded and an extracranial–intracranial shunt or other surgical procedure is contemplated, adequate ECA opacification and display of the existent collateral circulation to the ischemic cerebral hemisphere would be needed. This might entail filming of the ECA, contralateral ICA, and ipsilateral posterior circulation vessels. On the other hand, if a small plaque is found in the ICA, dictating only antiplatelet agglutinating treatment, no further studies are necessary. Thus, the decision on a second injection will depend on the results of the first; the further need and direction of subsequent opacification and filming will depend on the results of the prior studies. Do not routinely order four-vessel angiography.

Because these points are so crucial, I now examine a different clinical situation. Suppose that a patient had suffered a transient left hemiparesis that had cleared completely before he reached the hospital. The lesion might be within the right carotid or right vertebral artery territories. If a right carotid injection gave normal results, it would be logical to proceed with a right VA injection. Alternatively, a right brachial artery catheterization with injection of the innominate artery would allow opacification of both the right carotid and the vertebral artery territories.

Several critical rules for angiography should be emphasized:

1. *Tailor the procedure to the patient and the individual problem.* Avoid extra injections, catheterization, and dye because they increase the risk of the procedure.

2. *Follow Sutton's law.* Sutton robbed banks because that is where the money is—go after the highest-yield information first. Unfortunately, I have seen angiographers, after a catheter had flipped unexpectedly into a vessel that was not the primary focus of attention, take several films "while they were there," believing that the films might be necessary anyway. Too often, a complication or other unforeseen exigency then curtails the procedure before the important data are obtained. *First things first.*

3. *The clinician responsible for the patient and the angiographer must plan the procedure together.* Ideally, the procedure should be performed with both present and sequentially choosing together the next shot as the data accumulate. Because of the press of time and other commitments, this is not always possible. Telephone contact at critical decision points often is an acceptable substitute. If a clinician cannot be reached during the procedure, discussion of the plan of attack and treatment choices with the angiographer is a minimum requirement. In some circumstances, the relationship between angiographer and clinician is so well oiled by past experiences together that the angiographer learns how the clinician will approach most common situations. In that case, consultation during the procedure would occur only if the unusual were uncovered. Ideally, if the responsible clinician is not the surgeon who will perform an operative procedure, the surgeon also should be contacted when findings are uncovered that would dictate an operation. Surgeons may have their own demands for studies prior to surgery, and this is best accomplished during the angiography.

4. *Avoid an arch injection whenever possible.* The yield of arch opacification studies is very low. Akers and colleagues reviewed the results of 1000 consecutive patients who had arch angiography, followed by selective catheterization of both carotid and vertebral arteries.[57] Only 6 (0.6%) had intrathoracic vascular pathology that was hemodynamically significant, including 4 lesions at the CCA origin and 2 at the innominate artery origin. Three of these lesions (2 CCA and 1 innominate) still would have been discovered if only selective catheterization were performed.[57] Inability to selectively catheterize these arteries and fluoroscopy will identify most cases requiring arch injection. The absence of a significant lesion in the head or neck should alert the angiographer to opacify the origin of the artery on the way out. Arch injections usually require 40 to 50 ml of contrast material injected under pressure, so cardiac overload and renal toxicity can occur.[55,58] A large bolus of dye used for filming the arch limits the amount of dye that should be used during selective catheterization. Arch films are also not particularly easy to read because of overlapping of vessels. In my opinion, there is no reason to perform routine arch angiography. Only the major arteries of interest should be studied using the Seldinger technique of selective catheterization. In addition, intra-arterial DSA filming techniques allow use of less dye while retaining high-quality films.

5. *Use the least amount of dye and least number of injections that will allow sufficient information to arrive at a therapeutic decision.* In JH, I did not order contrast angiography. Often, the initial opacification provides enough information so that other injections are not needed. Preliminary CT or MRI and extracranial and intracranial ultrasound or MRA help limit the extent of angiography.

6.   *Talk to and examine the patient at least briefly after each dye injection,* to detect any complication that might dictate stopping the procedure. The examination will depend on the vessels studied. For example, after posterior circulation opacification, check vision and memory; after carotid artery injection, check speech and arm movement.

The advent of DSA has added new dimensions to the capability for opacification of the arterial system. DSA can be performed using a venous injection of dye, much like an intravenous pyelogram, or the computer equipment can be used during arterial injection ("arterial DSA").[59] The arterial technique is identical to the standard Seldinger system, but computer-subtraction filming techniques allow for better films with less dye. As with intravenous pyelography, renal complications of venous DSA occur, especially if the patient is dehydrated, has myeloma, or has reduced renal function. Opacification of the arch and proximal extracranial vessels is satisfactory in approximately 80 percent of individuals, but technical limitations make high-quality films unobtainable in about 20 percent of patients.[60,61] To obtain diagnostic-quality films, patients must be able to hold their breath and remain still during filming. Intracranial opacification with venous DSA is often poor. Thus, intravenous DSA has no advantages over MRA and, in my opinion, is no longer a useful diagnostic technique.

On the other hand, arterial DSA, by significantly decreasing the amount of dye required, helps to reduce complications and to improve the diagnostic quality of films. I have found arterial DSA especially helpful in studying the posterior circulation.

In JH, I did not perform contrast angiography. The concordance of the MRA and ultrasound data and the unlikelihood of a treatable lesion persuaded me not to pursue angiography. His clinical deficit was also severe and not reversible.

Cardiac evaluation

Cardioembolic mechanisms of ischemic stroke are very common. The proportion of ischemic strokes generally considered to have originated from cardioembolic sources has increased dramatically with the development of sophisticated technology that has the capability of defining cardiac and vascular lesions. A wide variety of different cardiac lesions are now known to be potential sources of embolism, while in the past, only acute myocardial infarction and rheumatic mitral stenosis with atrial fibrillation were generally accepted cardiac sources.

Cardiac emboli arise from a heterogeneous assortment of diseases that affect the heart valves, rhythm, endocardial surface, and myocardium. Pump failure can cause general cerebral hypoperfusion. In addition, many patients with cerebral ischemia due to atherosclerosis have coexisting coronary artery atherosclerosis. Late deaths in series of patients with ischemic stroke are most often due to coronary artery disease and myocardial infarction rather than to cerebrovascular disease. These facts should direct the physician's attention to the stroke patient's heart, as well as to the brain and its vascular supply.

The question is not whether to look at the heart but how thoroughly to do so. What is the yield of intensive cardiac investigation? Is it worth the cost? Most clinicians would agree that it is important to take a careful cardiac history, particularly seeking symptoms of arrhythmia, congestive heart failure, angina pectoris, and prior myocardial infarctions. The heart should be carefully examined, noting heart size, quality of sounds, rhythm, and presence of gallops, in addition to seeking and characterizing murmurs. An electrocardiogram and chest x-ray should also be obtained routinely because of their high screening value, safety, and low cost.

There has been an explosion of available cardiac noninvasive tests. Indiscriminate use of echocardiography has a low yield in large unselected series of stroke patients.[62-65] M-mode echocardiograms have a relatively low diagnostic yield. In contrast, 2D transthoracic and transesophageal echocardiography has a high yield in patients with ischemic stroke, in whom there is

1. known prior cardiac disease
2. a clinical course suggestive of cerebral embolism—that is, sudden onset of neurological deficit, while active, without prior TIAs
3. a history of peripheral embolism in the limbs or abdominal viscera
4. absence of a clear thrombotic explanation for cerebral ischemia

The fourth group is particularly important to emphasize. Young patients who have no apparent reason for atherosclerosis may harbor unexpected cardiac sources, such as cardiac tumors or cardiomyopathy. In other patients, the results of preliminary investigations include

1. absence of extracranial vascular disease on noninvasive testing
2. a superficial infarct on CT or MRI in the distribution of a peripheral branch of the MCA or PCA
3. CT or MRI showing infarcts in multiple vascular territories
4. normal arteriography in a patient whose clinical deficit and CT are not compatible with lacunar infarction
5. arteriographic documentation of distal cutoff of a cerebral artery branch or a luminal filling defect without severe proximal stenosis

In these circumstances, intensive cardiac testing is essential. Echocardiography should be done eclectically, choosing patients with a relatively high yield. Remember that echocardiography is also not perfect in detecting an embolic source because endocarditis (bacterial and marasmic), small mural thrombi, and thrombi that have left their cardiac resting places will be missed.[66] Routine 2D echocardiography also will not detect a patent foramen ovale or small intra-arterial septal defect associated with paradoxical embolism.[67] Introduction of bubbles of air while listening with a Doppler device over the cardiac septum is a good way of detecting shunting of blood across the septum. Transesophageal echocardiography has improved the yield of potential cardioembolic source detection.[68,69] Because the left atrium is directly anterior to the esophagus, atrial lesions, occult valvular disorders, and ulcerative lesions of the proximal aorta, often missed by 2D echocardiography, are detected by the transesophageal approach.[68,69]

When clinical suspicion is high and echocardiography is not diagnostic, CT, MRI,[70] or ultrafast CT[71] of the heart might image the cardiac clot, and platelet scintigraphy using radionuclides[72] might also indicate pooling of platelets on the surface of a mural thrombus or other cardiac lesion. Remember also that documentation of a possible cardioembolic source—such as mitral valve prolapse (MVP), mitral annulus calcification (MAC), or akinetic zones—does not mean that the patient has cerebral embolism. Coexistent atherosclerotic disease may be the culprit.

Many patients with atherosclerosis of the carotid and vertebral arteries in the neck have coexistent peripheral vascular occlusive disease and coronary artery disease. Because coronary artery disease, even when silent, can be life-threatening, screening of these patients for silent myocardial ischemia is important, especially if surgery is considered.[73,74] A variety of different radionuclide techniques can now detect regions of poor myocardial perfusion.[74-77] Imaging of the heart after the patient has been given dipyridamole (dipyridamole–thallium myocardial imaging) and some exercise often shows regions of silent ischemia.[76-78] In one study of 38 patients with severe cerebrovascular occlusive disease, 60 percent had reversible or fixed myocardial perfusion deficits using this radionuclide scintigraphic test.[78] Treadmill or supine exercise testing with electrocardiographic monitoring is another commonly used screening technique.[75-77] Radionuclide angiography can also be helpful in assessing left ventricular function and perfusion at rest and with exercise.[75-77] If severe coronary artery disease is suggested by screening, coronary angiography may be needed to localize and quantify the coronary artery disease to guide treatment.

The utility of routine Holter monitoring for cardiac rhythm disturbances is not clear. In patients suspected of cerebral embolism, as just outlined, the yield is probably high enough to dictate the use of monitoring. In patients with lacunar infarcts and those with a well-defined atherosclerotic extracranial vascular cause for their stroke, the yield is probably low. Holter monitoring should probably be done in any patient whose initial ECG suggests rhythm disturbance.

Computed tomography and magnetic resonance imaging

Some information about the brain vessels can often be gleaned from careful scrutiny of CT and MRI, especially after contrast infusion. On plain CT, an acutely thrombosed artery can sometimes be seen as a hyperdense image with the shape and distribution of an artery or vein. The MCA is the most frequently involved artery.[1,79] On the other hand, the hyperdense MCA sign is virtually diagnostic of an embolus to the MCA.[79,80] Calcific particles arising from calcific material in heart valves or a calcified atherostenotic plaque can also sometimes be identified within brain arteries on plain CT scans. Contrast enhancement can show large berry aneurysms and dolichoectatic fusiform aneurysms; absence of opacification of an artery can indicate the high probability of occlusion of that vessel. More recently, computer graphics have been used to reconstruct 3D images of the brain vessels, using data from contrast-enhanced CT.[81] CT can also suggest dural sinus thrombosis by showing thrombosed serpiginous cortical veins or the superior sagittal or other sinuses as high-density clots on plain CT scans.[82–85] After contrast enhancement, CT may show a filling defect, representing a clot within the sagittal sinus, the so-called empty delta sign.[84,85] Serial cross-sectional CT images of the neck after contrast infusion can also yield information about carotid artery plaques, occlusions, and plaque hemorrhages.[86] CT of the neck can also show spontaneous traumatic arterial dissections.

Flow within brain arteries can also be studied with MRI.[5] Vessels with high-velocity flow appear black (signal void) on MRI images, while arteries with slower flow may show as white hyperintensities. Occlusions can be inferred when a flow void is not seen on images that show cross-section views of arteries.[87] Aneurysms and dissections can also frequently be identified and followed by MRI scanning.

Other investigations

A wide variety of other tests have been used in the past to study arterial flow in the brain vessels. Most of these investigations have been superseded by newer ultrasound technology and neuroimaging techniques. These include oculoplethysmography and ophthalmodynamometry.

Oculoplethysmography. In oculoplethysmography (OPG), a sensing device is placed on the cornea and measures systolic ophthalmic artery pressure (Gee method)[88] or relative arrival time of the ocular pulse (Kartchner and McRae method).[89] These devices produce a quantitative measure of flow or pressure in the orbital vascular bed of the two eyes. A comparison of the measurements in the two eyes is used to predict disease in the proximal ICA–ophthalmic-artery system. The test is easy to perform, and the results are machine-generated, with little observer variation in the technique or the results. OPG should not be performed in patients with glaucoma or retinal tears. The technique will not reliably detect patients with lesions that are not hemodynamically important, and bilateral lesions may not be reconized.[90]

OPG is still useful in assessing whether carotid artery occlusive lesions are producing hemodynamically significant decreases in distal flow.[84] OPG and ophthalmodynamometry (ODM) measure flow in the ophthalmic artery, the first ICA branch, while TCD measures flow velocities in the other intracranial branches. OPG and ODM can aid in the evaluation of ophthalmic artery disease.

Ophthalmodynamometry. In ODM, a physician using an *ophthalmodynamometer*, a hand-held pressure sensor, measures systolic and/or diastolic retinal artery pressures. In the *direct method*, the ophthalmodynamometer is placed on the sclera, and external pressure is gradually increased while the observer is noting the retinal vessels through an ordinary ophthalmoscope.[90,91] When the external pressure applied exceeds ophthalmic artery diastolic pressure, the arteries visibly pulsate. The mechanism is identical to compression of the brachial artery by a sphygmomanometer; when diastolic pressure is reached, the arteries pulsate, producing Korotkoff sounds. When additional pressure is applied to the eye, systolic artery pressure is exceeded and the arteries blanch and stop pulsating. The pressures are read from the dynamometer. The external pressures needed to overcome diastolic and systolic pressure in the two eyes are then compared.

In the *indirect method*, the external pressure is applied to the upper eyelid.[92] The patient is asked to close the opposite eye and report the moment he or she detects a dimming of peripheral vision—a *grayout* (diastolic pressure)—and then a total loss of vision—a *blackout* (systolic pressure). The indirect method is helpful when the ocular fundus is difficult to visualize, but the results are less reproducible. In either method, the external pressure needed to overcome retinal artery pressure—that is, the ODM reading— varies with the intraocular pressure and the patient's systemic blood pressure. If intraocular pressure is high, relatively less extraocular pressure is required. When there is no proximal occlusion, high systemic blood pressure is, of course, directly reflected in higher retinal-artery pressure measurements. The ODM pressure only drops when there is a hemodynamically important lesion in the ICA or the ophthalmic artery. Ophthalmodynamometers have the great advantage of being portable. I still carry one in my doctor's bag and use it at the bedside.

Other so-called indirect noninvasive tests that yield information about flow in carotid artery branches—such as thermography, radionuclide angiography, and periorbital directional Doppler ultrasound (PDDU), discussed in the first edition of this book—are no longer useful. Carotid phonoangiography (CPA), a method of recording sound spectrum, was useful in studying patients with bruits and so was a direct test of the carotid bifurcation.[90] CPA has been superseded by duplex scanning, which yields both a sound analysis and a visual image in real time.

What If the Neuroimaging Tests Have Shown ICH?

The commonest cause of ICH is hypertension, either acute or chronic. When the blood pressure is high and CT or MRI shows a hematoma in a typical location for hypertensive ICH, a search for AVMs or aneurysms has a very low yield. However, in young patients with no hypertension or with intraventricular or lobar hematomas, studies of the intracerebral arteries often show vascular lesions. Patients with ICH after use of cocaine, especially the hydrochloride form, have a relatively high incidence of underlying vascular lesions.[93]

MR can often show AVMs and cavernous angiomas. Vascular channels, serpiginous arteries, mixed-density heterogeneous signals, and the presence of old bleeds containing hemosiderin are clues to the presence of vascular malformations. Contrast-enhanced CT,[1,94] and MR, plain or enhanced with gadopentetate dimeglumine-diethylenetriaminepentaacetic acid (Gd-DPTA), can show large aneurysms if they are in the plane of the sections taken.[5] MRA is quite good at showing AVMs and aneurysms.[52] In many patients, angiography using selective arterial catheterization by the Seldinger technique, with opacification of the arteries supplying the ICH, is needed for definitive exclusion of small aneurysms. Some AVMs and most cavernous angiomas are not detected by cerebral angiography.

What If Neuroimaging or Lumbar Puncture Show SAH?

Cerebral angiography is still mandatory for the study of patients with SAH not explainable by trauma or a known bleeding diathesis. Aneurysmal rerupture is such a potentially lethal event that clinicians must be sure an aneurysm is not present in patients with SAH. MRA may be useful in screening for aneurysms, but at present, the technique is probably not definitive enough for surgical exploration, and dye opacification is still mandatory. MR is helpful in looking for small AVMs near the ependymal and pial surfaces. MRA may be useful in following patients after surgical or endovascular treatment of aneurysms and AVMs and in following unruptured aneurysms and AVMs not treated surgically. TCD is very helpful in following patients with aneurysmal SAH in detecting and monitoring vasoconstriction in the basal intracranial arteries.[45,95,96]

Question 4: *Are Abnormalities in the Blood Causing or Adding to Brain Ischemia or Hemorrhage?*

Once the clinician has determined the nature, site, and severity of the vascular lesion, it is important to find out whether abnormalities of blood constituents are causing or contributing to brain ischemia or hemorrhage. Simply stated, *clinicians must not forget the blood.* Abnormalities of the clotting system can lead to hypercoagulability and thrombosis. Bleeding diatheses often cause intracranial bleeding. Abnormalities of the viscosity of blood can alter blood flow, especially in small arterioles and capillaries of the brain, and in patients with occlusive lesions. Increased viscosity can cause or contribute to regional decreases in cerebral blood flow and potentiate ischemia. Autoimmunity, which can be detected and monitored by blood tests, can lead to occlusive cerebrovascular disease.

What If the Problem Is Ischemia?

The formed cellular elements of the blood should always be studied carefully: erythrocytes, leukocytes, and platelets. In addition, other blood components may be analyzed, such as serum proteins, coagulation factors, antiphospholipid antibodies, and other measurements.

Erythrocytes

Quantitative and qualitative RBC abnormalities can affect blood flow and clotting. The level of the *hematocrit* (Hct) clearly affects blood viscosity and affects the rheological properties of blood. Physicians have long been aware that very high hematocrit levels, such as 60 percent or more, can cause clotting in normal young adults. In older patients with preexisting atherosclerosis and small-vessel disease, high hematocrits that are still within the normal range can compound the vascular disease and limit perfusion. Studies in animals[97] and humans[98-100] confirm that the hematocrit level can affect blood flow and prognosis even when hematocrit levels are not frankly polycythemic. The hematocrit also has a heavy impact on blood viscosity.[101,102] Lowering of the hematocrit from 45 to 32 results in doubling of cerebral blood flow (CBF).[103]

Sickle-cell disease and other hemoglobinopathies can lead to altered flow and hypercoagulability. Sickle-cell disease and spherocytosis are associated with multifocal brain infarcts. TCD documents abnormalities of flow velocities even in young patients with sickle-cell disease.[104] The hemoglobin and hematocrit certainly should be measured in every patient with stroke. Hemodilution has been advocated as a measure to augment blood flow during acute ischemia. Lowering of relatively high hematocrits by blood donations has been advocated as a measure to prophylactically reduce the risk of stroke in stroke-prone individuals.[103] Hemoglobin electrophoresis is important in those with racial and genetic predispositions to hemoglobinopathies, especially if anemia is present. Careful examination of a stained blood smear for the morphology of RBCs can suggest the possibility of a hemoglobinopathy. Very severe anemia also can compound brain ischemia, but very low hematocrits are rare in stroke patients.

Leukocytes

The white blood cell (WBC) count is often elevated in patients with myocardial infarction and is also often slightly elevated in patients with brain infarcts. Some have even correlated a high WBC count with the severity of carotid atherosclerosis, but the issue is complicated by the fact that cigarette smokers have high WBC counts. Leukemia with very high WBC counts can cause packing of capillaries and small arterioles with aggregates of large WBCs, causing multiple small infarcts and hemorrhages.[105] This happens when the leukocrit is obviously high in the capillary tube used to measure the hematocrit. Measurement of WBC count is usually a routine part of a complete blood count (CBC), which should be ordered on each stroke patient.

Platelets

Platelets are critical structures active in the initiation of blood coagulation. Quantitative and qualitative platelet abnormalities can cause hyper-coagulability and bleeding. Thrombocytosis, especially with platelet counts over 1 million/μl can cause hypercoagulability.[106] Platelet counts should be a routine part of the initial evaluation of patients with ischemic stroke because thrombocytosis can potentiate thrombosis, and low platelet counts can suggest the presence of other disorders, such as the antiphospholipid an-tibody syndrome,[107-109] consumptive coagulopathies, lupus erythematosis, and thrombotic thrombocytopenic purpura—all of which can be associated with brain ischemia. Platelet counts can fall during the course of illness (e.g., after use of heparin),[110] so that a baseline count before treatment is occasionally very useful for later comparison. Some patients with platelet counts in the normal range have increased aggregability or secretory function of their platelets or have qualitative abnormalities of platelet morphology and function. Tests of platelet function in vitro are usually now performed in hematological research laboratories,[111] and even experts disagree on their applicability to the in vivo state. The extent of platelet activation can also be studied by measuring the levels of β-thromboglobulin (BT6) in the blood.[112,113] BT6 is secreted during platelet-release reactions, and when op-timal venipuncture technique is used, the levels are good markers of in vivo platelet activation and secretion. Simultaneous measurement of platelet factor 4, which has a very short half-life, can help control for in vitro platelet changes.[113] Platelet production of thromboxane B_2 can be performed by radioimmunoassays and von Willebrand factor antigen can also be quantified.[114]

Serum proteins

Fibrinogen is a very important part of the coagulation system because fibrinogen is converted to fibrin monomers by the action of thrombin. Fibrinogen also contributes to blood viscosity because high levels of fibrinogen can increase blood viscosity. Under ordinary circumstances, the hematocrit and fibrinogen levels are the two most important single predic-tors of viscosity.[101,102]

Normal fibrinogen levels usually range from 250 to 450 mg/dl. High levels of fibrinogen have been considered risk factors for stroke in several prospective studies.[115,116] Fibrinogen levels can also rise as acute-phase reactants in the early period after stroke.[107] Recently, some have tried using *ancrod* (a defibrogenating enzyme of Malayan pit-viper venom), as a strategy to lower fibrinogen levels and to decrease fibrin formation and increase blood flow.[117] Omega 3 fish oil preparations containing eicosopentanoic acid may also act to decrease fibrinogen content.[118]

Patients with a predisposition to stroke recurrence seem to have a slightly lower serum albumin level and albumin/globulin ratio than those without recurrence.[116] Abnormally high levels of immunoglobulins IgA, IgG, and IgM can indicate autoimmune disease and can be a clue to diagnosis in patients with unexplained brain ischemia. Macroglobulins found in Waldenström's macroglobulinemia and multiple myeloma also can increase blood viscosity and cause or potentiate multiple loci of ischemia. At present, immunoglobulin measurements are not a routine evaluation in stroke patients because of their low yield. However, in selected patients with clinical and ophthalmoscopic suggestions of hyperviscosity, and in those with a high serum globulin level, serum immunoelectrophoresis can be helpful.

Studies of coagulation factors and coagulation

The prothrombin time (PT) and the activated partial thromboplastin time (aPTT) are excellent screening tests of coagulation function and are routinely available in nearly all hospital laboratories. Measurement of the PT and the aPTT should be a part of the evaluation of all stroke patients. Other tests are ordered if a hypercoagulable state is suspected by acceleration of the PT or aPTT, the presence of multiple vascular occlusions, a past history of recurrent thrombophlebitis or miscarriages, or the presence of known collagen vascular, rheumatological, or inflammatory diseases. Some serum proteins—such as antithrombin III, protein C, and protein S—are natural inhibitors of coagulation. A decrease in the level of these substances because of a familial inherited disorder or due to acquired disease can cause hypercoagulability. The level of coagulation Factors VII, VIII, IX, and X can be measured in most hematological laboratories but have not been well studied in large groups of stroke patients. Abnormal levels of Factor VIII can cause hypercoagulability and recurrent strokes.[119,120] Factor VIII elevation can be chronic, can precede and predispose to stroke,[119] can be elevated as an acute-phase reactant in systemic illnesses such as ulcerative colitis, and can be elevated secondary to thrombosis—in which case it is a marker and not the cause of the thrombosis.[120]

Recently, hemostatic markers of coagulation activity have been used to detect and monitor hypercoagulability. Thrombin acts as a catalyst of the proteolysis of fibrinogen to fibrin. During this reaction, *fibrinopeptide A (FPA)* is generated. The level of fibrin D-dimer is also an index of fibrin generation. Fibrinolysis involves the dissolution of fibrin by endogenous fibrinolytic mechanisms. Fibrinolytic activity can be estimated by the levels of *fibrinopeptide B-B1-42* (FPB) and of *tissue plasminogen activator* (tPA) and its *inhibitor* (tPAI). Thrombosis is favored when thrombin proteolysis of fibrinogen (increased FPA and D-dimer levels) exceeds plasmin proteolysis (increased FPB and tPA/tPAI ratio).[113,114,121] Several studies have monitored the levels of these substances in acute stroke patients and during follow-up.[113,114,121]

Antiphospholipid antibodies

Antiphospholipid antibodies (APLA) are usually IgG or IgM antibodies that bind to negatively charged phospholipids. *Phospholipids* are important constituents of vascular endothelium, heart proteins, platelets, and other cells. At present, the two most commonly measured APLAs are anticardiolipin antibody and the so-called lupus anticoagulant (LA). LAs are acquired immunoglobins that are associated clinically with thrombosis, not bleeding; most patients with LA do not have systemic lupus erythematosus. The laboratory hallmark of LA is a prolonged aPTT that does not correct when normal plasma is added. This indicates the presence of an inhibitor of clotting rather than the deficiency of a necessary coagulation factor.

LA can be sought using a sensitive phospholipid reagent or the kaolin clotting time or the Russell viper venom time.[107] Anticardiolipin antibody titers can also be measured. The screening tests for syphilis—the veneral disease reaction level (VDRL) and Reiter protein reaction (RPR)—depend on the activity of APLAs. False-positive serological tests for syphilis are often found in patients with APLAs, and thrombocytopenia is present in a third of these cases. The clinical syndrome consists of frequent venous and arterial thrombotic events, such as thrombophlebitis, pulmonary embolism, TIAs, strokes, myocardial infarctions, and recurrent fetal loss in women.[107,122–124] The mechanism of recurrent brain ischemia is likely to be excessive clotting. APLAs may be directed against the endothelium or platelet membranes and may alter coagulability and vascular functions. Insufficient information is now available to know the importance of these and other antibodies in ischemic stroke. APLAs should be measured in situations in which the usual risk factors for ischemic stroke are not present, and certainly in patients with livedo reticularis and strokes (Sneddon's syndrome) and those patients with clinical features matching the primary APLA syndrome.[123,124]

Other blood measurements

An elevated erythrocyte sedimentation rate is often an important clue to the presence of unsuspected vasculitis. It should be ordered in patients with unexplained stroke and in young and elderly patients.

After the demonstration that sugar administration could worsen experimentally induced brain ischemia,[125,126] Plum and colleagues[127,128] have noted a poorer prognosis in stroke patients with elevated blood sugars. Because *blood sugar* is a critical metabolite for the brain, there is no doubt that very abnormal levels can be deleterious to patients with stroke. Blood-sugar elevation can also be triggered by tissue damage with release of catecholamines and mobilization of sugar. Large infarcts and hemorrhages are often associated with elevations in the blood-sugar level. Patients with hypercalcemia due to hyperparathyroidism also have a higher frequency of stroke, probably due to the vascular or platelet effects of calcium.[129–131] Dehydration diminishes blood volume, thus potentially decreasing blood flow. Measurements of blood urea nitrogen (BUN) and electrolytes should be useful in deciding on the presence and degree of dehydration and would demonstrate any important electrolyte imbalance.

Every patient with stroke or TIA should have, at the minimum, measurements of hemoglobin, Hct, WBC count, platelet count, aPTT, fibrinogen, blood sugar, calcium, BUN, sodium, chloride, potassium, and carbon dioxide before proceeding with aggressive diagnostic or therapeutic interventions.

Patient JH had an Hct of 41 and had normal WBC and platelet counts. The PT and aPTT were also normal. Blood sugar on admission was 145, but levels returned to normal after a few days.

What If the Patient Has Hemorrhage—Either ICH or SAH?

Bleeding diatheses are important causes of intracranial bleeding. Probably the most common bleeding disorders are now iatrogenic, including the use of heparin, warfarin compounds, rtPA, and other fibrinolytic compounds, and possibly aspirin use. Usually, these clinical situations are known and are not diagnostic dilemmas. Measurement of the PT and partial thromboplastin time (PTT) are usually sufficient to screen for these disorders. Platelet counts detect thrombocytopenia, and the bleeding time is a useful screening procedure measuring platelet function, among other processes. Hemophilia and other lifelong bleeding diatheses are usually known before the intracranial bleed occurs. Measurement of antihemophilic globulin (AHG) and other coagulation factors is helpful in patients with previously uncharacterized bleeding disorders. A history of prior bleeding episodes (vaginal, dental, postoperative, etc.) and the presence of systemic purpura are the best clues to the presence of a bleeding diathesis.

The tests described so far help localize and quantify morphological structural abnormalities in the brain, in larger blood vessels, and in the blood.

Question 5: *Are There Abnormalities of Brain Function and Metabolism in Regions Not Shown to Be Damaged by CT or MRI Imaging? Are There Abnormalities of Blood Flow Not Detected by the Macro-Level Tests of Large-Artery Vascular Imaging (e.g., B-mode and Doppler Ultrasonography, TCD, MRA, Angiography)?*

At times, especially during the acute ischemic period, brain tissue is ischemic but not irreversibly damaged. Reduced regional cerebral blood flow (rCBF) in the range of 10 to 20 ml per 100 gm/minute can lead to stunning, with a decrease in electrical activity and reduced cerebral metabolism, but increased extraction of oxygen. The stunned brain region has usually been called the "ischemic penumbra," which borrows a term from astronomy to indicate the state of almost shadow that is characteristic of a partial solar eclipse.[132] There are now available clinical and research techniques that can yield information about brain function, metabolism, and blood flow. In this section of the chapter, I first describe the tests available and then comment on their possible present and future utility.

Positron-Emission Tomography

Positron-emission tomography (PET scanning) is a functional imaging technique that makes it possible to measure in vivo chemical reactions in body organs. Only a small number of suitable positron-emitting radionuclides—oxygen-15 ($^{15}O_2$), carbon-11 (^{11}C), fluorine-18 (^{18}F), and nitrogen-13 (^{13}N)—are available that are integral to most organic biological compounds. These radionuclides have very short half-lives, and so a dedicated medical cyclotron is required on site for synthesis, thereby making the equipment and its maintenance quite expensive.

The appropriate positron-emitting radionuclides are synthesized by a cyclotron and are tagged to physiologically active compounds and given to the patient at acceptably low radiation doses. With time, 2D or 3D CT studies of the distribution of these radionuclides allow for images of cerebral physiology and metabolism during life. CBF has been studied,[133,134] using $^{13}NH_3$ and continuous inhalation[135] of $C^{15}O_2$, and oxygen metabolism rate (CMRO$_2$) has been studied,[135–137] using $^{15}O_2$. The oxygen extraction function (OEF) can be derived from the measurements of CBF and CMRO$_2$, and it gives useful information about the metabolism and avidity for oxygen in the local region studied.[135] Metabolic function can also be studied[138,139] by using a deoxyglucose compound labeled with ^{18}F.

In the normal situation, flow and metabolism are coupled; however, flow and metabolism are often different in the core of infarcts, as compared with the peripheral zone (penumbra). When oxygen metabolism is markedly depressed, either in association with low rCBF or out of proportion to rCBF, the likelihood of useful return of function in the tissue is small.[135] On the other hand, if oxygen metabolism is preserved and there is a relatively high OEF, then the outlook for recovery may be better. Baron has dubbed the situation of avidity of the local tissue for oxygen in the presence of poor perfusion the "misery perfusion" syndrome.[140] In chronic infarcts, CT regions of hypodensity and PET images of rCBF, CMRO$_2$, and cerebral metabolic rate for glucose (CMRgl) are essentially congruous, showing dead tissue with both little flow and little metabolism. During some phases of a stroke, rCBF may be increased relative to metabolism, a phenomenon that has been called "luxury perfusion."[141] Luxury perfusion is usually temporary and customarily occurs at one of two time periods: Initially, shortly after the stroke ictus, augmented flow seems to be due to failure of normal cerebrovascular autoregulation;[142] a second phase of luxury perfusion is seen 10 to 20 days after infarction and probably is due to capillary hyperplasia.[143–145] These findings have now made neurologists aware of the limitations of conclusions based on rCBF studies alone.

More sequential PET scanning studies during the early phases of stroke are needed in order to demonstrate the utility of these measurements in estimating prognosis and in guiding therapy. PET is best used in conjunction with morphological evidence from CT and MRI.[146] Figures 4.14 and 4.15 illustrate examples of the data generated from PET examinations.

Metabolic depression can also occur at sites distant from the zones of infarction. This finding has sometimes been called diaschisis and is commonest in

1. the thalamus ipsilateral to a cerebral infarct[147]
2. the cortex ipsilateral to a thalamic lesion[147]
3. the cerebral hemisphere contralateral to a supratentorial infarct of the opposite hemisphere[148]
4. the cerebellar hemisphere contralateral to a cerebral lesion[148,149]
5. the cerebellar hemisphere ipsilateral to a pontine infarct[150]

These distant effects provide insight into brain pathways and help guide physiological approaches to rehabilitation. They also help in understanding previously confusing rCBF results associated with xenon inhalation.

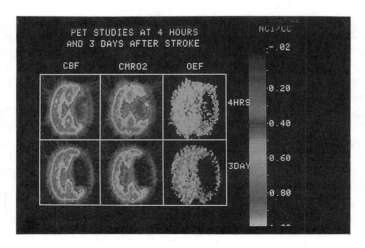

FIGURE 4.14 PET scans from a patient with an MCA-territory infarct (on right of scans); studies were taken at 4 hours (upper row) and at 3 days (bottom row). CBF = cerebral blood flow; $CMRO_2$ = cerebral metabolic rate for oxygen; OEF = oxygen extraction fraction. (Kindly supplied by Robert Ackerman, Massachusetts General Hospital.)

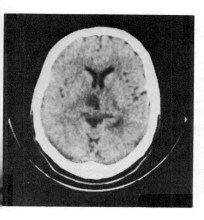
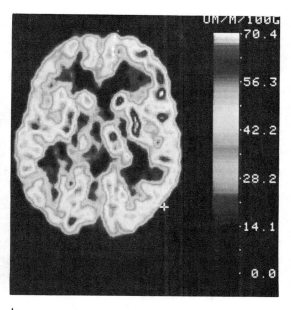

a   b

FIGURE 4.15   (a) CT scan of patient with small right thalamic infarct. (b) PET scan from same patient. Note diminished function in right thalamus and right frontal and parietal lobes. (Figure supplied by Michael Hennerici, Ruprecht-Karls Universitat Heidelberg, Mannheim, Germany.)

PET can also be used for studying changes in flow and metabolism after various types of stimulation.[145,151] Visual stimuli augment activity in the lateral geniculate body and striate regions,[152] while auditory stimuli activate the medial geniculate body and various temporal and parietal regions, depending on whether music, language, or other auditory stimuli are used and the content of the sound.[153] Speaking and right-limb movement activate parasylvian and frontal regions, predominantly in the left cerebral hemisphere. These studies give important insights into how the brain functions.[151] Also, in some circumstances, rCBF and metabolism might be adequate for baseline function but may fail to augment satisfactorily after stimulation. These functional studies also have the potential of telling how the damaged brain functions with sensory stimuli and how patterns of metabolism and flow change with recovery. Insight into reparative and adaptive mechanisms could ensue.

Without question, PET has opened up large vistas with potential insights into many brain functions and afflictions. Unfortunately, the expense of the equipment, the length of time required for testing, and the importance of ancillary physicists and chemists limit the applicability of the PET technique to large research centers funded for their studies. PET may become the "gold standard," such that if other less expensive, more readily available techniques become available, these techniques can be tested in large research centers in patients who receive concurrent PET scans. The results of the simpler technique then might be translated into comparable PET results.

Single Photon Emission Computed Tomography

One such newer technique is SPECT, which uses ordinary radionuclear camera equipment and does not require a cyclotron to generate the radionuclides. The equipment is thus less expensive than a CT or a PET scanner and will become more readily available in the future. The most commonly used radioisotopes are N-isopropyl-p-(I123) Iodoamphetamine (IMP)[154–156] and technetium-99M-labeled hexamethylpropylene amineoxime (HMPAO).[157,158] Regional radiotracer uptake can be imaged in three planes by the existing technology. The isotopes probably measure mostly rCBF rather than metabolic activity. SPECT is probably not as accurate or as definitive when compared to PET,[158] but practical considerations favor the use of SPECT. SPECT can be performed accurately and followed at intervals and is much less expensive to use. Like PET, it should be used in conjunction with standard neuroimaging (CT or MRI). The pattern of radiotracer uptake can suggest a stroke mechanism. Wedge-shaped regions of reduced uptake suggest embolism, while border-zone areas of decreased uptake suggest hemodynamically significant proximal arterial lesions.[159] Figures 4.16 and 4.17 show SPECT scans with different patterns of abnormal uptake. Interpretation of both PET and SPECT are greatly enhanced if the vascular lesion is defined.[160] To date, there are insufficient data about the utility of SPECT in the diagnosis and management of stroke patients, but the technique shows great promise when the proper questions are asked.[160,161]

Cerebral Blood Flow Measurements, Including
Xenon-Enhanced Computed Tomography

In 1944, Kety and Schmidt devised a technique based on the Fick principle that measured average blood flow to the brain.[162] After inhaling an inert gas—nitrous oxide—serial samples of arterial blood going to the brain and of jugular venous blood were analyzed for nitrous-oxide concentration. The integrated arteriovenous nitrous-oxide difference was calculated during 10 minutes of inhalation, and CBF was calculated. The normal average CBF was about 50 ml of blood per 100 gm of brain tissue.[162,163] This technique (or its modification by Scheinberg and Stead)[164] was used for many years, but it estimated only total or average blood flow and gave no regional information. In 1961, Lassen, Ingvar, and colleagues began to inject radioactive isotopes into the extracranial vessels at the time of angiography, and using local detectors, measured rCBF in humans.[165,166] Obrist and colleagues later introduced a method for measuring rCBF, using inhaled xenon-133 and extracranial recording devices[167,168] similar to those used by Lassen and

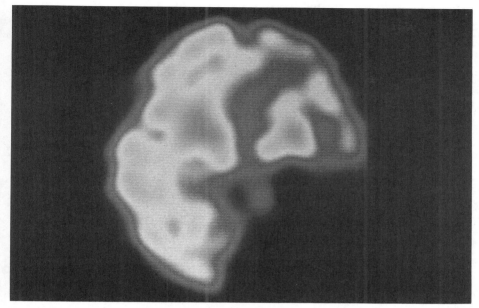

FIGURE 4.16 SPECT scan showing lack of isotope uptake in the left posterior part of the brain (on the lower right of the picture).

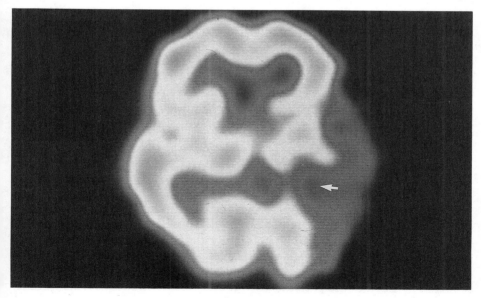

FIGURE 4.17 SPECT scan showing smaller areas of decreased isotope uptake in the left temporal-lobe region (white arrow).

colleagues in Denmark. The Obrist technique and its modifications[163,169] allow for a printout of quantitative rCBF under the probes. Both gray matter and white matter figures can be calculated.

The inhalation technique for rCBF was safe and could be performed on multiple occasions, thus allowing sequential determinations in individual patients. Technical problems limited the identification of some infarcts, and unfortunately, despite the fact that inhalation techniques had been in use for decades, few well-designed studies considered the utility of the technique in the diagnosis and management of individual stroke patients.

One of the major limitations of inhalation or injection rCBF techniques was the lack of anatomical definition. Because xenon is inert and is not metabolized by the brain, no metabolic data could be obtained. The development of XeCT has allowed the imaging of rCBF changes on sequential standard CT slices.[170-172] Xenon enhances or modifies the images, allowing visualization of relative rCBF in regions of interest. This technique facilitates comparison of infarction on CT with regions of reduced CBF. Of course, the technique, unlike PET, contains no metabolic information. In my opinion, XeCT and SPECT have replaced and superseded all of the prior CBF measurement techniques that used inhalation or injection of labeled gases.

Newer Magnetic-Resonance Techniques

A number of modern changes in MR capability have made it possible to begin to acquire functional information from MR. High-quality diagnostic images can be taken in 40 milliseconds ("ultrafast" imaging).[173,174] Ultrafast imaging after Gd-DTPA injection has been used to calculate regional cerebral blood volume and rCBF.[174] In experimental animals, other markers—such as intravascularly administered superparamagnetic iron oxides— have been used to study cerebral perfusion. Space- and time-specific resolution of images is likely to be better using MRI than is presently feasible using SPECT or XeCT. Undoubtedly, discovery and use of other paramagnetic agents and improvements in MR technology will allow MR to give clinicians new insights into functional changes in the brain in stroke patients.

Electrical Tests of Brain Function

The EEG is certainly the oldest available test of brain function and is clearly noninvasive. The test of time has revealed that the utility of EEG in stroke diagnosis and management is very limited. There are, however, occasional circumstances in which this test is quite helpful. In some patients with stroke or other CNS lesions, worsening of a neurological deficit is due to clinically inapparent or subtle seizure activity, which is usually dramatically captured by EEG. Some patients with recent-onset strokes, especially those due to subcortical ICHs or cerebral embolism, have seizures. In these patients, sequential EEGs can quantify seizure discharge and thereby guide anticonvulsant management. Because lacunar strokes are small and deep, they seldom influence the EEG, recorded primarily from superficial structures, whereas cortical lesions are usually more extensive and nearer the surface and so produce more effect on the EEG.[175] In patients with a clinical deficit due to ischemia and normal CT, the EEG may help the clinician decide whether the lesion is subcortical or cortical. A normal or symmetrical EEG suggests a deep subcortical locus, while an asymmetrical EEG, with the abnormality located on the side appropriate to the neurological symptoms and signs, suggests a cortical localization that has not produced enough irreversible damage to be visualized by CT. In patients with very severe vascular insults causing coma, the EEG can provide valuable data about the viability and residual electrical function of the brain.

Modern computer technology has more recently been used to create topographical maps of the distribution of scalp-recorded electrical activity. Frequency analysis and topographical EEG mapping is superior to standard EEG in localizing electrical abnormalities.[176,177] The color-coded maps are easier to read, and the results are more quantified and consistent.

EEGs can also be recorded during somatosensory, visual, and auditory stimuli and while the patient is performing various cognitive tasks. Computers then subtract the baseline electrical activity and generate a printout of that part of the electrical activity directly attributable to the stimulus or the task—the evoked potentials (EPs).[176,177] EPs can also be studied via topographic mapping techniques, to better localize the abnormalities. These techniques are particularly useful in unresponsive patients in whom it is impossible clinically to assess cognitive and sensory functions, and in patients under anesthesia. In patients with brainstem disease, both brainstem auditory evoked responses and quantified testing of the blink and masseter reflexes can help localize the functional abnormality to particular portions of the brainstem.[178]

These electrical tests are most helpful in answering the following questions: Is the patient having seizures? How much residual electrical activity is present in this comatose patient's cerebrum? Is this anesthetized patient now having cerebrovascular surgery suffering damage during the procedure? The clinical utility of topographic mapping and EP testing is still not clear and has not been well studied; that is, it is not known whether the tests give more information than a careful neurological examination.

In JH, I did not perform functional testing. His clinical deficit was severe, and morphological studies (CT) had shown a very extensive infarct. Moreover, his vascular lesion was not treatable.

References

1. Caplan LR. Computed tomography and stroke. In: McDowell F, Caplan L, eds. Cerebrovascular survey report for the National Institute of Neurological and

Communicative Disorders and Stroke (NINCDS), Washington, D.C. revised. 1985:61–74.

2. Norman D, Price D, Boyd D, et al. Quantitative aspects of computed tomography of the blood and cerebrospinal fluid. Radiology 1977;7:223–228.

3. Caplan LR, Flamm ES, Mohr JP, et al. Lumbar puncture and stroke: a statement for physicians by a committee of the Stroke Council of the American Heart Association. Stroke 1987;18:540–544A.

4. DeWitt LD, Buonanno FS, Kistler JP, et al. Nuclear magnetic resonance imaging in evaluation of clinical stroke syndromes. Ann Neurol 1984;16:535–545.

5. Kinkel P. Nuclear magnetic resonance imaging in clinical neurology. In: Baker AB, Joynt RJ, eds. Clinical neurology. vol. I. Philadelphia: Harper & Row, 1987:1–68.

6. Sipponen JT, Kaste M, Ketonin L, et al. Serial nuclear magnetic resonance (NMR) imaging in patients with cerebral infarction. J Comput Assist Tomogr 1983;7:585–589.

7. Kertesz A, Black SE, Nicholson L, et al. The sensitivity and specificity of MRI in acute stroke. Neurology 1987;37:1580–1585.

8. Walls S, Brant-Zawadzki M, Jeffrey R, et al. High frequency of CT findings within 24 hours after cerebral infarction. AJR 1982;38:307–311.

9. Salgado E, Weinstein M, Furlan A, et al. Proton magnetic resonance imaging in ischemic cerebral vascular disease. Ann Neurol 1986;20:502–507.

10. Becker H, Desch H, Hacker H, et al. CT fogging effect with ischemic cerebral infarcts. Neuroradiol 1978;18:185–192.

11. Skriver E, Olsen T. Contrast enhancement of cerebral infarcts: incidence and clinical value in different states of cerebral infarction. Neuroradiol 1982;23: 259–265.

12. Caplan LR. TIAs: we need to return to the question, "what is wrong with Mr. Jones?" Neurology 1988;38:791–793.

13. Nicolaides AN, Papadakis K, Grigg M, et al. Amaurosis fugax—data from CT scans. In: Bernstein E, ed. Amaurosis fugax. New York: Springer-Verlag, 1988:200–226.

14. Kelley R, Berger J, Scheinberg P, et al. Active bleeding in hypertensive intracerebral hemorrhage: computed tomography. Neurology 1982;32:852–856.

15. Chen ST, Chen SD, Hsy CY, et al. Progression of hypertensive intracerebral hemorrhage. Neurology 1989;39:1509–1514.

16. Adams HP Jr., Kassell NF, Turner JC, et al. CT and clinical correlations in recent aneurysmal subarachnoid hemorrhage: a preliminary report of the Cooperative Aneurysm Study. Neurology 1983;33:981–988.

17. Fishman RA. Cerebrospinal fluid in cerebrovascular disorders. In: Barnett JH, Mohr JP, Stein BM, Yatsu FJ, eds. Stroke: pathophysiology, diagnosis and management. New York: Churchill Livingstone, 1986:109–117.

18. Van der Meulen JP. Cerebrospinal fluid xanthrochromia: an objective index. Neurology 1966;16:170–178.

19. Soderstrom CE. Diagnostic significance of CSF spectrophotometry and computer tomography in cerebrovascular disease: a comparative study in 231 cases. Stroke 1977;8:606–612.

20. Lee MC, Heaney LM, Jacobson RL, et al. Cerebrospinal fluid in cerebral hemorrhage and infarction. Stroke 1975;6:638–641.

21. Chodosh EH, Foulkes MA, Kase CS, et al. Silent stroke in the NINCDS Stroke Data Bank. Neurology 1988;38:1674–1679.

22. Caplan LR. Reperfusion of ischemic brain: why and why not? In: Hacke W, delZoppo G, Hirschberg M, eds. Thrombolytic therapy in acute stroke. Berlin: Springer-Verlag, 1991:36–45.

23. Ropper AH. Lateral displacement of the brain and level of consciousness in patients with an acute hemispheral mass. N Engl J Med 1986;314:953–958.

24. Ropper AH. A preliminary MRI study of the geometry of brain displacement and level of consciousness with acute intracranial masses. Neurology 1989;39:622–627.

25. Weisberg LA, Stazio A, Shamsnia M, et al. Nontraumatic parenchymal brain hemorrhages. Medicine 1990;69:277–295.

26. Tyler K, Poletti C, Heros R. Cerebral amyloid angiopathy with multiple intracerebral hemorrhages. Neurology 1982;57:286–289.

27. Weisberg L. Multiple spontaneous intracerebral hematomas: clinical and computed tomographic correlation. Neurology 1981;31:897–900.

28. Kase C, Robinson R, Stein R, et al. Anticoagulant-related intracerebral hemorrhages. Neurology 1985;35:943–948.

29. Weisberg L. Computed tomography in aneurysmal subarachnoid hemorrhage. Neurology 1979;29:802–808.

30. Adams H, Kassell N, Torner J, et al. CT and clinical correlations in recent aneurysmal subarachnoid hemorrhage: a preliminary report of the cooperative aneurysm study. Neurology 1983;33:981–988.

31. van Gijn J, van Dongen K. Computerized tomography in subarachnoid hemorrhage: difference between patients with and without an aneurysm on angiography. Neurology 1980;30:538–539.

32. van Gijn J, van Dongen KJ, Vermeulen M, et al. Perimesencephalic hemorrhage: a non-aneurysmal and benign form of subarachnoid hemorrhage. Neurology 1985;35:493–497.

33. Rinkel GJ, Wijdicks EF, Vermeulen M, et al. Outcome in perimesencephalic (non-aneurysmal) subarachnoid hemorrhage: a follow-up study in 37 patients. Neurology 1990;40:1130–1132.

34. Kistler JP, Crowell R, Davis K, et al. The relation of cerebral vasospasm to the extent and location of subarachnoid blood visualized by CT scan: a prospective study. Neurology 1983;33:424–437.

35. Mohsen F, Pominis S, Illingworth R. Prediction of delayed cerebral ischemia after subarachnoid hemorrhage by computed tomography. J Neurol Neurosurg Psychiatry 1984;47:1197–1202.

36. O'Donnell TF, Erdoes L, Mackey W, et al. Correlation of B-mode ultrasound imaging and arteriography with pathologic findings at carotid endarterectomy. Arch Surg 1985;120:443–449.

37. Schenk EA, Bond G, Aretz T, et al. Multicenter validation study of real-time ultrasonography, arteriography and pathology: pathologic evaluation of carotid endarterectomy specimens. Stroke 1988;19:289–296.

38. Hennerici M, Freund H-J. Efficacy of CW-Doppler and duplex system examinations for the evaluation of extracranial carotid disease. J Clin Ultrasound 1984;12:155–161.

39. von Reutern GM, Budingen HJ. Ultraschalldiagnostik der hirnversorgenden arterien. Stuttgart: Georg Thieme Verlag, 1989.

40. Toole JF. Cerebrovascular disorders. 4th ed. New York: Raven Press, 1990: 174–211.

41. Steinke W, Kloetzsch C, Hennerici M. Carotid artery disease assessed by color

Doppler flow imaging: correlation with standard Doppler sonography and angiography. AJNR 1990;11:259–266.

42. Tegeler CH, Kremkau FW, Hitchings LP. Color velocity imaging: introduction to a new ultrasound technology. J Neuroimag 1991;1:85–90.

43. Hennerici M. New technical and clinical aspects for cerebrovascular applications of ultrasound methods. J Neurosci Methods 1990;34:169–177.

44. DeWitt LD, Weschler LR. Transcranial Doppler. Current Concepts of Cerebrovascular Disease (Stroke) 1987;22:31–36.

45. Caplan LR, Brass LM, DeWitt LD, et al. Transcranial Doppler ultrasound: present status. Neurology 1990;40:696–700.

46. Tettenborn B, Estol C, DeWitt LD, et al. Accuracy of transcranial Doppler in the vertebrobasilar circulation. J Neurol 1990;37:159.

47. Hennerici M, Rautenberg W, Sitzer G, et al. Transcranial Doppler ultrasound for the assessment of intracranial arterial flow velocity: I. examination of technique and normal values. Surg Neurol 1987;27:439–448.

48. Hennerici M, Rautenberg W, Schwartz A. Transcranial Doppler ultrasound for the assessment of intracranial arterial flow velocity: II. evaluation of intracranial arterial disease. Surg Neurol 1987;27:523–532.

49. Piepgras A, Schmiedek P, Leinsinger G, et al. A simple test to assess cerebrovascular reserve capacity using transcranial Doppler sonography and acetazolamide. Stroke 1990;21:1306–1311.

50. Teague SM, Sharma MK. Detection of paradoxical cerebral echo contrast embolization by transcranial Doppler ultrasound. Stroke 1991;22:740–745.

51. Masaryk TJ, Modic MT, Ross JS, et al. Intracranial circulation: preliminary clinical results with three-dimensional magnetic resonance angiography. Radiology 1989;171:793–799.

52. Ross JS, Masaryk TJ, Modic MT. Magnetic resonance angiography of the extracranial carotid arteries and intracranial vessels: a review. Neurology 1989;39:1369–1376.

53. Edelman RR, Mattle HP, Atkinson DJ, et al. MR angiography. AJR 1990;154:937–946.

54. Edelman RR, Mattle HP, O'Reilly GV, et al. Magnetic resonance imaging of flow dynamics in the circle of Willis. Stroke 1990;21:56–65.

55. Caplan LR, Wolpert SM. Angiography in patients with occlusive cerebrovascular disease: a stroke neurologist and neuroradiologist's views. AJNR 1991;12:593–601.

56. Caplan LR, Wolpert SM. Conventional cerebral angiography in occlusive cerebrovascular disease. In: Wood JH, ed. Cerebral blood flow: physiological and clinical aspects. New York: McGraw-Hill, 1987:356–384.

57. Akers DL, Markowitz IA, Kerstein MD. The value of aortic arch study in the evaluation of cerebrovascular insufficiency. Am J Surg 1987;154:230–232.

58. Martin-Paredero VM, Dixon SM, Baker JD, et al. Risk of renal failure after major angiography. Arch Surg 1983;118:1417–1420.

59. Little J, Furlan A, Modic M, et al. Digital subtraction angiography in cerebrovascular disease. Stroke 1982;13:559–566.

60. Celesia G, Strother C, Turski P, et al. Digital subtraction arteriography: a new method for evaluation of extracranial occlusive disease. Arch Neurol 1983;40:70–74.

61. Meaney T, Weinstein H, Buonocore E, et al. Digital subtraction angiography of the human cardiovascular system. AJR 1980;135:1153–1160.
62. Larson E, Stratton J, Pearlman A. Selective use of two-dimensional echocardiography in stroke syndromes. Ann Intern Med 1981;95:112–114.
63. Bergeron G, Shah P. Echocardiography unwarranted in patients with cerebral ischemic events. N Engl J Med 1981;304:489.
64. Greenland P, Knopman D, Mikell F, et al. Echocardiography in diagnostic assessment of stroke. Ann Intern Med 1981;95:51–54.
65. Robbins J, Sagar K, French M, et al. Influence of echocardiography on management of patients with systemic emboli. Stroke 1983;14:546–551.
66. Caplan LR. Of birds and nests and cerebral emboli. Rev Neurol 1991;147:265–273.
67. Jones HR, Caplan LR, Cone P, et al. Cerebral emboli of paradoxical origin. Ann Neurol 1983;13:314–319.
68. Lee R, Bartzokis T, Yeoh T-K, et al. Enhanced detection of intracardiac sources of cerebral emboli by transesophageal echocardiography. Stroke 1991;22:734–739.
69. Cujec B, Bolasek P, Voli C, et al. Transesophageal echocardiography in the detection of potential cardiac source of embolism in stroke patients. Stroke 1991;22:727–733.
70. Lockwood K, Sherman D, Gerza C, et al. Detection of left atrial thrombi by cardiac CT. Neurology 1984;34(1):205.
71. Helgason C, Chomka E, Louie E, et al. The potential role for ultrafast cardiac computed tomography in patients with stroke. Stroke 1989;20:465–472.
72. Ezekowitz M, Wilson D, Smith E, et al. Comparison of indium 111 platelet scintigraphy and two-dimensional echocardiography in the diagnosis of left ventricular thrombi. N Engl J Med 1982;306:1509–1513.
73. Adams HP, Kassel NF, Mazuz H. The patient with transient ischemic attacks: is this the time for a new therapeutic approach? Stroke 1984;15:371–375.
74. Rokey R, Rolak LA, Harati Y, et al. Coronary artery disease in patients with cerebrovascular disease: a prospective study. Ann Neurol 1985;16:50–53.
75. Gibbons RJ, Zinsmeister AR, Miller TD. Supine exercise electrocardiography compared with exercise radionuclide angiography in non-invasive identification of severe coronary artery diseases. Ann Int Med 1990;112:743–749.
76. Sirna S, Biller J, Skorton DJ, et al. Cardiac evaluation of the patient with stroke. Stroke 1990;21:14–23.
77. Verani M, Rokey R. Coronary artery disease: diagnosis and clinical features. In: Rolak L, Rokey R, eds. Coronary and cerebral vascular disease: a practical guide. Mt. Kisco, NY: Futura, 1990:19–49.
78. DiPasquale G, Andreoli A, Carini G, et al. Non-invasive screening for silent ischemic heart disease in patients with cerebral ischemia: use of dipyridamole-thallium myocardial imaging. Cerebrovasc Dis 1991;1:31–37.
79. G'Acs G, Fox A, Barnett H, et al. CT visualization of intracranial arterial thromboembolism. Stroke 1983;14:756–762.
80. Yock D. CT appearance of cerebral emboli. J Comput Assist Tomogr 1981;5:190–196.
81. Harbaugh R, Schusselberg DS, Cromwell LD, et al. Three dimensional computed tomographic angiography (3D-CTA) in the diagnosis of cerebrovascular disease. Stroke 1991;22:137.

82. Ford K, Sarwar M. Computed tomography of dural sinus thrombosis. AJNR 1981;2:539–543.
83. Brant-Sawadzki M, Chang G, McCarty G. Computed tomography in dural sinus thrombosis. Arch Neurol 1982;39:446–447.
84. Kingsley P, Kendall B, Moseley I. Superior sagittal sinus thrombosis, an evaluation of the changes demonstrated by computed tomography. J Neurol Neurosurg Psychiatry 1978;41:1065–1068.
85. Bousser M, Chiras J, Borris J, et al. Cerebral venous thrombosis, a review of 38 cases. Stroke 1985;16:199–213.
86. Culebras A, Leeson M, Cacayorin E, et al. Computed tomographic evaluation of cervical carotid plaque complications. Stroke 1985;16:425–431.
87. Biller J, Yuh WTC, Mitchell GW, et al. Early diagnosis of basilar artery occlusion using magnetic resonance imaging. Stroke 1988;19:297–306.
88. Gee W, Oiler D, Wylie E. Noninvasive diagnosis of carotid occlusion by ocular plethysmography. Stroke 1976;7:18–21.
89. Kartchner M, McRae L. Noninvasive evaluation and management of the asymptomatic carotid bruit. Surgery 1977;82:840–847.
90. Ackerman R. A perspective on noninvasive diagnosis of carotid disease. Neurology 1979;29:615–622.
91. Toole J. Ophthalmodynamometry. Arch Intern Med 1963;112:219–220.
92. Toole J, Janeway R. Diagnostic tests in cerebrovascular disorders. In: Vinken P, Bruyn G, eds. Handbook of clinical neurology: vol II, pt I. vascular diseases of the nervous system. Amsterdam: North Holland, 1972:208–266.
93. Levine SR, Brust JCM, Futrell N, et al. A comparative study of the cerebrovascular complications of cocaine—alkaloidal versus hydrochloride—a review. Neurology 1991;41:1173–1177.
94. Weisberg L. Direct visualization of intracranial aneurysm by computed tomography. Comput Tomogr 1981;5:191–199.
95. Sekhar L, Wechsler L, Yonas H, et al. Value of transcranial Doppler examination in the diagnosis of cerebral vasospasm after subarachnoid hemorrhage. Neurosurg 1988;22:813–821.
96. Sloan MA, Haley EC, Kassell NF, et al. Sensitivity and specificity of transcranial Doppler ultrasonography in the diagnosis of vasospasm following subarachnoid hemorrhage. Neurology 1989;39:1514–1518.
97. Pollock S, Tsitsopoulas P, Harrison M. The effect of hematocrit on cerebral perfusion and clinical status following occlusion in the gerbil. Stroke 1982;13:167–170.
98. Harrison M, Pollock S, Kindoll B, et al. Effect of hematocrit on carotid stenosis and cerebral infarction. Lancet 1981;2:114–115.
99. Thomas D, duBoulay G, Marshall J, et al. Effect of hematocrit on cerebral blood flow in man. Lancet 1977;2:941–943.
100. Tohgi H, Yamanouchi H, Murakami M, et al. Importance of the hematocrit as a risk factor in cerebral infarction. Stroke 1978;9:369–374.
101. Grotta J, Ackerman R, Correia J, et al. Whole-blood viscosity parameters and cerebral blood flow. Stroke 1982;13:296–298.
102. Thomas D. Whole blood viscosity and cerebral blood flow. Stroke 1982;13:285–287.
103. Kee DB Jr, Wood JH. Influence of blood rheology on cerebral circulation. In: Wood JH, ed. Cerebral blood flow: physiological and clinical aspects. New York: McGraw-Hill, 1987:173–185.

104. Brass LM, Prohovnik I, Pavlakis SG, et al. Middle cerebral artery blood velocity and cerebral blood flow in sickle cell disease. Stroke 1991;22:27–30.
105. Mercuri M, Bond MG, Evans G, et al. Leukocyte count and carotid atherosclerosis. Stroke 1991;22:134.
106. Wu K. Platelet hyperaggregability and thrombosis in patients with thrombocythemia. Ann Intern Med 1978;88:7–11.
107. Coull BM, Goodnight SH. Antiphospholipid antibodies, prethrombotic states, and stroke. Stroke 1990;21:1370–1374.
108. Bailey DP, Coull BM, Goodnight SH. Neurological disease associated with antiphospholipid antibodies. Ann Neurol 1989;25:221–227.
109. Levine SR, Welch KMA. The spectrum of neurologic disease associated with antiphospholipid antibodies: lupus anticoagulants, and anticardiolipin antibodies. Arch Neurol 1987;44:876–883.
110. Atkinson JLD, Sundt TM, Kazmier FJ, et al. Heparin-induced thrombocytopenia and thrombosis in ischemic stroke. Mayo Clin Proc 1988;63:353–361.
111. Uchyama S, Takeuchi M, Osawa M, et al. Platelet function tests in thrombotic cerebrovascular disorders. Stroke 1983;14:511–517.
112. Ludlam CA. Evidence for the platelet specificity of beta-thromboglobulin and studies on its plasma concentration in healthy individuals. Br J Haematol 1979;41:271–278.
113. Fisher M, Francis R. Altered coagulation in cerebral ischemia: platelet, thrombin, and plasmin activity. Arch Neurol 1990;47:1075–1079.
114. Landi G, D'Angelo A, Boccardi E, et al. Hypercoagulability in acute stroke: prognostic significance. Neurology 1987;37:1667–1671.
115. Kannel WB, Wolf PA, Castelli WP, et al. Fibrinogen and risk of cardiovascular disease. JAMA 1987;258:1183–1186.
116. Coull BM, Beamer NB, deGarmo PL, et al. Chronic blood hyperviscosity in subjects with acute stroke, transient ischemic attack, and risk factors for stroke. Stroke 1991;22:162–168.
117. Hossman V, Heiss WD, Berwermeyer H, et al. Controlled trial of ancrod in ischemic stroke. Arch Neurol 1983;40:803–808.
118. Radack K, Deck C, Huster G. Dietary supplementation with low-dose fish oils lowers fibrinogen levels: a randomized double-blind controlled study. Ann Int Med 1989;111:757–758.
119. Kosik KS, Furie B. Thrombotic stroke associated with elevated plasma Factor VIII. Arch Neurol 1980;8:435–437.
120. Estol C, Pessin MS, DeWitt LD, et al. Stroke and increased Factor VIII activity. Neurology 1989;39(1):225.
121. Feinberg WM, Bruck DC, Ring ME, et al. Hemostatic markers in acute stroke. Stroke 1989;20:592–597.
122. Levine SR, Welch KMA. The spectrum of neurologic disease associated with antiphospholipid antibodies, lupus anticoagulant, and anticardiolipin antibodies. Arch Neurol 1987;44:876–883.
123. Askerson RA. A "primary" antiphospholipid syndrome? J Rheumatology 1988;15:1742–1746.
124. DeWitt LD, Caplan LR. Antiphospholipid antibodies and stroke. AJNR 1991;12:454–456.
125. Myers R, Yamaguchi S. Nervous system effects of cardiac arrest in monkeys. Arch Neurol 1977;34:65–74.

148   *General Principles*

126. Pulsinelli W, Waldman S, Rawlinson D, et al. Hyperglycemia converts ischemic neuronal damage into brain infarction. Neurology 1982;32:1239–1246.
127. Plum F. What causes infarction in ischemic brain? Neurology 1983;33:222–233.
128. Pulsinelli W, Levy D, Sigsbel B, et al. Increased damage after ischemic stroke in patients with hyperglycemia with or without established diabetes mellitus. Am J Med 1983;74:540–544.
129. Walker G, Williamson P, Ravich R, et al. Hypercalcemia associated with cerebral vasospasm causing infarction. J Neurol Neurosurg Psychiatry 1980;43:464–467.
130. Gorelick PB, Caplan LR. Calcium, hypercalcemia, and stroke. Current Concepts of Cerebrovascular Disease (Stroke) 1985;20:13–17.
131. Yarnell P, Caplan LR. Basilar artery narrowing and hyperparathyroidism: illustrative case. Stroke 1986;17:1022–1024.
132. Lassen NA. Pathophysiology of brain ischemia as it relates to the therapy of acute ischemic stroke. Clin Neuropharm 1990;13(3):51–58.
133. Phelps M, Mazziotta J, Huang S. Study of cerebral function with positron computed tomography. J Cereb Blood Flow Metab 1982;2:113–162.
134. Kuhl D, Phelps M, Kowell A, et al. Effects of stroke on local cerebral metabolism and perfusion: mapping by emission computed tomography of ^{18}FDG and $^{13}NH_3$. Ann Neurol 1980;8:47–60.
135. Ackerman R, Correia J, Alpert N, et al. Positron imaging in ischemic stroke disease using compounds labeled with oxygen[15]. Arch Neurol 1981;38:537–543.
136. Baron JC, Sternling M, Tanaka T, et al. Quantitative measurement of CBF, oxygen extraction fraction (OEF), and $CMRO_2$ with the ^{15}O continuous inhalation technique and positron emission tomography (PET): experimental evidence and normal values in man. J Cereb Blood Flow Metab 1981;1(Suppl 1)55–56.
137. Frackowiak R, Lenzi G, Jones T, et al. Quantitative measurement of regional cerebral blood flow and oxygen metabolism in man using $^{15}oxygen$ and positron emission tomography: therapy, procedure, and normal values. J Comput Assist Tomography 1980;4:722–736.
138. Phelps M, Huang S, Hoffman E, et al. Tomographic measurement of local cerebral glucose metabolic rate in humans with F-18 2 fluoro deoxy D-glucose: validation of method. Ann Neurol 1979;6:371–388.
139. Reivich M, Kuhl D, Wolf A. The ^{18}F fluorodeoxyglucose method for the measurement of local cerebral glucose utilization in man. Circ Res 1979;44:127–137.
140. Baron JC, Bousser M, Rey A, et al. Reversal of focal misery-perfusion syndrome by extra-intracranial arterial bypass in hemodynamic cerebral ischemia. Stroke 1981;12:454–459.
141. Lassen N. The luxury perfusion syndrome and its possible relation to acute metabolic acidosis localized within the lesion. Lancet 1966;2:1113–1115.
142. Ackerman R. Positron imaging in stroke disease. In: Moosy J, Reinmuth O, eds. Cerebral vascular disease. 12th ed. New York: Raven Press, 1981:67–72.
143. Ackerman R, Alpert N, Correia J, et al. Correlations of positron emission scans with PET scans and clinical course. Acta Neurol Scand 1979;60(72):230–231.

144. Ackerman R, Alpert N, Correia J, et al. Importance of monitoring metabolic function in assessing the severity of a stroke insult (CBF: an epiphenomenon). J Cereb Blood Flow Metab 1981;1(Suppl 1):502–503.

145. Phelps M, Schelbert H, Mazziotta J. Positron computed tomography for studies of myocardial and cerebral function. Ann Intern Med 1983;98:339–359.

146. Heiss W-D, Herholz K, Bocher-Schwarz HG, et al. PET, CT and MR imaging in cerebrovascular disease. J Comput Assist Tomogr 1986;10:903–911.

147. Kuhl D, Phelps M, Kowell A, et al. Effects of stroke on local cerebral metabolism and perfusion: mapping by emission computed tomography of ^{18}FDG and ^{13}NH$_{13}$. Ann Neurol 1980;8:47–60.

148. Powers WJ. Cerebral hemodynamics in ischemic cerebrovascular disease. Ann Neurol 1991;29:231–240.

149. Martin W, Raichle M. Cerebellar blood flow and metabolism in cerebral hemisphere infarction. Ann Neurol 1983;14:168–176.

150. Bowler JV, Wade JP. Ipsilateral cerebellar diaschisis following pontine infarction. Cerebrovasc Dis 1991;1:58–60.

151. Powers WJ, Raichle ME. Positron emission tomography and its application to the study of cerebrovascular disease in man. Stroke 1985;16:361–376.

152. Phelps M, Kuhl D, Mazziotta J. Metabolic mapping of the brain's response to visual stimulation: studies in humans. Science 1981;211:1445–1448.

153. Mazziotta J, Phelps M, Carson R, et al. Tomographic mapping of human cerebral metabolism: auditory stimulation. Neurology 1982;82:921–937.

154. Holman BG, Hill TC, Lee RG, et al. Brain imaging with radiolabelled amines. In: Freeman LM, Weissman HS, eds. Nuclear medicine annual, 1983. New York: Raven Press, 1983:131–165.

155. Hill TC, Magistretti PL, Holman BL, et al. Assessment of regional cerebral blood flow (rCBF) in stroke using SPECT and N-isopropyl-(I 123)-P-iodoamphetamine (IMP). Stroke 1984;15:40–45.

156. Bushnell DL, Gupta S, Micoch AG, et al. Prediction of language and neurologic recovery after cerebral infarction with SPECT imaging using N-isopropyl-P (I123) iodoamphetamine. Arch Neurol 1989;46:665–669.

157. Giubilei F, Lenzi GL, DiPiero V, et al. Predictive value of brain perfusion single-photon emission computed tomography in acute ischemic stroke. Stroke 1990;21:895–900.

158. Heiss WD, Hirholz K, Podreka I, et al. Comparison of [^{99M}TC] HMPAO with [^{18}F] fluoromethane PET in cerebrovascular disease. J Cereb Blood Flow Metab 1990;10:687–697.

159. Pacia SV, Bose A, Fayad P, et al. Single-photon emission computed tomography in distal field hypoperfusion. J Neuroimag 1991;1:31–33.

160. Caplan LR. Question-driven technology assessment: SPECT as an example. Neurology 1991;41:187–191.

161. Fayad P, Brass LM. Single photon emission computed tomography in cerebrovascular disease. Stroke 1991;22:950–954.

162. Kety S, Schmidt C. The nitrous oxide method for the quantitative determination of cerebral blood flow in man: theory, procedure, and normal values. J Clin Invest 1948;27:476–483.

163. Lassen N, Ingvar D, Skinhoj E. Brain function and blood flow. Sci Amer 1978;239:62–71.

164. Scheinberg P, Stead E. The cerebral blood flow in male subjects as measured

by the nitrous oxide technique: normal values for blood flow, glucose utilization, and peripheral resistance. J Clin Invest 1949;28:1163–1171.

165. Ingvar D, Lassen N. Quantitative determination of regional cerebral blood flow in man. Lancet 1961;2:806.

166. Lassen N. Regional cerebral blood flow in man determined by krypton. Neurology 1963;13:719–727.

167. Obrist W, Thompson H Jr, King H, et al. Determination of regional cerebral blood flow by inhalation of ^{133}xenon. Circ Res 1967;20:124–135.

168. Obrist W, Thompson H Jr, Wang H, et al. Regional cerebral blood flow estimated by ^{133}xenon inhalation. Stroke 1975;6:245–250.

169. Meyer J, Ishihara N, Deshmukh V, et al. Improved method for noninvasive measurement of regional cerebral blood flow by ^{133}xenon inhalation. Stroke 1978;9:195–205.

170. Gur D, Wolfson S, Yonas H, et al. Progress in cerebrovascular disease: local cerebral blood flow by xenon-enhanced CT. Stroke 1982;13:752–758.

171. Segawa H, Wakai S, Tamura A, et al. Computed tomographic measurement of local cerebral blood flow by xenon enhancement. Stroke 1983;14:356–362.

172. Yonas H, Wolfson SK, Gur D, et al. Clinical experience with the use of xenon-enhanced CT blood flow mapping in cerebral vascular disease. Stroke 1984;15:443–450.

173. Belliveau JW, Rosen BR, Kantor HL, et al. Functional cerebral imaging by susceptibility-contrast NMR. Magn Reson Med 1990;14:538–546.

174. Belliveau JW, Cohen MS, Weisskoff R, et al. Functional studies of the human brain using high-speed magnetic resonance imaging. J Neuroimag 1991; 1:36–41.

175. Caplan LR, Young R. EEG findings in certain lacunar syndromes. Neurology 1972;22:403.

176. Nuwer MR, Jordan SE, Ahn SS. Evaluation of stroke using EEG frequency analysis and topographic mapping. Neurology 37:1153–1159.

177. Duffy FH. Clinical value of topographic mapping and quantified neurophysiology. Arch Neurol 1989;46:1133–1134.

178. Tettenborn B, Caplan LR, Krämer G, Hopf H. Electrophysiology in posterior circulation disease. In: Berguer R, Caplan LR, eds. Vertebrobasilar arterial disease. St. Louis: Quality Medical Publishing, 1991:124–129.

CHAPTER 5

Treatment

This chapter introduces the general principles that underlie treatment, outlining the various types of therapy available, the determinants or factors influencing treatment, and the diverse therapeutic strategies. More-specific treatments for patients with individual vascular pathologies and mechanisms—for example, stenosis of the ICA with TIAs, or lacunar infarction and progressing hemiparesis—are considered in the chapters in Part II of the book, which deal with these specific conditions.

Past Failure to Generate Useful Therapeutic Data

Few, if any, therapies have been scientifically proven effective in particular stroke subtypes. However, lack of certainty should not become an excuse for therapeutic nihilism but rather should promote caution. As in other illnesses, physicians should select the best available treatment based on their own past experience and on the published and shared advice and experiences of others. Stroke therapeutics have lagged far behind advances in knowledge of the basic pathology, pathophysiology, and diagnosis of stroke syndromes. Fortunately, solid therapeutic information is beginning to emerge from randomized trials of various medical and surgical therapeutic strategies. In my opinion, three major problems historically have limited the ability to provide clear answers to therapeutic dilemmas. Like the anxious patient on the psychiatrist's couch, we may have to purge ourselves however painfully of these past errors if we are to get on with studying and disseminating effective stroke treatment. The war against stroke has been held back because of (1) bad strategy, (2) insufficient ammunition and soldiers, and (3) a militia with inadequate interest and training.

Bad Strategy

Treatments have traditionally been evaluated in *large groups of patients* who were lumped together according to the *tempo of the stroke* and the *presence or extent of brain damage.* These groups include TIAs, partial stroke, reversible ischemic neurological deficit (RIND), stroke in progress, and completed stroke.[1]

While these designations were perhaps of some use in the past, there is no rational reason to continue to rely heavily on them now. After all, these terms concern only two factors: the time-sequenced course of the neurological symptoms at that particular moment and the present clinically detected degree of damage. The transient nature of a TIA may be the result of (1) relief of ischemia before significant neuronal damage, (2) small size of infarction, or (3) rapid compensation of function by other neuronal regions. In many patients with clinical TIAs and normal neurological examinations, CT and MRI show infarcts compatible with the clinical symptoms.[2] The classification of patients may change; today's stroke is yesterday's TIA. Accurate classification using this terminology relies on the ability to infallibly predict the future. In fact, the individual groups TIA, RIND, and completed stroke all share a high, relatively comparable risk of future stroke.[1-5] In other branches of medicine, physicians do not treat time courses. What would a nephrologist say when asked about treatment for transient or partial nephritis? He or she would probably ask, nephritis due to what? Physicians should *not treat time courses;* we should *treat patients with particular pathological and pathophysiological problems.* None of the time courses is specific for any single pathology or pathophysiology. In fact, most vascular pathologies and stroke mechanisms have the potential of producing most of the time-course designations mentioned. Stenosis of the ICA, the vasculopathy underlying lacunar infarction, and cardiogenic cerebral embolism can all cause TIAs, RIND, and progressing and completed strokes.

Investigators have not only designated groups in an irrational manner but also naively sought single remedies or cures for these groups. Even individual stroke-mechanism groups such as thrombosis and embolism are heterogeneous designations that join together fruits as divergent as grapes, watermelons, grapefruits, and mangoes. Would it make sense that divergent causes would respond the same way to a single treatment? If TIAs have many underlying causes, is it likely for one treatment to be effective for all or most underlying conditions? Despite the improbability of success, researchers have continued to seek a panacea that will prove effective for all ischemic strokes. Vasodilators, aspirin, endarterectomy, and warfarin are some of the hopes for omnipotence. Most such remedies have been hypothesized and then enthusiastically endorsed before the inevitable disenchantment.

Of course, physicians must consider how badly off the patient is: There is no profit in watering dead grass! The severity of the deficit is, however, not the only consideration. Grass that is now brown could turn green with proper nurturing. Clearly, in the future, physicians need studies of groups of patients with similar pathologies and stroke pathogenesis—for example, studies of patients with severe ICA stenosis with various degrees of brain damage.[2,6] This volume does not offer discussion of treatment of TIAs, strokes in progress, or completed strokes. Clinicians should be discouraged from using these designations to plan diagnosis or treatment. Instead, the book is organized by anatomy, pathology, and pathophysiology—the cornerstones of medicine. Clinicians must return to these foundations to successfully manage patients with cerebrovascular disease.

Inadequate Army and Equipment

Interest in stroke has lagged far behind other areas, such as heart disease and cancer. Despite the fact that stroke is the third leading cause of death in the United States, and an even more important cause of disability, it has been understudied, and its research and treatment have been underfunded. Until recently, there has been no diagnostic equipment capable of reliably separating stroke patients into meaningful etiological subgroups. That circumstance has now changed, as even a quick glance at Chapter 4, on laboratory diagnosis, will indicate. Testing equipment needs wider dissemination and perhaps concentration in regional centers specially interested in stroke and well stocked with trained personnel and the latest technology. Neurology has been an understaffed specialty, but that too is dramatically changing.[7]

Insufficient Interest and Training

An important problem is that nonstroke specialists frequently lack interest in stroke patients. "A stroke is a stroke" is an all-too-prevalent feeling. Having brilliantly concluded that a stroke has occurred, many physicians will attach a pseudoscientific set of meaningless initials, such as CVA (cerebrovascular accident), to the patient and rest on their laurels, not searching further along the diagnostic tree or suggesting anything but caregiver treatment. No wonder stroke treatment has been in such a bad fix! Practitioners must be encouraged to recognize that there are different stroke mechanisms and pathophysiologies, that diagnosis of these subtypes can be made without sophisticated knowledge of neuroanatomy, and that logical therapeutic strategies exist. Moreover, there are centers and clinicians interested and able to help the nonspecialists with stroke diagnosis and management. The brain is the most important organ in the body. The brain controls intelligence, behavior, personality, and character—those traits that make us human. It is the Rolls Royce organ. Brain illness, especially stroke, deserves the very best care and skills the medical system can offer.

Factors Influencing Treatment

Enough has been said about what has gone wrong in the past. I now turn to a discussion of what is known of treatment and some potentially useful strategies. First of all, what factors should the clinician consider when planning treatment of the individual stroke patient?

Socioeconomic and Psychological Factors

Some patients and their families will not and cannot pursue some treatments. A previously unreliable and noncompliant person cannot be depended on to take anticoagulants. Some patients do not have the economic resources that might allow particular therapies, and in other cases, a lack of caring family members or friends limits subsequent follow-up and treatment. One person might be disabled by fear of impending disability when informed of the presence of carotid artery disease and a threat of stroke, while another individual with a similar condition will weigh the alternatives more dispassionately.

Other Medical Conditions

Preexistent or coexistent illness may also limit or affect treatment. Physicians tend to be more conservative in suggesting surgery for stroke patients who have severe heart disease or advanced cancer. Particular concomitant conditions contraindicate some treatments. An active peptic ulcer or severe arterial hypertension make anticoagulation unwise. Other conditions, such as severe heart or lung disease, increase the risks of anesthesia and surgery. The patient's premorbid function and intellect are also critical. A hopelessly demented nursing-home resident with a new stroke should be treated humanely, but certainly not aggressively. An older widow, depressed and lonely for many years after the passing of her husband and friends, would be managed differently from a happy and pleasant but slightly demented grandmother who draws joy from her family and surroundings. Age is never an absolute contraindication to stroke therapy. Elderly patients tolerate medical and surgical treatments less well than younger patients, but they also rebound less well from strokes. They should be handled cautiously, but the same diagnostic and therapeutic strategies that apply to younger individuals should be considered for geriatric patients.

Nature of the Stroke

Nature of the arterial lesion

The pathology of ICA occlusion is different from severe ICA stenosis or carotid plaque without stenosis. These lesions differ greatly from lipohyalinosis of penetrating vessels caused by hypertension. The *nature, location,* and *severity* of the vascular lesions are the key factors in selecting possible therapeutic strategies.

The blood that courses through the vessels

Does the patient have a high Hct or platelet count? What is the blood viscosity? Are the platelets activated or sticky? Is there a bleeding diathesis? Abnormalities of blood constituents and coagulation functions might suggest some therapeutic strategies and might contraindicate other treatments.

Mechanisms and pathophysiology of the stroke

Was the ischemia due to local vascular thrombosis, embolism, or circulatory failure? For example, in the patient with ICA stenosis, was the cerebral ischemia caused by low flow or by embolism?

Extent and reversibility of the brain lesions

If the entire MCA territory is destroyed, there would be little point in increasing flow in the MCA because only dead brain would be irrigated. Reperfusion might even be harmful.[8,9] If, however, the MCA-territory ischemia is reversible and the neurons are stunned and dysfunctional but not knocked out completely, the argument for augmenting MCA flow would be greater. Functional tests discussed in Chapter 4 are now available that can help determine the potential reversibility of the ischemia. Also, even if the entire MCA territory is irreversibly damaged due to cardiac-origin embolism, the remainder of the brain would still be at risk for further damage—a factor that should be considered in planning treatment.

The size of the lesion, the degree of neurological deficit, and the length of time since the last worsening have traditionally been used to decide whether a stroke is completed.[1] The term *completed stroke* is variously defined and applied, and it should be discarded. Short of an infallible crystal ball or direct guidance from a deity, doctors cannot predict the future. The fact that a patient is stable today does not tell whether he or she will worsen tomorrow. Patients with so-called completed stroke have as high an incidence of further damage as those with TIA or RIND.[2] If, however, the vascular mechanism and pathology are known, the tissue at risk can be estimated. In a patient with penetrating vessel disease, a 5-mm basal-ganglionic lacune could represent infarction of the entire territory of that artery. If the same patient with a small basal-ganglia infarct had severe stenosis of the MCA, causing reduced flow in the lenticulostriate territory, the potential for further extensive damage would be much greater.

Similarly, *stroke in evolution* is a nonspecific term. Almost 30 percent of stroke patients worsen after entry into the hospital. These worsening deficits may be a result of numerous factors, including failure of collateral circulation, systemic hypotension, cardiac arrhythmias, embolization or propagation of thrombus, progressive occlusion of the vessel lumen, psychological depression, intercurrent infections, or seizures. Knowing that the patient is worsening should stimulate action, but the nature of the therapeutic action will depend on the pathophysiology of the patient's particular problem.

Pace of the stroke

I have decried the use of tempo of the illness as the only criterion for treatment. This does not mean, however, that it should not be considered at all. In fact, the pace of progression dictates the urgency and speed of evaluation and treatment. Table 3.6, in Chapter 3, depicts HSR data concerning timing of the first and last TIA prior to stroke in patients with severe ICA disease. A patient with a TIA this morning has a greater probability of stroke tomorrow than a patient with a single TIA 3 months ago. The patient with a single TIA a week ago differs from the patient with a flurry of 5 to 10 TIAs yesterday and today. Patients worsening while under immediate supervision will require more urgent management than patients stable for the past week. An improving patient would make the physician pause before deciding to tamper with natural forces that seem to be at least temporarily succeeding.

Personnel and Facilities Available for a Given Treatment or Evaluation

Complications and success rates vary widely from institution to institution and even within the same institution, depending on the personnel involved. Figures from Springfield, Illinois,[10] and Cincinnati, Ohio,[11] document striking variability in morbidity and mortality for the same surgical procedure—carotid endarterectomy. The risk/benefit ratio of carotid endarterectomy when the complication rate is 2 percent is quite different from the situation when it is 20 percent. The utility and complication rate for diagnostic tests such as cerebral angiography also vary with the skill, training, and experience of the angiographer and the available equipment. Especially in this era of limited resources, not all institutions will be economically able to specialize equally in all fields. Physicians owe patients the best possible care. Responsibility to the patient must exceed loyalty to one's colleagues and institution if physicians are to continue to deserve the respect of the community and patients. If a physician or a hospital has limited interest and capability in stroke management, and the patient's condition and socioeconomic status make it feasible for the patient to go elsewhere, then the physician should send the patient to where the best care is available. *The Golden Rule is the most important guide to treatment.*

Some therapeutic rules are general and apply to all stroke patients.[12] Other strategies depend on the problems and findings specific to the individual patient such as focal brain ischemia due to low flow, increased intracranial pressure (ICP) due to the mass effect of a hematoma or cerebral edema, a threatened second embolism, a threatened recurrence of subarachnoid hemorrhage. What treatment strategies are available to deal with these problems?

General Care

Important goals for physicians are to limit suffering, give comfort, and prevent complications. Even when no specific therapy seems warranted because of the severity of the deficit, the type of stroke, or severe comorbidities, patients deserve excellent nursing and general care. Stroke patients often are at least partially immobilized and may not be able to care fully for their bodily needs. Key goals are maintenance of adequate nutrition; prevention of contractures and painful stiff or apparently frozen joints, of decubiti, and of pressure-related peripheral nerve palsies; and prevention of thromboembolic, pulmonary, genitourinary, and skin complications. Table 5.1 lists some of these problems and general types of treatment. Perhaps just as important as these physical problems is maintenance of a positive but realistic outlook in patients and their families and significant others. Because depression is so common after stroke,[13,14] measures should be instituted early to prevent discouragement, and depression should be recognized and treated when it occurs.

Patients' visits to doctors and hospitals give physicians important opportunities to view the whole person and his or her environment. In the hurry to diagnose and treat acute stroke problems, preventive measures are often overlooked. The stroke patient of today, irrespective of cause, is at risk for future strokes and vascular disease in other important organs. Prevention strategies should be begun as early as possible. Patients get wrong messages when some factors are neglected. For example, arrival of food trays rich in red meats, cheese, and ice cream and equipped with a salt shaker tell the patient with hypertension and hypercholesterolemia that diet is not important. Nurses or aides helping the patient to smoke also convey approbation. While the specific stroke mechanism is being investigated and treated, begin to explore general health practices and stroke risk factors, and deal with them early in the care. Table 5.2 lists some of these risk factors. I explore these in more detail in Chapter 17.

While exploring diagnosis and treatment of the acute stroke, rehabilitation strategies should also begin. Restorative or rehabilitation therapy depends on the type of handicap and disability, not on the stroke etiology or mechanism. Limb weakness, gait abnormalities, language disturbances, dysphagia, neglect of the left side of space, and hemianopia are all quite different problems that require different rehabilitation and therapy strategies. To be maximally effective, rehabilitation should focus on the individual patient, taking past capabilities and activities and future needs and desires into consideration.

TABLE 5.1
General Problems and Treatments in Patients with Stroke

Problems	Treatments
1. Nutritional maintenance (especially if dysphagia is present)	Balanced diet that conforms to suggested calories and content (e.g., low cholesterol, low salt), vitamins when indicated, intravenous feeding, nasogastric tubes, gastrostomy
2. Pulmonary complications (aspiration, pneumonia atelectasis, pulmonary emboli)	Care or avoidance in oral feeding; in dysphagics, study of swallowing prior to oral feeding; respiratory therapy; early antibiotic treatment of infection; no smoking; anticoagulants (miniheparin or heparinoids); use of special leg boots to prevent phlebothrombosis
3. Immobility (body or one or more limbs)	Frequent full-range-of-motion exercises, frequent turning, prevention of pressure palsies and joint dislocations by slings and careful limb positioning
4. Urinary-tract complications (bladder distension, urinary retention, infection)	Catheterization using sterile technique when needed; avoidance, when possible, of indwelling catheters; early antibiotic treatment; urinary acidification
5. Skin (decubiti)	Careful, frequent turning; pillows and pads to protect pressure areas; water beds; skin surveillance
6. Psychological (apathy and depression)	Positive outlook; entire medical care personnel functioning as a team; antidepressants

Source: Modified with permission from Caplan LR. A general therapeutic perspective on stroke treatment. In: Dunkel R, Schmidley J, eds. Stroke in the elderly: new issues in diagnosis, treatment and rehabilitation. New York: Springer Publishing, 1987;60–69.

TABLE 5.2
Risk Factors and Potentially Unhealthy Practices

Smoking
Heart disease
Hypertension
Illicit drug use (especially cocaine, amphetamines)
Prescription drugs and their overuse
Overuse of alcohol
Abnormal blood lipids
Oral contraceptives
Sedentary life-style
Diabetes
Highly stressful work and home situations
Obesity

Rehabilitation involves an educational process, training patients to understand their handicaps and devising strategies for overcoming them. Recall that the word *doctor* is derived from the Latin word *docere,* "to teach" or "to lead." Sometimes well-learned routine tasks—such as walking, eating, or sitting on a toilet—must be performed in a different way, and patients must be instructed and trained to use new approaches. To be successful, the rehabilitation and education process must be shared with the family and others who will live with and help the patient. They must carry on and amplify the gains made in the hospital after the patient returns home. If they know the nature of the patient's disabilities, they can help modify the environment to make things easier, and they will be understanding when the patient fails at particular tasks. A kind, personal, understanding, unhurried approach by all personnel involved is needed. Rehabilitation, like prevention, should start early during the acute stroke period. Passive range-of-movement exercises, speech therapy, and explanation of the neurological dysfunction can begin during the first days after the stroke.

Unfortunately, in many medical centers and physician practices, the locations and personnel involved in stroke prevention, in acute treatment, and in rehabilitation are different. Usually, primary-care physicians encourage prevention when they see patients in their offices. Specialists treat acute strokes in acute-care facilities, sometimes even in special stroke or intensive-care units (ICUs). Other rehabilitation specialists manage the recuperative period in rehabilitation hospitals. Yet all phases of care should be a continuum, and ideally, the three types of practitioners should all be involved during the acute-care phase. Rehabilitation personnel must be aware of the preventive and acute treatment strategies used, so as to maintain them during rehabilitation. After being urged to avoid salt, refrain from smoking, and watch their diet in the acute-care hospital, what message do patients get if they are allowed to smoke and eat ad lib in the rehabilitation hospital?

Ischemic Stroke

Although mechanisms of ischemia vary, particular themes are applicable to all patients with brain ischemia. *Ischemia* means inadequate delivery of blood containing required nutrients. Maximizing blood flow to ischemic zones is clearly important. Can areas of vascular blockage in large arteries be opened or circumvented by medical or surgical treatments? Can local perfusion through the microcirculation supplying the ischemic zone be improved? Occlusive thrombosis and thromboembolism are important in most patients with ischemic stroke. Can the coagulation system be altered to diminish the development of so-called white platelet–fibrin clots and red thrombin-dependent clots? Metabolic changes within the ischemic zone are important in causing cell death. Can the brain be made more resistant to ischemia by manipulating its chemical environment? Edema and raised ICP can potentiate nerve-cell damage. Can they be controlled? I discuss these different issues separately.

Maximizing Blood Flow

Different medical and surgical strategies are available to try to improve circulation to a region distal to a vascular occlusive lesion.

Controlling position and activity

In some patients, sitting, standing, and even elevating the head of the bed increase ischemic symptoms.[15] The minor reduction in cephalad flow accompanying postural change decreases flow through the stenotic vessel or collateral channels just enough to decompensate a teetering and fragile equilibrium.[15,16] Physicians should note whether patients are sensitive to postural changes. Initially, after the acute stroke, patients should be observed when first sitting or standing, to ensure that blood pressure does not drop excessively or postural symptoms appear. Patients with progressive symptoms due to ischemia should be nursed supine, sometimes with the feet gently elevated.

Managing blood pressure, blood volume, and cardiac output

CBF increases with rising blood pressure until the pressure becomes very high, approaching the malignant range. For this reason, surgeons often give intravenous agents such as phenylephrine to raise blood pressure just prior to clamping the ICA during an endarterectomy. During the acute period of ischemic stroke, it is unwise to lower the systemic pressure unless it is extremely high—for example, above 200/120 torr. However, in some emergency rooms or ICUs, exposing physicians to an elevated blood pressure is like waving a red flag before a bull; they want to get all of the patient's numbers into the normal range, including blood pressure. Remember that physicians treat *patients*, not *numbers*. The patient's symptoms, signs, and neurological function are better guides to the appropriateness of a treatment than is the measured blood pressure. Blood volume also affects perfusion pressure and flow. Some patients who are not able to eat normally will become dehydrated and relatively hemoconcentrated. Other factors—such as vomiting, restrictions on eating because of concern for aspiration, or simply the rush of diagnostic testing occupying patients at mealtimes—all contribute to reduced fluid intake during the early hours and days after stroke onset. In general, it is wise to keep blood volume, especially plasma volume, high. Fluids must often be given intravenously or by nasogastric tube. Care, however, must be taken to avoid fluid overload and the complications of cardiac failure and brain edema. Careful monitoring of cardiac and cerebral function should accompany any therapeutic overload of volume.

Some patients have anoxic–ischemic brain damage due to cardiac malfunction; in others, a strong pump helps maximize CBF. Attention to cardiac rhythm and pump function is important, especially during the acute, fragile period of cerebral ischemia. Cardiac output can sometimes be improved by use of digitalis or vasodilators, use of pacemakers or medications to treat slow rhythms and heart block, adjustment of already prescribed drugs such as digitalis and diuretics, correction of abnormal serum K^+ and Ca^{++} levels, and control of tachyrhythmias. Now cardiac-ejection fractions and output can be monitored noninvasively by echocardiography.

Relieving vascular obstructions

The commonest method of unblocking a vessel is by direct surgery on that vessel—endarterectomy. This strategy differs from other techniques that augment flow because endarterectomy of a tightly stenotic vessel produces a sudden large increase in flow. During ischemia, capillaries and small arterioles, as well as neural substrate, can be damaged by ischemia. When flooded with blood under high pressure, these abnormal vessels then can bleed. The carotid sinus is also damaged during endarterectomy, leading to failure of the carotid sinus reflex and accelerated hypertension in the hours and days after carotid endarterectomy.[17,18] Elevated blood pressure and flooding of damaged vessels can lead to ICH following carotid endarterectomy.[19] Care must be taken in the timing of endarterectomy, and the blood pressure of patients undergoing carotid endarterectomy must be carefully monitored during the postoperative period. Usually, completely occluded vessels do not lend themselves to direct repair because, in the presence of low flow, clots form and propagate distally beyond the site of surgical access.

Recently, carotid endarterectomy has been shown to be more effective than medical therapy in patients with neurologically symptomatic severe (>70% luminal narrowing) carotid artery stenosis.[20,21] Endarterectomy not only removes the obstructing lesion, thus dramatically augmenting flow, but also removes the source of intra-arterial emboli.[22] However, patients must be carefully chosen because neurological and cardiac morbidity and mortality are significant risks.[23] Although trials are in progress, physicians still do not know whether endarterectomy is more effective than medical treatment in patients without neurological symptoms and in individuals with lesser degrees of stenosis.[23-25] Endarterectomy frequently also has been performed successfully in stenosing lesions of the extracranial innominate, subclavian, and vertebral arteries[26,27] and even on the intracranial VAs.[28,29] Insufficient cases have been studied to determine the indications and effectiveness of surgery versus medical therapy in patients with lesions at those sites. Emboli have also been removed directly from the MCA, but the procedure did not lessen stroke severity.[30]

In some systemic vessels, transluminal angioplasty has been performed.[31,32] This technique usually uses catheters or balloons to mechanically split plaques and dilate vessels. Vascular dilation has also been used to treat fibromuscular dysplasia. Angioplasty has occasionally been tried for cerebral vascular occlusive disease but is much more risky.[33,34]

Since the 1980s, interventional radiography has developed into a very important therapeutic alternative for many cerebrovascular conditions. To date, interventional techniques using coils, catheters, balloons, glues, and other devices have been applied mostly to treatment of patients with aneurysms and vascular malformations. Angioplasty is effective in dilating vasoconstricted intracranial arteries after SAH.[35] Percutaneous transluminal angioplasty using intra-arterial balloons has also occasionally been performed for stenosis of intracranial arteries the size of the MCA,[33] and even the basilar artery.[34] Technology is rapidly being developed. It may be possible in the future to open stenotic or occluded intracranial arteries by interventional intravascular techniques, but at present, the indications and risks and complication rates are unknown.

Clots can also be lysed chemically. In the body, thrombus formation stimulates an endogenous fibrinolytic mechanism for thrombolysis. Factor XII and the release of tissue plasminogen activator (tPA) and other substances promote conversion of plasminogen to plasmin, the active fibrinolytic enzyme.[36,37] Plasmin activity is concentrated at the sites of fibrin deposition. Endogenous formation of plasmin is probably responsible for some examples of spontaneous recanalization of thrombosed arteries.

Beginning in the late 1950s, clinicians have given stroke patients thrombolytic agents in an attempt to open thrombosed arteries. Early attempts used bovine or human thrombolysins or streptokinase.[37] During the early 1960s, Meyer and colleagues randomized 73 patients with worsening strokes to receive streptokinase intravenously and/or concomitant anticoagulants within 3 days of stroke onset.[37–39] Clots were lysed in some patients, but 10 patients treated with streptokinase died, and some patients had brain hemorrhages. After these studies, streptokinase was generally thought to be too dangerous to use, and in fact, the use of streptokinase for systemic and cardiac thromboembolism was considered contraindicated in the presence of brain lesions or past strokes.

During the 1980s, stimulated by the successful use of thrombolytic agents for the treatment of coronary artery thrombosis, clinicians turned again to these "clot busters" to treat cerebrovascular thromboembolism.[37,40,41] Streptokinase, urokinase, and rtPA have been the commonest substances used. These agents have been given intravenously or intra-arterially by catheter into the thrombosed artery. Both anterior and posterior circulation thromboembolism have been treated. Arteries have been successfully opened, especially MCA branches and vertebrobasilar thrombi.[42–45] Some treated patients have had hemorrhagic transformation of infarcts and frank intracerebral hematomas.[45] Trials are now underway to study the optimal dose, safety, and risk of rtPA and other thrombolytic agents. As in coronary artery disease, after occlusive thrombi are lysed, stenosing plaques remain, and rethrombosis is an imminent threat in the hours and days after thrombolytic treatment. Concomitant use of heparin, or use of heparin or aspirin or warfarin after thrombolytic agents, might prevent rethrombosis but clearly increase the risk of hemorrhage.

Surgically bypassing regions of blockage

A surgical bypass can be created, hooking one vessel to another just beyond an obstruction (for example, a CCA to VA connection) or intracranially creating an artificial conduit between ECA branches and intracranial vessels. An artery can be directly sewn to another, or a venous conduit can be interposed. When the vessel to be bypassed was stenotic but still patent, creation of a distal shunt has been shown to further reduce flow through the region of stenosis and to promote complete occlusion.[46,47] Clots that form at the site of occlusion could embolize distally, causing new ischemic damage.

Many anecdotal reports noted the effectiveness of extracranial (EC) to intracranial (IC) artery bypass, using the superficial temporal artery as the donor artery and an MCA branch as the recipient artery. A large, randomized study of the effectiveness of such EC–IC bypasses, however, proved beyond reasonable doubt that the surgery as it was customarily performed had no benefit, and in some circumstances, operated patients fared worse than patients treated medically.[48] The patients in this series had surgery about 6 weeks after stroke to prevent reperfusion hemorrhage in regions where the capillaries and arterioles might be ischemic and vulnerable to leakage. Several questions remain:

1. Might bypass earlier in the course, though more risky, be more effective?
2. Might a different recipient artery (e.g., the main stem MCA or a large conduit such as an interposed vein or larger artery) improve results?
3. Is posterior circulation bypass surgery effective?
4. Might there be some small groups of patients (e.g., those with misery perfusion, confirmed by PET scanning) who could benefit?

Bypass operations are still being performed in patients with critical flow-reducing intracranial occlusive disease in the vertebrobasilar system.[29] Most often, the occipital artery is anastomosed to the posterior inferior cerebellar artery (PICA) or to the anterior inferior cerebellar artery (AICA). Occasionally, the superficial temporal artery is used as the donor vessel and the superior cerebellar or posterior cerebral artery as the recipient.[29] Most bypass procedures now performed, however, involve the branches of the aortic arch and are performed by vascular surgeons.[27] These iatrogenic shunts are created to augment blood flow in the recipient arteries. During the procedure, at times, the proximal portion of the occluded or stenotic artery is ligated to prevent embolic material from traveling craniad into the brain.

*Increasing collateral circulation and perfusion
in the ischemic-zone capillary bed*

Vasodilating agents have long been prescribed to increase blood flow. These agents include cyclandelate, isoxsuprine, hydergine, papaverine, and nicotinic acid. Unfortunately, there is a woeful lack of information regarding the effect and utility of vasodilating agents on CBF in patients with TIAs or ischemic strokes.[49] Abnormal or even paradoxical responses of the cerebral circulation in stroke patients might theoretically render vasodilator treatment ineffective or even harmful.[49] Cerebral vessels have a scarcity of medial elastic fibers and are less responsive than systemic vessels to vasodilator stimuli. Vasodilator agents produce more systemic than cerebral vasodilation and thus could lead to hypotension or globally decreased CBF.

Some pharmaceutical agents have vasoconstrictive effects in some arteries and vasodilator effects in others. Even individual drugs sometimes have different effects on the same circulation, depending on dose and other factors. Recently, serotonin has been shown to dilate normal coronary arteries but to constrict coronary arteries in which the endothelium is diseased.[50] Of course, CO_2 is the oldest used vasodilator. Unfortunately, none of the available agents has been thoroughly studied in individuals with cerebrovascular disease. The technology to study rCBF and flow in the branch arteries is now available to do so: XeCT, PET scans, TCD,[51] and SPECT scans.[52]

Headache and faintness have been described after inhalation of glyceryl trinitrate, a known vasodilator. In situations such as SAH or migraine, when there is known vasospasm, agents that decrease vasoconstriction could have beneficial effects. Acetazolamide (Diamox) has been used as a provocative agent to acutely dilate brain arteries, to test the brain's vascular reserve capability to further augment blood flow.[53] Flow is measured in basal arteries by TCD before and after 1 gm of acetazolamide is given intravenously (IV).[53] In one study of patients with occlusive disease of intracranial or extracranial arteries, IV acetazolamide did increase rCBF, but mostly on the nonobstructed side.[54] Acetazolamide has not been extensively tried in stroke patients.

Calcium-channel blocking agents have been extensively tested since 1987 to determine whether they would improve function in patients with ischemic stroke and SAH. Calcium has a number of actions that could influence the outcome of ischemia.[55] These include promoting vasoconstriction by effects on vascular smooth muscle, altering coagulation (some of the reactions require Ca^{++}), killing cells when extracellular Ca^{++} passes through cell membranes into the intracellular compartment, and lowering systemic blood pressure.[55,56] Calcium-channel blocking agents may ameliorate migraine.[57]

A preliminary study of nimodipine in patients with SAH suggested some beneficial effects on cerebral vasospasm.[58] Later studies also showed some effects on morbidity and mortality and on prevention of delayed ischemic infarction in patients with SAH. It was not clear in these studies that nimodipine successfully increased blood flow or decreased the arterial vasoconstriction.[59-61] An early Dutch trial of oral nimodipine in ischemic stroke patients found that the drug reduced mortality in men and had a beneficial effect in reducing the clinical deficits in patients with moderate and severe neurological abnormalities.[62] However, a number of recent trials of the effectiveness of nimodipine in patients with ischemic stroke have had disappointing results,[63] although nimodipine may help in the most severe cases if given early enough.[64] Therapeutic benefits probably result more from blockage of extracellular-to-intracellular movement of Ca^{++} than from reversal of vasoconstriction.

Other, newer calcium-channel blockers might have more selective cerebral vasodilating effects. Newer technology now allows monitoring of blood flow both acutely and chronically and both focally and globally. Newer drugs and some untested older agents can now be studied in the laboratory and in the clinic.

Dextrans were introduced to clinical medicine about 50 years ago as acute volume expanders;[65] they are polysaccharide molecules made by the action of bacteria on sucrose. The most commonly used solution (10% dextran solution in normal saline or 5% dextrose) is called "dextran 40" and contains molecules ranging from 10,000 to 80,000 molecular weight (average 40,000). Infusion causes rapid volume expansion but rapid excretion in the urine of the dextran molecules of less than 50,000 molecular weight causes an osmotic diuresis with reduction in plasma volume. Dextran also coats RBCs, platelets, and endothelium, which is posited to decrease blood viscosity and prevent cellular aggregation and so improve microcirculatory flow. Dextran also has a potential antithrombotic action by its hemodiluting effect, erythrocyte coating, and decreased platelet aggregation. Early studies suggested a beneficial effect of dextran in decreasing the incidence of thrombotic disease in hip-surgery patients.[66] Dextran solutions have been used to treat stroke, either alone[66] or as part of hemodilution protocols.[67-69] Nonetheless, the utility of dextrans has not been properly analyzed by a study that would meet modern standards for adequately conceived therapeutic trials.

Hemodilution is another technique that has been used to augment CBF and microcirculatory flow. The two major determinants of blood viscosity within brain vessels are fibrinogen and Hct.[70] As flow falls, viscosity increases. Lowering the Hct by hemodilution dramatically reduces viscosity and increases flow.[71] The optimal Hct for blood flow and preservation of oxygen transport is around 33 percent.[68] Rapid hemodilution with reduction of the Hct theoretically could significantly improve blood flow to ischemic zones. Hemodilution may be *isovolemic* (that is, blood replaced with equivalent fluid volume), or replacement could be more (*hypervolemic*) or less (*hypovolemic*) than the original blood volume. Plasma, Ringer's solution, or colloid solutions such as dextran 40 or hydroxyethyl starch were usually used for fluid replacement.[72] Early studies of hemodilution showed some promise in relatively small numbers of patients.[69,73] Later studies did not show significantly better outcome in hemodiluted patients.[72,74] Optimally, the initial Hct should be over 40 percent, and the drop should be to a level that is 10 lower than the original Hct. Volume is also important because either hypovolemia with excessively reduced volume or hypervolemia with potential cardiac overload and brain edema can be problematic. Centers using hemodilution therapy must have experience in this technique.

Another means of reducing viscosity and also potentially altering blood coagulability is the use of substances that reduce fibrinogen levels. Fibrinogen contributes significantly to viscosity,[75] and high fibrinogen levels have been noted to predict stroke recurrence in high-risk patients.[76] *Ancrod*, a substance derived from the purified protein fraction of venom from the Malayan pit viper, has a thrombinlike enzymatic effect. Ancrod selectively acts on fibrinogen and inhibits formation of cross-linked fibrin.[77] Ancrod can reduce fibrinogen levels to about 100 mg and is being studied for its utility in patients with brain ischemia.[77,78] In one study, at onset, the mean plasma fibrinogen level was 385 mg/dl.[77] After IV infusions of ancrod, D-dimer levels rose, indicating clot lysis, and fibrinogen levels fell to a mean of 116 mg/dl at 6 hours and 52 mg/dl at 24 hours after start of treatment.[77]

Omega-3 fatty acids, especially eicosopentanoic acid (EPA), can also lower blood fibrinogen levels.[79] In a preliminary study, EPA also reduced blood viscosity, especially in those patients with high baseline viscosities.[80] EPA and omega-3 fatty acids, plentiful in various fish oils, have the potential to reduce platelet aggregability, in addition to their effects on fibrinogen and viscosity. Reduced incidence of atherosclerosis in Eskimos has been attributed by some to diets rich in fish and omega-3 fatty acids. To date, there have been no trials of these substances in stroke prevention or treatment.

Another strategy that has been used experimentally to improve microcirculatory flow and oxygen delivery is the use of perfluorochemicals. Perfluorochemicals are relatively small molecules—much smaller than erythrocytes—that can carry and release oxygen yet are not metabolized, remain chemically inert, and have low surface tension.[81] When patients or laboratory animals breathe 100 percent oxygen, these small molecules become saturated with oxygen. Animal experiments have shown promise that perfluorochemicals (e.g., Fluosol-DA) might be useful in ameliorating the extent of infarction in cats with transorbital ligation of an MCA.[82]

In humans, perfluorochemicals have been used mostly as so-called white blood, given to patients who are severely anemic but who refuse blood transfusions for religious reasons.[83] Theoretically, the smaller molecules can squeeze through vascular passages that block erythrocytes and thereby succeed in delivering needed oxygen to the ischemic stunned penumbral brain tissue. However, in clinical studies, investigators have not been able to attain concentrations of perfluorochemicals ("fluocrits") high enough to provide useful oxygen-carrying capabilities.[84] Still, the concept shows some future promise.

In patients with low flow, stagnation causes clot formation and embolization. Measures to prevent embolization, discussed in the next section, are thus also applicable to many low-flow situations.

Prevention of Clot Formation, Propagation, and Embolism

The formation of a thrombus depends on a number of interrelated factors that include local vascular injury or roughening, the number of platelets and their activation, and the presence of serum coagulant and anticoagulant substances. In general, so-called *red clots*—fibrin-dependent thrombi—tend to form in regions where there is low flow or stagnation, whereas smaller so-called *white platelet plugs* adhere to roughened places in faster-moving streams of blood.[85,86] Standard anticoagulants, such as heparin and warfarin, theoretically should be more useful in preventing red clots, and antiplatelet agglutinating agents should be better at preventing white platelet plugs.[85,86] Heparin and warfarin might work best in occlusive disease of large vessels, whereas agents that decrease platelet aggregation might have an advantage in plaque disease without stenosis. Some evidence documents the failure of aspirin, an antiplatelet agglutinating agent, in patients with severe carotid artery disease.[87]

Polycythemia and thrombocytosis increase the probability of clot formation. Frequent blood donations, removal of causes of secondary erythremia such as cigarette smoking, and specific antineoplastic treatment of polycythemia vera are therapeutic alternatives to reduce the Hct. In the acute situation, hemodilution also decreases viscosity and thrombotic tendencies.[73] Thrombocytosis can also cause a clotting tendency and usually accompanies hematological proliferative disorders that require specific therapy.

Heparin, a biological substance derived from tissues of various animals, has been used clinically since the 1940s. It decreases hyperlipemia and has a variety of different anticoagulant effects. The major anticoagulant activity occurs when heparin binds to and activates *antithrombin III,* a naturally occurring plasma inhibitor of coagulation. Activated antithrombin III slowly binds to thrombin and the other serum protease coagulation factors and neutralizes these compounds. Heparin also antagonizes thromboplastin and prevents thrombi from reacting with fibrinogen to form fibrin. Heparin is a heterogeneous mixture of sulfated mucopolysaccharides containing at least 21 compounds ranging in size from 3,000 to 37,500 daltons.[88,89] Commercial heparin is prepared from animal tissues, most often bovine lungs or porcine intestines. Heparin has customarily been used during the acute phase of thrombosis or embolism. The necessity of giving the drug parenterally has limited its long-term use. Heparin can be given as an IV bolus, a continuous-drip infusion, or—less effectively—subcutaneously. Dosage should be adjusted to keep the PTT at 1.5 to 2 times the normal control values.[90]

Customarily, heparin is given acutely to maintain anticoagulation until warfarin therapy produces therapeutic prolongation of the PT. Unfortunately, some patients treated with heparin develop a drop in their platelet count, thrombocytopenia, and new ischemic events.[91,92] There are two varieties of heparin-induced thrombocytopenia. The commonest variety involves a slight degree of thrombocytopenia, usually beginning 1 to 5 days after the start of heparin, which is caused by heparin-induced platelet aggregation.[92] Ischemia does not result, and platelet counts return to normal despite continued heparin use. In the more severe form of heparin-induced thrombocytopenia, antibodies of the IgG and IgM groups become bound to platelets, and platelet counts fall, usually during the second week of treatment. Often, thrombocytopenia is severe ($< 10,000$ mm^3), and thromboembolic and rarely hemorrhagic complications occur, presumably due to consumption of coagulation factors and platelets.[92] Occasionally, thrombosis seems to be precipitated by heparin without thrombocytopenia.[93]

The effectiveness of heparin in ischemic stroke has not been well studied. Ramirez-Lassepas and colleagues found good to excellent recovery in 81 percent of 136 patients treated with heparin and felt that the drug might reduce fluctuations and late deteriorations.[94] However, Duke and colleagues found no benefit.[95] Neither study was controlled, and for the most part, the arterial pathology and stroke mechanisms underlying the ischemia were not investigated. A 1989 survey of the present practice of neurologists shows wide variability in prescribing heparin for patients with acute ischemia.[96] Although some have argued vigorously against the use of heparin, citing the risk of bleeding and no proof of benefit,[97,98] my colleagues and I have taken the stance that the jury is still out.[99,100] Theoretical arguments support the use of heparin to prevent clot formation, and I continue to use it in patients with fresh thrombi in large arteries, with presumed cardiac thrombi, and with severe stenosis impeding flow in large arteries.

Unfortunately, the anticoagulant activities of various commercial preparations of heparin vary among sources and even within batches from the same source.[88,89] These variations lead to variability in clinical effectiveness and unexpected bleeding. Crude commercial preparations can be separated into low- and high-molecular-weight fractions. Some evidence suggests that low-molecular-weight (LMW) heparin has more anticoagulant effect and does not activate platelets.[89,101] Studies support the probability that the explanation for heparin's bleeding complications relate to effects on platelets, especially inhibition of platelet aggregation, mostly an action of the high molecular weight (HMW) components in heparin.[102] More recently, commercial companies have begun to supply extracts containing only LMW heparins and LMW heparinoids.[102] *Heparinoids* are heparin analogues prepared by tissue extraction or by blending various components that are structurally related to heparin and have similar biological functions, especially anticoagulant effects.[102] Preliminary studies have shown that LMW heparin is effective in preventing thromboembolism in patients with spinal-cord injury, and it caused less bleeding.[103] In another study, LMW heparin was more effective than standard heparin for prevention of deep-vein thrombosis and caused less bleeding.[104] Heparinoids have been used in stroke patients, and preliminary results show safety of the preparations used. Trials of ischemic stroke patients treated with heparinoids are now being pursued.[102]

Warfarin is a water-soluble derivative of coumaric acid, which is absorbed by the small intestine and transported in the blood, loosely bound to albumin. Its therapeutic effect is to inhibit the action of vitamin K, which is necessary for the biological synthesis of Factors II (prothrombin), VII, IX, and X.[105] By depressing these procoagulant factors, warfarin affects both the so-called intrinsic cascade and the extrinsic coagulation pathway.[105,106] Warfarin works quite differently from heparin. In some patients, who have continued transient spells or progressive ischemic symptoms despite warfarin, symptoms may almost miraculously stop when heparin is substituted for warfarin.

Customarily, in the past, PTs were maintained at 2 to 2.5 times the control value. This therapeutic range was selected as that level slightly below that at which bleeding occurred.[105,106] Wessler and Gitel provide data that persuasively show that the dosage at which warfarin protects against thrombosis is probably far below that needed to cause bleeding.[105] In one study of 96 patients with venous thromboses treated with various intensities of oral anticoagulation, higher intensity therapy (i.e., more prolonged PTs) caused more bleeding, and less intense therapy was equally effective in preventing recurrent thromboembolism.[107] Others have also corroborated the safety and effectiveness of less-intense warfarin anticoagulation.[108,109] I now aim at keeping the PT at about 1.3 to 1.5 times the control value. This translates to an international normalized ratio (INR) of 2.0 to 3.0. Because of the wide variation in thromboplastin reagents used, in 1977, the World Health Organization (WHO) designated a single batch of human brain thromboplastin as an international standard.[110] Manufacturers calibrate their reagent against the international standard and calculate an International Sensitivity Index (ISI), which relates their reagent to the international standard. Using the ISI and the PT, the INR can be readily calculated. Various expert groups have published recommendations for intensity of anticoagulation based on the international system.[110,111] Generally, two intensities of anticoagulation are used: a less intense range (INR 2.0–3.0, roughly equivalent to a PT of 1.3–1.5) and a more intense range (INR 3.0–4.5, about equivalent to a PT of 1.5–2.0 times control).[110]

Crystalline warfarin is given to patients to prevent red-clot formation. In some, warfarin is given for a period of 3 to 6 weeks until clots become organized and become adherent to the vascular wall. In other patients, mostly those with cardiac thrombi or arrhythmias or cardiac lesions promoting thrombus formation and those with severe stenosis of large arteries, warfarin is given indefinitely until the risk of thrombosis diminishes or anticoagulants become contraindicated. My present practice is to monitor vascular occlusive lesions by ultrasound. I stop warfarin about 1 month after stenotic lesions are shown to have become occluded, or after arteries recanalize. Warfarin is also used for some patients with congenital or acquired hypercoagulable states.

Agents that modify platelet adhesion and aggregation have been of great clinical interest in thrombotic disorders, particularly ischemic stroke. Perhaps the first clinical observations on aspirin as an anticoagulant were made by a practitioner, Craven.[112] Craven, observing that dental patients bled more if they had used aspirin, urged friends and patients to take one or two aspirin tablets a day. He later published the effectiveness of this strategy in preventing coronary and cerebral thrombosis in 8000 men in articles in the *Mississippi Valley Medical Journal*, not a periodical on every neurologist's bookshelf.[112–114] Twenty years later, case reports from the United States and Britain on the effectiveness of aspirin in preventing attacks of transient monocular blindness brought the subject to more general attention.[115,116] The American[117] and Canadian[118] aspirin trials soon ensued in the late 1970s. Aspirin and other nonsteroidal anti-inflammatory drugs such as indomethacin, phenylbutazone, and ibuprofen inhibit platelet release reactions, secondary ADP-induced platelet aggregation, and platelet adhesion to collagen, when tested in vitro.[119] Aspirin probably inhibits platelet aggregation and secretion by preventing the synthesis of prostaglandins and thromboxane A_2. This action is achieved by inhibiting the cyclo-oxygenase enzyme that converts arachidonic acid to prostaglandin G_2, the precursor of thromboxane A_2.[119–122] Aspirin, however, also inhibits the production of prostacyclin by endothelial cells. Prostacyclin has a potent platelet antiaggregant and vasodilator effect.[122,123]

The optimal therapeutic dose of aspirin is controversial. The American[117] and Canadian[118] therapeutic trials used four 5-grain aspirin tablets each day. Some have posited that smaller doses might produce the desired inhibition of platelet functions and yet not have the unwanted effect of inhibiting production of prostacyclin by endothelial cells.[124,125] In vitro studies of the effects of small- and larger-dose aspirin on prostaglandin and prostacyclin formation have used normal, young animal vessels, whereas in patients with extracranial vascular disease, the endothelium is frequently damaged and might no longer be able to synthesize prostacyclin. In the British UK-TIA Trial, one aspirin a day was as effective as higher doses,[126] and more recently, in a Dutch trial, even 30 mg was as effective and was better tolerated than 300 mg of aspirin a day.[127] In the Canadian trial, there were relatively few women, and benefit for women from aspirin could not be shown.[118] In subsequent trials, sex differences in responsiveness have not been prominent, but the issue is still often raised.

To complicate matters, some preliminary observations suggest that some patients who are given aspirin do not have significant effects on platelet functions, as measured in vitro.[128] It is not known whether this lack of aspirin response is idiosyncratic and possibly genetic, or whether it is dose dependent, some people simply requiring more aspirin to attain the desired effect on platelets. The last word has not been written on the biochemical aspects of platelet function, and aspirin dosage should be decided by future clinical trials (ideally in homogeneous subtypes of patients)[6,129] and by anatomical and functional tests of platelet vascular deposition in animals and humans.

A variety of other agents that decrease platelet aggregation are in clinical use. Sulfinpyrazone (Anturane) inhibits platelet prostaglandin synthesis and release; the usual dose is 200 mg four times per day.[118] Dipyridamole (Persantine) is a pyramidopyrimidine compound quite different chemically from the nonsteroidal anti-inflammatory drugs. Acting as a phosphodiesterase inhibitor, it also reduces platelet function. Dipyridamole might have a synergistic effect with aspirin.[130,131] In rabbits, a combination of aspirin and dipyridamole protected against thrombosis induced by combined chemical and electrical stimuli when neither drug did so separately.[130] Optimal dosage of dipyridamole is uncertain,[132] but 400 mg/day was used with warfarin to effectively inhibit embolization from prosthetic heart valves.[131] Even when combined with aspirin, doses below 200 mg/day might be ineffective.[132] In a large randomized trial, dipyridamole in doses of 300 mg/day had no demonstrable therapeutic effect when added to aspirin in patients with TIA or minor stroke.[133]

Ticlopidine hydrochloride is a thienopyridine derivative recently introduced as an effective platelet antiaggregant for use in patients with occlusive vascular disease.[134] Ticlopidine functions mostly as an inhibitor of the ADP pathway of platelet aggregation. The drug inhibits most known stimuli to platelet aggregation, but unlike aspirin, it does not inhibit the cyclooxygenase pathway.[134,135] Ticlopidine may also have the capability of reducing fibrinogen levels and of increasing erythrocyte deformability.[134,136] In a large, randomized trial, ticlopidine showed a relative risk reduction of about 30 percent in reducing the rate of stroke, myocardial infarction, and vascular death in men and women who had a previous minor stroke.[137] In a different study, ticlopidine (500 mg daily) was slightly more effective than aspirin (1300 mg daily) in reducing the rate of stroke in patients with TIAs or minor strokes.[135]

In each study, ticlopidine had a relatively high rate of side effects, especially diarrhea and skin rash. Neutropenia, sometimes severe, also was a serious, but infrequent complication of ticlopidine (about 1% of patients).[135,137] Patients taking ticlopidine had a slightly elevated cholesterol level.[135] Clearly, ticlopidine is an effective drug, but side effects, especially neutropenia, require careful monitoring. In most circumstances, neutropenia develops within the first 3 months of drug use, and WBC counts return to normal within days to weeks of stopping ticlopidine.

Some investigators have used a combination of warfarin anticoagulants and platelet antiaggregants, usually aspirin, in patients with severe atherosclerosis who had not responded to more conventional treatments.[138] This combination was effective but resulted in a higher bleeding-complication rate.[138,139] I have also used this strategy in patients in whom warfarin was indicated but was ineffective when used alone.

Interest is growing in the potential effects of natural substances such as EPA[140] and black-tree fungus, agents that could potentially affect platelet functions and are contained in natural foods.

A hypothetically useful strategy that I follow is to use platelet antiaggregants when there is no obstruction to flow but ischemia might be due to the process of platelet plugs and small white—or white and red—clots. Heparin and warfarin are reserved for situations of tight stenosis or clots within the heart. They are also used for 3 to 4 weeks in patients with a recent in situ occlusion within a large artery. This method is strictly hypothetical, and results to date are anecdotal and have not been tested scientifically.

Table 5.3 reviews present recommendations for the use of platelet antiaggregants and anticoagulants. The topic of anticoagulant use is very complex, and full discussion is beyond the scope of this book. The subject has been reviewed in detail elsewhere.[89]

Increasing the Brain's Resistance to Ischemia

Until now, I have discussed ways of improving the circulation. I now turn to means of helping the brain survive despite poor perfusion. Neuronal death probably depends on multiple factors, including level of activity (the more work that goes on, the more fuel is needed); presence of local metabolites such as lactic acid[141,142] and free radicals;[143-147] temperature of the system—at low temperatures, there is less metabolism and less need for fuel;[148] integrity of the neuronal cell membranes;[149] and influx of calcium into cells and the extracellular-to-intracellular gradient for calcium.[150-152] Preliminary evidence from experimental whole-brain ischemia in young animals indicates that hyperglycemia makes the brain more vulnerable to ischemia. Sugar increases metabolism and leads to the production of lactic acid. Acidosis can be destructive to brain tissue.[141,142] In the experimental animal, work can lead to increased vulnerability to ischemia, when compared to the resting state.[153] A high concentration of extracellular calcium can also contribute to final neuronal death.[149-152] Recent evidence suggests that some neurotransmitters released at sites of ischemia might overexcite neurons and cause toxic damage, increasing the effects of the initial ischemia.[154-159] This theory—often referred to as the "excitotoxin hypothesis"—has stimulated much recent research concerning neurotransmitters and ischemia.

These tentative early observations on factors influencing brain vulnerability to anoxic or ischemic insults have stimulated interest in many

TABLE 5.3
Present Recommended Use of Platelet Aggregants and Anticoagulants

---

Heparin (standard dose) (short-term, 2–4 weeks)
    Usually given by constant IV infusion, keeping aPTT between 60 and 100 seconds (1.5–2 × control aPTT)

1. immediate therapy of definite cardiac-origin cerebral embolism (large cerebral infarct, hypertension, bacterial endocarditis, or sepsis would delay or contraindicate this use)
2. for patients with severe stenosis or occlusion of the ICA origin, ICA siphon, MCA, VA, or basilar artery, with less than a severe clinical deficit—treatment then could be shifted to warfarin or surgery

Heparin (subcutaneous mini dose)
    For prophylaxis of deep-vein occlusion in patients immobilized by stroke (unless contraindicated)

Warfarin
    Usually overlapped with heparin, keeping PT around 1.5 times control (17–20 seconds) (INR 2.0–3.0)

1. long-term (greater than 3 months) in patients with cardiogenic cerebral embolization and rheumatic heart disease, atrial fibrillation with large atria or prior cerebral embolism, prosthetic valves, and some hypercoagulable states
2. long-term (greater than 3 months) in patients with severe stenosis of the ICA origin, ICA siphon, MCA stem, VA, basilar artery—used until studies show artery has been occluded for at least 3 weeks
3. shorter-term (3–6 weeks) in patients with recent occlusion of the ICA, MCA, VA, or basilar arteries

Platelet antiaggregants (aspirin, ticlopidine)

1. for patients with plaque disease of the extracranial and intracranial arteries without severe stenosis
2. for patients with polycythemia or thrombocytosis and related ischemic attacks

---

possible therapeutic regimens. Unfortunately, the field is quite new, and none of the strategies has been extensively investigated. *Reduction of blood sugar* by insulin might decrease brain lactate production in ischemic zones and thereby reduce necrosis.

Although early studies suggested that *hyperglycemia*, with or without diabetes mellitus, might aggravate ischemic brain damage,[160] more recent reviews indicate that the issues are complex.[161] Studies of glycosylated hemoglobin now allow an estimation of the adequacy of blood-glucose control in diabetics. Elevated fasting blood-sugar levels,[161,162] especially when accompanied by high levels of glycosylated hemoglobin,[161] do predict poor outcome. Others have related high glucose levels in stroke patients to a stress response;[163,164] large hemorrhages and infarcts induce catecholamine secretion, which in turn increases the WBC count and the blood-sugar levels.

At present, it seems prudent to avoid hyperglycemia and to treat very high blood-sugar levels with insulin. There are insufficient data to warrant reducing normal blood sugars to hypoglycemic levels.

Hypothermia and *barbiturate anesthesia* are nonspecific strategies that reduce cerebral energy and metabolism and thereby reduce the brain's requirements for fuel, oxygen, and blood.[165,166] Unfortunately, each can lead to circulatory changes and can complicate the examination and management of stroke patients. Some have hypothesized that ischemia and spinal injury can result in release of endogenous opiates (*endorphins*) that cause further injury.[167,168] Early reports suggested that *naloxone,* an opiate receptor antagonist, was effective in reducing stroke severity in gerbils[169] and humans,[170] but later studies showed an equivocal or lack of naloxone effect. In high doses, naloxone may be effective in reversing some clinical signs,[171] but this probably occurs mostly in patients with stunned brain regions and not in established infarcts. At present, naloxone is not being used in patients with ischemia.

Another strategy presently being tested for effectiveness in protecting neurons from the effects of ischemia is the use of *gangliosides.* The ganglioside compounds used are *glycosphingolipids,* normal components of plasma membranes that are particularly abundant in the cells of the CNS. Exogenous gangliosides are important chemical constituents of neurons. Monosialoganglioside GM^1 enters neural plasma membranes and might protect membranes from injury. Studies to date show promise but are inconclusive.[172,173] Clearly, ganglioside treatment is still experimental and not ready for use as an ordinary clinical stroke therapy.

Some have hypothesized that free radicals, found during hypoxic injury, may lead to further neuronal damage.[143-145] A *free radical* is an atom, group of atoms, or molecule having one or more unpaired electrons in its outermost orbit.[143,146,147] Covalent chemical bonds usually have paired electrons; free radicals are molecules with an open bond, which accounts for their extreme reactivity. The free radical types of importance in brain ischemia are superoxide (O_2^-) and hydroxyl (OH) radicals.[143] Hydrogen peroxide can generate OH radicals, in reaction with superoxide. Xanthine oxidase is the major enzyme that generates superoxide radicals. Free radicals can react with and damage proteins, nucleic acids, lipids, and other molecules and can initiate very destructive chain reactions.[143] Oxygen radicals can also damage blood vessels and cause vasodilation, increased permeability, endothelial and smooth muscle injury, and increased platelet aggregation.[174]

Strategies to prevent and neutralize oxygen free radicals have been attempted, mostly in experimental animals. Allopurinol inhibits xanthine oxidase but does not penetrate well into the brain, and inhibition has not proved effective. *Superoxide dismutase* is an enzymatic scavenger that could alter the oxygen radicals as they are formed. Mice that overexpress superoxide dismutase have reduced ischemic damage when exposed to glutamate neurotoxicity.[175] Another strategy is to scavenge the oxygen free radicals by using nonspecific antioxidants, such as vitamin E or a new class of compounds often called "lazaroids," which are usually 21-aminosteroids.[176,177] These compounds and strategies have been tried in experimental animals, but there are few data on their safety and effectiveness in humans.

The most novel and exciting advance in recent years has undoubtedly been the so-called excitotoxin hypothesis.[156,158,178] The concept was introduced by Olney and colleagues to describe the mechanism by which glutamate and some other acidic amino acids caused neuronal lesions in periventricular structures when given systemically to mice.[156,178] Electrophysiological studies showed that these compounds functioned as neuronal excitants and damaged the periventricular structures studied. Hypothetically, hypoxia and ischemia caused energy depletion and release of glutamate into the tissues. Glutamate then was taken up by receptors and excited the cells already depleted of blood supply, ultimately leading to neuronal death. Putative neurotoxins include glutamate, kainic acid, N-methyl-D-aspartate (NMDA), and homocysteic acid. By far, glutamate has been the most studied. These compounds have various receptor types, usually referred to as NMDA and non-NMDA receptors, including quisqualate and kainate receptors.

There is some experimental evidence supporting the role of excitotoxins in potentiating ischemia. When kainic acid is injected into the hippocampus of experimental animals, it causes a pattern of cell death similar to hypoxic–ischemic damage.[156,158,178] The concentration of glutamate in the extracellular compartment in ischemic brain is increased. Deafferentation of specific intrahippocampal excitatory pathways seems to protect against ischemic damage. Finally, drugs that block excitatory neurotransmission are sometimes protective when given early after experimentally induced ischemia.

Glutamate opens membrane sodium conductance, allowing a large influx of sodium to enter cells. Chloride ion and water follow the sodium, causing cytotoxic edema. Transmembrane influx of calcium into cells leads to a toxic increase in cytosolic free calcium, which kills the cells.[149,150] Experimentally, a number of competitive and noncompetitive NMDA receptor antagonists have been used, including MK 801, dextrorphan, dextromethorphan, ketamine, and phencyclidine. Adenosine and its agonists also seem to reduce glutamate release. Although the vast bulk of the work on excitatory neurotransmitters has been in laboratory animals, Choi and colleagues[159] have argued that NMDA antagonists are ready for trials in humans. Even if effective, their introduction into ordinary bedside clinical use is some years away.

The final common pathway of neuronal death in ischemia may well be calcium influx into cells. Excitotoxins, free radicals, acidosis, and other substances may ultimately kill cells by injuring membranes and allowing Ca^{++} into the cells. Calcium clearly does accumulate in the interstitial space and inside cells during ischemia.[179,180] A number of calcium-channel blockers have been used to attempt to block or alter the entry of calcium into cells. Unfortunately, early trials have shown inconsistent effects of nimodipine.[62-64] Perhaps newer pharmacological agents will provide more effective calcium-channel blockade within brain tissue in ischemic zones. This is an exciting time in stroke research because the idea of protection or salvage of ischemic brain is relatively new. At present, armchair ideas and theories abound and far outweigh the data, but this field of investigation may prove very fruitful in the near future.

Neurotransmitter Replacement and the Effect of Pharmacological Agents on Recovery

The previous sections discussed prevention and minimization of ischemic brain damage. What if damage has already occurred, and an infarct or hemorrhage is already present? Are there agents or strategies that might improve function or accelerate and promote maximum recovery? Injury to nerve cells affects their ability to secrete or respond to neurotransmitters. One strategy that has become popular since 1980 is to attempt to restore function by replacing neurotransmitters known to be active in the damaged region. L-Dopa is given to patients with Parkinson's disease to replace dopamine depleted because of nigrostriatal degeneration, and acetylcholinelike drugs have been tried, in an attempt to treat the hypothesized cholinergic deficit in Alzheimer's disease. Following this lead, a few clinicians have tried neurotransmitters in stroke patients. In one patient with bilateral paramedian thalamic infarcts, who was very apathetic and habitually assumed sleeping postures, *bromocriptine*—a dopamine agonist—led to improvement in spontaneity and less time in bed.[181] In a patient who had been aphasic since a left frontal-lobe hemorrhage 3½ years before study, bromocriptine led to an improvement in speech fluency and a reduction in hesitancy when talking.[182] Bromocriptine was also effective in a patient with neglect of the left side of space due to a right frontoparietal and striatal infarct.[183] Neglect and inattention were improved while taking bromocriptine and worsened after the drug was withdrawn. Bromocriptine and lisuride have been used effectively to treat abulia in four patients with degenerative diseases and strokes.[184] In all of these circumstances, bromocriptine presumably had no healing effect on the damaged tissues; it merely improved functional capacity.

Amphetamines have also been given to promote recovery and enhance function. Following the animal experiments of Feeney and colleagues,[185,186] who found that amphetamines coupled with motor activity accelerated recovery of beam-walking ability in rats,[187,188] some investigators began to try amphetamines in stroke patients. In rats, neither saline (if the rats had low blood volumes; also used as a control) nor amphetamine alone facilitated recovery after sensorimotor-cortex lesions; both a single 2 mg/kg injection of amphetamines and continued experience walking on the beam were needed.[187,188] In contrast, animals given haloperidol performed far worse than did controls.[187] Amphetamines were also effective in promoting recovery of function in cats with experimental sensorimotor-cortex lesions. In a very preliminary human study, 10 mg of D-amphetamine sulfate and physical therapy led to accelerated recovery when compared to patients given placebo and therapy.[187] Amphetamine had to be given early to be effective. From the available studies, it is not clear whether amphetamine has a very specific effect in promoting recovery or merely a generally pepped-up function when combined with physical activity. Might the drug lead to long-term potentiation of cell function[189] or merely to a nonspecific stimulation of less-than-normal cells?

Some pharmacological agents have the potential of retarding recovery. Haloperidol has a definite negative effect on recovery.[185-187] Similarly, drugs that enhance gamma amino butyric acid (GABA)[178] transmission, such as diazepam, might increase inhibition of function and also delay recovery.[190] Stroke patients are often exposed to polypharmacy.[191] Some drugs have been prescribed before the stroke, and others are given after the stroke, to treat various symptoms and general medical conditions. In general, the acute and chronic effects of concurrent drugs on recovery have been poorly studied but are clearly important. Sedatives, anticonvulsants, haloperidol, and opiates should be avoided when possible.

Increased Intracranial Pressure and Brain Edema and Their Control

Large ischemic and hemorrhagic strokes frequently alter the volume and pressure inside the cranium. Herniations, shifts in intracranial contents, and generalized increase in ICP are all common causes of death in patients with large strokes. Treatment of these patients often involves strategies to control changes in ICP.

The cranium can be thought of as a nearly completely closed structure within a rigid container. The brain and its interstitial fluid account for about 80 percent of the intracranial volume, while cerebrospinal fluid (CSF) and blood within vessels each account for about 10 percent of the volume.[181] When ICP rises, adaptation occurs mostly by altering the CSF and vascular compartments. Less CSF can be produced, or more can be absorbed. Blood volume inside the cranium can also be reduced. Most blood is contained in the low-pressure venous system, and this volume can be reduced.[192] ICP has a major effect on pressure and flow in the vascular bed. In order to maintain viability of brain tissue, there must be adequate cerebral perfusion pressure. In supine patients, cerebral perfusion pressure is approximately equal to the mean systemic arterial blood pressure minus the mean ICP.[192] Either an increase in ICP or a decrease in systemic blood pressure can further compromise rCBF to already ischemic brain regions. For practical purposes, there are only a few mechanisms of elevation of ICP in stroke patients. These include introduction of new contents into the cranium, such as a hematoma; edema in and around infarcts and hemorrhages; obstruction of the ventricular system, leading to hydrocephalus; and decreased absorption of CSF, due to subarachnoid bleeding. Each of these problems dictates different treatment strategies.

Reducing or Limiting the Size of an Intracerebral Hemorrhage

Unlike brain infarction, a hemorrhage always introduces extra volume into the closed cranial cavity. The larger the hemorrhage, the more the intracranial volume is expanded. In addition, the local blood collection induces surrounding edema, which further increases local volume. ICP is generally elevated, especially in the region of the hematoma; the pressure changes can lead to a shift of midline structures and herniation into other dural compartments. The aim of therapy is to limit the size of the hemorrhage. This can be accomplished by limiting the bleeding, treating the accompanying edema, or draining the hematoma. In the case of hemorrhage due to a vascular malformation or aneurysm, removing the offending vascular lesion would also prevent recurrent hemorrhage.

The most important method of stopping the bleeding is to reduce arterial tension. Overzealous blood pressure reduction, however, can be a problem because—to some degree—the elevated blood pressure helps to perfuse brain tissue remote from the hemorrhage. When ICP is elevated, venous and dural sinus pressures are also raised pari passu. In order to perfuse the brain, the arterial pressure must rise to produce an effective arteriovenous pressure differential. Excessive reduction in blood pressure may decrease perfusion. The patient's alertness and neurological findings must be carefully monitored as the blood pressure is lowered. When hemorrhage is due to a bleeding diathesis, correction of the coagulopathy is critical in containing the hemorrhage. Use of AHG in hemophiliacs and reversal of warfarin-induced hypoprothrombinemia by fresh frozen plasma or vitamin K are examples of such therapeutic interventions.

Drainage of hematomas can provide rapid decompression. Some patients may decompress their own lesions through spontaneous dissection of the clot into the ventricle or the subarachnoid space. Ease of surgical drainage will depend on the location of the lesion and its proximity to the surface. Lobar, putaminal, and cerebellar hemorrhages are easiest to drain surgically; thalamic and pontine hemorrhages are very difficult to drain effectively.[193] The purpose of drainage is to reduce critical volume expansion that threatens life. Drainage of the hematoma leaves a residual hole that disconnects brain pathways. Although allowing survival, drainage probably does noy reduce the neurological deficit. In comparable-sized infarcts, the cortex is invariably destroyed, whereas hematomas usually spare the cortex. For this reason, recovery from a hemorrhage is usually better than from an infarct of equal size. Surgical drainage should be performed if life is threatened by the volume of the lesion and the hematoma is accessible. The decision to operate must take into consideration the severity of the residual deficit and the patient's and family's wishes after they have been fully informed of the alternatives.

Cerebral edema surrounding the lesion can be treated with agents discussed in the next section.

Treatment of Brain Swelling

Vascular lesions can cause secondary effects that lead to swelling of the brain. The resulting increase in ICP contributes to reduction in consciousness and may further the likelihood of a bad outcome. There are three major processes that swell the brain: vascular congestion, so-called vasogenic cerebral edema, and cytotoxic edema. The potential volume of distended brain capillaries is great. When consciousness is reduced, the patient may hypoventilate, thus raising the partial pressure of arterial carbon dioxide. Carbon dioxide is a potent vasodilator. The potential importance of vascular congestion can be shown by the utility of mechanical hyperventilation in rapidly reducing elevated ICP.[194] Blood gases should be monitored in patients with reduced consciousness; inducing paralysis with a curare-like drug while mechanically hyperventilating the patient is a rapid means of temporarily reducing ICP. Reducing volume of blood in the head reduces ICP no matter what the cause, even if there is not "too much" blood there to begin with. Even when there is no important vascular dilation or congestion, decreasing the amount of venous blood volume in the cranium allows decompression of intracranial contents.

Infarcts and hematomas are frequently accompanied by considerable edema during the acute period. There are two basic types of cerebral edema: vasogenic and cytotoxic. Water in the interstitial or extracellular compartment has been traditionally called *vasogenic edema*, after Klatzo.[195] This type of edema responds to osmotic diuretics, such as mannitol or glycerol,[196,197] and can often be reduced by corticosteroids.[198–200] Vasogenic edema commonly surrounds hematomas. Most clinicians favor the use of corticosteroids and mannitol in patients with large hematomas,[193,201] although there is theoretical concern that hypertonic agents could diffuse into the hematoma during continued bleeding and that this ingress of fluid could increase the volume of the hematoma.

The second type, so-called *cytotoxic edema*,[195,200] is caused by swelling of the cells themselves, so that the water is intracellular. Most of the edema in patients with ischemia is intracellular and does not respond to corticosteroids. Ischemia can also produce some vasogenic edema, but this develops later, when brain cell necrosis has released substances that compromise the blood–brain barrier and lead to extracellular edema.[199] Both vasogenic and cytotoxic edema may be potentiated by reperfusion of brain tissue.[8,202] When the arterial supply to a brain region is blocked, the capillaries and small blood vessels may be damaged by the resulting ischemia. Then when this region is reperfused, the damaged capillaries leak fluid because of damage to the endothelium and basement membranes. The reperfused blood may also bring to the region or promote the circulation of substances such as excitotoxins and Ca^{++} ions, which might enhance cell damage, leading to more cytotoxic edema.[8] Clinical trials have not shown a general beneficial effect from corticosteroids in ischemic stroke,[203] and most authorities do not recommend their use in patients with infarction.[198] In most infarct patients, edema is not clinically important except when there is massive infarction and the prognosis is already very poor. There are, however, rare younger patients in whom dramatic edema develops despite seemingly limited infarction; in this circumstance, steroids are probably helpful.

Occasionally, surgical decompression with removal of infarcted and edematous brain has been performed in patients with herniations or increased ICP. Most often, the infarction has involved the cerebellum, with resultant compression of the brainstem and fourth ventricle.[204,205] The infarcted cerebellum acts very similarly to a hematoma, causing critical mass effect in a relatively small, enclosed compartment, the posterior cranial fossa. Large right temporal-lobe infarcts with edema have also been decompressed.[206] In that circumstance, the temporal lobe can herniate and compress the brainstem. Decompression has long been used to treat traumatic pulped temporal lobe, which acts as a middle fossa mass. The same strategy might apply to very edematous temporal lobe infarcts and large temporal lobe hematomas.

Hydrocephalus can be caused by blockage of the ventricular drainage system, most commonly the aqueduct or fourth ventricle, or by failure of CSF absorption due to plugging of the meninges by blood and blood products. In SAH, the ventricles may enlarge early in the course, and some patients develop persistent hydrocephalus.[207] Ventricular shunting is needed in only a minority of patients with SAH, because in many patients, the hydrocephalus is temporary, and others may respond to repeated LPs and the use of acetazolamide to decrease CSF production. Cerebellar infarcts and hemorrhages, when large, distort the fourth ventricle, leading to obstructive hydrocephalus.[208] Insertion of a ventricular drain or shunt can be life-saving in that situation and can allow recovery in some patients, without the need for direct surgery on the posterior fossa lesion.[209]

Summary and Rules

The field of stroke treatment is changing so quickly that, by necessity, I have included here much armchair theorizing and investigational strategies. Thus, I suggest the following rules, which clinicians should use now in approaching treatment in their patients with stroke:

1. *Begin preventive strategies early.* Education of patients and families about stroke risk factors and their control should occur early during the hospitalization.
2. *Treatment* of the acute stroke, *prevention* of the next stroke, and *rehabilitation should be concurrent* themes throughout hospitalization and recovery.
3. *Avoid common stroke complications,* such as deep-vein thrombosis, aspiration, hypovolemia, pressure sores, contractures, urinary tract infections. These problems are easier to prevent than to treat.
4. *Plan treatment of the acute stroke by analyzing the mechanism and pathophysiology in the individual patient.* The time course of the symptoms should never be the sole guide to treatment.
5. To treat logically, *the clinician should determine* (a) *the location and severity* of the vascular lesion; (b) *the blood constituents and coagulation functions;* and (c) *the state of the brain*—normal, stunned, or irreversibly damaged.
6. *Unblocking of occlusive arterial lesions* with endarterectomy or thrombolysis should mostly be considered when there is *no brain damage,* or when *ischemia is recent and possibly reversible.*
7. *Prevention of thrombus formation, propagation,* and *embolization* is often possible by using drugs that modify platelet aggregation and adhesion and by using anticoagulants of the heparin, heparinoid, and warfarin groups. I suggest using antiplatelet aggregants (e.g., aspirin) to prevent white clots and heparin and warfarin to counteract red clots.
8. When an artery is acutely occluded, anticoagulants are used for 3 to 6 weeks until the occlusive thrombus has organized and become adherent to the artery. In contrast, longer-term anticoagulants are warranted for severe stenosis in large arteries and for continued potential for embolism (e.g., in chronic cardiac lesions that represent a risk for cardiogenic embolism).
9. Try to maximize blood flow to ischemic regions during the acute stroke. Avoid excessive reduction of blood pressure and hypovolemia during the acute stage of infarction.
10. Cardiac disease and mortality are high in most stroke patients. Always consider the heart and its blood supply, in addition to the brain.

Discussion of these general treatments and strategies is expanded in the appropriate chapters in Part II, on the specific syndromes, and in Part III, on prevention, complications, and rehabilitation.

References

1. Caplan LR. Are terms such as *completed stroke* or *RIND* of continued usefulness? Stroke 1983;14:431–433.
2. Caplan LR. TIAs—we need to return to the question, what is wrong with Mr. Jones? Neurology 1988;38:791–793.
3. Matsumoto N, Whisnant J, Kurland L, et al. Natural history of stroke in Rochester, Minnesota, 1955–1969. Stroke 1973;4:20–29.
4. Whisnant J, Goldner J, Taylor W. Natural history of transient ischemic attacks. In: Moosy J, Janeway R, eds. Cerebral vascular disease: proceedings of the Seventh Princeton Conference. New York: Grune & Stratton, 1971:161–169.
5. Wiebers D, Whisnant J, O'Fallon W. Reversible ischemic neurologic deficit (RIND) in a community: Rochester, Minnesota, 1955–1974. Neurology 1982;32:459–465.
6. Caplan LR. Treatment of cerebral ischemia: where are we headed? Stroke 1984;15:571–574.
7. Menken M, Hopkins A, DeFriese GH. Norms of care in British and American neurologic practice. Arch Neurol 1988;45:94–98.
8. Caplan LR. Reperfusion of ischemic brain: why and why not? In: Hacke W, DelZoppo G, Hirschberg M, eds. Thrombolytic therapy in acute ischemic stroke. Berlin: Springer-Verlag, 1991:36–45.
9. Babbs C. Reperfusion injury of post ischemic tissue. Ann Emerg Med 1988;17:1148–1157.
10. Easton JD, Sherman D. Stroke and morbidity rate in carotid endarterectomy: 228 consecutive operations. Stroke 1977;8:565–568.
11. Brott T, Thalinger K. Carotid endarterectomy in Cincinnati 1980: indications and morbidity in 431 cases. Neurology 1983;33(Suppl 2):93.
12. Caplan LR. A general therapeutic perspective on stroke treatment. In: Dunkel R, Schmidley J, eds. Stroke in the elderly: new issues in diagnosis, treatment and rehabilitation. New York: Springer Publishing, 1987:60–69.
13. Robinson RG, Lipsey JR, Price TR. Diagnosis and clinical management of post-stroke depression. Psychosomatics 1985;26:769–778.
14. Wade DT, Leigh-Smith J, Hewer RA. Depressed mood after stroke. Br J Psychiatry 1987;151:200–205.
15. Caplan LR, Sergay S. Positional cerebral ischemia. J Neurol Neurosurg Psychiatry 1976;39:385–391.
16. Toole J. Effects of change of head, limb, and body position on cephalic circulation. N Engl J Med 1968;279:307–311.
17. Lehv M, Salzman E, Silen W. Hypertension complicating carotid endarterectomy. Stroke 1970;1:307–313.
18. Holton P, Wood J. The effects of bilateral removal of the carotid bodies and denervation of the carotid sinus in two human subjects. J Physiol 1965;181: 365–378.

19. Caplan LR, Skillman J, Ojemann R, et al. Intracerebral hemorrhage following carotid endarterectomy: a hypertensive complication. Stroke 1978;9:457–460.
20. North American Symptomatic Carotid Endarterectomy Trial Collaborators. Beneficial effect of carotid endarterectomy in symptomatic patients with high-grade carotid stenosis. N Engl J Med 1991;325:445–453.
21. MRC European Carotid Surgery Trial. Interim results for symptomatic patients with severe (70–99%) or with mild (0–29%) carotid stenosis. Lancet 1991;337:1235–1243.
22. Caplan LR, Pessin MS. Symptomatic carotid artery disease and carotid endarterectomy. Ann Rev Med 1988;39:273–299.
23. Caplan LR. Carotid artery disease [Editorial]. New Engl J Med 1986;315:886–888.
24. Therapeutics and Technology Assessment Subcommittee, American Academy of Neurology. Interim assessment: carotid endarterectomy. Neurology 1990;40:682–683.
25. Asymptomatic Carotid Atherosclerosis Study Group. Study design for randomized prospective trial of carotid endarterectomy for asymptomatic atherosclerosis. Stroke 1989;20:844–849.
26. Spetzler RF, Hadley MN, Martin NA, et al. Vertebrobasilar insufficiency: pt I. microsurgical treatment of extracranial vertebrobasilar disease. J Neurosurg 1987;66:648–661.
27. Lee RE. Reconstruction of the proximal vertebral artery. In: Berguer R, Caplan LR, eds. Vertebrobasilar arterial disease. St. Louis: Quality Medical, 1991:211–223.
28. Hopkins LN, Martin NA, Hadley MN, et al. Vertebrobasilar insufficiency: pt II. microsurgical treatment of intracranial vertebrobasilar disease. J Neurosurg 1987;66:662–674.
29. Ausman JI, Diaz FG, Pearce JE, et al. Endarterectomy of the vertebral artery from C2 to posterior inferior cerebellar artery intracranially. Surg Neurol 1982;18:400–404.
30. Meyer FB, Piepgras DG, Sundt TM, et al. Emergency embolectomy for acute occlusion of the middle cerebral artery. J Neurosurg 1985;62:639–647.
31. American College of Physicians, Health and Public Policy Committee. Percutaneous transluminal angioplasty. Ann Intern Med 1983;99:864–869.
32. Imparato AM. Vertebral artery reconstruction: a nineteen year experience. J Vasc Surg 1985;2:626–633.
33. Purdy PD, Devous MD, Unwin DH, et al. Angioplasty of an atherosclerotic middle cerebral artery associated with improvement in regional cerebral blood flow. AJNR 1990;11:878–880.
34. Piepgras D, Sundt T, Forbes G, et al. Balloon catheter transluminal angioplasty for vertebrobasilar ischemia. In: Buerger R, Bauer R, eds. Vertebrobasilar occlusive disease. New York: Raven Press, 1984:215–224.
35. Higashida RT, Hieshima GB, Tsai FY, et al. Transluminal angioplasty of the vertebral and basilar artery. AJNR 1987;8:745–749.
36. Collen D. On the regulation and control of fibrinolysis: Edward Kowalsky Memorial Lecture. Throm Haemost 1980;43:77–89.
37. Sloan MA. Thrombolysis and stroke, past and future. Arch Neurol 1987;44:748–768.

38. Meyer JS, Gilroy J, Barnhart ME, et al. Anticoagulants plus streptokinase therapy in progressive stroke. JAMA 1964;189:373.
39. Meyer JS, Gilroy J, Barnhart ME, et al. Therapeutic thrombolysis in cerebral thromboembolism: randomized evaluation of intravenous streptokinase. In: Millikan C, Siekert R, Whisnant JP, eds. Cerebral vascular diseases. New York: Grune & Stratton, 1964:200–213.
40. DelZoppo GJ. Thrombolytic therapy in cerebrovascular disease. Stroke 1988; 19:1174–1179.
41. Pessin MS, DelZoppo G, Estol CJ. Thrombolytic agents in the treatment of stroke. Clin Neuropharm 1990;13:271–289.
42. Zeumer H, Freitag HJ, Grzyska U, et al. Local intraarterial fibrinolysis in acute vertebrobasilar occlusion: technical developments and recent results. Neuroradiology 1989;31:336–340.
43. Hacke W, Zeumer H, Ferbert A, et al. Intraarterial thrombolytic therapy improves outcome in patients with acute vertebrobasilar occlusive disease. Stroke 1988;19:1216–1222.
44. DelZoppo G, the rtPA Acute Stroke Study Group. An open, multicenter trial of recombinant tissue plasminogen activator in acute stroke: a progress report. Stroke 1990;21(Suppl 4):174–175.
45. DelZoppo G. Fibrinolytic therapy in thromboembolic vertebrobasilar insufficiency. In: Berguer R, Caplan LR, eds. Vertebrobasilar arterial disease. St Louis: Quality Medical, 1991:179–192.
46. Furlan A, Little J, Dohn D. Arterial occlusion following anastomosis of the superficial temporal artery to middle cerebral artery. Stroke 1980;11:91–95.
47. Gumerlock M, Ono H, Neurvelt E. Can a patent extracranial–intracranial bypass provoke the conversion of an intracranial arterial stenosis to a symptomatic occlusion? Neurosurgery 1983;12:391–400.
48. The EC–IC Bypass Study Group. Failure of the extracranial–intracranial arterial bypass to reduce the risk of ischemic stroke. N Engl J Med 1985; 313:1191–1200.
49. Caplan LR. Use of vasodilating drugs for cerebral symptomatology. In: Miller R, Greenblatt D, eds. Drug therapy reviews. Amsterdam: Elsevier-North Holland, 1979:305–317.
50. Golino P, Pisclone F, Willerson JT, et al. Divergent effects of serotonin in coronary-artery dimensions and blood flow in patients with coronary atherosclerosis and control patients. N Engl J Med 1991;324:641–648.
51. Caplan LR, Brass LM, DeWitt LD, et al. Transcranial Doppler ultrasound: present status. Neurology 1990;40:696–700.
52. Caplan LR. Question-driven technology assessment: SPECT as an example. Neurology 1991;41:187–191.
53. Piepgras A, Schmiedek P, Leinsinger G, et al. A simple test to assess cerebrovascular reserve capacity using transcranial Doppler sonography and acetazolamide. Stroke 1990;21:1306–1311.
54. Hojer-Pedusen E. Effect of acetazolamide on cerebral blood flow in subacute and chronic cerebrovascular disease. Stroke 1987;18:887–891.
55. Braunwald E. Mechanism of action of calcium-channel blocking agents. N Engl J Med 1982;307:1618–1627.
56. Gorelick PB, Caplan LR. Calcium, hypercalcemia and stroke. Current Concepts of Cerebrovascular Disease (Stroke) 1985;20:13–17.

57. Solomon G, Steel J, Spaccevento L. Verapamil prophylaxis of migraine. JAMA 1983;250:2500–2502.
58. Allen G, Ahn H, Preziosi T, et al. Cerebral arterial spasm: a controlled trial of nimodipine in patients with subarachnoid hemorrhage. N Engl J Med 1983; 308:619–624.
59. Phillipon J, Grob R, Dagreou F, et al. Prevention of vasospasm in subarachnoid hemorrhage: a controlled study with nimodipine. Acta Neurochir (Wien) 1986;82:110–114.
60. Jan M, Buchheit F, Tremoulet M. Therapeutic trial of intravenous nimodipine in patients with established cerebral vasospasm after rupture of intracranial aneurysms. Neurosurg 1988;23:154–157.
61. Pickard JD, Murray GD, Illingworth R, et al. Effect of oral nimodipine on cerebral infarction and outcome after subarachnoid hemorrhage: British Aneurysm Nimodipine Trial. Br Med J 1989;298:636–642.
62. Gelmers HJ, Gorter K, deWeerdt C, et al. A controlled trial of nimodipine in acute ischemic stroke. N Engl J Med 1988;318:203–207.
63. TRUST study group. Randomized, double-blind placebo-controlled trial of nimodipine in acute stroke. Lancet 1990;336:1205–1209.
64. The American Nimodipine Study Group. Clinical trial of nimodipine in acute ischemic stroke. Stroke 1992;23:3–8.
65. Data JL, Nies AS. Dextran 40. Ann Int Med 1974;81:500–504.
66. Harris WH, Salzman EW, DeSanctis RW, et al. Prevention of venous thromboembolism following total hip replacement: warfarin vs. dextran 40. JAMA 1972;220:1319–1322.
67. Gilroy J, Barnhart MI, Meyer JS. Treatment of acute stroke with dextran 40. JAMA 1969;210:293–298.
68. Wood JH, Kee DB. Hemorheology of the cerebral circulation in stroke. Stroke 1985;16:765–772.
69. Strand T, Asplund K, Eriksson S, et al. A randomized controlled trial of hemodilution therapy in acute stroke. Stroke 1984;15:980–989.
70. Thomas DJ. Hemodilution in acute stroke. Stroke 1985;16:763–764.
71. Thomas DJ, duBoulay GH, Marshall J, et al. Effect of haemotocrit on cerebral blood flow in man. Lancet 1977;2:941–943.
72. Heros RC, Korosue K. Hemodilution for cerebral ischemia. Stroke 1989; 20:423–427.
73. Wood JH, Fleischer AS. Observations during hypervolemic hemodilution of patients with focal cerebral ischemia. JAMA 1982;248:2999–3004.
74. Scandinavian Stroke Study Group. Multicenter trial of hemodilution in acute ischemic stroke: results of subgroup analyses. Stroke 1988;19:464–471.
75. Grotta J, Ackerman R, Correia J, et al. Whole-blood viscosity parameters and cerebral blood flow. Stroke 1982;13:296–298.
76. Coull BM, Beamer NB, deGarmo PL, et al. Chronic blood hyperviscosity in subjects with acute stroke, transient ischemic attacks, and risk factors for stroke. Stroke 1991;22:162–168.
77. Olinger CP, Brott TG, Barsan TG, et al. Use of ancrod in acute or progressing ischemic cerebral infarction. Ann Emerg Med 1988;17:1208–1209.
78. Hossmann V, Dieter-Heiss W, Bewermeyer H, et al. Controlled trial of ancrod in ischemic stroke. Arch Neurol 1983;40:803–808.
79. Radack K, Deck C, Huster G. Dietary supplementation with low-dose fish oils

lowers fibrinogen levels: a randomized double-blind controlled study. Ann Int Med 1989;111:757–758.

80. Kobayashi S, Hirai A, Terano T, et al. Reduction in blood viscosity by eicosopentaenoic acid. Lancet 1981;2:197.

81. Geyer RP. Oxygen transport in vivo by means of perfluorochemical preparations. N Engl J Med 1982;307:304–306.

82. Peerless SJ, Nakamura R, Rodriguez-Salazar A, et al. Modification of cerebral ischemia with fluosol. Stroke 1985;16:38–43.

83. Tremper KK, Friedman AE, Levine EM, et al. The preoperative treatment of severely anemic patients with a perfluorochemical oxygen-transport fluid, Fluosol-DA. N Engl J Med 1982;307:277–283.

84. Gould SA, Rosen AL, Sehgal L, et al. Fluosol-DA as a red-cell substitute in acute anemia. N Engl J Med 1986;314:1653–1656.

85. Weksler B. Antithrombotic therapies in the management of cerebral ischemia. In: Plum F, Pulsinelli W, eds. Cerebrovascular diseases: proceedings of the Fourteenth Princeton Conference. New York: Raven Press, 1985:211–223.

86. Deykin D. Thrombogenesis. N Engl J Med 1967;276:622–628.

87. Carson S, Demling R, Esquivel C. Aspirin failure in symptomatic atherosclerotic carotid artery disease. Surgery 1981;90:1084–1092.

88. Wu K. New pharmacologic approaches to thromboembolic disorders. Hosp Pract 1985;20:101–120.

89. Caplan LR. Anticoagulation for cerebral ischemia. Clin Neuropharm 1986;9:399–414.

90. Salzman E, Deykin D, Shapiro R, et al. Management of heparin therapy. N Engl J Med 1975;292:1046–1050.

91. Ramirez-Lassepas M, Cipolle RJ, Rodvold KA. Heparin-induced thrombocytopenia in patients with cerebrovascular ischemic disease. Neurology 1984;34:736–740.

92. Becker PS, Miller VT. Heparin-induced thrombocytopenia. Stroke 1989;20:1449–1459.

93. Phelan BK. Heparin-associated thrombosis without thrombocytopenia. Ann Int Med 1983;99:637–638.

94. Ramirez-Lassepas M, Quinones MR, Nino HH. Treatment of acute ischemic stroke: open trial with continuous intravenous heparinization. Arch Neurol 1986;42:386–390.

95. Duke RJ, Bloch RF, Alexander GG, et al. Intravenous heparin for the prevention of stroke progression in acute partial stable stroke: a randomized controlled trial. Ann Intern Med 1986;105:825–828.

96. Marsh EE, Adams HP, Biller J, et al. Use of antithrombotic drugs in the treatment of acute ischemic stroke: a survey of neurologists in practice in the United States. Neurology 1989;39:1631–1634.

97. Scheinberg P. Heparin anticoagulation. Stroke 1989;20:173–174.

98. Philips SJ. Heparin anticoagulation in focal cerebral ischemia: an alternative view. Stroke 1989;20:295–298.

99. Estol CJ, Pessin MS. Anticoagulation: is there still a role in atherothrombotic stroke? Current Concepts Cerebrovasc Disease (Stroke) 1990;25:1–6.

100. Caplan LR. To heparinize or not: an unsettled issue. Stroke 1989;20:968.

101. Rosenberg R, Lam L. Correlation between structure and function of heparin. Proc Nat Acad Sci USA 1979;76:3198–3202.

102. Gordon DL, Linhardt R, Adams HP. Low-molecular weight heparin and heparinoids and their use in acute or progressing ischemic stroke. Clin Neuropharm 1990;13:522–543.
103. Green D, Lee MY, Lim AC, et al. Prevention of thromboembolism after spinal cord injury using low-molecular weight heparin. Ann Int Med 1990;113:571–574.
104. Levine MN, Hirsh J, Gent M, et al. Prevention of deep vein thrombosis after elective hip surgery. Ann Int Med 1991;114:545–551.
105. Wessler S, Gitel S. Warfarin: from bedside to bench. N Engl J Med 1984;311:645–652.
106. Deykin D. Warfarin therapy. N Engl J Med 1970;283:691–694.
107. Hull R, Hirsch J, Jay R, et al. Different intensities of oral anticoagulant therapy in the treatment of proximal-vein thrombosis. N Engl J Med 1982;307:1676–1681.
108. Taberner D, Poller L, Burslem R, et al. Oral anticoagulants controlled by the British cooperative: thromboplastin versus low dose heparin in prophylaxis of deep vein thromboses. Br Med J 1977;1:272–274.
109. Frances CW, Marder VJ, Evan CM, et al. Two-step warfarin therapy: prevention of post-operative venous thrombosis without excessive bleeding. JAMA 1983;249:374–378.
110. Hirsh J, Poller L, Deykin D, et al. Optimal therapeutic range for oral anticoagulants. Chest 1989;95(Suppl 5)S–11S.
111. Poller L. The effect of low-dose warfarin on the risk of stroke in patients with nonrheumatic atrial fibrillation. N Engl J Med 1991;325:129–130.
112. Fields WS, Lemak NA. A history of stroke: its recognition and treatment. New York: Oxford University Press, 1989:115–119.
113. Craven LL. Experiences with aspirin (acetylsalicylic acid) in the nonspecific prophylaxis of coronary thrombosis. Mississippi Valley Med J 1953;75:38–44.
114. Craven LL. Prevention of coronary and cerebral thrombosis. Mississippi Valley Med J 1956;78:213–215.
115. Mundall J, Quintero P, von Kaulla K, et al. Transient monocular blindness and increased platelet aggregability treated with aspirin—a case report. Neurology 1971;21:402.
116. Harrison MJG, Marshall J, Meadows JC, et al. Effect of aspirin in amaurosis fugax. Lancet 1971;2:743–744.
117. Fields WS, Lemak N, Frankowski R, et al. Controlled trial of aspirin in cerebral ischemia. Stroke 1977;8:301–306.
118. Barnett HJM. The Canadian Cooperative Study: a randomized trial of aspirin and sulfinpyrazone in threatened stroke. N Engl J Med 1978;299:53–59.
119. Moncada S, Vane J. Arachidonic acid metabolites and the interactions between platelets and blood vessel walls. N Engl J Med 1979;300:1142–1147.
120. Moskowitz M, Coughlin S. Basic properties of the prostaglandins. Stroke 1981;12:696–701.
121. Genton E, Gent M, Hirsh J, et al. Platelet-inhibiting drugs in the prevention of clinical thrombotic disease. N Engl J Med 1975;293:1174–1178.
122. Weiss H. Antiplatelet therapy. N Engl J Med 1978;298:1344–1346.
123. Moncada C. Biologic and therapeutic potential of prostacyclin. Stroke 1983;14:157–168.

124. Preston F, Whipps S, Jackson C, et al. Inhibition of prostacyclin and platelet thromboxane A_2 after low dose aspirin. N Engl J Med 1981;304:76–79.

125. Weksler B, Pelt S, Alonso D, et al. Differential inhibition by aspirin of vascular and platelet prostaglandin synthesis in atherosclerotic patients. N Engl J Med 1983;308:800–805.

126. UK-TIA Study Group. The UK-TIA Aspirin Trial: the interim results. Br Med J 1988;296:316–320.

127. The Dutch TIA Trial Study Group. A comparison of two doses of aspirin (30 mg vs 283 mg a day) in patients after a transient ischemic attack or minor stroke. N Engl J Med 1991;325:1261–1266.

128. Ackerman R, Helgason C. Unpublished observations, 1986–1990. Personal communication.

129. Caplan LR. Clinical trials in neurology, especially stroke: the clinician's role. In: Hachinski V, ed. Controversies and challenges in neurology. Philadelphia: FA Davis, (In press).

130. Honour A, Hochaday T, Mann J. The synergistic effect of aspirin and dipyridamole upon platelet thrombi in living blood vessels. Br J Exp Path 1977; 58:268–272.

131. Sullivan J, Harken D, Gorlin R. Pharmacologic control of thromboembolic complications of aortic valve replacement. N Engl J Med 1971;284:1391–1394.

132. Fitzgerald GA. Dipyridamole. N Engl J Med 1987;316:1247–1257.

133. Fields WS, Yatsu F, Conomy J, et al. Persantine–aspirin trial in cerebral ischemia: the American–Canadian Cooperative Study group. Stroke 1983; 14:97–103.

134. Ticlopidine [editorial]. Lancet 1991;337:459–460.

135. Hass WK, Easton JD, Adams HP, et al. A randomized trial comparing ticlopidine hydrochloride with aspirin for the prevention of stroke in high-risk patients. N Engl J Med 1989;321:501–507.

136. Ono S, Ashida S, Abiko Y. Hemorheological effect of ticlopidine in the rat. Thromb Res 1983;31:549–556.

137. Gent M, Easton JD, Hachinski V, et al. The Canadian American Ticlopinine Study (CATS) in thromboembolic stroke. Lancet 1989;1:1215–1220.

138. Miller A, Lees R. Simultaneous therapy with antiplatelet and anticoagulant drugs in symptomatic cardiovascular disease. Stroke 1985;16:668–675.

139. Chesebro J, Fuster V, Elveback L, et al. Trial of combined warfarin plus dipyridamole or aspirin therapy in prosthetic heart valve replacement: danger of aspirin combined with warfarin. Am J Cardiol 1983;51:1537–1541.

140. Dyerberg J, Bang H, Stofferson E, et al. Eicosopentanoic acid and prevention of thrombosis and atherosclerosis. Lancet 1978;2:117–119.

141. Plum F. What causes infarction in ischemic brain? Neurology 1983;33:222–233.

142. Myers R. Lactic acid accumulation as a cause of brain edema and cerebral necrosis resulting from oxygen deprivation. In: Korobkin R, Guilleminault C, eds. Advances in perinatal neurology. New York: Spectrum, 1979:88–114.

143. Schmidley JW. Free radicals in central nervous system ischemia. Stroke 1990;21:1086–1090.

144. Cord JM. Oxygen-derived free radicals in postischemic tissue injury. N Engl J Med 1985;312:159–163.

145. Fridovich I. Biological effects of the superoxide radical. Arch Biochem Biophys 1984;247:1–11.

146. McCord JM. Oxygen-derived free radicals in post ischemic tissue injury. N Engl J Med 1985;312:159–163.
147. Cross CE, Halliwell B, Borish C, et al. Oxygen radicals and human disease. Ann Int Med 1987;107:526–545.
148. Busto R, Dietrich WD, Globus MYT, et al. The importance of brain temperature in cerebral ischemic injury. Stroke 1989;20:1113–1114.
149. Siesjo BK. Brain energy metabolism. New York: Wiley, 1978.
150. Hass W. Beyond cerebral blood flow, metabolism, and ischemic thresholds: an examination of the role of calcium in the initiation of cerebral infarction. In: Meyer J, Lechner H, Reivich M, et al., eds. Cerebral vascular disease: proceedings of the Tenth International Salzburg Conference. Excerpta Medica (Amsterdam) 1981;3:3–17.
151. Siesjo BK, Bengtsson F. Calcium fluxes, calcium antagonists, and calcium-related pathology in brain ischemia, hypoglycemia and spreading depression: a unifying hypothesis. J Cereb Blood Flow Metab 1989;9:127–140.
152. Siesjo B. Historical overview: calcium, ischemia and death of brain cells. Ann NY Acad Sci 1988;522:638–661.
153. Dietrich W, Busto R, Ginsberg M, et al. Influence of functional activity on metabolic recovery following experimental ischemia. Neurology 1984;34(1): 261.
154. Simon RP, Swan JH, Griffiths T, et al. Blockade of N-methyl-D-aspartate receptors may protect against ischemic damage in the brain. Science 1984;226: 850–852.
155. Globus MY, Busto R, Dietrich WD, et al. Effect of ischemia on the in vivo release of striatal dopamine, glutamate and R-amino butyric acid studied by intracerebral microdialysis. J Neuro Chem 1988;51:1455–1464.
156. Olney JW. Excitotoxic mechanisms of neurotoxicity. In: Spencer PS, Schaumberg HH, eds. Experimental and clinical neurotoxicology. Baltimore: Williams & Wilkins, 1980:272–294.
157. Choi DW, Malulucci Gedde M, Kriegstein MR. Glutamate neurotoxicity in cortical cell culture. J Neurosci 1987;7:357–368.
158. Collins RC, Dobkin BH, Choi DW. Selective vulnerability of the brain: new insights into the pathophysiology of stroke. Ann Int Med 1989;110:992–1000.
159. Albers GW, Goldberg M, Choi D. N-methyl-D-aspartate antagonists: ready for clinical trial in brain ischemia? Ann Neurol 1989;25:398–403.
160. Pulsinelli WA, Levy DE, Sigsbee B, et al. Increased damage after ischemic stroke in patients with hyperglycemia with or without established diabetes mellitus. Am J Med 1983;74:540–544.
161. Helgason C. Blood glucose and stroke. Stroke 1988;19:1049–1053.
162. Adams HP, Olinger CP, Marler JR, et al. Comparison of admission serum glucose concentration with neurologic outcome in cerebral infarction. Stroke 1988;19:455–458.
163. Woo E, Ma JTC, Robinson JD, et al. Hyperglycemia is a stress response in acute stroke. Stroke 1988;19:1359–1364.
164. Woo E, Lam CWK, Kay R, et al. The influence of hyperglycemia and diabetes mellitus on immediate and 3-month morbidity and mortality after acute stroke. Arch Neurol 1990;47:1174–1177.
165. Safar P. Amelioration of post ischemic brain damage with barbiturates. Curr Concepts Cerebrovasc Dis (Stroke) 1980;15:1–5.

166. Black K, Weidler J, Jallad N, et al. Delayed pentobarbital therapy of acute focal cerebral ischemia. Stroke 1978;9:245–251.

167. Faden AI, Jacobs TP, Holaday JW. Opiate antagonist improves neurologic recovery after spinal injury. Science 1981;211:493–494.

168. Faden AI, Hallenbeck JM, Brown CQ. Treatment of experimental stroke: comparison of naloxone and thyrotropin releasing hormone. Neurology 1982;32: 1083–1087.

169. Hosobuchi Y, Baskins DS, Woo SK. Reversal of induced ischemic neurologic deficit in gerbils by the opiate antagonist naloxone. Science 1982;215:69–71.

170. Baskin DS, Hosobuchi Y. Naloxone reversal of ischemic neurological deficits in man. Lancet 1981;2:272–275.

171. Faden AI. Opiate antagonists in the treatment of stroke. Stroke 1984;15: 575–578.

172. Argentino C, Sacchetti ML, Toni D, et al. GM^1 ganglioside therapy in acute ischemic stroke. Stroke 1989;20:1143–1149.

173. Leon A, Lipartiti M, Seren MS, et al. Hypoxic–ischemic damage and the neuroprotective effects of GM^1 ganglioside. Stroke 1990;21(Suppl 3);95–97.

174. Kontos HA: Oxygen radicals in cerebral ischemia. In: Ginsberg MD, Dietrich WD, eds. Cerebrovascular disease. New York: Raven Press, 1989:365–371.

175. Chan PH, Chu L, Chen SF, et al. Reduced neurotoxicity in transgenic mice overexpressing human copper–zinc–superoxide dismutage. Stroke 1990;21 (Suppl 3):80–82.

176. Hall E, Pazara KE, Braughler JM, et al. Nonsteroidal lazaroid U78517F in models of focal and global ischemia. Stroke 1990;21(Suppl 3):83–87.

177. Hall ED, Pazara KE. Effects of novel 21-amino steroid antioxidants on post ischemic neuronal degeneration. In: Ginsberg MD, Dietrich WD, eds. Cerebrovascular disease. New York: Raven Press, 1989:387–391.

178. Meldrum B. Excitotoxicity in ischemia: an overview. In: Ginsberg MD, Dietrich WD, eds. Cerebrovascular diseases. New York: Raven Press, 1989:47–60.

179. Marcoux FW, Probert AW, Weber ML. Hypoxic neuronal injury in tissue culture is associated with delayed calcium accumulation. Stroke 1990;21 (Suppl 3):71–74.

180. Goldberg M, Choi DW. Intracellular free calcium increases in cultured cortical neurons deprived of oxygen and glucose. Stroke 1990;21(Suppl 3):75–77.

181. Catsman-Beirevoets C, Harskamp F. Compulsive pre-sleep behavior and apathy due to bilateral thalamic stroke: response to bromocriptine. Neurology 1988;38:647–648.

182. Albert ML, Bachman D, Morgan A, et al. Pharmacotherapy for aphasia. Neurology 1988;38:877–879.

183. Fleet WS, Watson RT, Valenstein E, et al. Dopamine agonist therapy for neglect in humans. Neurology 1986;36(Suppl):347.

184. Barrett K. Treating organic abulia with bromocriptine and lisuride: four case studies. J Neurol Neurosurg Psychiatry 1991;54:718–721.

185. Feeney DM, Gonzalez A, Law WA. Amphetamine, haloperidol and experience interact to affect the rate of recovery after motor cortex injury. Science 1982;217:855–857.

186. Houda DA, Feeney DM. Haldoperidol blocks amphetamine induced recovery of binocular depth perception after bilateral visual cortex abilities in the cat. Proc West Pharmacol Soc 1985;28:209–211.

187. Davis JN, Crisostomo EA, Duncan P, et al. Amphetamine and physical therapy facilitate recovery of function from stroke: correlative animal and human studies. In: Raichle ME, Powers W, eds. Cerebrovascular diseases. New York: Raven Press, 1987:297–304.

188. Goldstein LB. Amphetamine-facilitated functional recovery after stroke. In: Ginsberg MD, Dietrich WD, eds. Cerebrovascular diseases. New York: Raven Press, 1989:303–308.

189. Goldstein LB. Pharmacology of recovery after stroke. Stroke 1990;21(Suppl 3):139–142.

190. Hernandez TC, Kiefel J, Barth TM, et al. Disruption and facilitation of recovery of behavioral function: implication of the gamma-aminobutyric acid/benzodiazepine receptor complex. In: Ginsberg MD, Dietrich WD, eds. Cerebrovascular diseases. New York: Raven Press, 1989:327–334.

191. Goldstein LB, Davis JN. Physician prescribing patterns following hospital admission for ischemic cerebrovascular disease. Neurology 1988;38:1806–1809.

192. Ropper AH, Kennedy SK, Zervas NT, eds. Neurological and neurosurgical intensive care. Baltimore: University Park Press, 1983.

193. Caplan LR. Intracerebral hemorrhage. In: Tyler H, Dawson D, eds. Current neurology. Boston: Houghton Mifflin, 1979:185–205.

194. Zervas N, Hedley-White J. Successful treatment of cerebral herniation in five patients. N Engl J Med 1973;286:1075–1077.

195. Klatzo I. Neuropathological aspects of brain edema. J Neuropathol Exp Neurol 1967;26:1–14.

196. Newkirk T, Tourtellotte W, Reinglass J. Prolonged control of increased intracranial pressure with glycerin. Arch Neurol 1972;27:95–96.

197. Frank MS, Nahata MC, Hilty MD. Glycerol: a review of its pharmacology, pharmacokinetics, adverse reactions and clinical use. Pharmacotherapy 1981; 1:147–160.

198. Fishman R. Steroids in the treatment of brain edema. N Engl J Med 1982; 306:359–360.

199. Anderson D, Cranford R. Corticosteroids in ischemic stroke. Stroke 1979; 10:68–71.

200. O'Brien M. Ischemic cerebral edema: a review. Stroke 1979;10:623–628.

201. Langfitt T. Conservative care of intracranial hemorrhage. In: Thompson R, Green J, eds. Advances in neurology: vol 16. stroke. New York: Raven Press, 1977:169–180.

202. Kuroiwa M, Shibutani M, Okeda R. Blood–brain barrier disruption and exacerbation of ischemic brain edema after restoration of blood flow in experimental focal cerebral ischemia. Acta Neuropathol 1988;76:62–70.

203. Mulley G, Wilcox R, Mitchell J. Dexamethasone in acute stroke. Br Med J 1978;2:994–996.

204. Lehrich J, Winkler G, Ojemann R. Cerebellar infarction with brainstem compression: diagnosis and surgical treatment. Arch Neurol 1970;22:490–498.

205. Feeley MP. Cerebellar infarction. Neurosurg 1979;4:7–11.

206. Delashaw JB, Broaddus WC, Kassell NF, et al. Treatment of right hemispheric cerebral infarction by hemicraniotomy. Stroke 1990;21:874–881.
207. Fujita K, Kusonoki T, Noda M, et al. Normal pressure hydrocephalus (NPH) following subarachnoid hemorrhage (SAH): clinical considerations of CT and development of hydrocephalus after SAH. Brain and Nerve 1981;33:845–851.
208. Greenberg J, Shubick D, Shenkin H. Acute hydrocephalus in cerebellar infarct and hemorrhage. Neurology 1961;11:697–700.
209. Khan M, Polyzoidis K, Adegbite A, et al. Massive cerebellar infarction: "conservative" management. Stroke 1983;14:745–751.

PART II

Stroke Syndromes

CHAPTER 6

Large-Vessel Occlusive Disease of the Anterior Circulation

Occlusive lesions of the large extracranial and intracranial arteries share important epidemiological, etiological, and pathological features, and common therapeutic principles are applicable. Most of these general features are discussed in the introductory section of this book. In this chapter, the specific clinical and laboratory aspects of occlusive disease of each of the commonly involved arteries are analyzed. An example of a typical patient is usually included, to illustrate common findings.

Occlusion or Stenosis of the Internal Carotid Artery

Internal Carotid Artery Disease at Its Origin

The modern era in ischemic cerebrovascular disease began in 1951, with the key report of Fisher that called attention to the clinical findings associated with occlusion of the ICA in the neck.[1] Previously, ischemic strokes in the anterior circulation were invariably attributed to MCA occlusion. In this report, Fisher called attention to warning episodes preceding stroke, which he dubbed TIAs. At the time of Fisher's report, angiography required a surgical cutdown, and only single-frame hand-pulled films were available. The advent of safer and more widespread angiography led, during the next decades, to increased recognition of the frequency of disease of the ICA in the neck. Newer noninvasive techniques now make possible reliable detection of carotid artery lesions in outpatients.

Increased zeal for surgical correction has accompanied the improved diagnostic capability. Improved anesthesia, advanced surgical techniques, and more vascular surgeons have caused an explosion in the number of operative procedures performed on the carotid arteries. In 1983, an estimated 72,000 carotid endarterectomies were performed in the United States, making it one of the three most common surgical procedures. In 1984, more than

103,000 endarterectomies were performed in the United States.[2,3] After 1987, the number of endarterectomies began to decrease, probably in response to widespread concern about the indications, utility, and complications of the procedure.[4,5] Morbidity and mortality figures vary widely among surgeons and medical centers, even within the same city.[2,6,7] Many question whether too many surgeons are performing too many endarterectomies. In 1991, reports of the results of controlled trials[8,9] showed an important therapeutic benefit of endarterectomy in symptomatic patients with high-grade stenosis, which has given the procedure more credibility and will surely be an impetus for more vascular surgery in the future. Later in this chapter, I return to the important question of treatment after reviewing the epidemiological, clinical, and laboratory features of ICA occlusive disease in the neck.

> A 58-year-old man, HL, awakened with a numb and weak left hand. He had had a myocardial infarction six years earlier and continued to have angina pectoris on moderate exertion. When he walked more than two blocks, he developed pain in the left calf, which abated if he stopped to rest.

The major cause of ICA occlusive disease in the neck is atherosclerotic narrowing of the vessel. The lesion usually begins in the distal CCA and extends to the proximal few centimeters of the ICA and the ECA, almost always more severely narrowing the ICA. This lesion is found more often in whites than in blacks or Asians, and in men more than women.[10,11] Occlusive disease of the large systemic vessels, especially the coronary, iliac, and femoral arteries, often accompanies carotid atherosclerosis. Coexisting angina pectoris, myocardial infarction, and limb claudication are common.[12] Risk factors for the development of proximal ICA disease are similar to those for coronary artery disease and include hypertension, diabetes, and hypercholesterolemia. Mortality in patients with ICA disease is usually cardiac, so attention is appropriately focused on the heart, as well as on the brain and its circulation.

> Although HL failed to volunteer other symptoms, direct questioning revealed several important warning signs. In the months before presentation, he had two brief episodes of transient obscuration of vision in his right eye. A dark shade descended from above, rather quickly blocking vision completely on one occasion and obscuring only the upper half of vision during the other episode. The attacks were brief, lasting less than a minute each. He also had three episodes of transient neurological dysfunction, consisting of stumbling because of his left leg giving way, slurred speech associated with numbness of the left face, and numbness of the left arm, hand, and face, respectively. The initial episode was 3 months earlier, the most recent 3 days earlier. In the weeks before presentation, he noted unaccustomed frequent headaches.

Atherosclerotic plaques gradually narrow the ICA lumen. Ulceration, attachment of platelet nidi and clot to crevices in plaques, and hemorrhage into plaques all become more common as the artery becomes stenosed. Plugs of platelets and thrombin may detach from the vessel wall and embolize to distal vessels, causing transient or prolonged neurological dysfunction. Reduction in blood flow can also lead to periodic insufficiency in distal perfusion. For these reasons, TIAs often occur as the vessel narrows, thus warning of an impending stroke. Many times, when an artery occludes, adequate collateral circulation develops, and no permanent neurological damage ensues.

The single most important clue to an ICA localization of the occlusive process is an attack of transient monocular blindness. Most often, the visual loss is described as a dimming, darkening, or obscuration. An apparent shade or curtain usually falls from above but may move from the side like a theater curtain. After a brief period of seconds or a few minutes the curtain lifts or recedes, usually leaving no permanent visual loss. These attacks of transient visual obscuration are caused by decreased blood flow through the ophthalmic artery, the first tributary of the ICA. Amaurosis fugax occurs when the lesion affects the ICA proximal to the ophthalmic artery (in the neck or proximal carotid siphon) or affects the ophthalmic artery itself. Diminished flow or pressure in the ophthalmic artery is a clue to the presence of carotid artery disease. In migraine, the most common differential diagnostic consideration, patients usually describe brightness, glittering, flickering, and movement within the visual field that lasts 15 to 30 minutes and is seldom monocular. Occasionally, patients with severe ICA occlusive disease report unilateral spells of reduced vision after exposure to bright light, a type of retinal claudication.[13] In some patients with bilateral ICA disease, the transient visual loss can be bilateral. As in the patient described, individuals may not volunteer information about temporary loss of vision, thinking it completely unrelated to the present problem. The physician must *directly* and *repeatedly ask* about *specific symptoms* of ocular or brain ischemia.

Episodes of hemispheral ischemia are also usually brief. In some patients, attacks are quite varied and include different deficits in different limbs during individual attacks, while in other patients, the spells are quite stereotyped. In some patients with critical stenosis, the attacks are very frequent and may be precipitated by suddenly standing or by a drop in blood pressure.[14] Frequent, very brief machine-gun-like attacks usually mean low flow due to proximal severe stenosis, whereas emboli generally produce longer, less frequent attacks. In disease of larger vessels such as the ICA, TIAs may occur during a period of months, as compared to a briefer span of hours, days, or a week in patients with lacunar infarction due to disease of smaller blood vessels. As the ICA narrows, collateral circulation develops, leading to dilation of arteries and frequent headache. It is unusual, however, for headache to be the only symptom; in my experience, headache is usually accompanied by TIAs. The common symptoms of ICA disease in the neck are listed in Table 6.1.

On examination, HL had moderate weakness of the left arm, slight weakness of the left psoas muscle, and severe weakness of the left hand. Position sense was

TABLE 6.1
Symptoms of Internal Carotid Artery Disease

Attacks of transient monocular blindness
TIAs, sometimes variegated and occurring during a span of weeks or months
Frequent unaccustomed headache
Commonly associated history of coronary or peripheral vascular disease

decreased in the left hand, and HL could neither accurately localize left-limb touch stimuli nor recognize objects in the left hand. He drew a clock poorly (Figure 6.1, top) and also copied inaccurately (Figure 6.1, bottom). A soft high-pitched bruit was audible at the right carotid bifurcation in the neck. A right Horner's syndrome was noted.

Physical examination of the blood vessels and eyes may yield important clues to an ICA location of the lesion (Table 6.2). Palpation of the neck is not helpful unless the CCA is occluded, in which case there will be no carotid pulse on that side. Even when the ICA is occluded, the CCA pulse is usually transmitted to the ICA in the neck. The presence of a typical *bruit* (i.e., a high-pitched, long, very focal sound heard loudest over the carotid bifurcation) is virtually diagnostic of localized ICA disease. However, in many cases, flow is so severely diminished that no bruit is audible. When a bruit at the bifurcation is also audible over the ipsilateral eye, the physician can be confident that the bruit is of ICA origin and that the artery is patent. A bruit also can arise from the proximal ECA, in which case it usually radiates toward the jaw and can be diminished by pressure on ECA branches.[15]

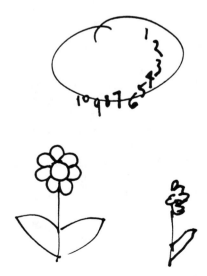

FIGURE 6.1   At top is a clock drawn by a patient with right parietal lobe lesion. At bottom is the patient's copy (right) of a daisy drawn by the examiner (left).

TABLE 6.2
Signs of Internal Carotid Artery Disease

Neck
  High-pitched, focal, long bruit at bifurcation
Face
  Increased angular, brow, cheek (ABC)[16] pulses
  Frontal artery sign[17]
  Increase in superficial temporal artery
Retina
  Cholesterol crystals[18]
  Platelet plugs[19]
  Retinal infarcts
  Reduced caliber of arteries
  Less severe hypertensive changes
  Venous stasis retinopathy[20,21]
  Reduced retinal-artery pressure

When the ICA is occluded or severely stenosed, ECA collaterals may feed into the orbit and may be palpable at the angular, brow, and cheek (ABC) regions (see Figure 1.1 in Chapter 1).[16,17]

Ischemia to the iris or retina on the side of the carotid lesion is another helpful clue. Retinal arteries on the side of the carotid lesion may be reduced in caliber or may show fewer hypertensive changes than their counterparts in the opposite retina. White, fluffy exudates or focal retinal atrophy can represent infarction. Small cholesterol crystal emboli are highly refractile bodies, which usually lodge at bifurcations of retinal arteries.[18] White platelet plugs can also be transiently seen within retinal arteries.[19] *Venous stasis retinopathy* is another descriptive term for the ophthalmoscopic appearance found in patients with ICA occlusion and is characterized by microaneurysms, small-dot retinal hemorrhages, and dilated dark retinal veins, sometimes of irregular caliber.[20,21] This disorder resembles diabetic retinopathy but can usually be distinguished by unilaterality, location in the midportion of the retina, and its association with low retinal arterial pressure, as measured by ODM, OPG, and diminished ophthalmic-blood-flow velocities by TCD. The presence of venous stasis retinopathy always means that flow reduction in the ophthalmic artery is severe and long-standing.

Neurological findings are caused by infarction of brain regions within the ICA circulation. Signs in patients with ICA disease are difficult to separate clinically from those in patients with intrinsic lesions of the MCA.[22] By far the commonest loci of infarction are within the MCA territory. Weakness is common and usually affects the contralateral hand and face more than the leg. When sensory loss is present, it usually is of the cortical type, with loss of position sense, point localization, and stereognosis on the opposite side of the body. Again, the hand and face often show more sensory abnormalities than the trunk or lower extremity. When bilateral simultaneous tactile stimuli are presented to the arms, the stimulus contralateral to the lesion is often not reported by the patient. Neglect of the opposite side of visual space and an attentional hemianopia are also common findings, especially when the infarct is in the right cerebral hemisphere. Poor drawing and copying, impersistence with tasks, diminished emotional responsiveness, and *anosognosia* (lack of awareness of the deficit) frequently also accompany right ICA territory infarction,[23,24] and aphasia is a common sequel to left-sided infarction. Occasionally, the infarct will be predominantly in the territory of the anterior cerebral artery (ACA), and foot, leg, and shoulder weakness will predominate. Very rarely, when the posterior cerebral artery (PCA) is supplied directly by the ICA, an infarct caused by ICA occlusion can lie solely within the PCA territory and can be manifested by a hemianopia without other signs.[25]

A duplex scan was performed first. B-mode showed some flat plaques within the distal right CCA and severe atherosclerotic disease at the right ICA origin, with near occlusion (Figure 6.2a). The Doppler frequencies also suggested high-grade stenosis of the right ICA (Figures 6.2b and 6.2c). The left carotid artery showed only minor disease. TCD examination revealed lower flow velocities in the right ICA siphon and the right MCA and ACA. CT showed a hypodensity in the cortical parietal lobe affecting the postcentral gyrus and superior parietal lobule (Figure 6.3). Cerebral angiography by femoral artery catheterization using the Seldinger technique demonstrated severe, irregular narrowing of the ICA at its origin, with a residual lumen of approximately 1 mm (Figure 6.4). The carotid siphon and MCA were normal, but there was a branch occlusion of one of the parietal branches of the superior trunk of the MCA. Echocardiography and Holter monitoring were normal.

Noninvasive diagnostic tests have been discussed in Chapter 4. In this patient, ultrasonography suggested a severe flow-reducing lesion at the ICA origin. Because of the likelihood that the lesion would require surgery and the necessity of opacifying the intracranial vessels, it was decided to proceed with standard angiography. Alternatively, magnetic resonance angiography (MRA) might have adequately shown the lesion. Angiography confirmed and further quantified the nature of the stenotic lesion.

In patients with ICA atherosclerotic disease, there are several frequent patterns of disease, which are diagrammed in Figure 6.5. When the ICA is occluded, the vessel may be absent angiographically or may show a pointed, tapering, or rounded stump.[26] Barnett and colleagues have called attention to embolization from the stump of previously occluded carotid arteries.[27] Stenotic lesions can be ulcerated, smooth, or very irregular, and the lesions may be long and tapered or may slope abruptly like a shelf. B-mode scans and color Doppler flow imaging (CDFI) studies of the carotid origin can help define the nature of plaques, the presence of ulceration, and the dynamics of

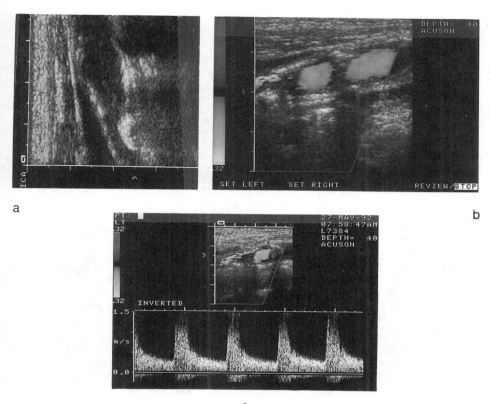

FIGURE 6.2   Ultrasound studies. (a) B-mode from Duplex scan, hard plaque is seen narrowing the ICA (arrow); in this view, the artery is narrowed about 60%; in other views, the narrowing is more severe. (b) Color Doppler flow imaging showing the stenosis and change in flow (arrow). (c) Doppler spectrum from Duplex scan corresponding to (a). High blood flow velocities through area of stenosis. (Figure kindly supplied by Professor Michael Hennerici.)

flow. Calcific smooth plaques are less often the source of intra-arterial emboli and usually do not show rapid progression, while irregular, ulcerated soft plaques often progress and are more often the source of emboli. When angiography is complete, it is often possible to detect embolic occlusion of the MCA or its branches, so-called occlusio supra occlusionem.[28]

Imaging Findings in Patients with ICA Disease

CT scans of patients with carotid occlusion or severe stenosis show several common patterns of distribution of infarction (Figure 6.6): watershed or border-zone infarction between the territories of the ACA and the MCA and between the MCA and the PCA; subcortical white-matter infarcts; wedge-

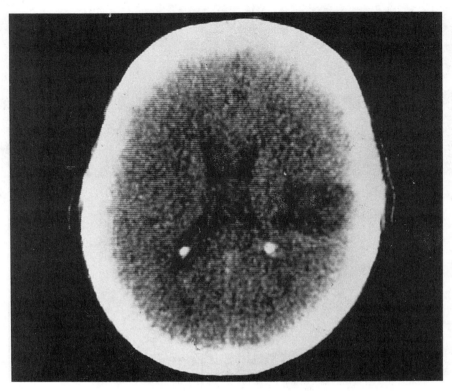

FIGURE 6.3   CT showing an infarct in the right parietal lobe (on right of figure).

shaped pial-artery territory infarcts; and infarction of the basal ganglia and lentiform nucleus.[28] The border zone and subcortical white-matter lesions are probably due to reduced flow, whereas the pial and basal ganglia infarcts are due to emboli to the main-stem MCA or its superior or inferior trunk or penetrating artery branches. In my experience, watershed infarction and large superficial infarcts in the MCA territory were the commonest lesions found on CT in patients with severe ICA obstructive disease.[22] The mechanism of stroke in the patient HL was a small superior parietal-lobe infarct caused by an embolus from the ICA stenosis in the neck. Cardiac testing failed to show an alternative embologenic donor source in the heart.

HL was placed on heparin therapy and after 1 week of treatment was switched to warfarin. PT was maintained at 1.5 times the normal control values. At 6 weeks, an uncomplicated carotid endarterectomy was performed. Blood pressure was carefully monitored postoperatively in an ICU, but it did not become elevated. The patient had minimal residual neurological signs of clumsiness and slight numbness of his left hand but was able to return to his former work.

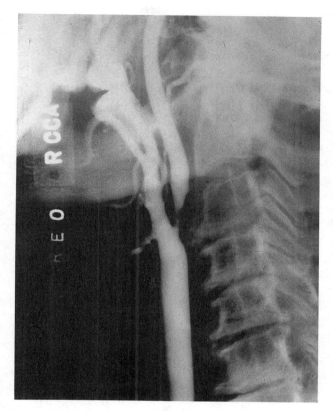

FIGURE 6.4 Right carotid angiogram: lateral view, showing very severe stenosis of the proximal ICA.

In my present practice, choice of treatment for patients with ICA disease in the neck depends on

1. severity of the stenosis
2. presence of a recent cerebral infarct, as determined either by a persistent clinical deficit or an appropriate CT or MRI lesion
3. general health of the patient, especially any contraindication to surgery, warfarin anticoagulation, or agents that decrease platelet agglutination
4. the morbidity and mortality record of the surgeon who would undertake surgery
5. the attitude of the patient and family toward the situation after the alternative courses of action have been discussed

I now consider symptomatic patients with TIA or small nondisabling strokes who have various ICA lesions.

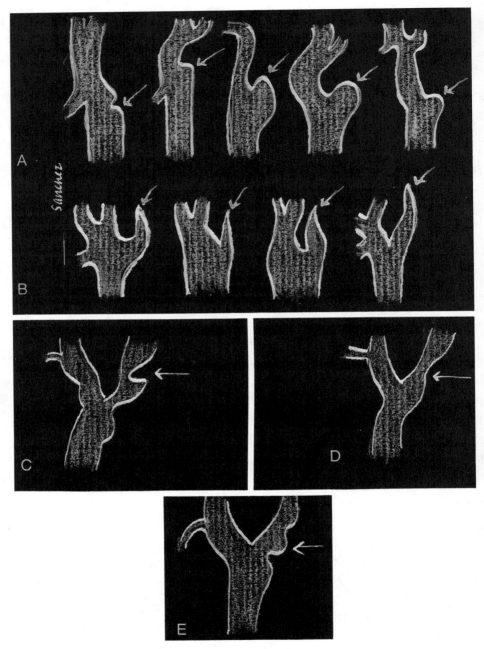

FIGURE 6.5   Examples of appearance on angiography of carotid artery lesions: (A) rounded stump, (B) pointed stump, (C) shelf plaque, (D) regular plaque, and (E) ulcerated plaque. (After Pessin MS, Duncan G, Davis K, et al. Angiographic appearance of carotid occlusion in acute stroke. Stroke 1980;11:485–487; reprinted with permission.)

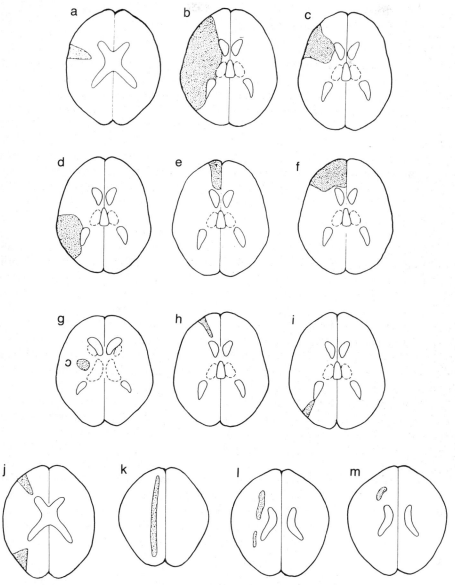

FIGURE 6.6   Most common CT locations of infarcts in the anterior circulation—infarcts are shown by hatched gray: (a) wedge-shaped MCA infarct, (b) entire MCA territory, (c) superior-division MCA, (d) inferior division MCA, (e) ACA, (f) ACA and MCA, (g) striatocapsular infarct, (h) wedge-shaped anterior watershed infarct, (i) wedge-shaped posterior watershed infarct, (j) anterior and posterior watershed infarcts, (k) linear watershed infarct, (l) ovular deep watershed infarct, (m) small white-matter watershed infarct. (From Caplan LR. Cerebrovascular disease: larger artery occlusive disease. In: Appel S, ed., Current Neurology, Vol 8, Chicago: Year-book Medical 1988, 179–226; reprinted with permission.)

*Complete Occlusion of the Internal Carotid Artery
in the Neck*

I do not suggest surgery. When the ICA occludes, clot propagates quickly high into the neck, often to the carotid siphon and beyond. Because there are no ICA branches in the neck, collateral flow patterns promote extension of clot toward the first branch, the ophthalmic artery. It is technically difficult to open the completely occluded ICA, and attempts to suction the clot can lead to distal embolization. If it were known that an occlusion had become complete minutes or a few hours before, as might happen after angiography, exploration of the neck would be reasonable. That circumstance is very rare in my experience. Angiography can yield clues as to the extent of the occlusive thrombosis. If opacification of the contralateral ICA shows retrograde filling of the occluded ICA down into the neck, it is more likely that the surgeon might be able to open the ICA surgically.

I treat patients with bed rest, keeping the head flat or slightly lower than the feet, to augment blood flow to the head. I try to avoid hypotension, and I have used agents such as ephedrine, which raise blood pressure in some patients. I avoid antihypertensive drugs during the first 1 to 2 weeks unless the blood pressure is in the malignant range—for example, greater than 225/125 torr. If the patient is normotensive and there is no contraindication to the use of anticoagulants, I use intravenous heparin, followed by warfarin for a short period (2 to 6 weeks), to attempt to prevent embolization of fresh clot and to discourage clot propagation. After this period, I do not use anticoagulants but do use aspirin in doses of one 300-mg tablet per day.

Caution must be exercised in the diagnosis of complete ICA occlusion because a severe reduction in flow can lead to collapse of the artery above the high-grade block. Angiography produces a picture that closely resembles occlusion, so called pseudo-occlusion,[29] but late films usually show a trickle of dye ascending anterograde toward the siphon. CT in cross-section of the high neck, after contrast, can show blood in the ICA, documenting preserved anterograde flow.[30] CDFI also sometimes visualizes flow through a pseudo-occlusion not seen with standard angiography. In pseudo-occlusion, the residual flow, albeit small, makes it possible for the surgeon to open the vessel. Patients with pseudo-occlusion are considered to have severe stenosis.

In patients with ICA occlusion, the deficit usually develops at or shortly after the time of occlusion, when embolization and low flow are maximal. A chronic low-flow state, so-called misery perfusion,[31] occurs but only rarely persists. Occasionally, patients with known ICA occlusion develop transient symptoms, especially if they become hypotensive from overzealous antihypertensive treatment or from dehydration or hypovolemia. The commonest symptoms are occular—transient obscuration of vision in the ipsilateral eye—or relate to the contralateral limbs. An unusual, but very characteristic, sign of hypoperfusion is a so-called limb-shaking

TIA.[32,33] Usually when standing or active, the patient develops a tremor with impressive shaking and oscillation of the arm and hand contralateral to the occluded ICA. Occasionally, the lower extremity is involved. The shaking stops when the patient sits or lies down and is due to ischemia rather than a seizure.[32] I have not referred patients with ICA occlusion for ECA–ICA bypass but would consider doing so if there were either persistent recurrent ischemic attacks or if PET, SPECT, or other new technology documented persistent misery perfusion. Sequential TCD studies of blood-flow velocity in the MCA and ACA, especially after acetazolamide infusion, also yield information about distal flow and the reserve capacity of the carotid tributaries to dilate. These laboratory techniques are discussed in Chapter 4.

Severe Stenosis of the Internal Carotid Artery in the Neck

In my opinion, this lesion, when symptomatic, requires surgery unless there is a severe disabling distal infarction. The 1991 reported results of the North American[8] and European trials[9] support this strategy. What constitutes a severe stenosis? There are two principal criteria: the degree of anatomical narrowing of the artery, and the presence of significant reduction in flow velocity or pressure in tributary vessels, as shown by TCD or OPG. Although it has been customary to report arterial narrowing in percentage, I prefer to think in terms of millimeters of residual lumen for two reasons. First, the size of arteries, especially the nuchal ICA, varies greatly, ranging from 7 to 15 mm in an arteriographic study.[34] Narrowing of a congenitally small lumen by 50 percent would be less well tolerated than reduction of a large lumen by the same percentage. By reporting percentage, the original size of the lumen is canceled. Second, to calculate percentage, the measured residual lumen in millimeters is divided by the projected or supposed normal-sized lumen at the same site. Using two numbers, one of which is not directly measured and admittedly is an approximation, is less reliable and less consistent than simply reporting the smallest residual luminal diameter. A residual lumen of less than 1.5 mm invariably represents severe stenosis and nearly always impedes distal flow. When the severely stenotic ICA is examined histologically, compound ulcers are often found. Although these lesions may also be found in nonstenosed vessels, they become more frequent as the artery narrows.

When patients have TIAs but no persistent neurological deficit and severe stenosis of the ICA with a residual lumen of less than 1.5 mm, I believe that carotid endarterectomy should be performed urgently. If there is evidence of infarction—either persistent abnormal neurological signs or symptoms, or a new infarct on CT—I prefer to wait 4 to 6 weeks before surgery because of the possibility of ICH following endarterectomy.[35–37] Many instances of postendarterectomy ICH are explained by hypertension following manipulation of the carotid receptors in the neck.[38–40] Careful postoperative monitoring of blood pressure in an ICU and careful treatment of hypertension if it develops should prevent ICH.

When there is a persistent deficit, I prefer to use heparin, then warfarin, keeping the PT at 1.5 times the normal, and then I wait 6 weeks, as long as the patient remains stable or improves. If, however, there are further attacks or worsening during this waiting interval, I suggest endarterectomy without further delay because, in my experience, severe deficits commonly develop if surgery is not performed in these instances. Also, if the patient appears to have a progressing stroke that worsens during observation in the hospital and continues to progress despite heparin therapy, I urge emergency correction of a critical ICA stenosis. Some patients improve dramatically immediately after surgery.

In patients with severe ICA stenosis, if surgery cannot be performed or if the patient refuses operation, I choose to anticoagulate with warfarin, keeping the PT about 1.5 times the control values. The duration of anticoagulation is uncertain and should be individualized. I have begun to use the results of sequential duplex scans to guide the duration of treatment. Arteries with tight stenosis often occlude on follow-up scans, most often without new symptoms.[41,42] During the 4 to 6 weeks after occlusion, thrombi become organized and adherent, after which embolization is rare. I switch from warfarin to one aspirin per day 4 to 6 weeks after scans show complete occlusion. While the lumen remains narrowed but patent, I continue warfarin. In some patients, plaques seem to regress and the lumen may become less narrowed. In these individuals, a switch to aspirin also seems logical. No studies have been undertaken to show the results of the strategy I have outlined.

Plaque Disease of the Internal Carotid Artery in the Neck, with Less Than Severe Stenosis

I suggest prophylactic treatment with agents that decrease platelet aggregation and avoid warfarin anticoagulation and surgery. While it is true that ulceration can occur in nonstenotic lesions and that ulcers can be the source of artery-to-artery embolization, this occurs less frequently in patients without severe stenosis. In the presence of a severe stenosing lesion, the physician can be more confident that this is the responsible lesion rather than another small plaque. Furthermore, the natural history of plaques has not been well studied. They may reendothelialize and heal. Plaques are ubiquitous in individuals over the age of 40 years, and present angiographic and noninvasive techniques do not infallibly predict the presence of ulceration on histological examination. Agents that decrease platelet aggregation would theoretically be most effective when there are nonstenosing plaques and high-velocity flow continues.

Because aspirin is likely to be safer and perhaps as effective for these lesions, at present, I prefer it to surgery. Aspirin also has theoretical advantages over warfarin, which probably works best in slow-moving vascular streams to prevent red thrombi. At present, I prefer aspirin to other agents. The dose of aspirin is as-yet uncertain. I use one 300-mg tablet per day but await better studies of the effectiveness of various dosages in patients with known carotid lesions. An accurate reproducible in vitro test of the effectiveness of the platelet antiaggregants might lead clinicians to titrate the dose in individual patients and so monitor effectiveness of the drug. I now reserve ticlopidine for those patients who cannot take aspirin or who have had recurrent ischemia while taking aspirin, and those in whom studies show that aspirin does not affect their platelet functions.

For these reasons, I presently choose aspirin or other platelet antiaggregants for nonstenosing plaque disease, but I believe that more data on the relative merits and complications of surgery, antiplatelet aggregants, and warfarin in patients with plaque disease are needed. When plaques are very shallow, the decision to use platelet antiaggregant agents is clear. However, as plaques become larger and more irregular or clearly ulcerated, and luminal narrowing approaches 3 to 1.5 mm, the therapeutic decision becomes more difficult and should be individualized. In a young patient with a lesion in this gray zone of near-critical stenosis with several TIAs, who is a good surgical candidate, I probably would choose surgery.

Clot

Some patients with atherosclerotic plaques in the neck, with or without severe stenosis, have thrombi that are grossly visible on angiography.[43,44] These patients should be treated urgently. In a review of prior cases of patients with intraluminal clot, both surgery and warfarin anticoagulation were effective in preventing further stroke,[43] but clot recurred in patients with coagulopathy after surgery.[44] The blood coagulation profiles of these patients should be carefully studied prior to treatment.

Asymptomatic Patients with ICA Disease in the Neck

The preceding discussion of treatment concerned symptomatic patients with TIA or stroke. In recent years, it has become commonplace to document ICA disease in the neck in patients who have no apparent CNS symptoms. The commonest circumstances provoking carotid artery investigation are an audible neck bruit or imminent surgical procedures on the aorta, coronary, or peripheral-limb vessels. Some cases are discovered at angiography for indications other than vascular disease or when angiographic study documents ICA disease on the asymptomatic side. Should these lesions be repaired before symptoms develop?

My present opinion is generally that asymptomatic patients should not undergo carotid endarterectomy. Present data indicate that these patients do not have an unusual risk of stroke during surgery on other major vessels. Furthermore, stroke is unusual without preceding TIAs. In most medical centers, the risk of surgery and angiography (probably about 6 percent combined morbidity and mortality)[45-47] is probably as great as, if not greater than, the risk of stroke without prior TIA.

Results of several studies of asymptomatic lesions are important to consider. In one series of 168 prospectively studied patients with known ICA stenosis, 26 patients (15 percent) had TIAs only; 3 had TIAs but refused surgery and had subsequent strokes; and just 1 patient developed sudden stroke without warning.[48] In another series of patients with carotid stenosis followed for 2 years, among 318 patients, 5 percent developed TIAs but only 2 patients had a stroke without a preceding TIA.[49] Sequential studies show that stenotic arteries often occlude without symptoms.[42]

In patients undergoing endarterectomy who have bilateral carotid artery stenosis, subsequent stroke on the unoperated side is also uncommon.[49] Even when a bruit is detected prior to elective surgery, the incidence of postoperative stroke is not increased.[50] Postoperative strokes are usually caused by cardiogenic emboli.

Treatment of asymptomatic patients, however, must be individualized. Some patients, when they are made aware of a definite risk of stroke, become quite anxious and psychologically tolerate the risk poorly. They would prefer the small gamble of an intraoperative complication to the sword that they sense hangs perpetually over them. In my opinion, the situation must be fully discussed with the patient and the benefits and risks of each possible therapy explained.

After such discussions, I usually advise the patient to join the Asymptomatic Carotid Artery Study (ACAS) presently in progress at our medical center.[51] Throughout North America, there are a number of other ongoing randomized trials of the utility of carotid endarterectomy in patients with ICA stenosis who have no associated symptoms. The American Academy of Neurology has urged physicians to enter all eligible patients in these trials.[52] If patients decline entry into trials, I advise them to take antiplatelet aggregants and do not use warfarin or suggest surgery unless ischemic symptoms develop. Mohr has reviewed the therapeutic dilemma of the patient with asymptomatic carotid disease in detail and has dispassionately outlined the factors to be considered in individual patients.[53] It is hoped that the anticipated results of the asymptomatic ICA stenosis trials will provide a more definitive guide to physicians and patients.

Internal Carotid Artery Occlusive Disease Intracranially

Narrowing and thrombotic occlusion of the ICA occur at the siphon far less frequently than at the ICA origin. The siphon includes the S-shaped portion of the carotid artery from its entry through the carotid foramen into the petrous bone to its exit from the cavernous sinus above the petrous clinoid.

The ophthalmic artery originates from the ICA within the siphon. Much less is known about the pathology of the artery in its entirely intraosseous course because the bone is seldom removed for study. Calcification of the ICA in the siphon is common.[54] Studies of groups of patients with ICA siphon disease document a high incidence of strokes, frequent coexistent extracranial vascular disease, and a high death rate from coronary disease.[55–58]

> RY, a 70-year-old man, had an attack of transient weakness of his right leg 1 week before awakening with weakness of the right foot and face, and with unaccustomed reluctance to speak. He repeated spoken language normally and comprehension of written and spoken language was good. There was a past history of angina pectoris, and a high-pitched focal bruit was audible over the right neck.

The epidemiology of carotid siphon disease is probably similar to ICA-origin disease, except that blacks have an unexpectedly high incidence of this lesion.[10] Accompanying disease at the ICA and VA origins is common. Tandem ICA origin and siphon disease occurred in 62 percent of the series of patients with siphon disease reported by Marzewski and colleagues.[55] TIAs are less frequent and fewer in number in patients with siphon disease, as compared to ICA-origin disease. The ratio of strokes to TIAs and of asymptomatic patients is higher in carotid-siphon disease.

The presence of amaurosis fugax depends on the level of the lesion in the siphon. In my experience, the occlusive lesion is most often distal to the ophthalmic artery origin, so that ICA siphon disease is an infrequent cause of transient monocular blindness. On examination, there are usually no signs of collateral circulation through the ECA vessels of the face, and the ocular and retinal pathologies discussed in ICA-origin disease are uncommon. I have, however, seen a number of patients with angiographically verified thrombotic occlusion of the carotid siphon who developed, days later, signs of decreased ophthalmic flow and reduced central retinal artery pressure—findings that were absent initially. The mechanism of delayed ophthalmic ischemia is retrograde extension of the clot below the ophthalmic branch, a phenomenon documented postmortem in patients with stenosis and thrombosis of the ICA siphon.[59] Retrograde extension of clot is, however, rare if the siphon occlusion is due to embolism.[59]

Too few patients have been well studied to allow a comparison of the topography and distribution of cerebral infarcts in patients with ICA-siphon disease, as compared to disease of the ICA origin or the MCA. My impression is that separate infarcts in portions of the ACA and MCA territories are more common in siphon disease. The leg is more often paretic in siphon disease, indicating ACA territory damage. Sometimes, the lesions affect the center of the ACA and MCA territories, causing weakness of the foot and face, with relative sparing of the hand, whereas in ICA-origin disease, upper-extremity weakness is most common.

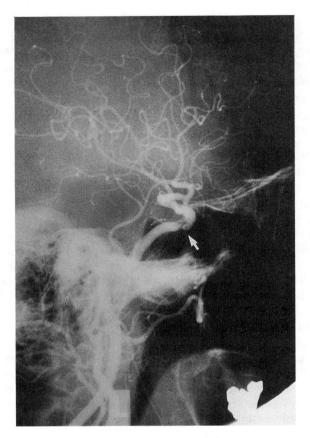

FIGURE 6.7   Carotid arteriogram: lateral view, showing stenosis of the left ICA in the siphon (white arrow).

In RY, a carotid duplex scan showed moderate stenosis (2.5 mm residual lumen) of the right ICA origin. TCD showed increased blood-flow velocities through the orbital window at the left carotid siphon and normal velocities in the MCA and ACA. Velocities in the right intracranial arteries were normal. Angiography by femoral catheterization revealed severe irregularity and stenosis of the left ICA siphon, the lesion beginning above the ophthalmic-artery origin (Figure 6.7). The left ICA origin had a shallow plaque, without stenosis. No definite distal-branch occlusion was seen. CT showed a small infarct in the paramedian frontal lobe.

The ultrasound studies confirmed severe siphon disease on the side appropriate to the symptoms and the CT lesion. The contralateral ICA-origin lesion was asymptomatic and not severe enough to reduce flow. The clinical signs of leg and foot weakness and transcortical motor aphasia were due to

ACA-territory ischemia. The infarct was due either to low flow with good MCA collaterals, or to embolism originating from the irregular siphon stenosis.

RY was given intravenous heparin and, after a slight increase in leg weakness during the first day, stabilized. Warfarin was begun on day 5, and on day 7, heparin was discontinued. The patient was maintained on warfarin therapy for 1 year, at which time he developed a fatal myocardial infarction.

Reviews in the 1980s confirm that ICA-siphon disease has a worse prognosis than ICA origin disease.[55–58] Late strokes and cardiac death are common. Lesions within the siphon cannot be approached surgically. Therapeutic alternatives include antiplatelet agglutinating agents, warfarin, and ECA–ICA bypass to MCA branches. There have been no prospective controlled studies to document fully the effectiveness or lack thereof of any medical treatment in patients with documented disease of the carotid siphon. In the ECA–ICA bypass study, there was no difference in outcome in patients with severe intracranial carotid artery occlusive disease who were treated by bypass or were treated medically.[60] ECA–ICA bypass shoud not be performed in patients with severe stenosis of surgically inaccessible vessels that still retain luminal patency. A patent shunt distal to an artery with low flow can further discourage flow through the stenosis, promoting thrombosis. Occlusion of stenotic vessels following a shunt has been documented in eight patients.[61,62] The thrombus could embolize distally, leading to cerebral infarction despite the presence of a shunt that delivers adequate flow. Since the results of the ECA–ICA bypass study have been published, I have not suggested bypass in patients with occlusion of the ICA siphon. There may rarely be patients with ICA siphon or MCA occlusion with chronic low perfusion and with stunned but not infarcted brain who might benefit from revascularization. Such could only be detected by sophisticated blood flow and metabolic studies using PET, SPECT, and TCD.

I suggest warfarin for those patients with tight ICA siphon stenosis and preserved anterograde flow who have no contraindication to anticoagulation. I reserve antiplatelet agglutinating agents such as aspirin for patients who have minor irregularity of the artery without severe impediment to flow. Recently, at the New England Medical Center, I have been entering patients with acute ICA-siphon occlusion into a research protocol using thrombolytic therapy (rtPA). I have no data to confirm or disprove the effectiveness of this therapeutic approach and welcome further studies of therapy in patients with ICA-siphon disease. As with disease of the ICA origin, attention should also be directed to the heart because of the high incidence of associated cardiac morbidity (as in the case of RY).

In some patients, there is associated severe disease of the ICA origin, in addition to the siphon stenosis. In these patients with tandem lesions, operation on the ICA in the neck is sometimes followed by apparent opening of the siphon lesion on follow-up angiography.[63] This could be explained by preoperative distal collapse or narrowing of the vessel due to diminished flow. In the face of complete occlusion of the ICA siphon, there is no point in opening an ICA origin stenosis. If, however, the ICA stenosis at the siphon is not critical, carotid endarterectomy of the more proximal ICA-origin lesion might greatly augment flow. In the presence of severe critical stenosis at both sites, often accompanied by stenosis of other vessels, I usually choose a trial of warfarin therapy before considering surgery.

Thrombotic occlusion of the supraclinoid carotid artery prior to its intracranial bifurcation into MCA and ACA branches (top of the carotid) does occur, but rarely. This portion of the ICA, often called the "T portion" because of its shape, is more often occluded by embolism.[64] In my experience, an unusual number of patients with a lesion at this site have had coagulation abnormalities, such as sickle-cell disease or circulating lupus anticoagulant (LA).[58]

Occlusion or Severe Stenosis of the Middle Cerebral Artery Stem or Its Major Upper and Lower Trunks

Occlusion of the MCA was a very common diagnosis in the era before angiography. After Fisher and others called attention to the high incidence of extracranial ICA disease[1] and angiography became prevalent, most patients who were formerly diagnosed as having MCA occlusion were found instead to have extracranial ICA disease. The vast majority of MCA occlusions were embolic, arising either from a proximal ICA plaque or from the heart.[12] These observations on the rarity of occlusive lesions in the intracranial anterior circulation were generated at hospitals with a predominance of white patients. Between the mid-1960s and early 1990s, studies of black[10,22,65-67] and Asian[65,68-72] patients have documented a higher incidence of intracranial occlusive disease of the MCA and its major trunk branches. Figure 6.8 shows the most common patterns of infarction in patients with MCA occlusions.

> A 48-year-old black woman, MR, awakened unable to speak and with weakness of her right face. These symptoms cleared during the day, but the next day, during the morning, she noted aphasia and weakness of her right limbs. She had a past history of slight hypertension but had no history of coronary or peripheral vascular disease.

In my experience, patients with MCA occlusive disease, when compared to patients with ICA disease, have more often been black, young, female, hypertensive, and diabetic.[10,22,65] They also have had a lower incidence of hypercholesterolemia and associated coronary and peripheral vascular disease. Patients of Japanese, Chinese, and Thai descent, as well as

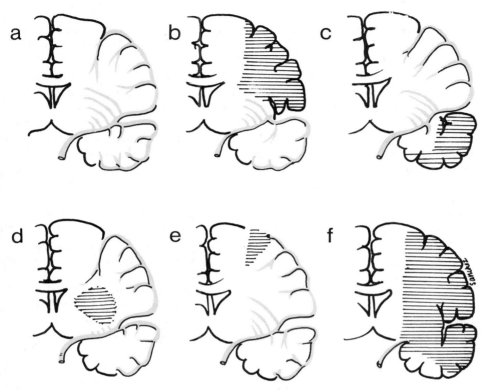

FIGURE 6.8 Common patterns of infarction with MCA occlusion: (a) diagram of the MCA in coronal section, (b) occlusion of the upper trunk of the MCA, (c) occlusion of the lower trunk of the MCA, (d) infarct of the deep basal ganglia, (e) wedge infarct in the pial territory, and (f) whole MCA occlusion.

diabetics and women taking contraceptive pills, probably share a propensity for MCA pathology with blacks. Although TIAs do occur in patients with MCA disease, they are probably less common than with ICA disease and occur during a shorter time span.[22] Of interest, the frequency of TIAs in patients with MCA disease seems also to vary with race. In four predominantly white patient series of cases of MCA occlusive disease, TIAs were a more frequent presentation than was stroke.[58,73-76] The TIA/stroke ratios in these studies were 15/1,[73] 15/6,[74] 13/11,[75] and 9/4.[76] In contrast, the TIA/stroke ratio in a predominantly black patient series was 4/16,[22] and it was 8/28 in a series of Japanese patients.[77] Smoking was a very important risk factor in the only study that reported its incidence.[72] In this study, 80 percent of patients with MCA occlusion and 72 percent of patients with MCA stenosis had a history of cigarette smoking.[72] Because the vascular lesion is intracranial and, of course, beyond the ophthalmic artery supply, transient monocular blindness does not occur.

During the first 3 days in the hospital, MR progressively worsened, gradually developing a complete right hemiplegia, minor tingling of the right limbs, and mutism. Examination revealed no bruits or facial or limb pulse abnormalities.

Patients with MCA disease often develop their deficits more gradually than comparable series of patients with ICA disease.[22] Patients with MCA disease frequently note their abnormalities on awakening in the morning or from a nap, and they have a high incidence of subsequent fluctuation or progression during the next 1 to 7 days. This gradual onset and progressive course support a low-flow mechanism for the ischemia. Deficits begin when flow is most sluggish, and collateral circulation then takes time to equilibrate. In contrast, patients with ICA disease more commonly have sudden-onset deficits while awake and thereafter remain stable, a course better explained by distal embolism from their ICA lesion than by low flow.

Because the occlusive process is intracranial, there are no important associated signs of extracranial disease. Neurological findings vary, depending on the location of the vascular occlusion and the brain ischemia. The next sections discuss the commonest patterns of neurological deficits seen in patients with MCA disease. Although these syndromes are discussed under the heading of intrinsic MCA occlusive disease, in fact, the patterns are more commonly due to embolism to the MCA territory. (Figure 6.9 shows the common patterns of MCA occlusion and their anatomical and clinical correlates.)

Occlusion or Stenosis of the Upper Trunk of the Middle Cerebral Artery

The superior trunk of the MCA supplies the frontal and superior parietal lobes. Occasionally, when the main-stem MCA is short, the lenticulostriate vessels arise from the proximal portion of the superior trunk.[22,78,79] In that case, the internal capsule and lateral basal ganglia will also be nourished by the superior trunk.

The findings include *hemiplegia,* more severe in the face and upper extremity, with relative sparing of the lower extremity; *hemisensory loss,* usually including decreased pinprick and position sense, again sometimes sparing the leg; *conjugate eye deviation,* the eyes resting toward the side of the brain lesion; and *neglect of the contralateral side of space,* especially to visual stimuli. Visual neglect is usually more severe with right-hemisphere lesions.

When the lesion is in the left, dominant hemisphere, there is invariably an accompanying aphasia. Verbal output is very sparse, and patients do not do what they are asked with either hand, though they may follow whole-body commands, such as turn over, sit, stand, and so forth. They may be able to nod appropriately to yes/no questions asked verbally, but comprehension of written material is poor. With time, a pattern of Broca's aphasia evolves,

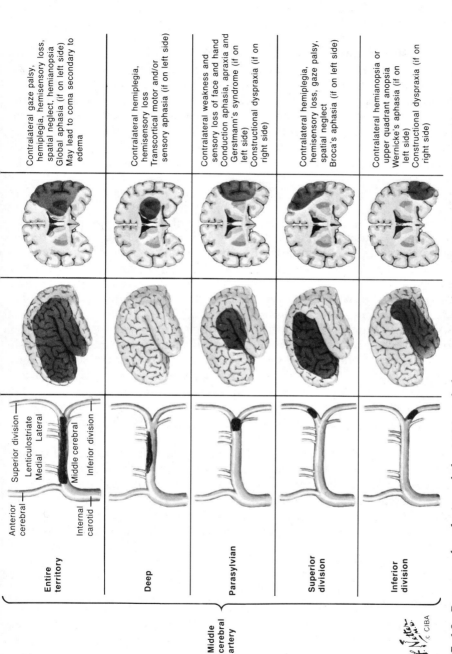

FIGURE 6.9 Patterns of occlusion of the MCA and their anatomical correlates. (© Copyright 1986 CIBA Pharmaceutical Company, Division of CIBA-GEIGY Corporation. Reprinted with permission from The Ciba Collection of Medical Illustrations, illustrated by Frank H. Netter, M.D. All rights reserved.)

with sparse effortful speech, poor pronunciation of syllables, and omission of filler words but preserved comprehension of spoken language.

In upper-trunk MCA infarcts in the right hemisphere, patients frequently seem unaware of their deficit (anosognosia) and may not admit that they are hemiplegic or impaired in any way.[23,80] Some patients are also impersistent, performing requested tasks quickly but they do not persevere, and they terminate tasks prematurely.[80,81] When asked to read, patients with right superior-trunk occlusions will often omit the left of the page or paragraph, and will fail to see people or objects to their left.

Occlusion of the Inferior Trunk of the Middle Cerebral Artery

This vessel usually supplies the lateral surface of the temporal lobe and inferior parietal lobule (Figure 6.9). The anterior, medial, and inferior portions of the temporal lobes are supplied by other vessels.

In contrast to patients with lesions of the upper trunk, these patients usually have no elementary motor or sensory abnormalities. They often have a visual field defect, either a hemianopia or an upper-quadrant anopsia, affecting the contralateral visual field.

When the left hemisphere is involved, patients have a Wernicke-type aphasia. Speech is fluent and syllables are well pronounced, but patients use wrong or nonexistent words, and what is said makes little sense. Comprehension and repetition of spoken language are poor. There may be relative sparing of written comprehension, with the patient preferring that words be written down.[82,83] When the right hemisphere is affected, patients draw and copy poorly and may have difficulty finding their way about or reading a map.

Behavioral abnormalities also frequently accompany temporal-lobe infarctions. Patients with Wernicke's aphasia are often irascible, paranoid, and may become violent. Patients with right temporal infarcts often have an agitated hyperactive state resembling delirium tremens.[84-86] The diagnosis of right inferior-trunk occlusion is sometimes difficult. The key findings are a left visual-field defect and poor drawing and copying in an agitated person.[86]

Deep Infarction of the Middle Cerebral Artery Territory

This pattern (Figure 6.9) is usually due to occlusion of the main-stem MCA before its lenticulostriate branches. There is excellent potential for collateral circulation over the convexities but poor collateral circulation in the deep basal gray nuclei. For this reason, some patients with MCA occlusion have selective ischemia of the deep lenticulostriate territory, but collateral circulation is adequate to prevent cortical infarction. On CT, the lesions can be confused with lacunes but are larger and often extend to the inferior brain surface. Some have called these lesions "giant lacunes,"[22,87] but the preferred term for these deep MCA lenticulostriate territory lesions is *striatocapsular infarcts.*[64,88,89]

These patients are invariably hemiparetic, but the distribution of weakness in face, arm, and leg is variable.[74] Sensory loss is usually minor because the posterior capsule is spared. When the lesion is in the left hemisphere, after a short period of temporary mutism, speech is sparse and dysarthric, but repetition of spoken language is preserved. Comprehension of spoken and written language depends on both the size and the anteroposterior extent of the lesion.[90,91] When the right hemisphere is involved, there is some neglect of contralateral visual and tactile stimuli, but this is usually more transient than with parietal cortical infarction.

Main-Stem Occlusion with Total Infarction of the Middle Cerebral Artery Territory

This lesion is most common in patients with embolism to the proximal MCA (Figure 6.9). In most patients with intrinsic occlusive disease of the MCA, there is sufficient collateral circulation to spare at least the outer borders of the territory.

These patients are usually devastated. Severe paralysis, hemisensory loss, attentional hemianopia, and conjugate eye deviation to the opposite side are found. When the left hemisphere is involved, there is a global aphasia. Right-hemisphere lesions produce severe neglect; anosognosia; disinterest, or poor motivation and apathy; and severe constructional apraxia.[23] Recovery to useful function is very unusual.[92]

Segmental Infarction in the Middle Cerebral Artery Territory

These lesions are caused by occlusion of the distal cortical branches of the upper or lower division of the MCA (Figure 6.9). They are almost invariably embolic and are seldom due to intrinsic atheromatous occlusion of a convexity branch. The syndromes are quite variable and will obviously depend on the branch affected.

Neck ultrasound in patient MR was normal. Blood-sugar levels were 240 on admission and remained elevated until insulin was begun. CT revealed a deep striatocapsular infarct. TCD showed an absence of flow velocities in the left

MCA, with normal ACA and right-sided values. Angiography showed occlusion of the left main-stem MCA after a tapered, irregular origin.

CT patterns of MCA infarction have already been described. In my experience, the commonest patterns are wedge-shaped pial-territory infarcts and subcortical deep basal ganglia and internal-capsule infarcts. TCD is a very useful technique for demonstrating MCA disease.[93] Stenosis often causes high velocities when insonating at the depth of the lesion. When the MCA is occluded, flow and velocities decline, and often, no signal can be obtained. MRA with concentration on intracranial views can also usually document severe MCA occlusive lesions. Using standard angiography, MCA occlusion is best seen on the anteroposterior view of a selective ICA injection. At times, the occlusion is near the MCA trifurcation, so that oblique views are needed. The area of poorest supply of MCA tributaries is best identified on the lateral view. At times, there is poor opacification of inferior and superior trunk arteries, but it is difficult to identify the precise point of narrowing or occlusion.

MR was treated with heparin, but nonetheless, the stroke progressed. She remained on warfarin for 2 months. Repeat angiography showed good collateral filling of the MCA from ACA and PCA branches. PET scanning at 2 months revealed no major disparity between perfusion and metabolism.

Therapy of intrinsic MCA disease is uncertain because there have been too few series of patients studied, and none has been studied in a controlled fashion. In patients with acute thrombotic or embolic MCA occlusion, thrombolytic treatment could be effective if given early enough. Warfarin might prevent total occlusion of a stenosed MCA and might decrease propagation of an MCA clot. In the series of Hinton et al., patients frequently stabilized while taking warfarin.[73] I use anticoagulation in patients with severe MCA stenosis, keeping the PT at 1.5 times the normal values. If the MCA is totally occluded and there is poorly functioning but not-yet-infarcted cortical MCA tissue, then an ECA–ICA bypass theoretically makes sense. It is also helpful to know the adequacy of collateral circulation, as seen angiographically, or as measured by TCD, SPECT, or PET. The poorer the circulation, the more one can presume a theoretical need for revascularization. There are few data about optimal timing of ECA–ICA bypass.

The results of the ECA–ICA bypass study have made me reevaluate my ideas because operated patients with severe MCA occlusive disease had poorer outcomes than did medically treated patients.[60] Although traditionally performed at least 6 weeks after the infarct, I wonder whether some patients might benefit from earlier shunting. I do not think that agents affecting platelet aggregation have an important role in the therapy of severe occlusive MCA disease. They may be useful, however, if there is only minor irregularity of the MCA, without stenosis.

Occlusion or Severe Stenosis of the Anterior Cerebral Artery

Intrinsic occlusive disease of the ACA is infrequently documented. Many patients with intrinsic disease of the ACA also have extensive ICA and MCA disease, often with multiple infarcts, making clinicopathological correlation of the ACA lesions difficult.[94] Some ACA-territory infarcts are due to occlusive disease of the ICA, and others are caused by vasospasm-related ischemia in patients with SAH due to aneurysms of the anterior communicating artery.[95] In a 1983 study of cerebral infarcts documented by CT, 13 of 413 (3%) were in the ACA territory.[96] Eight of the 13 patients with ACA-territory ischemia had angiography that showed 5 ACA occlusions. In an additional 3 patients, angiography showed ACA occlusion, but the CT showed no infarction in this territory. Nearly all patients in this series with occlusion of the ACA had severe occlusive disease at the origin of the ICA in the neck or in the carotid siphon on the side of the ACA lesion.[96] The most likely mechanism of ACA-territory infarction in this group of patients was intra-arterial embolism arising from the more proximal ICA lesions. In one patient, the authors postulated that intra-arterial embolic material traveled from an occluded ICA origin to the contralateral ACA through a widely patent anterior communicating artery. My own experience and that of others[94,96,97] leads me to the following opinions about the mechanisms of ACA-territory infarction: (1) ACA-territory infarction is most often embolic; (2) embolism is most often intra-arterial, arising from proximal ICA occlusive disease; (3) when intrinsic atherostenosis affects the ACA, patients usually have widespread extracranial and intracranial occlusive disease with multiple brain infarcts; (4) stenotic lesions of the ACA are not always in the horizontal first portion of the artery but can involve the pericallosal artery and other branches. Figure 6.10 depicts patterns of ACA occlusion and their anatomical correlates.

The ACA, after its brief horizontal A1 segment, gives off the artery of Heubner and medial striate arteries, which supply the caudate nucleus, internal capsule, and anterior perforated substance.[98–101] After reaching the midline, the ACA swings posteriorly and divides to form the pericallosal and callosomarginal arteries, which supply the paramedian frontal lobe above the corpus callosum. At times, the A1 segment of the ACA on one side may be atretic, so that both ACAs are supplied by one ICA. The extent of the infarction depends on the location of the obstruction and the pattern of the anterior circle of Willis.

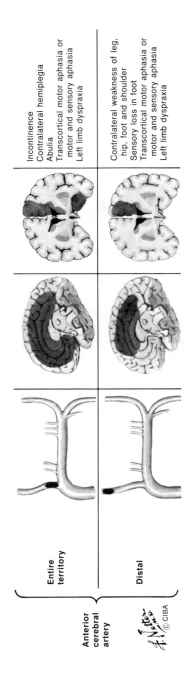

FIGURE 6.10 Patterns of occlusion of the ACA and their anatomical correlates. (© Copyright 1986 CIBA Pharmaceutical Company, Division of CIBA-GEIGY Corporation. Reprinted with permission from The Ciba Collection of Medical Illustrations, illustrated by Frank H. Netter, M.D. All rights reserved.)

A 75-year-old man, CF, awakened from a nap with paralysis of his left leg and foot. There was also slight tingling in his left toes. Examination confirmed complete paralysis of the left lower extremity. When asked to salute, to wave good-bye, or to pretend to throw a ball, he performed these functions normally with the right arm but used incorrect movements with the left arm, although these limbs were not weak or clumsy. The patient was surprised to find that, on occasion, the left hand would grasp the right hand in the midst of an activity and seemed to do things "without my will."

The single most important clue to an ACA-territory infarct is the distribution of motor weakness. Paralysis is usually greatest in the foot but is also severe in the proximal thigh. Shoulder shrug is weak on the involved side, but the hand and face are usually normal if the deep ACA territory is spared. Cortical sensory loss is also present in the weak limbs but is usually slight. The patient may have difficulty touching the spot on his lower extremity touched by the examiner, may be unable to identify numbers written on his foot with a blunt pencil, or may extinguish bilateral tactile stimuli on the paralyzed foot and leg.

Another very helpful sign is apraxia of the left arm. Normally, speech is received in the left posterior hemisphere. In order to communicate language to regions of the right hemisphere that control the left limbs, the information goes forward toward the left frontal region and then across the corpus callosum to the right frontal region. In ACA-territory infarcts, the callosum or its adjacent white matter is often infarcted, interrupting this pathway, no matter whether the right or the left ACA territory is infarcted.[102] This disconnection can be detected by simple bedside tests:

1. Ask the patient to perform spoken commands with the right and left arms. Patients with ACA infarction will usually be unable to perform with the left hand. The fact that they follow the commands normally with the right hand proves that they understand the commands.
2. Ask the patient to write or print with the right, then the left hand. Some patients with ACA infarction write aphasically with the left hand.
3. Ask the patient to name objects placed in the left and then the right hands. Patients with an ACA infarct may be unable to name objects in their left hand but they can select the same objects by vision or touch and can name them correctly when placed in the right hand.

This topic has been reviewed by Kaplan[102] and Geschwind[103] and has often been referred to as an "anterior disconnection syndrome."

When the lesion affects the left ACA territory and the supplementary motor cortex, a transcortical motor and sensory aphasia often results.[97,104–106] Despite reduced spontaneous speech, the patient can repeat spoken language well. Incontinence—characterized by inability to control micturition, although the urge to urinate is preserved—may occur, especially in patients with bilateral lesions. Patients with unilateral ACA infarcts or bilateral frontal infarcts are usually *abulic*—that is, they are apathetic, with decreased spontaneity, slow in responding to queries or commands, and use terse speech that is limited in amount.[107] These patients have difficulty in counting quickly from 20 to 1 or in persevering with any protracted task, such as crossing off all the letter "A"s in a paragraph or telling the examiner without prodding each time their finger is moved or touched. In some patients, the decreased activity is intermittent. At one moment, patients speak, and the next moment, they stare blankly and pay no heed to queries or conversation, as if the machine were temporarily shut off.[108]

Another phenomenon found in some patients with frontal-lobe infarction due to ACA disease has been called the "alien hand sign."[109,110] My patient, CF, had noticed that his left hand had a mind of its own, often doing things he did not will it to do. The sign is most common in the right hand, which interferes with willed movements of the left hand. One hand acts against the other or acts involuntarily. Similar findings occur in patients with epilepsy after callosal sections, making it likely that the phenomenon is due to defective interhemispheric connections. Forced grasping and a heightened grasp reflex, found often contralateral to frontal-lobe lesions may also play a role in causing this sign.

> CT revealed a moderate-sized right medial frontal infarct in CF (Figure 6.11a,b) and angiography documented severe stenosis of the right ACA before it formed the callosomarginal artery (Figure 6.11c). After physical therapy, he was able to walk with a brace.

Little is known about treatment for intrinsic ACA disease. I elected not to expose this older gentleman with an already sizable infarct to the risk of anticoagulation because little additional damage would ensue even if the rest of the right ACA territory were infarcted.

Occasionally, patients have the sudden development of bilateral ACA territory infarction (Figure 6.12). This is explained by hypoplasia or absence of the A1 segment of the ACA on one side. In that circumstance, the territories of the ACA on both sides are supplied by one ACA. On angiography, dye instillation into one ICA produces bilateral ACA opacification. Occlusion of the ICA or ACA supplying both sides leads to bilateral frontal-lobe infarction. The resulting clinical picture is that of sudden apathy, abulia, and incontinence. When the paracentral lobule is involved, there is weakness on one or both sides, predominantly affecting the lower extremities. The sudden onset of dementia presents a striking clinical picture, especially to those unfamiliar with this rare syndrome.

Caudate Infarcts

One of the major branches of the ACA is the recurrent artery of Heubner, which supplies the head of the caudate nucleus and the anterior limb of the

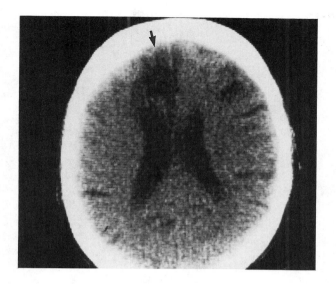

a

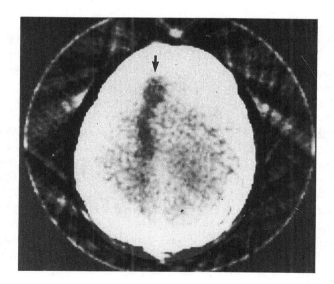

b

FIGURE 6.11 (a) CT showing infarct in the right frontal lobe (black arrow); (b) CT showing linear infarct in the right ACA territory (black arrow); (continued)

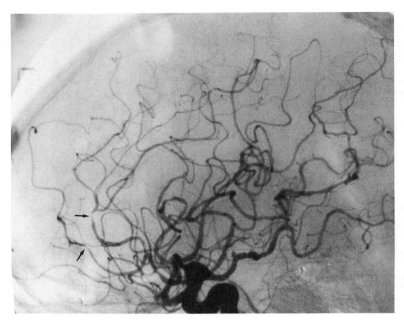

c

FIGURE 6.11 continued. (c) carotid arteriogram, lateral intracranial view, showing stenosis of branches of the right ACA (arrows).

internal capsule.[98–100] Although older descriptions spoke of a single vessel, more recent dissections show that there usually are multiple parallel penetrating arteries arising from the ACA near the anterior communicating artery junction. In about 25 percent of individuals, there is a single Heubner's artery; more often, there are two, three, or even four recurrent arteries.[99,100] Occlusion of one of these penetrating arteries or of the parent ACA before the origin of the perforators leads to infarcts in the head of the caudate nucleus. Frequently, the infarction also involves the anterior limb of the internal capsule and the most anterior part of the putamen. Lateral lenticulostriate artery branches of the MCA also supply the caudate nucleus, anterior limb of the internal capsule, and the putamen. Figure 6.13 shows a montage of the findings from CT scans from my colleagues' and my recent series of caudate infarcts.[100]

The clinical signs of caudate infarction are quite variable. Motor weakness is not prominent, although some patients have slight but usually transient hemiparesis. Dysarthria is a more common finding and was present in 11 of 18 (61%) patients with caudate infarcts in our series.[100] Most important are changes in behavior. The most common behavioral change in my experience has been abulia.[100,107] Families describe the patients as more apathetic, uninterested, inert, laconic, and inactive. Slowness is a frequent

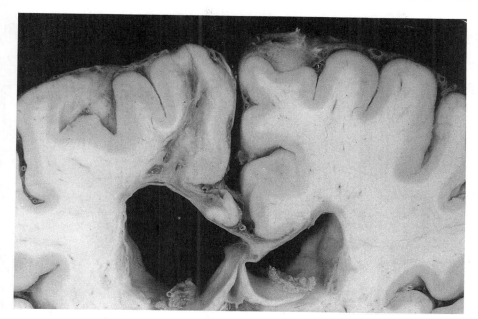

FIGURE 6.12   Postmortem necropsy coronal slice of brain showing a large ACA-territory infarct above the very enlarged left lateral ventricle. The corpus callosum is necrotic, and the infarct extends toward the right cingulate gyrus.

theme; each activity takes longer and requires more concentration and effort. Another frequent abnormality, especially in patients with right-caudate infarcts, is restlessness and hyperactivity. Some patients speak incessantly, call out, and appear very agitated, confused, and delirious, closely resembling patients with right-temporal-lobe infarcts.[86,100] In some patients with caudate infarction, restlessness and agitation alternate with apathy and inertia. Slight aphasia can be found in left-caudate infarcts, and some patients with right-caudate lesions have left visual neglect.[100]

The cognitive and behavioral changes found in patients with caudate infarcts closely resemble the clinical signs found in patients with lesions in the medial thalamus and the frontal and temporal lobes. Recent anatomical and physiological studies have shown strong interconnections both between the caudate nucleus and various cortical regions and between the caudate nucleus and the thalamus, the globus pallidus, and the substantia nigra.[111,112] Caudatonigrothalamocortical circuits are intimately related to planning, thinking, acting, and other higher cortical functions.[100,111]

The causes of caudate infarction are probably diverse. The most lateral portion is supplied by the medial striate penetrators of the proximal MCA. Occlusion of these branches or of the parent proximal MCA can lead to striatocapsular infarction, including the caudate nucleus. Occlusion of the ACA, either by intrinsic atherosclerosis or more often by embolism, is a

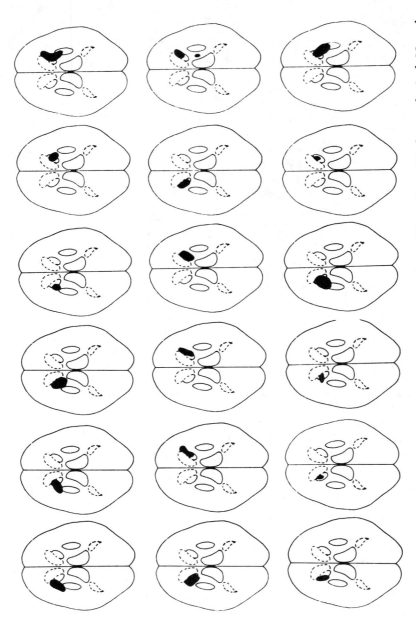

FIGURE 6.13 Montage of drawings of CTs showing caudate-nucleus infarcts. (From Caplan et al., Arch Neurol, 1990;47:134, reprinted with permission.)

more frequent mechanism of caudate infarction than is MCA disease. In most patients, the lesions probably are due to atheromatous branch disease at the origins of these penetrating arteries.[100,113] In a 1990 series of patients with caudate infarcts, risk factors for small-artery disease were prevalent. Among the 18 patients, hypertension (77%) and diabetes (33%) were common; 5 patients had both diabetes and hypertension; and only 3 of 18 had neither hypertension nor diabetes. Only 1 of the 18 had confirmed large-artery disease (ICA siphon stenosis), and 1 had a cardiac source of embolism (mitral stenosis).[100] These data suggest that most caudate infarcts are due to atheromatous branch disease, but this conclusion must be tentative without more clinical and necropsy data. At present, I suggest screening patients with caudate infarcts with cardiac testing and ultrasound or MRA before diagnosing a small-artery etiology.

Occlusion of the Anterior Choroidal Artery

Neuroimaging (CT and MRI) now often shows infarction limited to the territory of the anterior choroidal artery (AChA). This vessel originates from the ICA after its ophthalmic and posterior communicating branches, and it courses posteriorly and laterally to supply the globus pallidus, lateral geniculate body, posterior limb of the internal capsule, and medial temporal lobe.[114,115] Before CT, occlusion of the anterior choroidal artery had seldom been diagnosed during life. Cooper, at first inadvertently and later purposefully, tied this vessel in Parkinsonian patients to stop tremor. The results were variable.[116]

A recent series of mine and my colleagues[117] and series by others[115,118,119] have led me to conclude that the syndrome of the anterior choroidal artery includes

1. hemiparesis affecting face, arm, and leg
2. a rather prominent hemisensory loss, which is often temporary
3. in cases when the lateral geniculate body is infarcted, an unusual hemianopia, with sparing of a beak-shaped tongue of vision within the center of the hemianopic visual field[120]
4. absence of important persistent neglect, aphasia, or other higher-cortical-function abnormalities

The diagnosis is verified by CT (Figure 6.14), or MRI, showing infarction in the pallidum and in the lateral geniculate body adjacent to the temporal horn,[115,121] and by occlusion of the AChA demonstrated angiographically. Many of the patients with necropsy-proven AChA-territory infarcts have been diabetic or hypertensive.[113,117]

The PCA occasionally is supplied directly through the posterior communicating branch of the ICA, but because it more often arises from the

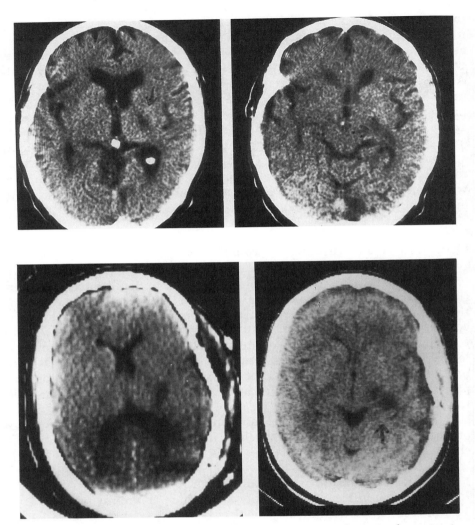

FIGURE 6.14   Four CT scans, all showing AChA-territory infarcts in the region just above the temporal horn, and in the region of the posterior limb of the internal capsule, and the globus pallidus; all of the infarcts are on the right of the figures.

basilar artery, this vessel is considered in the chapter on the posterior circulation, which follows.

References

1. Fisher CM. Occlusion of the internal carotid artery. Arch Neurol Psychiatry 1951;65:346–377.

2. Brott TG, Labutta RJ, Kempczinski RF. Changing patterns in the practice of carotid endarterectomy in a large metropolitan area. J Am Med Assoc 1986; 255:2607–2612.

3. Dyken M. Carotid endarterectomy studies: a glimmering of science. Stroke 1986;17:355–358.

4. Barnett HJ, Plum F, Walton J. Carotid endarterectomy—an expression of concern. Stroke 1984;15:941–943.

5. Caplan LR. Carotid-artery disease. N Engl J Med 1986;315:886–888.

6. Easton JD, Sherman D. Stroke and morbidity rate in carotid endarterectomy: 228 consecutive operations. Stroke 1977;8:565–568.

7. Brott T, Thalinger K. Carotid endarterectomy in Cincinnati, 1980: indications and morbidity in 431 cases. Neurology 1983;33(Suppl 2):93.

8. NASCET Collaborators. Beneficial effect of carotid endarterectomy in symptomatic patients with high-grade carotid stenosis. N Engl J Med 1991;325: 445–453.

9. European Carotid Surgery Trialists Collaborative Group. Interim results for symptomatic patients with severe (70–99%) or with mild (0–19%) carotid stenosis. Lancet 1991;337:1235–1243.

10. Gorelick PB, Caplan LR, Hier DB, et al. Racial differences in the distribution of anterior circulation occlusive disease. Neurology 1984;34:54–59.

11. Caplan LR, Gorelick PB, Hier DB. Race, sex, and occlusive cerebrovascular disease: a review. Stroke 1986;17:648–655.

12. Mohr JP, Caplan LR, Melski J, et al. The Harvard Cooperative Stroke Registry: a prospective registry. Neurology 1978;28:752–754.

13. Furlan A, Whisnant J, Kearns T. Unilateral visual loss in bright light. Arch Neurol 1979;36:675–676.

14. Caplan LR, Sergay S. Positional cerebral ischemia. J Neurol Neurosurg Psychiatry 1976;39:385–391.

15. Reed C, Toole J. Clinical technique for identification of external carotid bruits. Neurology 1981;31:744–746.

16. Fisher CM. Facial pulses in internal carotid artery occlusion. Neurology 1970;20:476–478.

17. Caplan LR. The frontal artery sign. N Engl J Med 1973;288:1008–1009.

18. Hollenhorst R. Ocular manifestations of insufficiency or thrombosis of the internal carotid artery. Am J Ophthalmol 1959;47:753–767.

19. Fisher CM. Observations of the fundus oculi in transient monocular blindness. Neurology 1959;9:333–347.

20. Kearns T, Hollenhorst R. Venous stasis retinopathy of occlusive disease of the carotid artery. Mayo Clin Proc 1963;38:304–312.

21. Carter JE. Chronic ocular ischemia and carotid vascular disease. In: Bernstein EF, ed. Amaurosis fugax. New York: Springer-Verlag, 1988:118–134.

22. Caplan LR, Babikian V, Helgason C, et al. Acclusive disease of the middle cerebral artery. Neurology 1985; 35:975–982.

23. Stein R, Hier DB, Caplan LR. Cognitive and behavioral deficits after right hemisphere stroke. Curr Concepts Cerebrovasc Dis (Stroke) 1985;20:1–5.

24. Hier DB, Mondlock J, Caplan LR. Behavioral abnormalities after right hemisphere stroke. Neurology 1983;33:337–344.

25. Pessin MS, Kwan E, Scott RM, Hedges TR. Occipital infarction with hemianopsia from carotid occlusive disease. Stroke 1989;20:409–411.

26. Pessin M, Duncan G, Davis K, et al. Angiographic appearance of carotid occlusion in acute stroke. Stroke 1980;11:485–487.

27. Barnett HJM, Peerless S, Kaufmann J. "Stump" of internal carotid artery: a source for further cerebral embolic ischemia. Stroke 1978;9:448–452.

28. Ringelstein E, Zeumer H, Angelou D. The pathogenesis of strokes from internal carotid artery occlusion: diagnostic and therapeutic implications. Stroke 1983;14:867–875.

29. Sekhar L, Heros R. Atheromatous pseudo-occlusion of the internal carotid artery. J Neurosurg 1980;52:782–789.

30. Riles T, Posner M, Cohen W, et al. Rapid sequential CT scanning of the occluded internal carotid artery. Stroke 1982;13:124.

31. Baron JC, Bousser M, Comar D, et al. Human hemispheric infarction studied by positron emission tomography and the ^{15}O continuous inhalation technique. In: Caille J, Salamon C, eds. Computerized tomography. Berlin: Springer-Verlag, 1980:231–237.

32. Baquis GD, Pessin MS, Scott RM. Limb shaking—a carotid TIA. Stroke 1985;16:444–448.

33. Yanigahara T, Piepgras DG, Klass DW. Repetitive involuntary movement associated with episodic cerebral ischemia. Ann Neurol 1985;18:244–250.

34. Caplan LR, Baker R. Extracranial occlusive disease. Does size matter? Stroke 1980;11:63–66.

35. Caplan LR, Skillman J, Ojemann R, et al. Intracerebral hemorrhage following carotid endarterectomy: a hypertensive complication. Stroke 1978;9:457–460.

36. Bruetman M, Fields W, Crawford E, et al. Cerebral hemorrhage in carotid artery surgery. Arch Neurol 1963;9:458–467.

37. Wylie E, Hein M, Adams J. Intracranial hemorrhage following surgical revascularization for treatment of acute stroke. J Neurosurg 1964;21:212–215.

38. Wade J, Larson C, Hickey R, et al. Effect of carotid endarterectomy on carotid chemoreceptor and baroreceptor function in man. N Engl J Med 1970;282:823–829.

39. Holton P, Wood JB. Effects of bilateral removal of the carotid bodies and denervation of the carotid sinus in two human subjects. J Physiol 1965;181:365–378.

40. Countee R, Sapru H, Vijayanathan T, et al. "Other syndromes" of the carotid bifurcation. In: Smith RR, ed. Stroke and the extracranial vessels. New York: Raven Press, 1984:345–357.

41. Hennerici M, Rautenberg W, Struck R. Spontaneous clinical course of asymptomatic vascular processes of the extracranial cerebral arteries. Klin Wochenschr 1984;62:570–576.

42. Hennerici M, Hulsbower HB, Hefter K, et al. Natural history of asymptomatic extracranial disease: results of a long term prospective study. Brain 1987;110:777–791.

43. Caplan LR, Stein R, Patel D, et al. Intraluminal clot of the carotid artery detected angiographically. Neurology 1984;34:1175–1181.

44. Pessin MS, Abbott BF, Prager R, et al. Clinical and angiographic features of carotid circulation thrombus. Neurology 1986;36:518–523.

45. Toronto Cerebrovascular Study Group. Risks of carotid endarterectomy. Stroke 1986;17:848–852.

46. Fode NC, Sundt T, Robertson J, et al. Multicenter retrospective review

of results and complications of carotid endarterectomy. Stroke 1986;17: 370–376.

47. Caplan LR, Pessin MS. Symptomatic carotid artery disease and carotid endarterectomy. Ann Rev Med 1988;39;273–299.

48. Humphries A, Young J, Santilli P, et al. Unoperated asymptomatic significant carotid artery stenosis: a review of 182 instances. Surgery 1976;80:694–698.

49. Durward Q, Ferguson G, Barr H. The natural history of asymptomatic carotid bifurcation plaques. Stroke 1982;13:459–464.

50. Ropper A, Wechsler L, Wilson L. Carotid bruits and the risk of stroke in elective surgery. N Engl J Med 1982;307:1387–1390.

51. Asymptomatic Carotid Atherosclerosis Study Group. Study design for randomized prospective trial of carotid endarterectomy for asymptomatic atherosclerosis. Stroke 1989;20:844–849.

52. Caplan LR, Easton JD. Position statement: Carotid endarterectomy—report of the therapeutics and technology assessment subcommittee American Academy of Neurology. Neurology 1990;40:682–683.

53. Mohr JP. Asymptomatic carotid artery disease. Stroke 1982;13:431–433.

54. Fisher CM, Gore I, Okabe N, et al. Calcification of the carotid siphon. Circulation 1965;32:538–548.

55. Marzewski D, Furlan A, St Louis P, et al. Intracranial internal carotid artery stenosis: long-term prognosis. Stroke 1982;13:821–824.

56. Craig D, Meguro K, Watridge G, et al. Intracranial internal carotid artery stenosis. Stroke 1982;13:825–828.

57. Wechsler LR, Kistler JP, Davis KR, et al. The prognosis of carotid siphon stenosis. Stroke 1986;17:714–718.

58. Caplan LR. Cerebrovascular disease: larger artery occlusive disease. In: Appel S, ed. Current neurology. vol 8. Chicago Yearbook Medical, 1988:179–226.

59. Castaigne P, Lhermitte F, Gautier JC, et al. Internal carotid artery occlusion: a study of 61 instances in 50 patients with postmortem data. Brain 1970; 93:231–258.

60. The EC-IC Bypass Study Group. Failure of extracranial–intracranial arterial bypass to reduce the risk of ischemic stroke. N Engl J Med 1985;313:1191–1200.

61. Gumerlock M, Ono H, Neuwelt E. Can a patent extracranial–intracranial bypass provoke the conversion of an intracranial arterial stenosis to a symptomatic occlusion? Neurosurgery 1983;12:391–400.

62. Furlan A, Little J, Dohn D. Arterial occlusion following anastomosis of the superficial temporal artery to middle cerebral artery. Stroke 1980;11:91–95.

63. Day A, Rhoton A, Quisling R. Resolving siphon stenosis following endarterectomy. Stroke 1980;11:278–281.

64. Bladin PF, Berkovic SF. Striatocapsular infarction. Neurology 1984;34:1423–1430.

65. Caplan LR, Gorelick PB, Hier DB. Race, sex, and occlusive cerebrovascular disease: a review. Stroke 1986;17:648–655.

66. Russo L. Carotid system transient ischemic attacks: clinical, racial, and angiographic correlations. Stroke 1981;12:470–473.

67. Bauer R, Sheehan S, Wechsler N, et al. Arteriographic study of sites, incidence,

and treatment of arteriosclerotic cerebrovascular lesions. Neurology 1962;
12:698–711.

68. Kieffer S, Takeya Y, Resch J, et al. Racial differences in cerebrovascular disease: angiographic evaluation of Japanese and American populations. AJR 1967; 101:94–99.

69. Brust R. Patterns of cerebrovascular disease in Japanese and other population groups in Hawaii: an angiographic study. Stroke 1975;6:539–542.

70. Kubo H. Transient cerebral ischemic attacks: an arteriographic study. Naika 1968;22:969–978.

71. Feldmann E, Daneault N, Kwan E, et al. Chinese–white differences in the distribution of occlusive cerebrovascular disease. Neurology 1990;40:1541–1545.

72. Bogousslavsky J, Barnett JHM, Fox AJ, et al., for the EC–IC bypass study group. Atherosclerotic disease of the middle cerebral artery. Stroke 1986;17:1112–1120.

73. Hinton R, Mohr JP, Ackerman R, et al. Symptomatic middle cerebral artery stenosis. Ann Neurol 1979;5:152–157.

74. Corston RN, Kendall BE, Marshall J. Prognosis in middle cerebral artery stenosis. Stroke 1984;15:237–241.

75. Moulin DE, Lo R, Chiang J, et al. Prognosis in middle cerebral artery occlusion. Stroke 1985;16:282–284.

76. Feldmeyer JJ, Merendaz C, Regli F. Stenosis symptomatiques de l'artere cerebrale moyenne. Rev Neurol (Paris) 1983;139:725–736.

77. Naritomi H, Sawada T, Kuriyama Y, et al. Effect of chronic middle cerebral artery stenosis on the local cerebral hemodynamics. Stroke 1985;16:214–219.

78. Jain K. Some observations on the anatomy of the middle cerebral artery. Can J Surg 1964;7:134–139.

79. Kaplan H. Anatomy and embryology of the arterial system of the forebrain. In: Vinken P, Bruyn G, eds. Handbook of clinical neurology: vol 11, pt 1. vascular diseases of the nervous system. Amsterdam: North Holland, 1972:1–23.

80. Hier DB, Gorelick PB, Shindler AG. Topics in behavioral neurology and neuropsychology. Boston: Butterworth, 1987.

81. Fisher CM. Left hemiplegia and motor impersistence. J Nerv Ment Dis 1956;123:201–218.

82. Hier DB, Mohr JP. Incongruous oral and written naming: evidence for a subdivision of the syndromes of Wernicke's aphasia. Brain Lang 1977;4:115–126.

83. Sevush S, Roeltgen D, Campanella D, et al. Preserved oral reading in Wernicke's aphasia. Neurology 1983;33:916–920.

84. Awada A, Poncet M, Signoret J. Confrontation de la Salpetriere 4 Mai 1983: troubles des compartement soudains avec agitation chez un homme de 68 ans. Rev Neurol (Paris) 1984;140:446–451.

85. Schmidley J, Messing R. Agitated confusional states in patients with right hemisphere infarctions. Stroke 1984:15;883–885.

86. Caplan LR, Kelly M, Kase CS, et al. Infarcts of the inferior division of the right middle cerebral artery. Neurology 1986;36:1015–1020.

87. Adams H, Damasio H, Putnam S, et al. Middle cerebral artery occlusion as a cause of isolated subcortical infarction. Stroke 1983;14:948–952.

88. Weiller C, Ringelstein EB, Reiche W, Thron A, Buell U. The large striatocap-

sular infarct: a clinical and pathological entity. Arch Neurol 1990;47:1085–1091.

89. Caplan LR. The large striato-capsular infarct: a clinical and pathophysiologic entity: critique. Neurology Chronicle 1991;1:12–13.

90. Damasio A, Damasio H, Rizzo M, et al. Aphasia with nonhemorrhagic lesions in the basal ganglia and internal capsule. Arch Neurol 1982;89:15–20.

91. Naesser M, Alexander M, Estabrooks N, et al. Aphasia with predominantly subcortical lesion sites. Arch Neurol 1982;39:2–14.

92. Hier DB, Mondlock J, Caplan LR. Recovery of behavioral abnormalities after right hemisphere stroke. Neurology 1983;33:345–350.

93. Caplan LR, Brass CM, DeWitt LD, et al. Transcranial Doppler ultrasound: present status. Neurology 1990;40:696–700.

94. Critchley M. The anterior cerebral artery, and its syndromes. Brain 1930;53:120–165.

95. Uihlein A, Thomas R, Cleary J. Aneurysms of the anterior communicating artery complex. Mayo Clin Proc 1967;42:73–87.

96. Gacs G, Fox A, Barnett HJM, et al. Occurrence and mechanisms of occlusion of the anterior cerebral artery. Stroke 1983;14:952–959.

97. Brust JC. Anterior cerebral artery. In: Barnett HJM, Mohr JP, Stein B, Yatsu F, eds. Stroke: pathophysiology, diagnosis and management. New York: Churchill Livingstone, 1986:351–375.

98. Rhoton AL, Sacki N, Pearlmutter D, Zeal A. Microsurgical anatomy of common aneurysm sites. Clin Neurosurg 1978;26:248–306.

99. Gorczyca W, Mohr G. Microvascular anatomy of Heubner's recurrent artery. J Neurosurg 1976;44:359–367.

100. Caplan LR, Schmahmann JD, Kase CS, et al. Caudate infarcts. Arch Neurol 1990;47:133–143.

101. Dunker R, Harris A. Surgical anatomy of the proximal anterior cerebral artery. J Neurosurg 1976;44:359–367.

102. Geschwind N, Kaplan E. A human cerebral deconnection syndrome. Neurology 1962;12:675–695.

103. Geschwind N. Disconnection syndromes in animals and man. Brain 1965;88:237–294,585–644.

104. Rubens A. Aphasia with infarction in the territory of the anterior cerebral artery. Cortex 1975;11:239–250.

105. Alexander M, Schmitt M. The aphasia syndrome of stroke in the left anterior cerebral artery territory. Arch Neurol 1980;37:97–100.

106. Ross E. Left medial parietal lobe and receptive language functions: mixed transcortical aphasia after left anterior cerebral artery infarction. Neurology 1980;30:144–151.

107. Fisher CM. Abulia minor versus agitated behavior. Clin Neurosurg 1983;31:9–31.

108. Fisher CM. Intermittent interruption of behavior. Trans Am Neurol Assoc 1968;93:209–210.

109. Brion S, Jedynak C-P. Trouble du tranfer inter-hemispherique a propos de trois observations de tumeurs du corps calleux. Le signe de al main etrangere. Rev Neurol 1972; 126:257–266.

110. Goldberg G, Mayer NH, Toglia JU. Medial frontal cortex infarction and the alien hand sign. Arch Neurol 1981;38:683–686.
111. Alexander GE, DeLong MR, Strick PL. Parallel organization of functionally segregated circuits linking basal ganglia and cortex. Ann Rev Neurosci 1986;9:357–381.
112. Alexander GE, Delong MR. Microstimulation of the primate neostriatum: I. physiological properties of striatal microexcitable zones. J Neurophysiol 1985;53:1417–1432.
113. Caplan LR. Intracranial branch atheromatous disease. Neurology 1989;39:1246–1250.
114. Rhoton A, Fuji K, Fradd B. Microsurgical anatomy of the anterior choroidal artery. Surg Neurol 1979;12:171–187.
115. Mohr JP, Steinke W, Timsit SG, et al. The anterior choroidal artery does not supply the corona radiata and lateral ventricular wall. Stroke 1991;22:1502–1507.
116. Cooper I. Surgical occlusions of the anterior choroidal artery in Parkinsonism. Surg Gynecol Obstet 1954;99:207–219.
117. Helgason C, Caplan LR, Goodwin V, et al. Anterior choroidal territory infarction: case reports and review. Arch Neurol 1986;43:681–686.
118. Ward T, Bernat J, Goldstein A. Occlusion of the anterior choroidal artery. J Neurol Neurosurg Psychiatry 1984;47:1046–1049.
119. Masson M, DeCroix JP, Henin D, et al. Syndrome de l'artere choroidienne anterieure: etude clinique et tomodensitometrique de 4 cas. Rev Neurol (Paris) 1983;139:553–559.
120. Frisen L. Quadruple sector anopia and sectorial optic atrophy: a syndrome of the distal anterior choroidal artery. J Neurol Neurosurg Psychiatry 1979;42:590–594.
121. Damasio H. A computed tomographic guide to the identification of cerebral vascular territories. Arch Neurol 1983;40:138–142.

CHAPTER 7

Large-Vessel Occlusive Disease of the Posterior Circulation

Following the suggestion of American[1-3] and British[4] authors in the late 1950s and early 1960s, physicians lumped all posterior circulation ischemia under the catchall terms *vertebrobasilar insufficiency* (VBI) or *vertebrobasilar infarction.* Various treatments were tried in groups of patients with VBI.[5] Unfortunately, as in the case of large heterogeneous groups of patients with anterior and posterior circulation disease, lumped under the categories of TIA or progressing or so-called completed stroke, no single treatment strategy proved helpful for the group as a whole. With the advent of more angiography, better surgery, and, finally, safe noninvasive diagnostic techniques, physicians and surgeons began to consider treatment of individual patients with anterior circulation disease, depending on the nature, severity, and location of their vascular lesions; the degree of infarction; the hematological findings; and the general health.

I have proposed that the same strategy be applied to vertebrobasilar disease because it probably is even more heterogeneous than anterior-circulation ischemic disease.[6] This chapter follows that idea and categorizes posterior-circulation occlusive disease, depending on the causative vascular lesions. Remember that in the posterior circulation, considerably more tissue is fed by small penetrating arteries, and so the proportion of small-artery to large-artery disease is higher than it is in the anterior circulation. Lacunes and penetrating branch territory infarcts within the vertebrobasilar system are considered in Chapter 8, "Penetrating and Branch Artery Disease."

Occlusion or Severe Stenosis of the Proximal Subclavian Artery

The VA arises from the proximal subclavian artery, so disease of the subclavian or innominate arteries before the VA origin can lead to changes in VA flow. Reivich et al.[7] and others[8–10] brought this practical fact to the attention of physicians when they recognized the *subclavian-steal syndrome*. In this syndrome, obstruction to the proximal subclavian artery led to a low-pressure system within the ipsilateral VA and in blood vessels of the ipsilateral upper extremity. Blood from a higher-pressure system, the contralateral VA and basilar artery, was diverted and flowed retrograde down the ipsilateral VA into the arm (Figure 7.1). In the nearly 3 decades since the description of this syndrome, knowledge of its natural history, diagnosis, and treatment has greatly expanded.

Now, most often, subclavian artery disease is detected when patients with coronary or peripheral vascular occlusive disease in the legs are referred to the ultrasound laboratories for noninvasive testing. Most patients with subclavian artery disease are asymptomatic. In those with symptoms, the majority of complaints relate to arm ischemia. Fatigue, aching after exercise, and coolness are described. In a large series of patients with subclavian steal studied in 1988 by Hennerici and colleagues, one third of patients reported pain, numbness, or fatigue in the arm, but only 15 of 324 (4.8%) had objective physical signs of brachial ischemia or embolism.[11] Neurological symptoms are not common unless there is accompanying carotid artery disease. Among 155 patients, 116 (74%) who had a unilateral subclavian steal shown by ultrasonography had no neurological symptoms.[11]

JK, a 53-year-old laborer, noted occasional dizziness, sometimes with diplopia and fuzzy vision, when he worked. The attacks were brief and always went away within seconds of his stopping work. For 6 months, he also realized that his left hand felt cool and occasionally ached after he exercised.

The most frequent symptoms of subclavian artery disease relate to the ipsilateral arm and hand. Coolness, weakness, and pain on use of the arm are common but may not be severe enough for the patient to consult a doctor. When there is impairment of VA flow (either decreased antegrade flow or retrograde flow), patients may report spells of dizziness. Dizziness is by far the commonest neurological symptom of the subclavian-steal syndrome and usually has a spinning or vertiginous character. Diplopia, decreased vision, oscillopsia, and staggering all occur, but less frequently, often accompanying the dizziness. The attacks are brief and occasionally may be brought on by exercising the ischemic arm, a diagnostic point that sometimes can be used during examination. In most patients, however, exercise of the ischemic limb does not provoke neurological symptoms or signs.

On examination of JK, the left radial pulse was smaller in volume and delayed relative to the carotid and right radial pulses. Blood pressure was 160/90 in the right arm and 120/50 in the left. The left hand felt cool. There was a loud bruit in the left supraclavicular region, which decreased slightly as the blood pressure cuff on the left arm was inflated to a pressure exceeding 120 torr. There also

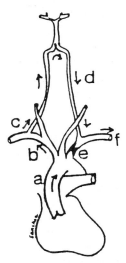

FIGURE 7.1   Subclavian steal: (a) aortic arch, (b) innominate artery, (c) right VA, (d) left VA, (e) occlusion of subclavian artery proximal to the left VA, (f) subclavian artery. Arrows represent direction of flow.

was a loud, high-pitched focal bruit at the right carotid bifurcation. Neurological examination was normal.

The diagnosis of subclavian-artery occlusive disease can usually be made by physical examination. Invariably, there is a difference in the wrist and the antecubital pulses in the two arms. The pulse in the affected limb is of smaller volume and is delayed relative to the contralateral arm. Blood pressure is also reduced asymmetrically, but in my experience, the pulse asymmetry has usually been more obvious. I am not aware of a single case of subclavian-steal syndrome in which the pulse was symmetrical and a blood pressure difference was prominent. I believe that it is more important to carefully feel both wrist pulses simultaneously than it is to routinely measure blood pressure in both arms. A supraclavicular bruit may be present. When the bruit originates from a VA stenosis without subclavian narrowing, inflating a blood pressure cuff above systolic pressure may augment the bruit by directing more blood into the VA. When the bruit is caused by subclavian stenosis, inflating the cuff reduces flow into the arm, so the bruit becomes softer.

Atherosclerosis of the proximal subclavian artery is usually associated with evidence of occlusive disease in other large arteries, typically the coronary, lower extremity, and other extracranial arteries. In this patient, the loud, focal right-carotid bruit probably indicates important concomitant right-ICA disease. Other diseases, especially Takayasu's disease and temporal arteritis,[12] can lead to subclavian stenosis. Baseball pitchers and cricket bowlers are also at risk for developing innominate or subclavian artery disease, in relation to their arm mechanics during throwing. A cervical rib or chronic use of an arm crutch can also lead to stenosis or aneurysmal dilation of the subclavian artery. Clot can form in the diseased vessel and periodically embolize to individual finger arteries, causing a syndrome that can be confused with unilateral Raynaud's syndrome. When the lesion affects the innominate artery, signs and symptoms of decreased carotid artery flow also can occur. Innominate artery disease is much less common than subclavian disease.[13]

A high proportion of patients with innominate disease are cigarette smokers. In series of patients with innominate disease, women are more often affected than men, in contrast to series of patients with carotid, subclavian, and peripheral vascular occlusive disease, in which there is a male preponderance.[13] Although right subclavian steal is much less frequent than left, it is more serious and more important to treat. Two early cases reported by Symonds describe right subclavian-artery occlusion with spread of clot into the innominate and carotid arterial systems.[14]

A more recent case report described the events in a well-known professional baseball pitcher.[15] Symptoms began when the pitcher noted his throwing arm suddenly went what he called "dead," and his first three digits felt numb. Angiography showed complete occlusion of the right subclavian artery just proximal to the medial edge of the first rib. Five days later, while exercising, he suddenly developed a left hemiplegia and confusion.[15] Subsequent angiography showed that the clot had propagated proximally to block the innominate artery and had embolized into ICA branches intracranially.[15]

Though frequent spells of posterior-circulation ischemia may occur in patients with subclavian steal, development of a posterior-circulation stroke is rare.[11,16] There is usually much smoke but little fire. I could find only two documented examples of serious brainstem or cerebellar infarction in patients with subclavian steal, and both followed severe hypotension.

Noninvasive testing of JK's arms showed reduced left forearm blood flow, as measured by oscillography. Continuous-wave (CW) Doppler examination at C2 revealed a reversal of flow in the left VA. TCD blood-flow velocities were normal. MRI was normal. Angiography confirmed a high-grade stenosis of the left subclavian artery, with retrograde flow down the left VA on delayed films. There was also a moderately severe stenosis (2.5 mm residual lumen) of the right ICA and slight stenosis of the left ICA at their origins. Intracranial vessels were normal. He was treated with aspirin (300 mg daily) and urged to try to decrease vigorous exercising of the left arm. The episodes of dizziness persisted for 3 months and then stopped. He has been followed carefully for symptoms of anterior-circulation ischemia.

Noninvasive testing of flow in the arm should allow the diagnosis of subclavian stenosis. Helpful are oscillographic measurements of forearm blood flow, venous occlusive plethysmography of the arm,[17] and analysis of the relative velocities of pulse-wave propagation in the two arms.[18]

Doppler sonography gives an accurate indication of flow in the proximal VA system. Hennerici et al. studied the accuracy of CW Doppler in detecting innominate and subclavian artery lesions.[19] All 21 patients with Doppler-detected innominate artery stenosis and all 66 with subclavian steal had angiography that confirmed the ultrasound findings.[19] In patients with slight or moderate subclavian-artery stenosis, reduction of flow was found in the VA during systole, but flow was usually antegrade. With increasingly severe subclavian stenosis, flow reversed during systole but remained cephalad in diastole, or flow was persistently decreased.[11,20,21] TCD recordings give information about the intracranial effects of the proximal arterial disease. Hennerici et al. reported the TCD findings in 50 patients with subclavian steal: 47 unilateral and 3 bilateral.[11] Most patients had normal brachial artery flow velocities and retrograde flow, irrespective of the flow pattern in the proximal VA.

When angiography is performed, it is especially important to obtain delayed films of VA flow; otherwise, the retrograde phase of flow might be missed. It is also important to assess the carotid arteries carefully because there so often is associated occlusive disease in other vessels.

Treatment of subclavian steal remains controversial. I feel that in most circumstances, the disease is relatively benign. The spells of posterior-circulation ischemia and the arm symptoms often improve with time, as collateral circulation to the arm develops. Operations on the proximal subclavian or innominate artery, when performed by thoracotomy, are more serious operative procedures than vascular surgery involving only a neck incision. In some circumstances, the intriguing radiological demonstration of reversal of VA flow has seduced the surgeon into repairing the subclavian disease (either by repair of the subclavian artery or ligation of the proximal VA) but neglecting the more serious concomitant ICA disease. When the patient is incapacitated by arm ischemia—for example, if the syndrome occurs in a golfer or a pitcher—repair is clearly indicated. When the disease affects the right innominate or subclavian artery, serious carotid-territory infarction can ensue, so that repair is in order. In most other patients, I suggest watchful waiting. I do try to reduce risk factors—such as smoking, hypertension, and hyperlipidemia—and observe the patient carefully for attacks related to the anterior circulation.

Occlusion or Severe Stenosis of the Vertebral Artery

Proximal Vertebral Artery Disease in the Neck

The most frequent location for atherosclerotic disease of the VAs is at their origin from the subclavian arteries. Atherosclerosis at this site shares epidemiological features with its close cousin, atherosclerosis of the ICA origin. In fact, the two sites are frequently affected in the same individuals.[22,23] My colleagues and I have found that the incidence of stenosis of the VA origin was much lower in blacks than in whites.[24]

LM, a 63-year-old white man, complained of repeated attacks of spinning dizziness during the past 2 weeks. In some spells, the only symptom was dizziness, but in others, diplopia and staggering occurred. In one attack, his right limbs felt transiently weak. The attacks were brief, lasting 30 seconds to 4 minutes. They tended to occur while he was quietly resting and never occurred during exertion. He also had occasional left-occipital headaches.

The most frequently reported symptom during TIAs due to VA origin disease is dizziness. The attacks are indistinguishable from those described by patients with subclavian steal, except that VA TIAs are not precipitated by effort or by arm exertion. Although dizziness is the commonest symptom, it is seldom isolated. Usually, in at least some attacks, dizziness is accompanied by other more definite signs of hindbrain ischemia. Diplopia, oscillopsia, weakness of both legs, hemiparesis, or numbness are often mentioned if the patient is closely questioned. Fisher stated that he had not seen a patient with spells of unaccompanied dizziness lasting 6 weeks or more that were due to documented VA disease.[25] In the years since this report, I also have not seen such a patient. Because dizziness is such a frequent neurological symptom and is in most cases not caused by cerebrovascular disease, I prefer not to diagnose VA disease in patients with repeated unaccompanied dizziness. True vertigo present only on rising and retiring and true positional vertigo are never due to VA-origin disease. In patients with risk factors for stroke and unaccompanied spells of dizziness, I usually order ultrasound or MRA to detect lesions of the VA in the neck or intracranially.

VA atheromas often originate in the subclavian artery and spread to the proximal few centimeters of the VA, or they may arise at the origin of the VA itself. Little has been written about the morphology of VA-origin lesions. While ulceration and plaque hemorrhage are commonly recognized when carotid endarterectomy specimens are examined, VA lesions are said to be fibrous and smooth, and they seldom ulcerate.[26,27] Unfortunately, there are very scant pathological data about VA-origin lesions, because VA surgery is usually performed by using a bypass, and so the vessel is not available for pathological examination. Careful necropsy examinations of the VAs have not been reported subsequent to recognition of the importance of plaque ulceration and hemorrhage. It cannot be assumed the ICA- and VA-origin lesions are morphologically identical. The geometry of the two origins is quite different. The VA takes off at nearly 90 degrees from the subclavian artery, whereas the ICA is almost a direct 180-degree extension of the common carotid artery (CCA). There are also caliber and flow disparities between the ICA and VA origins. Only a small fraction of subclavian flow goes into the VA, a much smaller vessel, whereas a high proportion of CCA blood goes into the ICA, a vessel of nearly the same size.

In 1989, Pelouze reported a man with multiple attacks of vertigo and brainstem ischemia that continued despite prescription of aspirin.[28] Angiography showed irregular stenosis near the VA origin, and a B-mode scan suggested an ulcerative plaque. A VA endarterectomy was performed, and the surgical specimen showed an ulcerative irregular plaque.[28] The question of the presence of VA-origin plaque ulceration is of great importance but will remain unsolved until more necropsy or surgical specimens are carefully examined. Do small platelet-fibrin and thrombin emboli arise frequently from the proximal VA and embolize to distal arteries in the posterior circulation? Would agents that reduce platelet aggregability be effective for VA-origin TIAs?

Two very important anatomical facts explain why VA-origin lesions seldom cause chronic hemodynamically significant low flow to the vertebrobasilar system: (1) The VAs are paired vessels that unite to form a single basilar artery; only rarely is there complete atresia of one VA, although asymmetries are frequent. (2) The VA gives off numerous muscular and other branches as it ascends in the neck. In contrast, there are no nuchal branches of the ICA. In the VA system, there is much more potential for development of adequate collateral circulation. Even when there is bilateral occlusion of the VAs at their origins, patients usually do not develop posterior-circulation infarcts.[29] VA-origin disease is thus much more benign than ICA-origin disease from a hemodynamic aspect.

A series of patients with VA stenosis in the neck studied in 1984 had a relatively low incidence of brainstem strokes at presentation or during follow-up.[30] There are, however, examples of embolization from recently thrombosed VAs in the neck.[31-34] In 1991, during a period of 2 weeks at the New England Medical Center in Boston, I cared for three patients with intra-arterial posterior-circulation embolism arising from an occlusive lesion at the VA origin.[34] The similar situation is well known in the anterior circulation. A patient is admitted with a small MCA-territory infarct, and ultrasound or angiography shows an occlusion at the ICA origin. The recently formed occlusive thrombus has fragmented and embolized distally. Clearly, intra-arterial embolism to the intracranial posterior-circulation arteries occurs more often than is presently recognized.

Neurological examination of LM was normal. A high-pitched focal bruit was audible in the left supraclavicular fossa, and a soft bruit was heard over the right posterior mastoid region. MRI was normal. Noninvasive testing confirmed a reduction in flow in the left VA. Angiography showed a tight stenosis of the left VA origin (Figure 7.2). Intracranial films showed good basilar artery filling. The right VA was normal. He was treated with warfarin and had no further attacks. Six months later, B-mode, CW Doppler, and color Doppler flow imaging (CDFI) suggested complete occlusion of the proximal VA, with no antegrade flow. Warfarin was stopped a month later, without subsequent spells.

In patients with proximal VA disease, a bruit can often be heard over the supraclavicular region. The physician should auscultate by moving the stethoscope bell, listening over the posterior cervical muscles and the mastoid. Sometimes, as in the patient LM, a bruit is heard over the con-

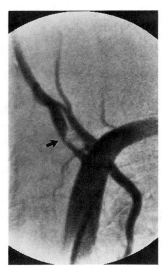

FIGURE 7.2   Subclavian angiogram showing severe stenosis of the left VA origin (arrow).

tralateral side because of increased collateral flow.[35] B-mode scans can image the proximal VA in the segment between the origin of the artery until its entrance into the foramen transversara of the cervical vertebrae. CDFI is also very helpful in showing VA flow patterns. CW Doppler insonation in the low neck and at the C2 region is the most effective means of monitoring VA flow. Perhaps MRA will prove effective in imaging disease of the VA origin, obviating the need for invasive catheter angiography.

Data about the natural history of disease of the VA origin and the response of patients with this lesion to various treatments are insufficient to warrant firm conclusions as to the best therapy. Moufarrij and colleagues reviewed their experience with VA lesions. Long-term follow-up of their series of more than 80 patients with greater than 75 percent stenosis of the VA origin showed that only 2 had brainstem strokes, and these 2 patients also had basilar artery stenosis.[30]

Vascular surgeons have shown that they can bypass VA-origin lesions with low morbidity and mortality.[27,34-37] There are no data about the effectiveness or lack thereof of antiplatelet aggregating agents or of warfarin in patients with proximal VA disease. In the preceding case of LM, I chose warfarin, to prevent thrombosis and subsequent embolization in a vessel with low antegrade flow. If the lesion had been less stenotic, I would have chosen aspirin, to prevent fibrin or platelet emboli. I did not choose surgery because the surgeons with whom I work have had little past experience with this lesion, and I believe that this condition is relatively benign. Clearly, more data are needed regarding the natural history of VA-origin disease and its response to medical and surgical treatment. Perhaps the advent of MRA and wider application of noninvasive techniques to the VA circulation will provide groups of patients with VA-origin disease, who can be followed prospectively and studied, to determine the relative utility of various therapies.

Intracranial Vertebral Artery (ICVA) Disease

Severe atherosclerotic narrowing is rare in the cervical portions of the VAs, except at their origins. Plaques are relatively routinely observed opposite osteophytes, but they rarely narrow the vessel.[26] The distal extracranial VA is vulnerable to trauma, spontaneous dissection,[38] and fibromuscular dysplasia. The distal cervical VA is occasionally severely narrowed in patients with temporal arteritis[39] and in women taking high-estrogen-content contraceptive pills.[40] Atherosclerosis of the ICVA is usually most severe in the portions of the artery that supply the posterior inferior cerebellar artery (PICA) and the anterior spinal artery branches. Narrowing often extends to the origin of the basilar artery. Less often, stenosis involves the VA just after it penetrates the dura to enter the cranium. In contrast to patients with proximal VA disease, there is no single typical patient with ICVA occlusive disease. Therefore, four different patient examples are presented and discussed herein.

Patient 1

A 57-year-old white man, WA, had a transient attack of dizziness and diplopia when he arose from a nap. The next day, on awakening, he felt dizzy, as if the room were rocking or wavering like a ship. He felt a series of sharp painful jabs in his left eye, and his left face felt strangely numb. When he tried to sit or stand, he veered to the left. His left arm was clumsy. His voice was hoarse, and he gagged as he tried to swallow water. Vomiting and hiccups developed as the morning progressed, and he went to the hospital. Examination there showed diminished pain and temperature sensitivity on the left face and right body, including the limbs; nystagmus worse on looking leftward; diminished left corneal reflex; left ptosis and a smaller left pupil; clumsiness of the left hand and foot; and decreased palatal motion on the left.

The most frequent findings in patients with ICVA occlusion are related to ischemia of the lateral medulla, the lesion illustrated by this patient. In patients with lateral medullary infarction, the most common vascular lesion is occlusion of the VA intracranially proximal to its PICA branch.[41] Less often, lateral medullary infarction is caused by occlusion of medullary branches or the PICA. Important symptoms and signs of lateral medullary infarction can be understood best by recalling the anatomical nuclei and tracts in the lateral medulla (Figure 7.3).

1. *Nucleus and descending spinal tract of V*—Symptoms include sharp jabs or stabs of pain in the ipsilateral eye and face and a feeling of numbness of the face; examination usually confirms decreased recognition of

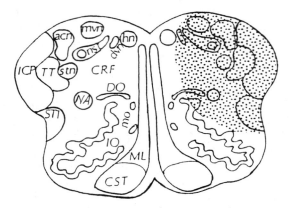

acn = accessory cuneate nucleus, CRF = central reticular formation, CST = corticospinal tract, DO = dorsal accessory olivary nucleus, dvn = dorsal vagal nucleus, hn = hypoglossal nucleus, ICP = inferior cerebellar peduncle, IO = inferior olivary nucleus, ML = medial lemniscus, mo = medial accessory olivary nucleus, mvn = medial vestibular nucleus, nst = nucleus of the solitary tract, STT = spinothalamic tract, stn = spinal trigeminal nucleus, TT = trigeminal tract, NA = nucleus ambiguus.

FIGURE 7.3   Dorsal lateral medullary infarct (Wallenberg's syndrome).

pinprick and temperature on the ipsilateral face and a reduced corneal reflex.

2. *Vestibular nuclei and their connections*—Feelings of dizziness, or instability of the environment result from dysfunction of the vestibular system and may invoke vomiting; careful examination usually documents nystagmus with coarse rotatory eye movements when looking to the ipsilateral side and small-amplitude faster nystagmus when looking contralaterally; sometimes, the eyes forcibly deviate to the side of the lesion, so-called *lateral pulsion.*[42,43]

3. *Spinothalamic tract*—Lesions of this structure usually produce diminished recognition of pinprick and temperature in the contralateral limbs and body; this loss of function is seldom spontaneously recognized or reported by patients and is usually noticed only after detection on examination; at times, the pinprick and temperature loss extends to the contralateral face because of involvement of the crossed quintothalamic tract, which appends itself medially to the spinothalamic tract.

4. *Restiform body (inferior cerebellar peduncle)*—Symptoms include veering or leaning toward the side of the lesion and clumsiness of the ipsilateral limbs; on examination, there is frequently hypotonia and exaggerated rebound of the ipsilateral arm, but frank intention tremor is not common; on standing or sitting, patients may lean or tilt to the side of the lesion.

5. *Autonomic nervous system nuclei and tracts*—The descending sympathetic system traverses the lateral medulla in the lateral reticular for-

mation; dysfunction causes an ipsilateral Horner's syndrome; the dorsal motor nucleus of the vagus is sometimes affected, leading to tachycardia and a labile increased blood pressure.

6. *Nucleus ambiguus*—When the infarct extends medially, it often affects this nucleus, causing hoarseness and dysphagia. The pharynx and palate are weak on the side of the lesion, sometimes causing patients to retain food within the piriform recess of the pharynx. A crowlike cough represents an attempt to extricate food from this area. At times, there is also ipsilateral facial weakness, perhaps related to ischemia of the caudal part of the VII-nerve nucleus just rostral to the nucleus ambiguus or involvement of corticobulbar fibers going toward the VII-nerve nucleus.

7. *Abnormal respiratory control*—Initiation and control of respiration are known to involve the lateral pontine and medullary tegmentum. Poliomyelitis and bilateral medullary infarcts are well known to cause decreased respiratory drive.[44] Levin and Margolis described a single patient with failure of automatic respirations ("Ondine's curse"—sleep-related apnea) due to a one-sided lateral medullary infarct.[45] Bogousslavsky et al. described in detail the clinical and autopsy findings in two patients with one-sided lateral medullopontine infarction.[46] Hypoventilation is probably related to involvement of the nucleus of the solitary tract, the nucleus ambiguus, the nucleus retroambiguus, and the nuclei parvocellularis and gigantocellularis.[46]

When infarction is limited to the lateral medulla, prognosis for recovery is good,[47] with three important exceptions:[48] (1) Some patients have infarction in the ipsilateral inferior cerebellum, a region fed by the PICA; when the infarct is large, headache, head tilt, and stupor can result. A posterior fossa pressure cone can develop and can cause death from medullary compression. Also, (2) some patients with lateral medullary infarcts die suddenly; although the etiology of sudden death is uncertain, it could be due to sudden increase in vagal tone (secondary to involvement of the dorsal motor nucleus of the vagus) or to involvement of the automatic respiratory center.

In addition, (3) some patients with a one-sided lateral medullary infarct have occlusive lesions in both ICVAs. Development of symptomatic ischemia in the lateral medulla that is contralateral to the infarct has a serious prognosis because of the frequency of autonomic dysfunction and loss of automatic control of respiration. Bilateral ICVA disease has a poor prognosis once symptoms develop.[49] Because of these important problems, it has been my practice to watch patients carefully for cerebellar pressure and to monitor respiration early in the course of the illness.

In some patients with ICVA occlusion, ischemia of the medial medulla accompanies the lateral medullary infarct. This phenomenon is explained by a vertebral occlusion that blocks both the PICA and the anterior spinal artery orifices.[50] In addition to the signs already mentioned, a hemiparesis affects the contralateral arm and leg because of ischemia to the medullary pyramid. Ipsilateral weakness of the tongue and contralateral loss of position sense are less frequent findings and are explained by involvement of the hypoglossal nerve and the medial lemniscus.

In WA, B-mode and CW Doppler of the neck VA were normal. TCD showed an increase in blood-flow velocities in the left VA. Right VA pressures were normal. MRA showed severe stenosis of the left VA just after the artery entered the cranium.

TCD can give accurate indications of occlusive lesions involving the ICVAs, using insonation through a suboccipital foramen magnum window.[51,52] Because of the TCD and MRA results, the patient was treated with warfarin. The arterial stenosis is being followed by serial TCD examinations.

Patient 2

A 48-year-old woman, AD, suddenly felt dizzy and unsteady on her feet. She vomited and felt unable to walk. When examined, the only positive findings were gait ataxia and slight conjugate gaze paresis to the left. CT was normal. The next morning, she was sleepy and complained of severe headache. Her neck was stiff, and she preferred to stay stationary in bed. There was a complete left conjugate gaze paresis to oculocephalic maneuvers, and the left corneal reflex was reduced. Both plantar responses were extensor. CT now confirmed a large area of hypodensity in the left cerebellum. The fourth ventricle was not visible, and the lateral ventricles were enlarged. MRI confirmed a very large PICA-territory cerebellar infarct (Figure 7.4). She became stuporous and difficult to arouse. She was treated with IV steroids and mannitol but did not awaken. Soft necrotic cerebellar tissue was removed through a left posterior fossa craniotomy, after which she made an excellent recovery.

The commonest vascular lesion found in patients with cerebellar infarction is occlusion or severe stenosis of the ICVA.[53-55] Often, the occlusion is due to embolism, the thrombus arising in the heart or proximal vascular system.[55] The syndrome of cerebellar infarction is often difficult to diagnose. Symptoms can resemble labyrinthitis and can appear deceptively slight. Gait ataxia and vomiting are often accompanied by dizziness, closely mimicking the findings in cerebellar hemorrhage.[56] There are frequently no signs of lateral medullary ischemia. Initial CT scan, as in this case, is often normal. It is very important to make certain that the fourth ventricle is of normal size and in normal position. In retrospect, this was not done in this case. Review of the initial films revealed slight rightward deviation and tilting of the fourth ventricle. MRI is more accurate in detecting early cerebellar ischemia. Especially important for localization are T2-weighted sagittal sections. On sagittal films, localization of the vascular territory involved is relatively easy. Lesions above the horizontal fissure are in the

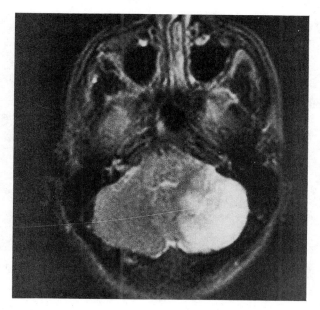

FIGURE 7.4   MRI T2-weighted axial image showing large PICA-territory infarct.

superior cerebellar artery (SCA) territory, and lesions below the fissure are localized to anterior inferior cerebellar artery (AICA) or PICA territories, depending on anterior or posterior localization on the inferior surface of the cerebellum. Figure 7.5 shows a PICA-territory infarct on a T2-weighted sagittal section.

Swollen cerebellar lesions may compress the cerebellopontine angle, leading to involvement of the ipsilateral fifth, sixth, seventh, and eighth cranial nerves. Compression of the medulla and pons is the probable cause of conjugate-gaze paresis to the ipsilateral side. This finding is especially important because the presence of a conjugate-gaze palsy without contralateral hemiplegia is virtually diagnostic of a cerebellar space-taking lesion. With more severe compression, the plantar responses become extensor, systolic pressure rises, diastolic pressure falls, the pulse may slow, and respiration may cease.

As the cerebellum swells, hypodensity usually appears on repeat CT. Posterior fossa cisterns are compressed, and the ventricles become enlarged because of compression of the fourth ventricle. On MRI, compression of the contralateral vermis and brainstem are usually evident. Without treatment, death often ensues.[57,58] Preferred therapy is decompression of the swollen cerebellum. In some patients, medical decompression using steroids and osmotic agents has been helpful; success has also been achieved in some patients by placing a ventricular drain in the lateral ventricles.[59] It is often difficult to separate brainstem pressure due to cerebellar infarction from

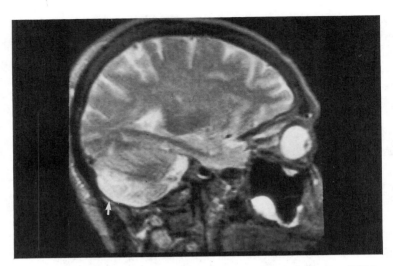

FIGURE 7.5   MRI T2-weighted sagittal view: white arrow points to PICA-territory infarct.

brainstem ischemia due to the propagation of clot into the basilar artery. MRI scans are helpful in making this distinction, but angiography is often necessary to visualize the vascular lesion.

Patient 2, AD, is an example of a large cerebellar infarct. In other patients, cerebellar infarcts are quite small and cause little or no abnormal neurological signs. Embolism from the heart or proximal VA can cause cerebellar infarction by blocking the ICVA, the PICA, or the SCA. Cardiac evaluation and MRA or standard angiography can usually delineate the nature of the offending vascular process.

Patient 3

A 65-year-old white man, BE, had transient headache and dizziness on two occasions, 7 and 10 days before admission. On the day of admission, he suddenly became blind and agitated. When examined, 5 hours later, he could not recall events of the past 3 weeks. He could make no new memories and had a complete right hemianopia. There were no other abnormalities of brainstem or CNS function. CT revealed infarcts of the left occipital and temporal lobes in the distribution of the left PCA. MRI also showed a small infarct in the left cerebellum in PICA territory. Angiography revealed occlusion of the left ICVA and embolic amputation of the left PCA. All other vessels were normal or showed only minor atheroma. Cardiac evaluation was normal.

This patient had an ICVA occlusion, followed by an embolus to the distal basilar system. In retrospect, the two episodes of dizziness probably represented transient cerebellar or medullary ischemia. When the vertebrobasilar system has been studied at necropsy, embolic occlusions are common in the PCAs.[60] These emboli may arise from recent occlusion within the proximal or the intracranial VAs.[34] Koroshetz and Ropper systematically studied 12 patients with both PCA infarcts and brainstem symptoms.[61] They found that 3 patients had donor sites for intra-arterial embolism in the ICVA, and 3 others had lesions of both the IC and EC VAs. All of the patients had intra-arterial embolism as the cause of PCA infarction.[61] Documentation of artery-to-artery emboli from freshly occluded VAs has made me wonder whether heparin or warfarin is indicated for all such patients during the time it takes for the clot to solidify and attach to the vessel (2 to 4 weeks). There are at present insufficient arteriographic or pathological data to conclude how often this occurs and what the risk/benefit ratio would be of using anticoagulants for preventing this.

Patient 4

A 60-year-old hypertensive, diabetic black man, EO, noted diplopia and dizziness after arising from a nap. The symptoms were transient, but 2 days later, he staggered and again saw double. On examination, there was gait ataxia, nystagmus, and a slight left facial weakness. When he stood, he became dizzy, felt weak, and his vision dimmed. He was treated with heparin and bed rest but 6 days later gradually became stuporous and quadriplegic. He died soon after of pneumonia. Necropsy revealed bilateral occlusion of the ICVAs and extensive necrosis of the cerebellar hemispheres, medulla, and pons.

The diagnosis of bilateral ICVA occlusion is difficult.[49] Early symptoms may be deceptively mild and are usually referable to the cerebellum and lateral medulla, like those seen in Patients 1 (WA) and 2 (AD). Because of a low-flow system, the symptoms are often positionally sensitive, worsening when the patient sits or stands or when blood pressure falls either spontaneously or after treatment. Usually, symptoms and signs gradually progress. Heparin is most often ineffective because the progressive ischemia is due to low flow. Cerebellar and pyramidal signs and symptoms predominate. At times, also, ischemia of the PCA territories leads to abnormalities of vision, memory, and behavior. Bilateral ICVA occlusive lesions are most common in hypertensive and diabetic patients. Death due to extensive hindbrain ischemia has been invariable in my experience, unless an artificial posterior circulation conduit is created. Sundt,[62] Ausman,[63] and Roski and colleagues,[64] among others, have noted the success of this treatment for patients with bilateral VA lesions. A variety of different shunts have been used, depending on the location of the blockage. The most common procedures involve anastomosis of the occipital artery to the PICA or the superficial temporal artery to the AICA, SCA, or PCA. Before such a shunt is performed, angiography with full visualization of the VAs is critical. ICA injections should also be made to detect retrograde flow from the posterior communicating arteries into the basilar system.

Patients 1 through 4 are illustrative of serious posterior-circulation infarction caused by ICVA disease. In some patients, undoubtedly, this vascular lesion is tolerated without symptoms or with only minor TIAs. As a general rule, however, the more distally located a vascular lesion is along the path from the proximal subclavian–vertebral junction to the distal basilar artery, the more likely it is to cause infarction. The more proximal the lesion, the more likely it is to be benign.

Little is known about optimal treatment of lesions of the ICVA. Allen and others have performed direct endarterectomies on the ICVA, usually in its proximal portion.[65] Interventional radiologists now have the capability to perform angioplasties on the ICVA. Thrombolytic treatment also could lyse VA thrombi if given early enough after occlusion. In the patient examples and discussion, I have already emphasized the need for vigilance to detect large cerebellar infarcts and the need to decompress these lesions. I have reserved surgically created vascular shunts for patients with bilateral ICVA disease (or unilateral disease with a very hypoplastic contralateral VA). I often use short-term heparin or warfarin therapy for patients with angiographically documented VA occlusion, in an attempt to prevent clot propagation and embolization. In some patients, with severe ICVA stenosis, I have used longer-term warfarin (6 months to 1 year), keeping the PT at 1.5 times the control values. I follow patients with ICVA stenosis with serial TCD and MRA examinations for progression of the lesion to complete occlusion, or for recanalization with disappearance of critical stenosis. I stop anticoagulants about a month after either documented occlusion or reestablishment of wide patency. I have absolutely no data that support these choices of treatment, but they make good sense to me at present. I anxiously await careful prospective studies of treatment of patients with ICVA disease.

Occlusion or Severe Stenosis of the Basilar Artery

In a landmark report, Kubik and Adams called attention to the clinical and pathological features of occlusion of the basilar artery.[66] Characterized by quadriparesis and cranial nerve abnormalities that allowed for accurate diagnosis during life, the disorder was then considered invariably fatal. We now know that the outcome of patients with basilar-artery occlusive disease is quite variable. Some patients succumb or are left severely disabled, but others survive with little or no deficit.[31] Prognosis depends on the rapidity of the occlusion, the location and extent of the thrombosis, and the development of adequate collateral circulation.

A 63-year-old man, OL, was unable to rise from bed because of weakness of both his legs. He had had a myocardial infarction 5 years earlier. During the past 2 weeks, he had had two transient episodes of diplopia, one accompanied by momentary buckling of the legs. During the past month, he had occasional severe occipital headaches.

Atherosclerosis commonly affects the first few centimeters of the basilar artery, although stenosis can also occur in the middle and distal segments.[67] Patients with basilar-artery atherosclerosis have a high incidence of atherosclerosis elsewhere, especially in the coronary, carotid, and iliofemoral arteries. In Kubik and Adams's original report,[66] most patients developed signs abruptly without previous warnings, but their paper preceded recognition of the frequency and importance of TIAs and emanated from the pathology laboratory. Careful questioning of most patients with basilar-artery occlusive disease elicits descriptions of attacks of temporary brainstem dysfunction prior to their strokes. The commonest symptoms during these TIAs are diplopia; dizziness, most often without true spinning; weakness of both legs; or weakness alternating between different limbs in different attacks. As in occlusive disease of other large extracranial and cranial arteries, some patients develop prominent headache during the weeks before and during development of a critical decrease in blood flow. With basilar-artery occlusive disease, the headache is usually occipital, often spreading to the vertex of the head.

On examination, OL's limbs were very weak, more so on the left. He could not move his right arm and leg but could lift the left heel off the bed to a height of 15 cm for 5 seconds before it would fall. He could adduct the left shoulder toward him by sliding it along the bed but could not lift the arm or move his fingers. Both plantar responses were extensor. Pinprick and touch perception were normal. He could not look to the right. On gaze to the left, only the left eye moved, but it exhibited abducting nystagmus. There was no adduction of the right eye on attempted left gaze. The voice was very dysarthric, and secretions pooled in the back of his throat.

The basilar artery forms from the merging of the two VAs at the medullopontine junction. The basilar artery ends at the junction of the pons and the midbrain. The major territory of supply of the basilar artery is the pons, especially the basis pontis. The tegmentum of the pons has a rich collateral supply of vessels but depends primarily on the SCAs, vessels that originate from the rostral basilar artery just before it bifurcates. Occlusion of the basilar artery often causes ischemia in the pontine base bilaterally, sometimes extending into the medial tegmentum on one or both sides. Figure 7.6 contains an example of the distribution of ischemia in basilar-artery occlusion, patterned after Kubik and Adams.[66] Note that the medulla and cerebellar hemispheres are usually spared, in contrast to the situation when one or both VAs are blocked. Blockage of the midbasilar artery at the orifice of the AICAs often is accompanied by infarction in the anterior inferior cerebellum on one or both sides.[68]

Visualizing the anatomical regions of damage helps in predicting and understanding the usual neurological signs and symptoms that accompany basilar-artery occlusion:

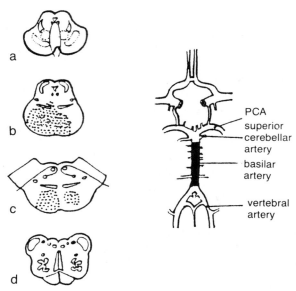

FIGURE 7.6   Pons with infarct caused by occlusion of the basilar artery: (a) mid-brain, (b) upper pons, (c) lower pons, (d) medulla. (Redrawn after Kubik C, Adams R. Occlusion of the basilar artery: a clinical and pathological study. Brain 1946;69: 73–121.)

1.   *Paralysis of the limbs*—Weakness is usually bilateral but may be asymmetric, as in the patient OL's presentation; stiffness, hyperreflexia, and extensor plantar reflexes are found on examination of the weak limbs.

2.   *Bulbar or pseudobulbar paralysis of the cranial musculature*—The infarct can directly involve cranial motor nuclei, causing paralysis of the face, palate, pharynx, neck, or tongue on one or both sides. The IX to XII nerve nuclei are located within the medullary tegmentum, which is usually below the level of the infarct. Weakness of the cranial musculature innervated by these nuclei causes dysarthria, dysphonia, hoarseness, dysphagia, and lingual weakness, all common findings in patients with basilar occlusion and pontine infarction. The pontine lesion interrupts corticofugal descending fibers destined for these cranial-nerve nuclei. The resulting weakness is called "pseudobulbar" because it involves the descending pathways controlling the bulbar nuclei rather than the nuclei themselves. Exaggerated jaw and facial reflexes, increased gag reflex, and easily induced emotional incontinence, with excessive laughing or crying accompany the weakness. In some cases, the limb and bulbar paralysis is so severe that the patient cannot communicate either verbally or by gesture. Such patients have been called "locked-in" because of their loss of motor function. Eye movement or eye-blinking signals can sometimes be arranged that clearly prove that the patient is alert and intellectually preserved despite the paralysis.

3. *Absence of sensory or cerebellar abnormalities*—The infarct usually affects the midline and paramedian structures in the basis pontis. Collateral circulation is generally through the circumferential vessels that supply the lateral base and tegmentum and the cerebellum. The cerebellar hemispheres are mostly nourished by the PICA, which originates before the basilar artery, and the SCA, which is preserved when the basilar-artery clot does not extend to the distal basilar artery. The spinothalamic tracts and the cerebellum are often spared from the ischemia.

4. *Abnormalities of eye movement*—The sixth-nerve nuclei, medial longitudinal fasciculi (MLF), and pontine lateral gaze centers are all located in the paramedian pontine tegmentum and therefore are vulnerable to ischemia in this region. Lesions of the sixth nerve or nucleus cause paralysis of abduction of the eye. An MLF lesion produces a defect in adduction of the ipsilateral eye, on gaze directed to the opposite side, and it produces nystagmus of the contralateral abducting eye. This syndrome, called an internuclear ophthalmoplegia (INO), can be bilateral. Lesions of the paramedian pontine tegmentum may also affect the paramedian pontine reticular formation (PPRF), the so-called pontine lateral gaze center, which mediates gaze to the same side. A lesion of this region causes an ipsilateral conjugate-gaze paresis. A unilateral lesion can affect both the PPRF and the MLF on the same side. The resulting syndrome was present in the patient described and has been called the "one and one-half syndrome" by Fisher[69] because only one-half of gaze (scoring 1 for gaze to each side) is preserved. The patient described had paralysis of right gaze due to a lesion of the right PPRF and paralysis of the adducting right eye on gaze to the left, caused by involvement of the right MLF.

5. *Nystagmus*—The vestibular nuclei and their connections are also commonly affected, causing vertical and horizontal nystagmus.

6. *Other eye signs*—Ptosis, small pupils, and ocular skewing are also commonly found in patients with basilar-artery occlusion.

7. *Coma*—If the lesion interrupts function of the medial pontine tegmentum bilaterally, coma may supervene.[70] Reduced consciousness is a very poor prognostic sign, but care must be taken in differentiating reduced alertness from the locked-in state.

CT of OL was normal. MRI showed ischemia in the mid and lower pons bilaterally in the basis pontis. The basilar-artery flow void was absent in the lower pons. Heparin was given intravenously in a continuous-drip infusion. During the first 24 hours, the patient developed increased weakness of the right leg. He remained stable thereafter, and by day 10, he could lift both arms and speak more clearly. Angiography showed slight irregularity without stenosis of the VAs at their origins. The basilar artery was completely occluded just after its origin (Figure 7.7). An ICA injection opacified the rostral basilar artery through the posterior communicating artery. By day 14, he could sit with help and had no blood pressure drop or increased weakness when he did so.

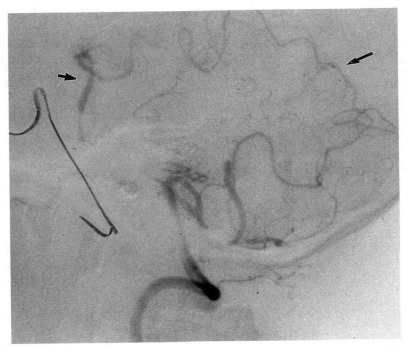

FIGURE 7.7 Vertebral angiogram, lateral view: Basilar artery is occluded; rostral basilar artery is filled (small arrow, upper left) from collaterals going around the cerebellum (long arrow, upper right) from PICA to SCA branches.

Heparin was stopped. He recovered partially during rehabilitation and had no further worsening of signs or symptoms.

CT has not been very sensitive in imaging brainstem infarcts, although this capability has improved with newer-generation scanners.[71,72] CT is, however, very reliable in excluding primary brainstem hemorrhage, one of the differential diagnostic considerations. MRI provides better imaging of brainstem and cerebellar infarcts.[73–75] In the patient described and in others with bilateral abnormalities of brainstem function, the principal differential diagnosis is between basilar-artery obstruction and obliteration of basilar branch arteries bilaterally despite a patent basilar artery.[76] This distinction can usually be made by angiography.

In this patient, OL, the lack of a history of prior stroke and the extensive nature of the bilateral signs made it highly probable that the lesion involved the main basilar artery. Because the early course is often unstable, I usually administer heparin intravenously after excluding hemorrhage. Even though preceding TIAs and the absence of hypertension made brainstem hemorrhage very unlikely, I still obtained a CT and MRI scan early in the course. I prefer not to do invasive studies early in the course of fluctuating brainstem ischemia, performing angiography only when the diagnosis is quite uncertain. Reduced perfusion of the brainstem is the major problem, so attention must be given to maximizing blood flow. I prefer to keep patients at bed rest, with the head flat. Blood pressure should not be lowered unless it is in the malignant range, and cardiac failure should be treated. Dehydration and hypovolemia should be avoided. During the initial course of the ischemia (up to 2 weeks), patients may develop additional symptoms when they sit, stand, or are merely propped up in bed.[77] It is my practice to observe patients carefully when they sit or stand, checking the pulse and blood pressure and noting any change in neurological function. Ambulation should be very gradual and carefully supervised. Unfortunately, TCD is not very accurate in showing basilar-artery disease because the lesion is often beyond the range of the suboccipital probe.[52] MRI can suggest basilar-artery occlusion by the absence of the usual basilar-artery-flow void. MRA shows great promise in defining basilar-artery disease.[78,79]

When there is a strong clinical suspicion that the vascular lesion affects the main basilar artery, or when the clinical picture is confusing and preliminary studies do not clarify the nature of the vascular lesion, I use angiography to help decide on the next therapeutic step. Angiography is usually deferred 8 to 13 days, while the patient continues to receive heparin, until the clinical course appears stable. If the patient with ischemia has not stabilized and continues to deteriorate despite heparin, then I suggest angiography earlier. I feel that long-term warfarin therapy is more dangerous than is angiography. If angiography reveals a complete basilar-artery occlusion, I continue heparin for a total of 3 weeks and use aspirin thereafter or no treatment. If there is a tight stenosis of the basilar artery without occlusion, I usually use long-term warfarin treatment, in an attempt to prevent occlusion. If there is only minor plaque disease in the major basilar artery, I select agents such as aspirin or ticlopidine, which decrease platelet aggregation and agglutination.

In patients with no obvious intrinsic lesions by angiography, it is important to think of the possibility of embolism and to be certain that studies are adequate to exclude a cardiogenic embolus or embolism from the aorta or proximal VA. I consider the use of surgically created extracranial to intracranial artery shunts for patients with bilateral VA or severe basilar-artery occlusive disease whose clinical course is progressive or who continue to have transient attacks despite adequate anticoagulation and efforts to augment blood flow.

A 31-year-old man, PG, was discovered to be comatose by his son. That morning, he had been normal, according to his wife, who recalled no recent signs of ill health in her husband. He had no history of heart or vascular disease. On examination, his pupils were dilated and fixed at 8 mm each, and the eyes were each deviated down and outward. Lateral motion in each eye was obtained by oculocephalic maneuvers. There were no abnormal motor signs.

The bilateral III-nerve dysfunction and coma suggested a lesion intrinsic to the midbrain. This could be caused by a large supratentorial space-taking lesion, with midbrain compression, or by an intrinsic lesion within the midbrain. Because of the lack of history, absence of stroke risk factors, and limitation of the neurological examination by coma, I felt it mandatory to order urgent neuroimaging tests.

The CT in patient OL was normal with and without contrast. MRI could not be performed urgently, but the next day, T2-weighted images showed infarction in the paramedian thalamus and midbrain tegmentum. MRA was normal. An echocardiogram showed a left atrial myxoma.

In most patients with basilar artery occlusion, the thrombus is limited to the proximal basilar artery. In some patients, the occlusion extends to the distal basilar-artery segment; in other patients, more often in blacks, occlusion or severe stenosis can affect predominantly the distal basilar artery.[24,67] Occlusion of the distal basilar artery is most often due to embolism from the heart or the proximal VA system. Emboli small enough to pass through the VAs will not usually lodge in the proximal basilar artery, a vessel larger than each VA, but they will travel to the distal basilar artery or to PCA branches. The distal basilar artery supplies the midbrain and diencephalon through small vessels that pierce the posterior perforated substance. Signs of dysfunction in this territory include[80–82]

1. *Pupillary abnormalities*—The lesion may interrupt the afferent reflex arc by interfering with fibers going toward the Edinger-Westphal nucleus. The III-nerve nucleus can also be involved, as well as the rostral descending sympathetic system. The pupils are usually abnormal and can be small, midposition, or dilated, depending on the level and extent of the lesion. Decreased pupillary reactivity and eccentricity of the pupil are also found.[83,84]
2. *Eye movement abnormalities*—Vertical gaze abnormalities are common in patients with rostral brainstem lesions. Paralysis of upward or downward gaze is common. The eyes may also be skewed and may be deviated at rest, most often downward and inward. Hyperconvergence, retractory nystagmus, and pseudo VI-nerve paresis[80,82] are other oculomotor features.
3. *Altered level of alertness*—Hypersomnolence or frank coma can result from bilateral paramedian rostral brainstem dysfunction. After the acute phase, the patient may remain relatively inert and apathetic.[80]
4. *Amnesia*—Memory loss can accompany thalamic infarction. Patients are unable to make new memories and may have no recall of events just preceding their stroke. There may be an array of other behavioral abnor-

malities, including agitation, hallucinations, and abnormalities that mimic lesions of the frontal lobe.

In OL, the bilateral III-nerve palsies identified the midbrain lesion, which was confirmed by MRI. Because the most frequent cause is embolic, the cardiac and vascular investigations are very important. Identification of the left atrial myxoma led to later successful removal of the lesion. The patient awakened on day 4 after his stroke and was left with a bilateral III-nerve palsy as his only important neurological disability.

Occlusion or Severe Stenosis of the Posterior Cerebral Arteries

The PCAs are the major tributaries of the basilar artery. In approximately 30 percent of patients, one basilar communicating segment is hypoplastic, and so the PCA is derived primarily from the ipsilateral ICA through its posterior communicating artery branch. (Figure 7.8 illustrates the fetal-type PCA and also a retained primitive ICA–basilar artery communication, the trigeminal artery.) Intrinsic atheromatous disease of the PCA most often affects the origin of the vessel, and its epidemiology is similar to disease of the proximal MCA. Most often, infarcts in the PCA territory are due to emboli to the posterior circulation.[60,83] Castagne and colleagues, in a necropsy study, identified 30 infarcts within PCA territory.[60] The most common mechanism of infarction was embolism from a proximal occlusive lesion within the vertebrobasilar system (15/30, 50%). In 8 patients, clot propagated from the basilar artery into the PCA. Only 3 patients had thrombosis of the PCA engrafted on previous atherosclerotic narrowing.[60]

Pessin and I and our colleagues studied the mechanism of infarction in 35 patients with hemianopia and a unilateral infarct on CT limited to the PCA territory on one side.[83] Figure 7.9 is a montage of the CT lesions from that study. The most frequent mechanism of infarction was embolism. A cardiac source of embolism was present in 10 patients (28.5%), and intra-arterial embolism arising from proximal posterior circulation lesions was found in 6 patients (17%). In 11 other patients, the clinical and angiographic findings suggested embolism, but no definite donor site was established. Among the 35, 27 patients (77%) had embolic occlusion of PCA branches.[83]

An analogy can be drawn between the two brain circulations. In the anterior circulation, emboli usually lodge in MCA branches, leading to cortical infarcts; in the posterior circulation, emboli traverse the vertebral and basilar arteries and ultimately lodge in PCA branches, producing cortical infarcts. Intrinsic disease of the MCA and PCA does occur but is far less common than cardiogenic or artery-to-artery embolization. When intrinsic atherosclerosis of the PCA is present, the clinical presentation usually consists of transient hemianopic visual symptoms, sometimes accompanied by transient hemisensory symptoms on the same side.[84]

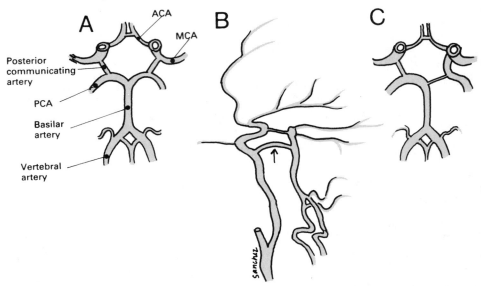

FIGURE 7.8   (a) Normal circle of Willis, basal view; (b) primitive trigeminal artery (arrow), lateral view; (c) origin of posterior communicating artery from the ICA.

A 64-year-old black woman, MA, awakened with the realization that she could not see to her left. She was able to read and could clearly identify objects in the room but felt it necessary to turn to the left to "see better." She also noted a dull pain behind her right eye. She was not aware of any difficulty with her limbs, walking, or thinking. On examination, there was a left homonymous hemianopia, with slight sparing of the most central portion of the left visual field. The patient could read, note the color and nature of objects and pictures, draw common objects, copy drawings, and accurately bisect lines scattered on a page. Motor, sensory, reflex functions, and gait were normal.

After giving off penetrating branches to the midbrain and thalamus, the PCA supplies branches to the occipital lobes and supplies the medial and inferior portions of the temporal lobes. Headache in patients with PCA disease is often retro-orbital or above the eye, probably reflecting the fact that the upper surface of the tentorium is innervated by the first division of the Vth nerve. Infarction in the cerebral territories of the PCA most often affects vision and somatic sensation but seldom causes paralysis.

Visual-Field Abnormalities

The single most common finding in patients with PCA territory infarction is a *hemianopia*. Hemianopia is due to infarction of the striate visual cortex on the banks of the calcarine fissure, a region supplied by the calcarine branch of the PCA, or it is due to interruption of the geniculocalcarine tract as it nears the visual cortex. If just the lower bank of the calcarine fissure is involved—the lingual gyrus—a superior-quadrant field defect results. An

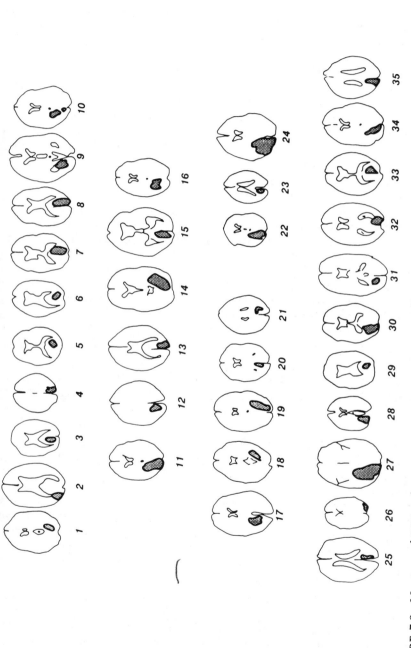

FIGURE 7.9 Montage of PCA infarcts on CT. (From Pessin MS, Lathi E, Cohen M, et al. Clinical features and mechanism of occipital infarction, Ann Neurol 1987;21:290–299; reprinted with permission.)

inferior quadrantanopia results if the lesion affects the cuneus on the upper bank of the calcarine fissure.

When infarction is restricted to the striate cortex and does not extend into adjacent parietal cortex, the patient is fully aware of the visual defect. Usually described as a void, a blackness, or a limitation of vision to one side, patients usually recognize that they need to focus extra attention to the hemianopic field. When given written material or pictures, patients with hemianopia due to occipital infarction are able to see and interpret the stimuli normally, although it may take them a bit longer to explore the visual field. Hemianopia and visual neglect are not synonymous, nor is visual neglect merely a more or less severe form of hemianopia. In patients with occipital lobe infarcts, physicians can reliably map out the visual fields by confrontation. At times, the central or medial part of the field is spared—so-called macular sparing. Optokinetic nystagmus is normal. Some patients, although they accurately report motion or the presence of objects in their hemianopic field, cannot identify the nature, location, or color of that object.

In contrast, patients with infarction in the parietal lobe, most often in MCA territory, who have preservation of geniculocalcarine fibers and the striate cortex have *visual neglect*, and their findings are quite different from those in patients with medial occipital infarction. Patients with visual neglect are usually unaware of their visual-field defect; ignore and do not heed objects in the abnormal visual field; fail to notice words in their impaired field, often reading only half of a headline or paragraph; miss objects in pictures in the neglected field; and have reduced optokinetic nystagmus to the side of the visual defect. Poor drawing and copying are also commonly associated with visual neglect. When the parieto-occipital and temporal branches of the PCA are involved, leading to large infarcts in the entire PCA territory, both a hemianopia and visual neglect are present. More often, in isolated infarcts of the striate cortex, patients have a hemianopia without neglect. In my experience, visual neglect without a hemianopia is always due to infarction within the MCA territory.

Somatosensory Abnormalities

The lateral thalamus is the site of the major somatosensory relay nuclei, the ventroposteromedial and -lateral (VPM and VPL) nuclei. Ischemia to these nuclei or to the white-matter tracts carrying fibers from the thalamus to somatosensory cortex (postcentral gyrus and the Sensory 2 region in the parietal operculum) produces changes in sensation, usually without paralysis. Patients complain of paresthesias or numbness in the face, limbs, and the trunk. On examination, their touch, pinprick, and position senses are reduced. The combination of hemisensory loss with hemianopia without paralysis is virtually diagnostic of infarction in the PCA territory. Rarely, occlusion of the very proximal portion of the PCA can cause a hemiplegia.[85–88]

Penetrating branches from the most proximal portion of the PCA penetrate into the midbrain to supply the cerebral peduncle. PCA-origin occlusions cause hemiplegia due to midbrain peduncular infarction, accompanied by a hemisensory loss due to lateral thalamic infarction and hemianopia due to occipital-lobe infarction. The resultant neurological deficit is not easily distinguished clinically from MCA and anterior choroidal artery (AChA) territory infarcts, but separation is made readily by CT or MRI results. Figure 7.10, from Hommel,[87] shows the proximal branches of the PCA.

Cortical Function Abnormalities

When the left PCA territory is infarcted, several additional findings may occur:

1. *Alexia without agraphia*—Infarction of the left occipital lobe and splenium of the corpus callosum have been associated with a remarkable clinical syndrome first described by Dejerine[89] and later amplified by Geschwind and Fusillo.[90] Because the left visual cortex is infarcted, patients see with their right occipital lobe and their left visual field. In order to name what they see, the information must be communicated from the right occipital cortex to the language region in the left temporal and parietal lobes. Infarction of the corpus callosum or adjacent white matter paths interrupts communication between the right occipital cortex and the left hemisphere. Patients have difficulty naming what they see. The most conspicuous abnormality is in reading. Although usually able to name individual letters or numbers, the patient cannot read words or phrases. Because the speech cortex is normal, they retain the ability to speak, repeat speech, write, and spell aloud. Although they are able to write a paragraph, they often cannot read it back moments later. Usually accompanying the dyslexia is a defect in color naming.[90] Patients can match colors and shades, proving that their perception of colors is normal. They can also describe the usual color of familiar objects and can even color correctly when given an array of crayons. Nonetheless, they are unable to give a color its correct name.
2. *Anomic or transcortical sensory aphasia*[91]—Some patients with left-PCA-territory infarction have difficulty naming objects, and others can repeat but not understand spoken language.
3. *Gerstmann's syndrome*—PCA-territory infarction can undercut the angular gyrus, leading to a host of findings, usually lumped together as Gerstmann's syndrome.[92] These findings include difficulty telling right from left; difficulty in naming digits on their own or on others' hands; constructional dyspraxia; agraphia; and difficulty in calculating.

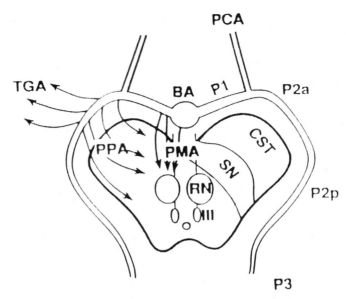

FIGURE 7.10   Axial diagram of the midbrain arteries. BA = basilar artery; PCoA = posterior communicating artery; P1 = proximal segment of the PCA; P2a = anterior segment of the P2 part of the PCA; P2p = posterior segment of the P2 part of the PCA; P3 = P3 part of the PCA; TPA = thalamoperforating arteries; TGA = thalamogeniculate arteries; PPA = peduncular perforating arteries; PMA = paramedian arteries; CST = corticospinal tract in the cerebral peduncle; SN = substantia nigra; RN = red nucleus; III = oculomotor nucleus. (From Hommel M, Besson G, Pollak P, et al., Hemiplegia in posterior cerebral artery occlusion, Neurology 1990;40: 1496–1499; reprinted with permission.)

In any single patient all features may appear together or one or more may occur in isolation.

4.   *Altered memory*—A defect in acquisition of new memories is common when both medial temporal lobes are damaged[93] but also occurs in lesions limited to the left temporal lobe.[92,94] The memory deficit in unilateral lesions is not permanent but has lasted up to 6 months.[90,92,95] Patients cannot recall what has happened recently, and when given new information, they cannot recall it moments later. They often repeat statements and questions spoken only minutes before.

5.   *Associative visual agnosia*[91,92,96]—Some patients with left-PCA infarction have difficulty in understanding the nature and use of objects presented visually. They can trace with their fingers and copy objects, demonstrating that visual perception is preserved. They often can name objects if the objects are presented in their hand and explored by touch or when verbally described. One patient, when shown a pair of scissors, had no idea what it was. When the instrument was placed in her

hand, she called it, "scissors." When asked to list five objects that might be used for cutting, she included scissors, indicating that the name of the object was available to the patient.[92]

Infarcts of the right-PCA territory are often accompanied by *prosopagnosia*, difficulty in recognizing familiar faces.[97] At times, patients cannot recognize their own spouses, their children, or even their own images in a mirror. Despite the seeming inability to recognize or match or identify faces, physiological tests of autonomic function are consistent with familiarity on a subconscious level.[98] Patients with right PCA lesions also may have difficulty revisualizing what a given object or person should look like. Dreams may also be devoid of visual imagery. Visual neglect is much more common after lesions of the right than of the left PCA territory.

When the PCA territory is infarcted bilaterally, the commonest findings are cortical blindness, amnesia, and agitated delirium. Most often, bilateral PCA infarction is due to embolism, with blockage of the distal basilar bifurcation. Cortically blind patients cannot see or identify objects in either visual field but have preserved pupillary light reflexes.[99] Some patients with cortical blindness do not volunteer or admit that they cannot see and seem to avoid barriers in their way. Amnesia due to bilateral medial temporal-lobe infarction may be permanent and closely resembles Korsakoff's syndrome. Also, infarcting the hippocampus, fusiform, and lingual gyri, usually bilaterally, leads to an agitated hyperactive state that could be confused with delirium tremens.[80,100,101] When infarction is limited to the lower banks of the calcarine fissures bilaterally, the major findings are prosopagnosia and defective color vision.[102,103]

CT demonstrated an infarct in MA in the medial occipital lobe on the right. Angiography was not performed. Noninvasive Doppler examination at C2 did not show reversed VA flow on either side. TCD showed a focal region of increased blood-flow velocity in the right PCA. Cardiac echo and Holter monitoring were normal. She was discharged on aspirin therapy. The findings did not change during the ensuing years of follow-up.

CT can accurately reflect the vascular territory involved. In this patient, it confirmed that the lesion was in the territory of the calcarine branch of the right PCA.[104,105] CT also verified that the lesion was ischemic and not due to ICH. MRI is probably better able to image small associated lesions in the thalamus, midbrain, and more proximal brainstem and cerebellum, thus helping to localize the offending vascular lesion. Sagittal T2-weighted MRI sections through the medial occipital lobes also can identify the location of the lesions in relation to the calcarine fissure and the optic radiations and thereby can help prognosticate recovery in visual-field defects. The occipital lobe is a site of predilection for amyloid angiopathy. Hemmorhage from amyloid angiopathy often occurs in the absence of hypertension and can mimic an ischemic stroke. Little is known at present about optimum therapy for patients with intrinsic disease of the PCA. When infarction is limited to branches of the PCA, cardiogenic embolism should be considered and appropriate investigations performed to exclude it.

In MA, there was no clinical or laboratory evidence to suggest cardiac-origin embolism. Noninvasive studies gave no evidence for VA occlusion in the neck, a potential source of intra-arterial embolism to the PCA. If VA occlusion had been suggested by noninvasive tests or if epidemiological and ecological factors had favored a VA-origin lesion, an MRA examination or standard angiography would have been ordered. She was black and had no history of coronary or peripheral vascular disease and did not have hyper-cholesterolemia. These factors weighed against the likelihood of a proximal VA lesion.[24] The absence of brainstem symptoms, and normal VA blood-flow velocities on TCD examination argued against an ICVA occlusion, although that diagnosis was certainly not excluded. The available evidence favored an intrinsic right PCA lesion. The TCD findings of a focal increase in blood-flow velocity strongly suggested this diagnosis. Even if more extensive infarction were to occur in the right PCA territory, the likelihood of serious disability was small. The risk to the patient of further serious neurological disability did not, in my opinion, warrant invasive diagnostic procedures or hazardous therapy. I elected to prescribe aspirin.

Advances in technology, especially the introduction of MRI, echocardiography, ultrasound and TCD, and MRA, have now made it possible to investigate noninvasively patients with posterior-circulation infarction and to often identify the causative vascular mechanism. It is hoped that in the near future, trials of various therapies in patients with documented vascular lesions will shed more light on treatment.

References

1. Millikan C, Siekert R. Studies in cerebrovascular disease. The syndrome of intermittent insufficiency of the basilar arterial system. Mayo Clin Proc 1955;30:61–68.
2. Denny-Brown D. Basilar artery syndromes. Bull N Engl Med Center 1953; 15:53–60.
3. Fang H, Palmer J. Vascular phenomena involving brainstem structures. Neurology 1956;6:402–419.
4. Williams D, Wilson T. The diagnosis of the major and minor syndromes of basilar insufficiency. Brain 1962;85:741–774.
5. Millikan C, Siekert R, Shick R. Studies in cerebrovascular disease: the use of anticoagulant drugs in the treatment of insufficiency or thrombosis within the basilar arterial system. Mayo Clin Proc 1955;30:116–126.
6. Caplan LR. Vertebrobasilar disease: time for a new strategy. Stroke 1981; 12:111–114.

7. Reivich M, Holling E, Roberts B, et al. Reversal of blood flow through the vertebral artery and its effects on cerebral circulation. N Engl J Med 1961; 265:878–885.

8. Heyman A, Young W, Dillon M, et al. Cerebral ischemia caused by occlusive disease of the subclavian or innominate arteries. Arch Neurol 1964;10:581–589.

9. North R, Fisher W, DeBakey M, et al. Brachial–basilar insufficiency syndrome. Neurology 1962;12:810–820.

10. Patel A, Toole J. Subclavian steal syndrome: reversal of cephalic blood flow. Medicine 1965;44:289–303.

11. Hennerici M, Klemm C, Rautenberg W. The subclavian steal phenomenon: a common vascular disorder with rare neurologic deficits. Neurology 1988;38: 669–673.

12. Pollock M, Blennerhassett J, Clark A. Giant cell arteritis and the subclavian steal syndrome. Neurology 1973;23:653–657.

13. Brewster DC, Moncure AC, Darling C, et al. Innominate artery lesions: problems encountered and lessons learned. J Vasc Surg 1985;2:99–112.

14. Symonds C. Two cases of thrombosis of subclavian artery with contralateral hemiplegia of sudden onset, probably embolic. Brain 1927;50:259–260.

15. Fields WS, LeMak NA, Ben-Menachem Y. Thoracic outlet syndrome: review and reference to a stroke in a major league pitcher. AJNR 1986;7:73–78.

16. Baker R, Rosenbaum A, Caplan L. Subclavian steal syndrome. Contemp Surg 1974;4:96–104.

17. Ekestrom S, Eklund B, Liljequist L, et al. Noninvasive methods in the evaluation of obliterative disease of the subclavian or innominate artery. Acta Med Scand 1979;206:467–471.

18. Berguer R, Higgins R, Nelson R. Noninvasive diagnosis of reversal of vertebral artery blood flow. N Engl J Med 1980;302:1349–1351.

19. Hennerici M, Aulich A, Sandmann W, et al. Incidence of asymptomatic extracranial arterial disease. Stroke 1981;12:750–758.

20. Von Reutern GM, Pourcelot L. Cardiac cycle-dependent alternating flow in vertebral arteries with subclavian artery stenosis. Stroke 1978;9:229–236.

21. Liljequist L, Ekestrom S, Nordhus O. Monitoring direction of vertebral artery blood flow by Doppler shift ultrasound in patients with suspected subclavian steal. Acta Chir Scand 1981;147:421–424.

22. Fisher CM, Gore I, Okabe N, et al. Atherosclerosis of the carotid and vertebral arteries: extracranial and intracranial. J Neuropathol Exp Neurol 1965;24: 455–476.

23. Hutchinson E, Yates P. Caratico-vertebral stenosis. Lancet 1957;1:2–8.

24. Gorelick PB, Caplan LR, Hier DB, et al. Racial differences in the distribution of posterior circulation occlusive disease. Stroke 1985;16:785–790.

25. Fisher CM. Vertigo in cerebrovascular disease. Arch Otolaryngol 1967;85: 529–534.

26. Moosy J. Morphology, sites, and epidemiology of cerebral atherosclerosis. Res Publ Assoc Res Nerv Ment Dis 1966;51:1–22.

27. Imparato A, Riles T, Kim G. Cervical vertebral angioplasty for brainstem ischemia. Surgery 1981;90:842–852.

28. Pelouze GA. Plaque ulcerie de l'ostium de l'artere vertebrale. Rev Neurol 1989;145:478–481.

29. Fisher CM. Occlusion of the vertebral arteries. Arch Neurol 1970;22:13–19.
30. Moufarrij N, Little JR, Furlan AJ, et al. Vertebral artery stenosis: long term follow-up. Stroke 1984;15:260–263.
31. Caplan LR. Occlusion of the vertebral or basilar artery. Stroke 1979;10:277–282.
32. Caplan LR, Rosenbaum A. Role of cerebral angiography in vertebrobasilar occlusive diease. J Neurol Neurosurg Psychiatry 1975;38:601–612.
33. George B, Laurian C. Vertebrobasilar ischemia with thrombosis of the vertebral artery: report of two cases with embolism. J Neurol Neurosurg Psychiatry 1982;45:91–93.
34. Caplan LR, Tettenborn B. Embolism in the posterior circulation. In: Bergner R, Caplan LR, eds. Vertebrobasilar arterial disease. St. Louis: Quality Medical Publishers, 1991:50–63.
35. Callow A. Surgical management of varying patterns of vertebral artery and subclavian artery insufficiency. N Engl J Med 1964;270:546–552.
36. Roon A, Ehrenfeld W, Cooke P, et al. Vertebral artery reconstruction. Am J Surg 1979;138:29–36.
37. Berguer R. Surgical indications for reconstruction of the vertebral artery. In: Berguer R, Caplan LR, eds. Vertebrobasilar arterial disease. St.Louis: Quality Medical Publishers, 1991:201–210.
38. Caplan LR, Zarins C, Hemmatti M. Spontaneous dissection of the extracranial vertebral arteries. Stroke 1985;16:1030–1038.
39. Wilkinson I, Russel R. Arteries of the head and neck in giant cell arteritis. Arch Neurol 1972;27:378–391.
40. Bickerstaff E. Neurological complications of oral contraceptives. Oxford: Clarendon Press, 1975.
41. Fisher CM, Karnes W, Kubik C. Lateral medullary infarction: the pattern of vascular occlusion. J Neuropathol Exp Neurol 1961;20:323–379.
42. Kommerall G, Hoyt W. Lateropulsion of saccadic eye movements. Arch Neurol 1973;28:313–318.
43. Meyer K, Baloh R, Krohel G, et al. Ocular lateropulsion: a sign of lateral medullary disease. Arch Opthalmol 1980;98:1614–1616.
44. Devereaux M, Keane J, Davis R. Automatic respiratory failure associated with infarction of the medulla: report of two cases with pathologic study of one. Arch Neurol 1973;29:46–52.
45. Levin B, Margolis G. Acute failure of automatic respirations secondary to a unilateral brainstem infarct. Ann Neurol 1977;1:583–586.
46. Bogousslavaky J, Khurma R, Deruaz JP, et al. Respiratory failure and unilateral brainstem infarction. Ann Neurol 1990;28:668–673.
47. Currier R, Giles C, Westerberg M. The prognosis of some brainstem vascular syndromes. Neurology 1958;8:664–668.
48. Caplan LR, Pessin M, Scott RM, et al. Poor outcome after lateral medullary infarcts. Neurology 1986;36:1510–1513.
49. Caplan LR. Bilateral distal vertebral artery occlusion. Neurology 1983;33:552–558.
50. Hauw J, Der Agopian P, Trelles L, et al. Les infarctes bulbaires. J Neurol Sci 1976;28:83–102.
51. Caplan LR, Brass LM, DeWitt LD, et al. Transcranial Doppler ultrasound: present status. Neurology 1990;40:696–700.

52. Tettenborn B, Estol C, DeWitt LD, et al. Accuracy of transcranial Doppler in the vertebrobasilar circulation. J Neurol 1990;237:159.

53. Sypert G, Alvord E. Cerebellar infarction: a clinicopathological study. Arch Neurol 1975;32:351–363.

54. Amarenco P, Hauw JJ, Henin D, et al. Les infarctus du territoire de l'artere cerebelleuse postero-inferieure: etude clinico-pathologique de 28 cas. Rev Neurol 1989;145:277–286.

55. Amarenco P, Hauw JJ, Gautier JC. Arterial pathology in cerebellar infarction. Stroke 1990;21:1299–1305.

56. Fisher CM, Picard E, Polak A, et al. Acute hypertensive cerebellar hemorrhage: diagnosis and surgical treatment. J Nerv Ment Dis 1965;140:38–57.

57. Lehrich J, Winkler G, Ojemann R. Cerebellar infarction with brainstem compression: diagnosis and surgical treatment. Arch Neurol 1970;22:490–498.

58. Fairburn B, Oliver L. Cerebellar softening: a surgical emergency. Br Med J 1956;1:1335–1336.

59. Seelig J, Selhorst J, Young H, et al. Ventriculostomy for hydrocephalus in cerebellar hemorrhage. Neurology 1981;31:1537–1540.

60. Castagne P, Lhermitte F, Gautier J, et al. Arterial occlusions in the vertebral–basilar system. Brain 1973;96:133–154.

61. Koroshetz WJ, Ropper AH. Artery-to-artery embolism causing stroke in the posterior circulation. Neurology 1987;37:292–296.

62. Sundt T, Whisnant J, Piepgras D, et al. Intracranial bypass grafts for vertebral–basilar ischemia. Mayo Clin Proc 1978;53:12–18.

63. Ausman J, Diaz F, de los Reyes R, et al. Anastomosis of occipital artery to AICA for vertebrobasilar junction stenosis. Surg Neurol 1981;16:99–102.

64. Roski R, Spetzler R, Hopkins L. Occipital artery to posterior–inferior cerebellar artery bypass for vertebrobasilar ischemia. Neurosurgery 1982;10:44–49.

65. Allen G, Cohen R, Preziosi T. Microsurgical endarterectomy of the intracranial vertebral artery for vertebrobasilar transient ischemic attacks. Neurosurgery 1981;81:56–59.

66. Kubik C, Adams R. Occlusion of the basilar artery: a clinical and pathologic study. Brain 1946;69:73–121.

67. Pessin MS, Gorelick PB, Kwan ES, et al. Basilar artery stenosis: middle and distal segments. Neurology 1987;37:1742–1746.

68. Amarenco P, Hauw JJ. Cerebellar infarction in the territory of the anterior inferior cerebellar artery: a clinicopathological study of 20 cases. Brain 1990;118:139–155.

69. Fisher CM. Some neuro-ophthalmological observations. J Neurol Neurosurg Psychiatry 1967;30:383–392.

70. Chase T, Moretti L, Prensky A. Clinical and electroencephalographic manifestations of a vascular lesion of the pons. Neurology 1968;18:357–368.

71. Tsai F, Teal J, Heishima G, et al. Computed tomography in acute posterior fossa infarcts. Am J Neuroradiol 1982;3:149–156.

72. Hinshaw D, Thompson J, Hasso A, et al. Infarction of the brainstem and cerebellum: a correlation of computed tomography and angiography. Radiology 1980;137:105–112.

73. Kistler J, Buonanno F, DeWitt D, et al. Vertebral–basilar posterior cerebral ter-

ritory stroke: delineation by proton nuclear magnetic resonance imaging. Stroke 1984;15:417–426.

74. Simmons Z, Biller J, Adams HP, et al. Cerebellar infarction: comparison of computed tomography and magnetic resonance imaging. Ann Neurol 1986;19:291–293.

75. Biller J, Yuh W, Mitchell GW. Early diagnosis of basilar artery occlusion using magnetic resonance imaging. Stroke 1988;19:297–306.

76. Fisher CM. Bilateral occlusion of basilar artery branches. J Neurol Neurosurg Psychiatry 1977;40:1182–1189.

77. Caplan LR, Sergay S. Positional cerebral ischemia. J Neurol Neurosurg Psychiatry 1976;39:385–391.

78. Edelman RR, Mattle HP, Atkinson DJ, et al. MR angiography. AJR 1990;154: 937–946.

79. Roether J, Wentz KW, Rautenberg W, Hennerici M. Preliminary results of MR-angiography in vertebrobasilar infarction. J Neurol 1991;238:124.

80. Caplan LR. Top of the basilar syndrome: selected clinical aspects. Neurology 1980;30:72–79.

81. Mehler MF. The rostral basilar artery syndrome: diagnosis, etiology, prognosis. Neurology 1989;39:9–16.

82. Mehler MF. The neuro-ophthalmologic spectrum of the rostral basilar artery syndrome. Arch Neurol 1988;45:966–971.

83. Pessin MS, Lathi E, Cohen M, et al. Clinical features and mechanism of occipital infarction. Ann Neurol 1987;21:290–299.

84. Pessin MS, Kwan E, DeWitt LD, et al. Posterior cerebral artery stenosis. Ann Neurol 1987;21:85–89.

85. Benson DF, Tomlinson EB. Hemiplegic syndrome of the posterior cerebral artery. Stroke 1971;2:559–564.

86. Caplan LR, DeWitt LD, Pessin MS, et al. Lateral thalamic infarcts. Arch Neurol 1988;45:959–964.

87. Hommel M, Besson G, Pollak P, et al. Hemiplegia in posterior cerebral artery occlusion. Neurology 1990;40:1496–1499.

88. Hommel M, Moreaud O, Besson G, Perret J. Site of arterial occlusions in the hemiplegic posterior cerebral artery syndrome. Neurology 1991;41:604–605.

89. Dejerine J. Contribution a l'etude anatomo-pathologique et clinique des differnetes varietes de cecite verbale. Memoires de la Societe Biologique 1892;4:61–90.

90. Geschwind N, Fusillo M. Color naming defect in association with alexia. Arch Neurol 1966;15:137–146.

91. Kertesz A, Sleppard A, MacKenzie R. Localization in transcortical sensory aphasia. Arch Neurol 1982;39:475–479.

92. Caplan LR, Hedley-White T. Cueing and memory dysfunction in alexia without agraphia. Brain 1974;97:251–262.

93. Victor M, Angevine J, Mancall E, et al. Memory loss with lesion of hippocampal formation. Arch Neurol 1961;5:244–263.

94. Benson F, Marsden C, Meadows J. The amnestic syndrome of posterior cerebral artery occlusion. Acta Neurol Scand 1974;50:133–145.

95. Mohr JP, Leicester J, Stoddard L, et al. Right hemianopia with memory and color deficits in circumscribed left posterior cerebral artery territory infarction. Neurology 1971;21:1104–1113.

96. Rubens A, Benson F. Associative visual agnosia. Arch Neurol 1971;24:305–316.
97. Damasio A, Damasio H, Van Hoesen G. Prosopagnosia: anatomic basis and behavioral mechanisms. Neurology 1982;32:331–341.
98. Tranel D, Damasio AR. Autonomic recognition of familiar faces by prosopagnosics: evidence of a knowledge without awareness. Neurology 1985;35(Suppl 1):119–120.
99. Symonds C, McKenzie I. Bilateral loss of vision from cerebral infarction. Brain 1957;80:415–455.
100. Medina J, Rubino F, Ross E. Agitated delirium caused by infarctions of the hippocampal formation and fusiform and lingual gyri: a case report. Neurology 1974;24:1181–1183.
101. Horenstein S, Chamberlain W, Conomy J. Infarction of the fusiform and calcarine regions: agitated delirium and hemianopsia. Trans Am Neurol Assoc 1962;92:357–367.
102. Meadows J. Disturbed perception of colors associated with localized cerebral lesions. Brain 1974;97:615–632.
103. Damasio A, Yamada T, Damasio H, et al. Central achromatopsia: behavioral, anatomic,and physiologic aspects. Neurology 1980;30:1064–1071.
104. Kinkle W, Newman R, Jacobs L. Posterior cerebral artery branch occlusions: CT and anatomical considerations. In: Berguer R, Bauer R, eds. Vertebrobasilar arterial occlusive disease. New York: Raven Press, 1984:117–133.
105. Goto K, Tagawa K, Uemma K, et al. Posterior cerebral artery occlusion. Radiology 1979;132:357–368.

CHAPTER 8

Penetrating and Branch Artery Disease

Occlusions or stenoses of large extracranial and intracranial arteries are traditional lesions generally recognized by all physicians and surgeons caring for stroke patients. Abnormalities in larger vessels are easily corroborated by angiography and noninvasive tests and are readily verified by gross inspection of vessels removed at surgery or necropsy. In contrast, lesions in microscopic-sized intracranial arteries, although acknowledged as genuine pathological findings, are a more controversial cause of stroke. Fisher (Chapter 1, Figure 1.2) reviewed the history of lacunar infarctions,[1] defined the nature and etiology of the vascular pathology causing lacunes,[2] and described many clinical syndromes that can be readily and reliably diagnosed as lacunar. Fisher almost single-handedly brought this disorder to the attention of the neurological community. Yet many still fail or refuse to integrate the concept of lacunar infarction into their differential diagnosis of stroke, and others are skeptical that lacunes can be diagnosed clinically. Even in the 1990s, lacunes remain controversial.

Durand-Fardel first introduced the term *lacunes* in 1843, to describe small holes, usually found in the striatum, that contain fine meshwork of tissues and vessels.[3] The clinical findings in patients with lacunar infarction were first described by Ferrand, working in the laboratory of Pierre Marie,[4] and by Marie himself.[5] These authors found that lacunes were most often located in the lentiform nuclei, thalamus, pons, internal capsule, and cerebral white matter. Hemiplegia was the major finding in acute lacunar infarction. The clinical condition of multiple lacunes was termed *etat lacunaire* by Marie and was characterized by pseudobulbar palsy and an abnormal small-stepped gait. Foix and colleagues added clinical details about the findings in capsular and pontine lacunar infarcts.[6-8] Little was added after Foix until Fisher's work on the pathology and clinical findings in lacunar infarction.

Pathology

Lacunes are small, discrete, often irregular lesions, ranging from 1 to 20 mm in size. Only 17 percent of lacunes are smaller than 1 cm.[1] Inspection of the tiny cavities usually reveals fine strands of connective tissue resembling cobwebs. Marie recognized that true lacunes had to be differentiated from dilated perivascular spaces (so-called *etat crible*) and from postmortem holes produced by gas bacilli (*etat vermoulu*).[5] Gas cavities are usually numerous, perfectly round, have no cobwebs, and often retain a characteristic bad smell. These distinctions are very important today because recent studies show that MRI often shows the dilated perivascular *etat crible* lesions as discrete loci of increased signal.[9] The commonest locations of lacunar infarcts are the putamen and the pallidum, followed by the pons, the thalamus, the caudate nucleus, the internal capsule, and the corona radiata. More rare are lacunes in the cerebral peduncles and pyramids, and in cerebral white matter. These lesions are not found in the cerebral or cerebellar cortices.

Serial sections of the penetrating arteries that supply the territory of lacunar infarcts reveal a characteristic vascular pathology.[2] These tiny vessels often have focal enlargements and small hemorrhagic extravasation through the walls of the arteries. Subintimal foam cells sometimes obliterate the lumens, and pink-staining fibrinoid material lies within the vessel walls (Figure 8.1). The vessels in spots are often replaced by whorls, tangles, and wisps of connective tissue that obliterate the usual vascular layers. Fisher called these processes segmental arterial disorganization, fibrinoid degeneration, and lipohyalinosis. Fisher also recognized that sometimes larger deep infarcts, which he dubbed "giant lacunes," could be caused by occlusion of parent vessels, such as the MCA stem, causing obstruction of the orifices of lateral lenticulostriate vessels.[10]

Fisher,[11,12] Cole and Yates,[13] and Rosenblum[14] recognized that small aneurysmal dilations of these lipohyalinotic penetrating arteries could rupture, causing intracerebral hemorrhage (ICH). These lesions were probably similar to those recognized by Charcot and Bouchard[15] as the cause of parenchymatous bleeding. The distribution of deep hypertensive hemorrhages was the same as the locations of lacunes (putamen, capsule, thalamus, and pons). Lipohyalinotic arteries could either occlude, leading to lacunar infarction, or rupture, causing ICH.[7] Fisher reviewed the charts of 114 patients who had lacunes at necropsy. All but 3 had hypertension, as defined by a history of hypertension, elevated blood pressure recorded on examination, or heart weight exceeding 400 gm without other explanation.[1] Fisher attributed segmental arterial disorganization and lipohyalinosis to hypertension.

Foix and Hillemand,[7,8,16–18] Stopford,[19,20] and Düret[21,22] defined the territories of arteries that branched from the parent cerebral and basilar arteries. Foix recognized that infarcts were often limited to the territories of one of these branches. Fisher and Caplan,[23] Fisher,[24] and Caplan[25] defined the

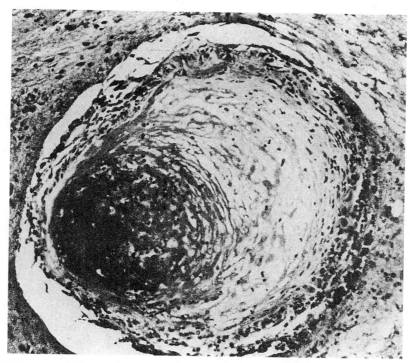

FIGURE 8.1 Small penetrating artery showing lipohyalinosis and fibrinoid necrosis; lumen is considerably compromised. (Courtesy of Dr. C. Miller Fisher.)

vascular pathology in these branches. Fisher and Caplan[23] reported vascular lesions causing ischemia limited to the territory of basilar branches, separating this vasculopathy from lipohyalinosis. This pathology is referred to as "intracerebral branch atheromatous disease" (Figures 8.2–8.4).[25] The orifices of the penetrating branches could be blocked by atheroma in the parent artery; atheroma could originate in the parent artery and extend into the branch (so-called junctional plaques), or microatheroma could arise at the origin of the branch itself. Thrombus was often superimposed on the atheromas. This vasculopathy could be called "microatheroma" and is clearly distinct on pathological grounds from the arteriopathy underlying lacunes. Pontine infarcts are the most frequent pathological lesion found in necropsies of diabetics and must, in some cases, be caused by microatheromatous branch disease.[26] Microatheromas, parent-artery plaques, and occlusion of parent arteries by in-situ thrombosis or embolism probably explain deep infarcts in normotensive patients. Although lipohyalinosis and microatheroma are readily separated by meticulous pathological examination, the distinction is nearly impossible clinically. Boiten categorized 100 patients with lacunes into two separate groups.[27] One group had atherosclerotic risk factors and single symptomatic lacunes; the other group had hypertension, multiple

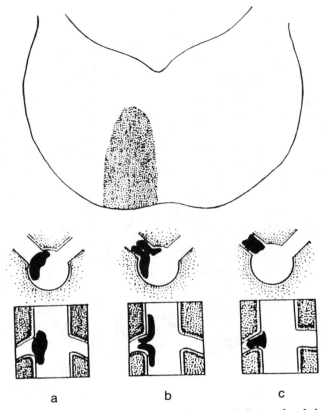

FIGURE 8.2 Top drawing shows an infarct (stippled) in the left basis pontis. Bottom drawings show (a) plaque within parent artery, blocking the orifice of the branch; (b) plaque within the parent artery, extending into the branch (junctional plaque); (c) microatheroma, formed within the branch and blocking it.

lacunes—some of which were asymptomatic—and white-matter lucency. He posited that the former group had microatheromatous branch disease and the latter group had lipohyalinosis.[27] Because the prognosis for branch occlusions and lacunes is probably identical, and at present, treatment is similar, there is little practical reason to separate clinically the lacunes from the branch infarcts.

General Clinical Findings

A 56-year-old black man, RB, awakened with weakness of his right arm. As he stood to go to the bathroom, he became aware that his right leg was weak. He called to his wife, who noted that his voice was slightly thick. He had no headache, nor did he feel dizzy or otherwise unwell. As the day progressed,

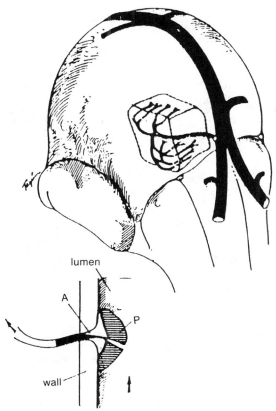

FIGURE 8.3 Basilar-branch occlusion: The diagram at the bottom shows a close-up of the artery shown within the cube above; A = atheroma, P = plaque; a plaque is seen extending into the branch. (From the original Fisher and Caplan paper, Basilar artery branch occlusion: a cause of pontine infarction, Neurology 1971;21:900–905; reprinted with permission.)

the weakness in his arm and leg seemed to fluctuate, but by nightfall, he could not move the right arm or the right leg. He had no prior history of stroke, heart disease, or claudication and recognized no warnings in the days before. Two months earlier, a physician had told him that his blood pressure was high and "bore watching" but prescribed no medication.

Fisher emphasized repeatedly in his writings that hypertension was the major cause of fibrinoid degeneration and lipohyalinosis, the arteriopathy that leads to lacunar infarcts. Others have noted a lower frequency of hypertension in patients with a CT-verified diagnosis of lacunar infarcts (52.5%,[28] 57%,[29] 65%,[30] 72%[31]). Seventy-five percent of patients clinically diagnosed as having lacunar infarcts in the Harvard Stroke Registry (HSR)

Middle Cerebral

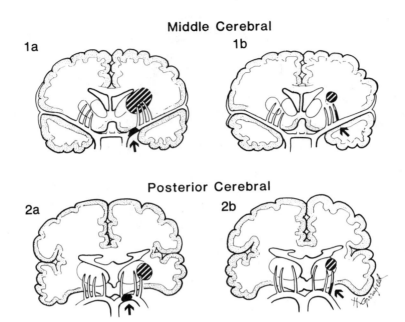

FIGURE 8.4   Mechanisms of deep infarction: (1a) basal ganglionic capsular infarct due to MCA occlusion (arrow); (1b) smaller deep capsular infarct due to lenticulostriate artery occlusion (arrow); (2a) lateral thalamic infarct due to PCA occlusion (arrow); (2b) lateral thalamic infarct due to thalamogeniculate artery occlusion (arrow). (Reprinted from Caplan LR, DeWitt LD, Pessin MS, et al. Lateral thalamic infarcts. Arch Neurol 1988;45:959–964, with permission.)

had hypertension.[32] In a necropsy study, 64 percent of patients with lacunes at postmortem had a history of hypertension.[33] For a more thorough evaluation, Fisher used pathological criteria to diagnose lacunes and hypertension (heart weight greater than 400 gm, with no other cause) and carefully searched hospital and doctors' notes for past blood-pressure recordings. Although clearly not all patients with deep infarcts are hypertensive, a diagnosing physician should be wary of attributing a lesion to small-vessel occlusive disease if there is no past or current evidence of hypertension or diabetes. We have also seen normotensive patients with elevated hematocrits (Hcts) who have a clinical picture of lacunar infarction, possibly due to clotting within small vessels. Fisher found severe large-vessel atherosclerosis in 64 percent of the 114 patients with lacunes, a frequency far exceeding the usual 9 percent found in a population without lacunes.[1] Thus, hypertension definitely predisposes patients to premature atherosclerosis of both larger extracranial and intracranial arteries. Large- and small-vessel diseases frequently coexist, so the mere presence of clinical, noninvasive, or angiographic evidence of atherosclerotic stenosis does not exclude a lacunar etiology of a stroke.

Lacunes are small and deep. Because there is no accompanying over-distension of superficial arteries, and deep arteries have no pain fibers, headache due to vascular distension does not occur in patients with lacunes. These small lesions produce no mass effect that might cause headache or decreased alertness. Lacunes are far from the cortex and do not produce seizures[32] or affect the surface-recorded EEG.[34] The presence of decreased alertness, unaccustomed headache, or seizures argue against a lacunar etiology of a stroke.

The course of illness of patients with lacunar infarction is also different from patients with large-vessel occlusive disease and cerebral embolism.[32,35] Prior TIAs occur in about 20 percent of patients with lacunes,[35–37] a frequency far below that for large-vessel disease but more than in cerebral embolism. When TIAs do occur in patients with lacunar infarcts, they span a shorter time interval and are more stereotyped than in other ischemic etiologies. The deficit often evolves gradually in patients with lacunar infarcts, with frequent fluctuations and progression during the initial 72 hours of the stroke. Sudden deficits, maximal at onset, are less frequent than with other etiologies of ischemic stroke. Gradual worsening of paralysis over a few days is a characteristic course in some patients with pure motor hemiparesis due to lacunar infarction.

> On examination of RB, the blood pressure was 165/95. The patient was alert and understood, repeated, and used language normally. He read, wrote, and spelled words correctly. His voice was slightly slurred. The right face, shoulder, arm, hand, thigh, and foot were moderately weak. Deep tendon reflexes were exaggerated on the right, and the right plantar response was extensor. He felt touch normally in his right limbs and could identify accurately the nature of objects in his right hand and could localize spots touched on his right limbs. Visual fields were normal.

Lacunes have a predilection for particular anatomical sites—those nourished by penetrating vessels. Some of these deep lesions produce characteristic clinical syndromes, while others are clinically silent or produce findings difficult to distinguish from superficial infarction. In a necropsy series of 167 patients with lacunes, 93 (56 percent) patients had no reported related symptoms.[33] Anatomical localization is probably most helpful in the diagnosis of lacunes. RB had paralysis of face, arm, and leg with exaggerated reflexes and an extensor toe sign. A lesion of the motor cortex causing these findings would have to extend from the face area, near the sylvian fissure—a region fed by the MCA—to the paramedian frontal lobe foot area, which is fed by the ACA. Such a lesion would invariably affect language, sensation, or vision. A sizable superficial or deep frontal-lobe lesion not only would produce motor dysfunction but also could cause conjugate-eye deviation to the side of the lesion and abulia. Marie emphasized hemiplegia as the sign of lacunar infarction.[5] Fisher termed the syndrome of isolated weakness of face, arm, and leg "pure motor hemiplegia"[10] and taught that these findings are diagnostic of lacunar infarction in the pons or internal capsule. Some authors,[30,38,39] using radioisotope studies or CT, found lesions other than lacunes in patients with pure motor hemiplegia. Remember that Fisher examined the patients intensively. When he called the patient's syndrome "pure motor," he had compulsively tested sensation, visual fields, and cortical function and had found them normal. Fisher also demanded that weakness include face, arm, and leg and that hypertension be present to make the diagnosis of a pure motor stroke. Were patients with CT lesions other than lacunes examined in the same compulsive and thorough manner as an important requisite for the clinical diagnosis of lacunes in these other radiographic studies? I advise a strategy similar to that taught in high school geometry: Try to prove your original diagnostic impression wrong. Seek out features—for example, sensory, visual, or intellectual abnormalities—that would disprove your diagnosis. Mental-status testing is key because most pure-motor patients with lesions other than lacunes have some aberration in alertness, behavior, or intellect that suggests frontal-lobe disease.

Even when the lacunar syndromes are apparently pure, some patients will have a very small hematoma as the cause of the syndrome. Small putaminal, capsular, and pontine hematomas are known to cause pure motor hemiparesis and other syndromes most often caused by lacunar infarction.[35,37,40,41] Miller emphasized the need for confirming the clinical diagnosis of lacunar infarction by a CT scan.[36] Before clinicians can be secure in their diagnosis of lacunar infarction, I believe that neuroimaging (CT or MRI) tests that either show a lacune or exclude parenchymatous hemorrhage and surface infarction are mandatory.

Loci of Lesions and Clinical Syndromes

Hemispheral Lesions within the Anterior Circulation

Probably the most commonly recognized clinical syndrome in patients with lacunes in the cerebral hemispheres is *pure-motor hemiparesis*. The patient, RB, had this syndrome. The causative lesion is usually found in the internal capsule. Rascol and colleagues were able to distinguish three types of capsular lesions causing pure-motor hemiparesis: (1) large lesions spanning the anterior and posterior limbs of the capsule, due to occlusion of large lateral lenticulostriate arteries; (2) capsulopallidal infarcts located predominantly in the posterior limb of the capsule in the territory of medial lenticulostriate arteries; and (3) lesions in the anterior limb and caudate nucleus, in the supply region of the recurrent artery of Heubner.[35,37] MRI studies show that patients with pure-motor hemiparesis can also have lesions in the midbrain, pons, and medulla, affecting descending corticospinal fibers in the cerebral peduncle, basis pontis, or pyramid.[42,43]

Motor weakness does not always equally affect the face, arm, and leg. Often the face is at least partially spared.[35] At times almost a pure monoparesis of the arm or leg is present with only minimal weakness or hyperreflexia of the other limb on that side. In the Stroke Data Bank (SDB) the clinical findings related to the degree of involvement of face, arm, and leg did not correlate with the location of the lesion in the internal capsule.[35,44] Mohr summarized, "There no longer seems much reason to adhere to the older dogma[35] that the motor fibers occupy the anterior half of the posterior limb of the internal capsule. . . . Further, the available case material does not document a series of cases with an homunculus whose face is anterior and whose leg is posterior in the plane of the internal capsule."[35]

In some patients with lacunar infarction, the clinical picture includes a combination of weakness, pyramidal signs, and cerebellar-type ataxia and incoordination in the limbs on one side of the body. This syndrome was first called "homolateral ataxia and crural paresis" in patients in whom the predominant involvement was in the lower limbs.[46] Later, Fisher dubbed the syndrome *ataxic hemiparesis,* indicating that the arm and leg could be variously involved, but the major signature of the syndrome was the combination of cerebellar and motor signs on the same side of the body.[47] In some patients, there are also sensory symptoms ipsilateral to the motor abnormalities.[48] The relative severity of ataxia compared to weakness varies considerably, as does the relative involvement of arm compared to leg. Localization of lesions causing ataxic hemiparesis varies widely. Many lesions are in the posterior limb of the internal capsule, but lacunes in the midbrain and pons can also cause this clinical syndrome.

At times, the clinical findings show abnormalities of motor function on one side of the body, but there is no true paralysis, reflexes are not exaggerated, and the plantar response is flexor. I refer to these findings as a "nonpyramidal hemimotor syndrome." Some lesions effecting these changes involve the striatum and the globus pallidus. Decreased spontaneous and associated movements, clumsiness, slight increased resistance to passive movement, slowness of the affected limbs, and forced grasping are often found. Some patients have a minor degree of hemi-Parkinsonism. Others have a movement disorder with choreic features. Some patients with hemichorea have had striatal infarcts.[49,50]

Sometimes, the predominant dysfunction in patients with hemispheral lacunes seems to be bulbar. Dysarthria, dysphagia, and even mutism may occur, due to interruption of corticobulbar fibers in the white matter underlying the motor cortex, capsule, striatum, or pons. Limb symptoms may be minor or absent. Tapping the corner of the mouth may show heightened contraction of the orbicularis oris and orbicularis oculi on the side of the bulbar dysfunction. Often, the tongue and face are weak on one side. In patients with predominantly bulbar signs, the lesions are often bilateral, and the syndrome is pseudobulbar.[51] The initial lesion sometimes produces no symptoms or only minor hemimotor signs. When the contralateral side becomes involved, the bilateral disturbance in corticobulbar fibers causes predominantly bulbar abnormalities, especially dysarthria and dysphagia, sometimes with exaggerated laughing and crying.

In Chapter 6, on large-artery anterior-circulation lesions, I have discussed both caudate[52] and AChA territory infarcts.[53-55] Infarcts in these regions can be quite small, readily qualifying as lacunes, or they can be more extensive deep infarcts. Caudate lesions can be limited to the caudate nucleus or can extend into the anterior limb of the internal capsule and the anterior putamen.[53] AChA-territory infarcts can involve the palladum, or the posterior limb of the internal capsule.[51,53-55] Infarcts in these areas are probably due to intracranial-branch atheromatous disease affecting one or more of Heubner's arteries and the AChA.[25]

Involvement of small penetrating branches of these arteries is probably most often due to microatheromas or lipohyalinosis. Unfortunately, neuropathological studies of patients with lesions in the distribution of Heubner's artery and the AChA are too scanty to document or refute this hypothesis.[25] Some patients with caudate infarcts have prominent dysarthria and cognitive and behavioral abnormalities, especially abulia and restlessness.[52] Some patients have aphasia, usually slight and transient. In a necropsy series of patients with lacunes found at postmortem, aphasia with right hemiparesis was one of the most frequent clinical syndromes correlating with lacunar infarction.[33] The responsible lesions were in the striatum and anterior limb of the internal capsule or the thalamus.

Posterior Circulation—Brainstem and Thalamic Lacunes and Branch Occlusions

Pons and Medulla

Lacunes and branch-territory infarcts are often found in the pons.[42,43] In a 1990 prospective study of MRI in 100 patients hospitalized with lacunar infarcts in Grenoble, France, 38 (25%) of the lesions were in the pons.[42] Among 12 patients in another series studied acutely with MRI, 6 of 11 lesions were located in the pons and had symptoms appropriate to that localization.[56] The commonest site of the pontine lesions is in the basis pontis on one side, most often medially in the distribution of one of the paramedian branches of the basilar artery. Few necropsy specimens of patients with infarcts in this location have been studied. The pathology in some has been lipohyalinosis and segmental arterial disorganization of penetrating arteries within the basis pontis.[2,10]

In three patients, the arterial lesion involving basilar-artery branches was studied in more detail by serially sectioning the pons, with the basilar artery and its branches still attached to the pons.[23,24] In one patient, an atheromatous plaque within the basilar artery obstructed the intramural part of the 0.5-mm-diameter basilar artery branch.[23] Distally, in the blocked branch, there was a mass of agglutinated platelets, which either arose as a tiny intra-arterial embolus from the lesion in the parent artery or formed in situ because of the reduced flow. In another patient, a plaque arising in the lumen of the basilar artery extended into the mouth of a 0.5-mm-diameter branch, forming a junctional plaque.[23] In a third patient, basilar-artery branches were blocked bilaterally.[24] At the orifice of a basilar branch in this patient, a microdissection made a crevice in a plaque, and a superimposed thrombus obstructed the branch. The mechanisms of blockage of branches are depicted in Figures 8.2 to 8.4. Flat or elevated plaques in the parent basilar artery can either block branches or provide the nidus for small embolic fragments that extend into the branches. A dilated dolichoectatic basilar artery can also distort branch orifices.

Infarction of the medullary pyramid can give rise to a *pure-motor hemiparesis,* sparing the face.[10,57,58] Lesions are baso-medial in the territory of anterior spinal artery branches. In the pons, there are three syndromes related to infarcts in the basis pontis. Pure-motor hemiplegia is probably the most common of the syndromes. In some patients, additional findings help identify the pontine locus. An ipsilateral VI-nerve palsy or intranuclear ophthalmoplegia (INO) are occasionally associated with the contralateral hemiparesis.[23] Involvement of the tegmentum and base can include the PPRF, causing a conjugate-gaze palsy toward the side of the lesion, accompanied by contralateral limb weakness and pyramidal signs. At times, although there is no gaze palsy, conjugate-gaze movements are asymmetric, with slight abnormalities of ipsilateral conjugate gaze. Involvement of the medial lemniscus, as well as the pyramidal fibers, leads to some sensory symptoms and signs on the side of the hemiparesis. Usually, these are minor paresthesias and slight loss of vibration sense, with preserved pinprick and temperature sensation.

The basis pontis carries fibers crossing into the brachium pontis, traveling toward the cerebellum. Interruption of pontocerebellar fibers can cause cerebellar-type incoordination and ataxia. *Ataxic hemiparesis* is often caused by a pontine lesion.[46,47] Subtle minor incoordination of the ipsilateral limbs can provide a clue to this localization because pontocerebellar crossing fibers are involved bilaterally, to some extent. The *dysarthria–clumsy-hand syndrome* is usually due to a small lacune in the more dorsal portion of the basis pontis, affecting corticobulbar fibers near the medial lemniscus.[59] Often, the associated facial and tongue weakness is severe, but examination of the hand and arm is nearly normal, despite the patient's report of awkwardness.

Occasionally, lacunes are located in the lateral tegmentum, in the distribution of branches that penetrate horizontally from long circumferential arteries.[60] These lacunes are the ischemic counterpart of lateral tegmental brainstem hematomas.[61] These lesions usually involve the sensory lemniscus, which has formed from the joining of the medial lemniscus and lateral spinothalamic tracts in the rostral pons. A pure sensory strokelike syndrome occurs, with subjective paresthesias in the contralateral face, arm, and leg. Ataxia, dysarthria, and nystagmus are variable. Helgason and Wilbur identified 10 patients with hemisensory symptoms and pontine lacunes, in whom the anatomical locale was confirmed by MRI.[60]

Midbrain

In the midbrain, penetrating-artery lesions involve primarily the cerebral peduncle and the paramedian zones. Very few examples have been reported in detail.[62] Some infarcts in this distribution are caused by occlusion of the parent PCA. The distribution of the penetrating branches of the PCA has been diagrammed in Figure 7.10 in the preceding chapter. One clinical syndrome includes a III-nerve palsy ipsilaterally, due to involvement of the fascicles of the IIIrd nerve within the midbrain, accompanied by a contralateral hemiparesis (Weber's syndrome). In some patients, involvement of the red nucleus, as well as the cerebral peduncle on the same side, gives rise to a combination of *motor weakness and tremor*. The tremor usually develops as the hemiparesis improves and is present both at rest and on intention. The affected arm is usually also quite incoordinated and ataxic. Few cases of midbrain branch lesions with neuropathological confirmation have been reported.[63,64]

Thalamus

Thalamic lacunes are quite common. In the MRI study of Hommel and colleagues, thalamic lesions accounted for 14 percent of the lacunes.[42] Penetrating-artery territory infarcts are localized paramedially in the distribution of the various thalamoperforating arteries or laterally in the distribution of the thalamogeniculate artery and its lateral thalamic branches. The two most important and consistent paramedian thalamoperforating arteries are the polar (tuberothalamic) artery and the thalamic–subthalamic arteries.[64-70] The polar artery arises on each side from the middle third of the posterior communicating artery and supplies the anteromedial and anterolateral thalamic nuclei. At times, this vessel is absent, in which case its territory is also supplied by the thalamic–subthalmic arteries. The predominant findings in infarcts fed by the thalamoperforating arteries are cognitive and behavioral, but the syndromes do differ, depending on the artery involved.[65,68,70] Unilateral anterolateral thalamic infarction in the distribution of the polar artery on the left or right side usually causes abulia, facial asymmetry, transient minor contralateral motor abnormalities, and—at times—aphasia (left lesions) or visual neglect (right lesions). Abulia with slowness, decreased amount of activity and speech, and long delays in responding to queries or conversation is the predominant abnormality. Some patients have been disorganized and dressed in a slovenly manner.[65,69,70] Usually, in patients with unilateral lesions, the abulia and cognitive and behavioral changes improve after 3 to 6 months. Occasionally, bilateral infarcts are found in the territory of the polar artery of each side.[71] This probably means that bilateral arteries occasionally arise from a single vessel or a common rete or loop artery. When the polar artery is affected bilaterally, the behavioral abnormality is more severe and more persistent. Memory may also be affected.[71] The behavioral effects are probably explained by the synaptic cortico-thalamic relationship with the frontal lobe and other cortical regions.

The thalamic–subthalamic arteries originate from the proximal PCAs and supply the most posteromedial portion of the thalamus near the posterior commissure. The right- and left-sided arteries may arise separately but are known often to originate from a single unilateral artery or a common pedicle.[64] Unilateral lesions are usually characterized by some degree of paresis of vertical gaze (upward or both upward and downward) and by amnesia. Motor and sensory signs and symptoms are absent. The pathway for vertical gaze includes the rostral interstitial nucleus of the MLF, and connections between the two eyes for vertical eye movements travel through the commissures at the diencephalic–mesencephalic junction. A unilateral lesion interrupts these commissural fibers, thus causing conjugate vertical-gaze palsy.[72] Memory loss may be severe, with profound difficulty in making new memories or encoding recent events. The amnesia often improves in 6 months in unilateral-infarct patients. Bilateral butterfly-shaped paramedian posterior thalamic infarction can result from a branch occlusion of a single supplying artery or pedicle, although scant necropsy data are available from well-studied cases.[64,69,73] Hypersomnolence and bilateral IIIrd nerve palsies can occur in patients with bilateral infarcts.[73] The same syndrome can result from occlusion of the rostral basilar artery, as discussed in Chapter 7.

Lacunes and branch-territory infarcts are especially common in the lateral thalamus. This region—including the somatosensory nuclei (VPL and VPM) and the ventral lateral and ventral anterior nuclei—is supplied by the thalamogeniculate group of arteries. These vessels arise from the PCA and are the posterior-circulation counterpart of the lenticulostriate branches of the MCA. Occlusion of these arteries or these branches leads to a variety of different clinical syndromes.[74]

Larger lateral thalamic infarcts were first described by Dejerine and Roussy, and the clinical findings have long been referred to as "le syndrome thalamique."[75] The essential features of this syndrome, almost always caused by atheromatous-branch disease in my experience, are contralateral hemisensory symptoms, accompanied by contralateral limb ataxia. At times, there are jumpy adventitious hemichoreic movements of the contralateral arm, and the hand may tend to assume a fisted posture. Some patients have a transient hemiparesis at onset, which improves quickly.

Usually, the sensory phenomena are mostly paresthesias, which involve the face, neck, trunk, and limbs. Sensory loss is usually slight. The sensory signs relate to ischemia of the somatosensory nuclei. The ataxia is due to interruption of cerebellofugal fibers going to the ventral anterior and ventral lateral nuclei. Also interrupted are fibers from the striatum (the ansa lenticularis), which are also projected toward these motor nuclei. Dystonia, chorea, and hemi-Parkinsonian-like features are probably due to interruption of these extrapyramidal-system projections. Pain in the affected limbs and trunk may develop months after the original stroke and was one of the cardinal features mentioned by Dejerine and Roussy.[75] Many patients never have pain, and pain is almost never noted at or shortly after the onset.

Occlusion of branches of the thalamogeniculate arteries supplying the somatosensory nuclei is responsible for the vast majority of patients with so-called pure sensory stroke.[76–79] In this condition, the patient has somatosensory complaints, without other signs or symptoms. Most often, the patient describes numbness, tingling, or pins-and-needle sensations in the face, limbs, or trunk. All hemicorporeal sensations are represented in the thalamic somatosensory relay nuclei. In somatosensory cortex, the hand and face have very large representations, while little space is accorded the trunk, scalp, and other regions not capable of fine sensory distinctions; thus, numbness of the inner mouth, eye, ear, scalp, chest, back, abdomen, and genitalia is much more common in thalamic lacunes than in superficial lesions of parietal cortex.[77]

After a few days, the somatic sensations may take on an unpleasant quality and may be characterized as burning, tightness, or soreness.[77] Sensory symptoms may be transient or permanent, even when lacunar infarction has been documented. Usually, subjective sensory complaints are more prominent than objective loss of sensation. Many patients with pure sensory stroke have no detectable loss of threshold to any sensory modality, while others show only a minimal qualitative or quantitative difference between the two sides of the body. Motor, visual, and intellectual functions are normal. Occasionally, pure sensory stroke can be caused by a lateral tegmental pontine or midbrain infarct.[60,80]

Occlusion of thalamogeniculate branches, on occasion, can cause a syndrome referred to as *sensory-motor stroke*.[81] This condition is characterized by the sensory symptoms and signs described in relation to pure sensory stroke, and these are also accompanied by paresis and pyramidal signs in the same limbs as the sensory symptoms. Very few such cases have been studied at necropsy. In one well-studied case, the responsible infarct involved the somatosensory nuclei, and there was pallor of the adjacent posterior limb of the internal capsule.[81] Careful review of the drawings from the original Dejerine-Roussy article clearly shows that lateral thalamic infarcts often affect the adjacent internal capsule.[74,75] The thalamogeniculate arteries must supply this zone, contrary to the teachings in some neuroanatomy texts. Ischemia of the capsule is probably responsible for the transient paresis found in some patients with lateral thalamic infarcts, and for the motor abnormalities in patients with sensory-motor stroke.

Laboratory Investigations in Patients Suspected of Having Lacunar Stroke

Having described the known lacunar syndromes and their usual responsible lesions I now return to patient RB, with hypertension and the clinical findings of pure motor hemiparesis.

In RB, complete blood count (CBC) was normal. EEG showed minor symmetrical slowing. CT showed a small infarct in the posterior limb of the internal capsule on the left and a tiny lesion in the right putamen. MRI also showed these lesions and another tiny lacune in the right thalamus. Ultrasound of the carotid and vertebral arteries was normal.

Because lacunes are small and deep in the hemisphere or are located in the brainstem, they usually do not have a major influence on the EEG recorded from the convexity.[34] CT findings depend on the location and size of the lesion. Pontine lacunes are seldom imaged by CT but can be seen on high-quality MRI examinations.[42,43,79,80,82,83] Pure motor hemiplegia probably has the highest frequency of CT positivity among the lacunar syndromes. Rascol et al. found hypodense lesions on CT in 29 of 30 patients with pure motor stroke.[37] They divided the lesions into large capsulo-putamino-caudate infarcts and smaller capsulo-pallido or capsulo-caudate infarcts.[37] Some patients with larger infarcts had angiographic abnormalities in the lenticulostriate arteries. Others have verified MCA-occlusive disease in patients with large basal ganglionic and capsular infarctions.[25,84–87] In contrast, patients with pure sensory stroke seldom have lesions visible on CT.[77]

MRI is undoubtedly superior to CT in imaging small brainstem and thalamic infarcts.[42,43,56,82,83,88] Rothrock and colleagues evaluated 31 patients with the clinical diagnosis of lacunar infarction, and 23 (74%) had appropriate lesions on MRI.[56] When both CT and MRI were performed, MRI was superior in imaging lesions appropriate to the symptoms. In another study, among 110 patients, MRI was very effective in imaging one or more possibly responsible lacunar infarcts in 89 patients.[42] When gadolinium-diethylene-triamine penta-acetic acid (Gd-DTPA) enhancement is given, acute lacunar infarcts generally are enhanced.[88] Use of enhancement may be helpful when the clinicians find more than one lesion and are uncertain of the age of the lesions. Generally, only acute lesions are enhanced. CT or MRI is essential for excluding small hemorrhages from the differential diagnosis; such hemorrhages can cause findings identical to lacunar syndromes. By imaging hemosiderin, MRI is more effective than CT in determining whether old lesions were small hematomas or were lacunar infarcts.

Angiographic abnormalities have been discovered in some patients with lacunar infarcts and include carotid-artery and MCA disease.[87] Some are probably incidental and unrelated to the cause of the stroke. Necropsy studies have shown that most patients with hypertension and lacunes have a high incidence of coexisting atherosclerosis. Angiography in apparently normal prisoners[89] also documents a high incidence of atherosclerosis. Thus, the finding of atherosclerotic occlusive disease in larger extracranial and intracranial arteries does not prove an etiological relationship to the lacunar infarct. In some cases, blockage of parent arteries can produce infarction in territories of lenticulostriate, thalamogeniculate, and pontine penetrating vessels. Figure 8.4 depicts diagrammatically the vascular lesions in occlusion of penetrating and parent arteries. The lesion in the parent artery can be a plaque, an in situ thrombosis, or an embolism.[25] Parent-vessel lesions are especially important to consider in patients with lacunes exceeding 20 mm, which involve the basal ganglia and capsule. In my experience, the clinical syndrome usually includes more features than the usual lacunar syndrome.[25,86] Echocardiography and cardiac rhythm monitoring are also important in some cases, to exclude cardiac-origin embolism to parent arteries. The larger deep infarcts are less often caused by lipohyalinosis.

Miller emphasized the importance of confirming the clinical impression of lacunar infarction by laboratory and imaging tests.[36] Neuroimaging with CT—or preferably with MRI—is especially important. The need for thorough laboratory testing will depend on (1) the presence of appropriate risk factors, such as hypertension or diabetes; (2) the typicality of the neurological findings; and (3) the thoroughness of the neurological examination and experience of the examining physician. If the patient has no evidence of past or present hypertension, physicians should be skeptical of lipohyalinosis as the cause of infarction. Atypical neurological findings or the presence of unaccustomed headache, reduced alertness, or seizures all argue for more complete laboratory investigations. At times, unexpected superficial infarcts, small hemorrhages, and even nonvascular conditions such as tumors are discovered by CT or MRI.

When the clinical diagnosis is uncertain, MR or standard angiography may be indicated. Generally, after preliminary evaluation, which should include a detailed history and examination, blood studies, EEG, and either CT or MRI, physicians will be able to place the patient with brain ischemia into one of three categories: (1) high certainty of lacune, (2) lesion consistent with but not diagnostic of lacune—that is, atypical; or (3) findings not compatible with a lacunar etiology. Examples of possible findings in these three groups are listed in Table 8.1. Patients in categories 2 and 3 will require more evaluation.

RB was kept at bed rest. Weakness began to improve during the second week, when he was transferred to a rehabilitation hospital. During the rehabilitation hospitalization, he was referred to an internist, who carefully followed the patient while in the hospital, and who will later institute antihypertensive treatment.

Treatment

No treatment has been shown to modify the course of lacunar infarction. The morphological nature of lipohyalinosis and fibrinoid degeneration, both of which involve lesions of the wall of the vessel and not really intimal disease, would make it theoretically unlikely that anticoagulants or agents

TABLE 8.1
Findings in Patients with Suspected Lacunar Infarction

	Diagnosis Highly Probable	Diagnosis Likely but Uncertain	Lacune Unlikely or Excluded
Ecology	Hypertension	Diabetic Mild hypertension	No hypertension
Neurological signs	Paralysis (R) face, arm, leg No other findings	Paralysis (R) arm > leg No other signs	Paralysis of (R) hand Aphasia
Accompanying symptoms	None	Slight unaccustomed headache	Severe headache Seizure at onset
Laboratory	Compatible small deep infarct on MRI or CT	Normal CT	Hypodensity (L) frontal region or other cortical zone on CT; hemorrhage on CT or MRI

that decrease platelet aggregation would be effective. Anecdotal reports indicate that they are not.[90] The disease is also beyond the reach of the surgeon's knife. Because the lesion is caused by hypertension, the most logical therapy to prevent new lipohyalinotic disease is careful control of the blood pressure; however, overzealous reduction of blood pressure during the acute ischemia can decrease flow in collateral arteries and can expand the region of infarction.[23,25] I prefer to wait until after the first 2 to 3 weeks of the stroke to institute major reductions in blood pressure. I try to maximize blood flow during the first days and to keep the patient at rest with the head flat, to augment cranial flow, but I know of no evidence that shows that this is effective or important. If the vascular etiology of the lesion is parent-vessel disease and not lipohyalinosis, then treatment of that condition should be considered.

Some authors and physicians fail to include lacunar infarction in their differential diagnosis of cerebral ischemia because they feel that clinical recognition of the disorder is unreliable. I feel that its inclusion is very important for two reasons: (1) The disorder is very common; to omit a lesion found in 10 percent of all brains is foolhardy. (2) Recognition of this etiology has a direct behavioral result—that is, no aggressive diagnostic testing and no anticoagulant or surgical treatment is prescribed. The investigation and treatment of other causes of cerebral ischemia—large-vessel occlusive disease, cerebral embolism, and systemic hypotension—are quite different. In addition, technological advances, especially CT and MRI, have greatly improved the clinical diagnosis of lacunar infarction.

Chronic Small-Vessel Disease

The disorder that leads to single lacunar infarcts often involves multiple penetrating arteries. As a result, multiple lacunar infarcts are often found in the brain at necropsy or are visible on MRI scan. In the necropsy study of Tuszynski and colleagues, 169 patients had 327 lacune, an average of 1.9 per patient.[33] Less than half (46%) had only one lacune, 16 percent had two, and 38 percent of patients had three or more lacunes. Others[1,2,5] have found an even higher frequency of multiple lesions, but now more widespread control of blood pressure may have altered this tendency. Most often, lacunes involve the striatum, capsule, thalamus, cerebral white matter, and pons. When extensive, they give the deeper portions of the brain a Swiss-cheese-like appearance. This condition was labeled *etat lacunaire* after Marie.[5] Traditionally, the clinical findings have been described as including pseudobulbar abnormalities of speech and swallowing and emotional control; small stepped gait; Parkinsonianlike rigidity; hyperreflexia; extensor plantar reflexes; dementia with slow thinking and responses; and variable weakness and sensory signs and symptoms. More-recent experience, especially from CT and MRI, raises questions about this traditional view. First, many patients with multiple lacunes seem quite well preserved and function normally. Second, patients with the syndrome described almost always have associated rather severe changes in the cerebral white matter and ventricular enlargement. Most clinicians and investigators are now inclined to ascribe the dementia and clinical signs more to the white-matter disease (dubbed leuko-araiosis by Hachinski)[91] than to the lacunes. The combination of lacunes and white-matter gliosis and atrophy almost invariably occur together and are associated with widespread abnormalities of penetrating small arteries.[92] The combination should be considered a *chronic microvasculopathy*.

The chronic white-matter changes were initially described by Binswanger.[89] Olszewski, in a review of the history and pathology of the condition, used the term *subcortical arteriosclerotic encephalopathy*.[93,94] In 1987, Babikian and Ropper reviewed the pathological features in over 40 cases described in the literature.[95] Grossly visible in the cerebral white matter are confluent areas of soft, puckered, and granular tissue. These areas are patchy and emphasize the occipital lobe and periventricular white matter, especially anteriorly and close to the ventricles.[95-97] The cerebellar white matter is also often involved. The ventricles are enlarged, and at times, the corpus callosum is small. The volume of white matter is reduced, but the cortex is generally spared. There are nearly always some lacunes. These were present in 39 of 42 necropsy cases of Binswanger's disease.[95] Microscopic study shows myelin pallor. Usually, the myelin pallor is not homogeneous, but islands of decreased myelination are surrounded by normal tissue. At times, the white-matter changes are so severe that necrosis and cavitation occur. Gliosis is prominent in zones of myelin pallor. The walls of penetrating arteries are thickened and hyalinized. Occlusion of the small arteries is rare.[96] Occasional cases of Binswanger white-matter changes have had amyloid angiopathy as the underlying vascular pathology.[98–100]

The clinical picture is quite variable. Most patients have some abnormalities of cognitive function and behavior.[95,101] Most often, the condition is characterized by slowness and abulia. Memory loss, aphasic abnormalities, and visuospatial dysfunction are also found. Pseudobulbar palsy, pyramidal signs, extensor plantar reflexes, and gait abnormalities are also common. The clinical findings often progress gradually or stepwise, with worsenings during periods of days to weeks. Often, there are long plateau periods of stability of the findings.[97]

CT often shows periventricular hypodensity. On MRI, the findings are more obvious and dramatic, with zones of periventricular increased density on T2-weighted images and of patchy white-matter changes. Figure 8.5 is an MRI of a patient with Binswanger white-matter abnormalities. I prefer not to use the term *leuko-araiosis* for these white-matter changes because I feel that it is a general term, and there are several different patterns of white-matter change: Caps occur around the ventricular system, especially in the region of the anterior horns and occipitally; a rim of abnormal white-matter signal often surrounds the ventricle diffusely or more focally; discrete small foci or patchy or confluent regions of abnormal signal are also noted and vary from single to many lesions. Awad and colleagues have attempted to correlate these various lesions with the neuropathology.[9] In general, diffuse, periventricular rims represent gliosis that is probably due to transependymal flow of CSF.[9] Very tiny foci often are due to *etat crible*. Lesions in the centrum semiovale and corona radiata are generally regions of chronic partial ischemia.[9] Some recent studies indicate that hemorrheological changes in the blood, with increased viscosity, may be prevalent in this condition.[102] Increased blood viscosity and slow flow through the microvasculature could compound the vascular lesions, leading to hypoperfusion in the territory of deep penetrating arteries.[102,103]

Treatment of this chronic microangiopathic condition is unknown. Impressed by the preliminary data about hyperviscosity, I have begun to treat these patients by attempting to reduce their Hcts (by blood donation and stopping smoking) and by reducing their fibrinogen levels by prescribing eicosopentanoic-rich fish-oil preparations.

This microvasculopathy must be differentiated from multiple infarcts due to large-artery occlusive disease and from multiple cerebral emboli, as causes of vascular dementia. In these two other conditions, most of the infarcts are cortical or cortical and subcortical, and the history usually includes a history of episodes of acute strokes. To differentiate among these,

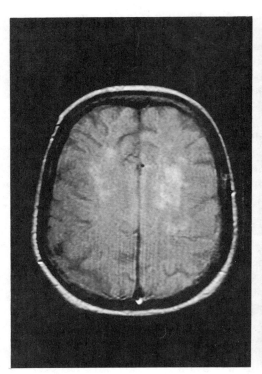 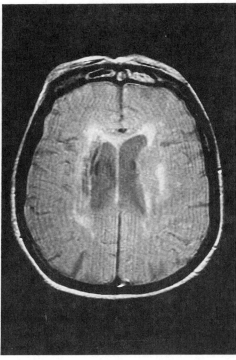

a   b

FIGURE 8.5   MRI T2-weighted images: Axial sections (a) and (b) show increased signal around the ventricles and punctate and large areas of abnormal signal in the white matter of the centrum semiovale in a patient with Binswanger's disease.

extracranial and transcranial ultrasound, echocardiography, cardiac rhythm monitoring, and angiography usually show a cardiac-origin embolic source or multiple large-artery occlusive disease.

References

1.   Fisher CM. Lacunes, small deep cerebral infarcts. Neurology 1965;15:774–784.
2.   Fisher CM. The arterial lesions underlying lacunes. Acta Neuropathol 1969;12:1–15.
3.   Durand-Fardel M. Traite des ramollisements du cerveau. Paris: Bailliere, 1843.
4.   Ferrand J. Essai sur l'hemiplegie des vieillards: les lacunes de desintegration cerebrale. Paris: Thesis, 1902.
5.   Marie P. Des foyers lacunaires de desintegration et des differents autres etats cavitaires du cerveau. Rev Med (Paris) 1901;21:281.

6. Foix C, Levy M. Les ramollissements sylviens. Rev Neurol 1927;43:1–51.
7. Foix C, Hillemand P. Contribution a l'etude des ramollisements protuberantiels. Rev Med 1926;43:287–305.
8. Caplan LR. Charles Foix—the first modern stroke neurologist. Stroke 1990;21:348–356.
9. Awad I, Johnson PC, Spetzler RF, Hodak JA. Incidental subcortical lesions identified on magnetic resonance imaging in the elderly: II. postmortem pathological correlations. Stroke 1986;17:1090–1097.
10. Fisher CM. Pure motor hemiplegia of vascular origin. Arch Neurol 1965;13: 30–44.
11. Fisher CM. Pathological observations in hypertensive cerebral hemorrhage. J Neuropathol Exp Neurol 1971;30:536–550.
12. Fisher CM. Cerebral miliary aneurysms in hypertension. Am J Pathol 1972; 66:313–324.
13. Cole F, Yates P. Intracerebral microaneurysms and small cerebrovascular lesions. Brain 1966;90:759–767.
14. Rosenblum WJ. Miliary aneurysms and "fibrinoid" degeneration of cerebral blood vessels. Hum Pathol 1977;8:133–139.
15. Charcot J, Bouchard C. Nouvelles recherches sur la pathogenie de l'hemorrhagie cerebrale. Arch Phys Norm Pathol 1868;1:110–127, 643–665.
16. Foix C, Hillemand P. Irrigation de la protuberance. Compt Rendu Soc Biol (Paris) 1925;42:35–37.
17. Foix C, Hillemand P. Les arteres de l'axe encephalique jusqu'a diencephale inclusivement. Rev Neurol 1925;41:705–739.
18. Foix C, Hillemand P. Irrigation du bulbe. Compt Rendu Soc Biol (Paris) 1924;42:33–35.
19. Stopford J. The arteries of the pons and medulla oblongata: I. J Anat Physiol 1915;50:131–164.
20. Stopford J. The arteries of the pons and medulla oblongata: II. J Anat Physiol 1916;50:255–280.
21. Düret H. Conclusion d'un memorie sur la circulation bulbaire. Arch Phys Norm Pathol 1873;50:88–89.
22. Düret H. Recherches anatomiques sur la circulation de l'encephale. Arch Phys Norm Pathol 1874;1:60–91, 316–353.
23. Fisher CM, Caplan LR. Basilar artery branch occlusion: a cause of pontine infarction. Neurology 1971;21:900–905.
24. Fisher CM. Bilateral occlusion of basilar artery branches. J Neurol Neurosurg Psychiatry 1977;40:1182–1189.
25. Caplan LR. Intracranial branch atheromatous disease: a neglected, understudied and underused concept. Neurology 1989;39:1246–1250.
26. Peress N, Kane W, Aronson S. Central nervous system findings in a tenth-decade autopsy population. Prog Brain Res 1973;40:473–484.
27. Boiten J. Lacunar stroke: a prospective clinical and radiologic study. Maastricht Thesis 1991.
28. Norrving B, Cronqvist S. Clinical and radiologic features of lacunar versus nonlacunar minor stroke. Stroke 1989;20:59–64.
29. Pullicino P, Nelson R, Kendall B, et al. Small deep infarcts diagnosed on computed tomography. Neurology 1980;30:1090–1096.
30. Weisberg L. Computed tomography and pure motor hemiparesis. Neurology 1979;29:490–495.

31. Donnan G, Tress B, Bladin P. A prospective study of lacunar infarction using computed tomography. Neurology 1982;32:47–56.
32. Mohr JP, Caplan LR, Melski J. The Harvard Cooperative Stroke Registry: a prospective registry. Neurology 1978;28:754–762.
33. Tuszynski MH, Petito CK, Levy DB. Risk factors and clinical manifestations of pathologically verified lacunar infarctions. Stroke 1989;20:990–999.
34. Caplan LR, Young R. EEG findings in certain lacunar stroke syndromes. Neurology 1972;22:403.
35. Mohr JP. Lacunes. Stroke 1982;13:3–11.
36. Miller V. Lacunar stroke, a reassessment. Arch Neurol 1983;40:129–134.
37. Rascol A, Clanet M, Manelfe C, et al. Pure motor hemiplegia: CT study of 30 cases. Stroke 1982;13:11–17.
38. Nelson R, Pullicino P, Kendall B, et al. Computed tomography in patients presenting with lacunar syndromes. Stroke 1980;11:256–261.
39. Richter R, Bruse J, Bruun B, et al. Frequency and course of pure motor hemiparesis: a clinical study. Stroke 1977;8:58–60.
40. Gobernado JM, de Molina AR, Gimeno A. Pure motor hemiplegia due to hemorrhage in the lower pons. Arch Neurol 1980;37:393.
41. Mori E, Tabuchi M, Yamadori A. Lacunar syndrome due to intracerebral hemorrhage. Stroke 1985;16:454–459.
42. Hommel M, Besson G, LeBas JF, et al. Prospective study of lacunar infarction using magnetic resonance imaging. Stroke 1990;21:546–554.
43. Besson G. Les infarctus lacunaires: evaluation clinique et par l'imagerie par resonance magnetique. These, Grenable, France, 1989.
44. Kase CS, Wolf PA, Hier DB, et al. Lacunar infarcts: clinical and CT aspects: the Stroke Data Bank experience. Neurology 1986;36:178–179.
45. Dejerine J, Dejerine-Klumpke H. Anatomie des Centres Nerveux Vol 2, Paris Rueff 1901:128–157.
46. Fisher CM, Cole M. Homolateral ataxia and crural paresis, a vascular syndrome. J Neurol Neurosurg Psychiatry 1965;28:48–55.
47. Fisher CM. Ataxic hemiparesis. Arch Neurol 1978;35:126–128.
48. Helgason CM, Wilbur AC. Capsular hypesthetic ataxic hemiparesis. Stroke 1990;21:24–33.
49. Goldblatt D, Markesbury W, Reeves AG. Recurrent hemichorea following striatal lesions. Arch Neurol 1974;32:51–54.
50. Kase C, Maulsby G, DeJaun E. Hemichorea–hemiballism and lacunar infarction in the basal ganglia. Neurology 1981;31:452–455.
51. Helgason C, Wilbur A, Weiss A, et al. Acute pseudobulbar mutism due to discrete bilateral capsular infarction in the territory of the anterior choroidal artery. Brain 1988;111:507–524.
52. Caplan LR, Schmahmann JD, Kase CS, et al. Caudate infarcts. Arch Neurol, 1990;47:133–143.
53. Fisher FM. Capsular infarcts. Arch Neurol 1979;36:65–73.
54. Helgason C, Caplan LR, Goodwin J, Hedges T. Anterior choroidal artery territory infarction: case reports and review. Arch Neurol 1986;43:681–686.
55. Mohr JP, Steinke W, Timsit SG, et al. The anterior choroidal artery does not supply the corona radiata and lateral ventricular wall. Stroke 1991;22:1502–1507.

56. Rothrock JF, Lyden PD, Hesselink JF, et al. Brain magnetic resonance imaging in the evaluation of lacunar stroke. Stroke 1987;18:781–786.

57. Leestra JE, Noronha A. Pure motor hemiplegia, medullary pyramid lesion, and olivary hypertrophy. 1976;39:877–884.

58. Ropper AH, Fisher CM, Kleinman GM. Pyramidal infarction in the medulla: a cause of pure motor hemiplegia sparing the face. Neurology 1979;29:91–95.

59. Fisher CM. A lacunar stroke, the dysarthria–clumsy hand syndrome. Neurology 1967;17:614–617.

60. Helgason CM, Wilbur AC. Basilar branch pontine infarctions with prominent sensory signs. Stroke 1991;22:1129–1136.

61. Caplan LR, Goodwin J. Lateral tegmental brainstem hemorrhages. Neurology 1982;32:252–260.

62. Ho K-L. Pure motor hemiplegia due to infarction of the cerebral peduncle. Arch Neurol 1982;39:524–526.

63. Hommel B, Besson G, Pollak P, et al. Hemiplegia in posterior cerebral artery occlusion. Neurology 1990;40:1496–1499.

64. Castaigne P, Lhermitte F, Buge A, et al. Paramedian thalamic and midbrain infarcts: clinical and neuropathological study. Ann Neurol 1981;10:127–148.

65. Caplan LR. Posterior cerebral arteries. In: Vinken P, Bruyn G, Klawans H, Toole J, eds. In: Handbook of clinical neurology: vol. I. cerebrovascular disease. rev. Amsterdam: Elsevier Scientific, 1989:409–415.

66. Percheron G. Les arteres du thalamus humain: II. arteres et territoires thalamique paramedians de l'arterie basilarie communicante. Rev Neurol 1976;132: 309–324.

67. Bogousslavsky J, Miklossy J, Deruaz J, et al. Unilateral left paramedian infarction of thalamus and midbrain: a clinicopathological study. J Neurol Neurosurg Psychiatry 1986;49:686–694.

68. Graff-Radford NR, Damasio H, Yamada T, et al. Non haemorrhagic thalamic infarction. Brain 1985;108:495–516.

69. Bogousslavsky J, Regli F, Assal G. The syndrome of tuberothalamic artery territory infarction. Stroke 1986;17:434–441.

70. Bogousslavsky J, Regli F, Uske A. Thalamic infarcts: clinical syndromes, etiology, and prognosis. Neurology 1988;38:837–848.

71. Kaplan RF, Estol CJ, Damasio H, et al. Bilateral polar artery thalamic infarcts. Neurology 1991;41(Suppl 1):329.

72. Wall M, Slamovits TL, Weisberg LA, Trufant SA. Vertical gaze ophthalmoplegia from infarction in the area of the posterior thalamo-subthalamic paramedian artery. Stroke 1986;17:546–555.

73. Meissner I, Sapir S, Kokmen E, Stein SD. The paramedian diencephalic syndrome: a dynamic phenomenon. Stroke 1987;18:380–385.

74. Caplan LR, DeWitt LD, Pessin MS, et al. Lateral thalamic infarcts. Arch Neurol 1988;45:959–964.

75. Dejerine J, Roussy G. Le syndrome thalamique. Rev Neurol 1906;14:521–532.

76. Fisher CM. Pure sensory stroke involving face, arm, and leg. Neurology 1965;15:76–80.

77. Fisher CM. Thalamic pure sensory stroke: a pathologic study. Neurology 1978;28:1141–1144.

78. Fisher CM. Pure sensory stroke and allied conditions. Stroke 1982;13:434–447.

79. Fisher CM. Lacunar strokes and infarcts: a review. Neurology 1982;32: 871–876.

80. Hommel M, Besson G, Pollak P, et al. Pure sensory stroke due to a pontine lacune. Stroke 1989;20:406–408.

81. Mohr JP, Kase C, Meckler R, et al. Sensorimotor stroke. Arch Neurol 1977; 34:734–741.

82. Dewitt D, Wray S, Kistler P, et al. Nuclear magnetic resonance imaging in neuro-ophthalmologic syndromes. Neurology 1984;34(Suppl 1):96–97.

83. Kistler JP, Buonano F, Dewitt D, et al. Vertebral-basilar posterior cerebral artery territory stroke: delineation by proton nuclear magnetic resonance imaging. Stroke 1984;15:417–425.

84. Adams H, Damasio H, Putnam S, et al. Middle cerebral artery occlusion as a cause of isolated subcortical infarction. Stroke 1983;14:948–952.

85. Maki G, Mihara H, Shizuka M, et al. CT and arteriographic comparison of patients with transient ischemic attacks: correlation with small infarcts of basal ganglia. Stroke 1983;14:276–280.

86. Caplan LR, Babikian V, Helgason C, et al. Occlusive disease of the middle cerebral artery. Neurology 1985;35:975–982.

87. Bogousavsky J, Regli F, Maeder P. Intracranial large-artery disease and "lacunar" infarction. Cerebrovas Dis 1991;1:154–159.

88. Miyashita K, Naritomi H, Sawada T, et al. Identification of recent lacunar lesions in cases of multiple small infarction by magnetic resonance imaging. Stroke 1988;29:834–839.

89. Faris A, Poser C, Wilmore D, et al. Radiologic visualization of neck vessels in healthy men. Neurology 1963;13:386–396.

90. Dobkin B. Heparin for lacunar stroke in progression. Stroke 1983;14:421–423.

91. Hachinski V, Potter P, Merskey H. Leuko-araiosis. Arch Neurol 1987;44:21–23.

92. Okeda R. Morphometrische Vergleichsuntersuchungen an Hirnarterien bei Binswangerscher Encephalopathie und Hochdruckencephalopathie. Acta Neuropathol (Berlin) 1973;26:23–43.

93. Olszewski J. Subcortical arteriosclerotic encephalopathy. World Neurol 1965;3:359–374.

94. Blass JP, Hoyer S, Nitsch R. A translation of Otto Binswanger's article: the delineation of the generalized progressive paralysis. Arch Neurol 1991;48: 961–972.

95. Babikian V, Ropper AH. Binswanger disease: A review. Stroke 1987;18:1–12.

96. Fisher CM. Binswanger's encephalopathy: a review. J Neurol 1989;236:65–79.

97. Caplan LR, Schoene WC. Clinical features of subcortical arteriosclerotic encephalopathy (Binswanger's disease). Neurology 1978;28:1206–1215.

98. Gray F, Dubas F, Roullet E, Escourolle R. Leukoencephalopathy in diffuse hemorrhagic cerebral amyloid angiopathy. Ann Neurol 1985;18:54–59.

99. Dubas F, Gray F, Roullet E, Escourolle R. Leukoencephalopathies arteriopathiques. Rev Neurol 1985;141:93–108.

100. Loes D, Biller J, Yuh WT, et al. Leukoencephalopathy in cerebral amyloid angiopathy: MR imaging in four cases. AJNR 1990;11:485–488.

101. Caplan LR. Binswanger's disease. In: Vinken PJ, Bruyn GW, Klawans HL, eds. Handbook of clinical neurology: vol 46. neurobehavioral disorders. New York: Elsevier, 1985:317–321.

102. Schneider R, Ringelstein EB, Zeumer H, et al. The role of plasma hyperviscosity in subcortical arteriosclerotic encephalopathy (Binswanger's disease). J Neurol 1987;234:67–73.
103. Caplan LR. Binswanger's disease. Current opinion in neurology and neurosurgery. Gower Acad J 1988;1:57–62.

CHAPTER 9

Nonatherosclerotic Ischema

Many different nonatherosclerotic vascular diseases cause brain ischemia. Some have been very well characterized, while in others, information about pathogenesis and clinical features is meager. Herein, I discuss the most frequent and most important conditions not covered elsewhere in this book.

Arterial Dissection

Dissection of extracranial arteries was once considered rare. The reports of Fisher, Ojemann, and colleagues clarified the clinical and radiological features in patients with dissection of the ICA.[1,2] Since then, the disorder has been recognized more often. The extracranial ICA is the most commonly affected vessel and is usually involved in its pharyngeal and distal extracranial segments, well above the carotid origin. This location is unusual for atherosclerosis, which almost invariably affects the carotid origin or the carotid siphon. Dissections of the extracranial VA affect the vessel in its distal segment, between its emergence from the vertebral column and its dural penetration, or in the first segment of the artery, above the VA origin but before entrance into the transverse foramina.[3,4] The pharyngeal ICA and the first and third segments of the VA are more mobile and less firmly anchored than the origins and intracranial penetration sites of these arteries.

   Most dissections probably involve some trauma or mechanical stress. Trauma may be severe but can be trivial—for example, twisting the neck to avoid a falling tree branch, lunging for a Ping-Pong ball, or turning abruptly while skiing. Many examples of so-called spontaneous dissection may actually have been triggered by minor trauma—forgotten or deemed inconsequential by the patient. Congenital changes in the media or elastica of the arteries and edema of the arterial wall could promote dissection because Marfan's syndrome, cystic medial necrosis, fibromuscular dysplasia, and migraine are disorders found more commonly than expected in patients with dissection.[3]

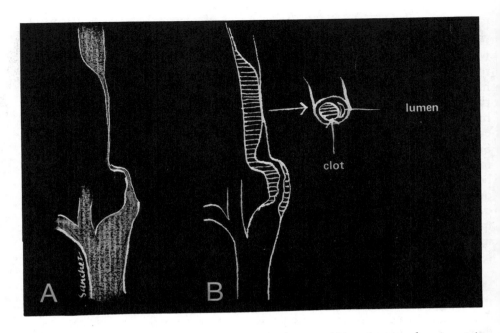

FIGURE 9.1   Dissection of the internal carotid artery: (A) angiogram showing string sign; (B) lumen compromised by intramural clot.

A tear within the arterial wall leads to bleeding. Blood dissects, usually within the media, along the longitudinal course of the artery. Dissection in the plane between the media and adventitia probably causes aneurysmal out-pouching of the vessel. The dissection can also produce an intimal tear, allowing the blood clot within the media to reenter the lumen (Figure 9.1). The expanded arterial wall encroaches on the lumen. Clot is often present within the lumen, either as a result of reentry or because of stasis of blood flow from luminal compromise. The intramural expansion probably also stimulates the endothelium to release factors promoting thrombosis. The luminal clot is usually loosely adherent to the intima and can readily embolize distally. In the weeks following dissection, the intramural blood is absorbed and the lumen usually returns to its normal size. Aneurysmal pouches may remain as a mark of the healed lesion.

In carotid dissection, often, the most impressive feature is pain. Ipsilateral throbbing headache and sharp pain locally in the neck, jaw, pharynx, or face may be noted, separating dissection from ordinary atherosclerotic occlusion.[1-10] The sympathetic fibers traveling along the wall of the ICA are usually disturbed, leading to an ipsilateral partial Horner's syndrome, characterized by ptosis and meiosis. Facial sweat function is preserved because the sympathetic innervation of the sweat glands travels along the ECA.

TIAs are common and may involve both the ipsilateral eye and the brain. The spells often come more frequently than in atherosclerotic ischemia, which led Fisher to coin the term *carotid allegro*.[1] Some patients with ICA dissection have visual scintillations and bright sparkles very reminiscent of migraine, even though many have had no personal or family history of migraine. Some patients complain of hearing a pulsatile noise in the head or ear. TIAs are probably due to luminal compromise, with distal hypoperfusion, but most patients with severe strokes have evidence of embolization of clot to the MCA from thrombus at the site of the dissection. Stroke, when it occurs, is usually noted shortly after the ICA dissection but may occur during the days and weeks following. Late stroke is rare but has been reported after traumatic ICA dissection.[11] At times, dissection may occur in steps. Pain in the neck may be present for days, and then days or even weeks later, the pain may recur and be accompanied by ischemic attacks or strokes. Undoubtedly, the initial tear has extended and more intramural bleeding developed when the symptoms worsened.[7] At times, both carotid arteries and even the VAs are dissected at the same time.

Ultrasound testing can suggest the presence of dissection. B-mode can show tapering of the ICA lumen, beginning well above the ICA origin; an irregular membrane crossing the lumen; and even demonstration of true and false lumens.[12] CW Doppler can show a typical pattern characterized by a high-amplitude signal, with markedly reduced systolic Doppler frequencies and alternating flow directions over the region of luminal narrowing.[13] This Doppler signal probably results from abnormal vessel-wall pulsations and some bidirectional movement of the blood column. Duplex scans of the VAs in the neck can also suggest dissection.[14] Typical findings are increased arterial diameter, decreased pulsatility, intravascular abnormal echoes, and hemodynamic evidence of decreased flow. Color Doppler flow imaging (CDFI) can also show the regions of dissection within the neck. Diminished flow in the high neck at the level of the atlas detected by CW Doppler and decreased flow in the intracranial VA shown by transcranial Doppler (TCD) help in the recognition of distal extracranial VA dissections. In patients with extracranial ICA dissections, TCD may show diminished intracranial velocities in the ICA siphon and the MCA. When this occurs in young patients without risk factors for atherosclerosis or embolism, who have normal ICA bifurcations in the neck, the diagnosis of dissection is quite likely.

The diagnosis of arterial dissection has traditionally been made by evaluating the results of standard catheter angiography. (Figure 9.2 illustrates various arteriographic features of carotid dissections.) The most common angiographic finding is a string sign (Figure 9.1), consisting of a long, narrow column of contrast material that begins distal to the carotid bifurcation and can extend to the base of the skull.[1,2] There may also be total occlusion of the ICA. This occlusion differs from the typical atherosclerotic occlusion, beginning more than 2 cm distal to the origin of the ICA, sparing the siphon, and having a gradually tapering segment that ends in the occlu-

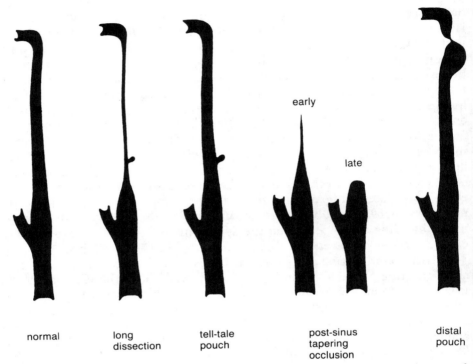

FIGURE 9.2 Drawings of various abnormal carotid arteriograms in patients with carotid-artery dissection (From Fisher CM, Ojemann RG, Robertson GH, Spontaneous dissection of cervicocerebral arteries, Can J Neurol Sci 1978;5:9–19; reprinted with permission.)

sion. There may also be localized aneurysmal sacs or outpouchings, both proximal and distal, along either a narrowed, a normal, or an unusually dilated portion of the artery. More recently, CT—taken as axial sections through the area of dissection—and MRI can visualize the intramural bleeding and expansion and can confirm the diagnosis of dissection. MRA can also show dissections, but it is too early to determine the sensitivity and specificity of this new imaging technique in patients with dissection.

ECA dissection or a pharyngeal aneurysm related to a large ICA dissection can also lead to dysfunction of the lower cranial nerves at the skull base. Dysgeusia, Horner's syndrome, and weakness and atrophy of the tongue are perhaps the commonest cranial-nerve signs. The lingual weakness and atrophy are due to compression of the hypoglossal nerve as it lies adjacent to the carotid sheath. At times the IX, X, XI, and XII cranial nerves are involved.

Extracranial VA dissections had initially been recognized in patients who had either trauma or chiropractic manipulation,[6,15,16] but VA injuries also have been reported in patients who manipulate their own necks[17,18] or who have maintained their necks in a fixed position for some time.[19–22] These lesions most often involved the distal extracranial—third segment— of the VA. Spontaneous dissections clinically and radiologically closely mimic those related to trauma.[4,6] Pain in the posterior neck or occiput is common, as is generalized headache.

Pain often precedes neurological symptoms by hours, days, and— rarely—weeks. Some patients with dissection have only neck pain and do not develop neurological symptoms or signs. TIAs most often include diz- ziness, diplopia, veering, staggering, and dysarthria. TIAs are less common in VA dissections than in ICA dissections. Infarcts usually cause signs that begin suddenly. The commonest patterns of ischemic brain damage are cerebellar infarction in PICA distribution and lateral medullary infarction. As in extracranial ICA dissections, infarcts are invariably explained by em- bolization of fresh thrombus to the intracranial VA. Occasionally, the dissec- tion begins intracranially and extends directly into the intracranial VA. Sometimes, emboli reach the superior cerebellar arteries (SCAs), the main basilar artery, or the posterior cerebral arteries (PCAs).

Many patients with extracranial carotid artery and VA dissections have headache, pain, and TIAs without lasting neurological deficits. Intracranial dissection is less common but is more serious and is almost invariably associated with severe deficits or death unless the dissection has a very limited extent. Intracranial dissections can cause infarction, subarachnoid bleeding, or mass effects.[4,23–26] When the dissections are between the media and the intima, vascular occlusions usually occur and lead to infarction in the regions of supply. In the anterior circulation, the supraclinoid ICA and main-stem MCA are most often involved.[26] In the posterior circulation, the intracranial VAs and the basilar artery are most often affected.[4,24] The resulting brainstem infarcts usually have proven fatal in reported cases. When dissections extend between the media and the adventitia, both aneurysms and tears through the adventitia may lead to subarachnoid hemorrhage (SAH), which can be repeated. At times, dissections lead to prominent aneurysmal masses, which can present as space-taking lesions that compress adjacent cranial nerves or brain parenchyma.

Occasionally, patients have apparently chronic dissections, with bilateral aneurysms and multifocal regions of dissection of various ages.[4,24] These patients usually have very abnormal arterial media and elastic mem- branes, and the arteries show healing intramural hematomas and tears of dif- ferent ages. I have cared for two such patients, one who had recurrent SAH, and the other recurrent posterior-circulation TIAs and strokes.[24] In the lat- ter patient, thrombus was visible within each bilateral intracranial VA- dissecting aneurysm, and symptoms stopped after treatment with warfarin and aspirin combined. Some patients with chronic or recurrent dissections have fibromuscular dysplasia. When intracranial vessels are involved, hemorrhage and local mass effect can be prominent.

Most extracranial dissections heal spontaneously with time. Their location high in the neck usually makes surgical repair difficult or impossible. When complete occlusion has occurred, the arteries often do not recanalize, and they remain occluded. Arteries that retain some residual lumen invariably heal and normalize. Intracranial dissections have been repaired surgically in patients with SAH, although the incidence of spontaneous healing and recurrent bleeding is not known. Though there have been no controlled trials of medical therapy, I am struck with the many anecdotal reports and my own positive experience with anticoagulants. Prevention of embolization of clot at or shortly after the dissection should prevent stroke. Anticoagulants have not seemed to increase the extent of the dissections, a major theoretical concern. Because the risk of embolization is only during the acute period, I use heparin, followed by warfarin, but I stop all anticoagulants after 6 weeks. I now follow patients with dissections using MRI, MRA, and ultrasound, and I seldom perform repeat standard angiography. I also try to maximize cerebral blood flow (CBF) during the acute period, to augment collateral circulation.

Fibromuscular Dysplasia

First recognized in the renal circulation, fibromuscular dysplasia is now known to affect many other systemic arteries, including extracranial and cerebral arteries. It is a nonatheromatous multifocal disease that can involve any or all of the three layers in the vessel wall. In the cerebral circulation, it is reported in only 0.6 percent of nonselected consecutive cerebral arteriograms.[27,28] There are no data on its true incidence in patients evaluated for stroke. This blood vessel abnormality is most commonly described in middle-aged women.[28] Bilateral ICA involvement is common (86%); changes usually extend from the level of C1 proximally 7 to 8 cm, with sparing of the carotid bifurcation and the intracranial carotid artery. Twenty percent of patients have coexistent VA disease.[28]

The most common form of fibromuscular dysplasia affects the media. Constricting bands, composed of fibrous dysplastic tissue and proliferating smooth-muscle cells in the media, alternate with areas of luminal dilation related to medial thinning and disruption of the elastic membrane.[29,30] These changes produce the characteristic string-of-beads appearance on arteriography (Figure 9.3). Additionally, hypertrophy of fibrous tissues in the adventitia or intima can cause segmental areas of stenosis.

Although most fibromuscular-dysplasia vascular lesions are asymptomatic, this vascular abnormality can cause brain ischemia. There is a frequent association of fibromuscular dysplasia with aneurysms of the intracranial vessels. In one series of 37 patients with fibromuscular dysplasia, 19 patients had a total of 25 aneurysms.[31] The diagnosis of fibromuscular dysplasia is occasionally made at the time of evaluation of SAH.

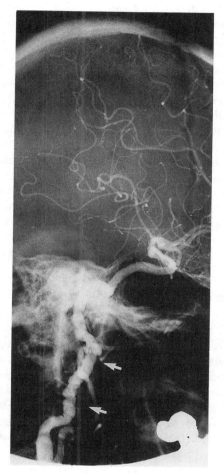

FIGURE 9.3   Carotid arteriogram, lateral view, showing typical sausagelike string-of-beads effect (white arrows) in a patient with fibromuscular dysplasia.

Fibromuscular dysplasia can also predispose the patient to arterial dissections with related stroke syndromes. In other patients, fibromuscular dysplasia affecting an artery appropriate to explain the CT and clinical findings is the only abnormality uncovered, but the lumen is not drastically compromised. The exact mechanism of the distal ischemia in this circumstance is unknown. Functional changes in vessel constriction could lead to distal hypoperfusion. Any medium-sized muscular intracranial artery can be affected. The most prominent clinical features are TIAs and strokes, usually of minor or moderate degree; fatal or very severe strokes are unusual. Headache, syncope, and Horner's syndrome are also frequent accompanying symptoms.

Most research and clinical interest has been directed at atherosclerotic disease of the intima and subintima of arteries. Little is known about the other portions of the arterial wall. Clearly, disease of the walls of arteries can lead to altered contractility, dilation with aneurysm formation, and tears with intramural hematomas. The disorder now called "fibromuscular dysplasia" is pathologically heterogenous and may occur as a result of a variety of different etiologies that share abnormalities of connective tissue. Knowledge of these disorders is now very rudimentary.

In a series of patients with stroke presumably due to fibromuscular dysplasia, the recurrence rate is quite low, even with no therapy.[29] Insufficient data are available to warrant rational therapeutic suggestions. I sometimes prescribe antiplatelet aggregating agents but rarely, if ever, use anticoagulants or recommend surgical repair or mechanical dilation of the vessels. If the patient is hypertensive, the renal arteries should be studied. When fibromuscular dysplasia is found on angiography, arch or neck, either standard arteriography or MRA is warranted, to exclude associated intracranial aneurysms.

Heritable Disorders of Connective Tissue

These are a group of hereditary disorders that are usually recognizable in childhood and involve the skin, vascular system, and skeletal tissues. The full spectrum of these disorders is still unraveling, and little in-depth analysis has been made of the neurological and cerebrovascular features.

Pseudoxanthoma elasticum (PXE) has an estimated prevalence of about 1 in 160,000 and has both autosomal dominant and recessive hereditary patterns.[32] The most easily recognized abnormalities are the skin changes.[32–34] The skin of the face and neck and in the axilla, antecubital, inguinal, and periumbilical regions first becomes thickened and grooved. Yellowish papules and plaques are seen in these areas and also on the mucosa of the lips, palate, buccal area, vagina, and rectum. Later, the skin becomes lax and redundant. Angioid streaks, which are reddish brown or gray, radiate from the optic disc and are usually wider than veins. The abnormality of connective and elastic tissue causes tortuosity of vessels, premature vascular calcification, intimal thickening, microaneurysms, and fusiform aneurysms. Gastrointestinal bleeding is common and is a result of the vascular changes.[33] Premature occlusive vascular disease affects the coronary, peripheral vascular, and cerebral arteries. The degenerative vascular changes begin with fragmentation and calcification of the internal elastic lamina, followed by extensive intimal and medial calcification.[33] The arteries of the aortic arch and the intracranial arteries are involved. One patient had occlusion of both ICAs at the skull base and a carotid-cavernous fistula.[35] Hypertension and mitral valve prolapse (MVP) are common,[32] and both SAH and ICH occur.

The *Ehlers-Danlos syndrome* (EDS) describes a group of clinically and genetically heterogenous conditions that share defects in collagen. The skin is hyperextensible and easily bruised, and the joints show hypermobility. Cardiac and cerebrovascular lesions are common and include MVP and tricuspid valve prolapse, septal defects, and dilation of the aortic root and pulmonary arteries.[36] Aneurysms, carotid-cavernous fistulae, and arterial dissections have been reported.[37,38] Rupture of various systemic and cerebral vessels leads to frequent bleeding and SAH.

Marfan's syndrome is an autosomal-dominant hereditary disorder that is probably more common than the other hereditary disorders, occurring in about 4 to 6 per 100,000 individuals.[39] The underlying nature of the condition is not known but is assumed to relate to abnormal collagen and elastin. The phenotype of long limbs, pectus chest deformity, arachnodactyly, and joint laxity is easily recognizable. Subluxation of the lens occurs in more than half of the patients, and ophthalmological examination is very helpful at times in diagnosis. The diameter of the aortic root is invariably enlarged, and aortic regurgitation and MVP are very common. Aortic aneurysms and aortic dissections are also very frequent clinical problems in patients with Marfan's syndrome.

Dilatative Arteriopathy

Some patients are prone to elongated, ectatic, tortuous intracranial arteries. This abnormality can be found in children and often involves multiple arteries.[40-42] When the abnormality is severe, the elongated dilated arteries are called "dolichoectatic" or "fusiform aneurysms." The most frequent location is in the posterior fossa, where the basilar artery or one or both VAs are involved.[43-47] The anomaly is readily recognized on CT as curvilinear calcified enhancing channels that usually cross the cerebellopontine angle.[43,44] The MCAs are also often involved, and some patients have dolichoectatic changes in both circulations.[43,45]

Extensive atherosclerotic plaques—often with calcification, encroachment on the lumen, and thrombus formation—are often found at necropsy. On microscopic examination, there are often fibrotic changes in the vessel wall, with reduced muscularis and attenuated, fragmented, or absent elastica.[48] Clinically, the commonest symptoms are due to brain ischemia. Mass effect with compression or displacement of cranial nerves or brain parenchyma is also common. Some patients have had hydrocephalus, possibly related to the effects of the dolichoectatic aneurysms on the third ventricle.

Ischemia is most often found in penetrating arteries to the brainstem and basal ganglia. Ischemia is related to the effects of the disease in the parent arteries on the branches. Plaques or clot may obliterate or obscure the orifice of branches or can embolize into the branches. Angiography may show thrombi within the dolichoectatic aneurysms.[43] In other patients, distortion and elongation of the branches may reduce blood flow, without obliteration of the branch ostia or lumens. Occasionally, clot within the aneurysm can embolize to the larger distal branches.[43,49] Rupture of these aneurysms, with resulting subarachnoid bleeding, is unusual but does occur.[43,48]

CT, MRI, and MRA should suffice to identify the aneurysmally dilated, ectatic arteries and may suggest the presence of clot within the vessels. TCD is very helpful in diagnosis and may show reduced mean flow velocities, with relatively preserved peak flow velocities.[50] In patients with recurrent ischemia and thrombi within the dolichoectatic arteries, warfarin may prevent strokes. Agents that modify platelet function have not been studied in patients with dilatative arteriopathy.

Cerebral Amyloid Angiopathy

Cerebral congophilic or amyloid angiopathy (CAA) is also discussed in Chapter 13 on ICH because the major clinical feature is recurrent lobar ICH. The disorder is characterized by a cellular thickening of the walls of small- and medium-sized arteries, by an amorphous eosinophilic-staining material, with a smudged appearance on light microscopy.[51] The material within the vessel wall shows a yellow-green birefringence when stained with Congo red and viewed under a polarizing microscope—hence the term *congophilic*. The changes usually involve many arteries, especially those in the leptomeninges and cerebral cortex of the cerebral lobes. The brainstem, basal gray nuclei, hippocampi, and subcortical white matter are spared.[52] The changes are most prevalent in the parietal and occipital lobes, but ICH is often frontal and central.[52-55] Affected arteries, especially those in the leptomeninges have a distinctive double-barrel lumen, with amyloid found in either the outer or the inner media.[51]

The most common clinical syndromes now recognized are ICH, usually multiple and subcortical lobar, and SAH.[51-55] Senile plaques containing amyloid and Alzheimer changes are also prevalent in brains of patients harboring CAA. Many patients with CAA are or become demented with time, due to multiple strokes and to Alzheimer pathology. Early studies also noted that scattered small infarcts were also prevalent in brains of patients with amyloid-related ICH.[53-55] TIAs can occur.[56] Recent studies have now shown that some patients with CAA have multiple infarcts and a prominent leukoencephalopathy with periventricular, subcortical, and corona radiata lucencies on CT, and with signal changes on MRI.[57-59] The clinical picture is that of Binswanger's disease. In fact, CAA may be a very important, often unrecognized, cause of this chronic ischemic microangiopathy.

The cause of CAA is unknown. Familial CAA has been identified—especially in Icelandic, Dutch, and German families—and is usually inherited as an autosomal-dominant trait, with high penetrance. The Icelandic variety has been attributed to abnormal metabolism of a gamma-trace protein.[60]

At times, there are prominent inflammatory changes in relation to the amyloid-staining arteries,[51,61] and there have been some reports of patients who seemed to have both CAA and granulomatous arteritis (or the CAA evoked a granulomatous reaction in these patients).[51] No specific treatment is known. Although it was formerly thought that drainage of CAA-related hematomas might be hazardous, recent data show that surgical results are not very different from other causes of ICH.[62] Treatment aimed at improving the hemorrheology of flow (see Chapter 5) might forestall ischemic damage and is worth trying.

Vasculitis and Other Possibly Inflammatory Vascular Disorders

Arteritis is mentioned as a cause of stroke in the differential diagnosis of nearly every medical student, nonneurologist, and some neurologists. Although often considered, documented arteritis is a very, very rare cause of stroke. Most often, CNS vasculitis presents as an encephalopathy with headache, seizures, decreased alertness, and cognitive and behavioral abnormalities, often with multifocal signs. Recognition of those rare instances in which arteritis is due to a specific microbial infection is critical for effective treatment. Patients with allergic hypersensitivity and systemic vasculitis may respond to corticosteroids or other treatments used to control systemic autoimmune diseases.

Bacterial, Spirochetal, and Fungal Arteritis

In patients with acute *bacterial meningitis* (e.g., pneumococcal or meningococcal), the pial arteries and veins are often surrounded by pus. Vascular occlusions and strokes may complicate the clinical picture, which is invariably dominated by headache, fever, stiff neck, and decreased alertness. *Listeria monocytogenes* may produce a characteristic inflammatory disorder involving predominantly the medulla and the pontine tegmentum.[63–65] Multiple lower cranial-nerve palsies and vestibular and oculomotor signs develop. At times, onset of symptoms is abrupt, and subsequent necropsy shows an arteritis, with multiple infarcts, as well as focal encephalitis. The CSF shows a pleocytosis.

In patients with *syphilis*, the spirochete probably invades cerebral arteries at the time of the meningitis of secondary lues. Meningovascular syphilis results and is characterized by apoplectic attacks of hemiplegia, headache, seizures, and CSF pleocytosis. The serology is always positive in

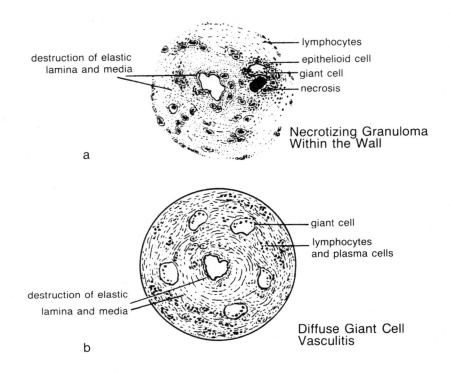

FIGURE 9.4   Changes in the vessel wall in (a) tuberculosis; (b) giant cell arteritis.

patients with meningovascular syphilis. The spinal arterial circulation can also be affected. All forms of syphilis are more common and more severe in patients with AIDS.

Lyme borreliosis mimics syphilis in many ways.[66] Meningitis, multiple cranial-nerve palsies, and root- and peripheral-nerve syndromes predominate.[67–69] Strokes have been described but are unusual and are not as common as a syndrome of headache, fatigue, and difficulty concentrating.[69] The CSF invariably shows some abnormalities, and specific antibodies to borrelia are present in the blood and CSF.

Chronic basal meningitis, usually caused by the *tubercle bacillus* or particular fungi—for example, *Cryptococcus, Histoplasma,* or *Coccidioides*—is frequently complicated by inflammation of the arteries within the exudate.[70,71] The proximal MCA and the arteries in the posterior perforated substance are most often involved. The exudate surrounds the arteries, producing thickening and inflammation of the walls of the arteries, usually called "Heubner's arteritis" (Figure 9.4A). Infarcts in the basal ganglia and midbrain result and can develop even after sterilization of the microbial agent. Other fungi, especially *Mucor* and *Aspergillus,* cause a necrotizing arteritis, with regions of cerebral infarction and necrosis. *Mucor* is usually spread from the paranasal sinuses, and *Aspergillus* reaches the cerebral circulation by hematogenous spread, usually without meningitis.[72] *Aspergillus* infections are especially common in patients who take corticosteroids or are immunosuppressed.[72]

Viral Infections

Viruses may be responsible for many cases of vasculitis that we now consider idiopathic. Hepatitis B surface antigen, immunoglobulin, and complement are found in the vessel walls of patients with polyarteritis nodosa who have hepatitis B antigenemia.[73] The varicella-zoster virus is also known to directly invade CNS vessels, sometimes without causing much visible inflammatory reaction. Viruses can cause vasculitis, either by direct invasion or by triggering an immune response to components of vessels. Alternatively, immune-complex deposition can injure arteries and cause inflammation.

Herpes varicella-zoster virus (HVZ) is the most well known and best documented of the viral arteritides. The most common clinical syndrome is delayed brain infarction, usually causing hemiplegia contralateral to herpes zoster ophthalmicus.[74–76] The symptoms begin days to weeks (average 6–8 weeks)[74,75] after onset of the painful rash. Infarctions are usually hemispheral and cause hemiparesis, hemisensory loss and aphasia, or right-hemispheric types of cognitive and behavioral changes. Usually, the infarct is ipsilateral to the rash. Angiography has shown occlusion of the carotid siphon, MCA, or ACA and sometimes stenosis of these vessels.[74–76] At times, TIAs may precede the stroke, but most often, the onset is abrupt and the neurological signs develop immediately. Some patients have an accompanying encephalitis. Recurrent ischemia and multiple infarcts have been reported. The mortality has been estimated at about 25 percent, higher than for comparable-sized infarcts caused by atherosclerosis.[75] The CSF usually shows some cells and immunoglobulins, and IgG indices may be elevated.[74,75] Rarely, the rash involves other divisions of Vth nerve (maxillary or mandibular) and can occur in the back of the neck and upper cervical dermatomes.[77–79] Rarely, the PCA and the vertebrobasilar territory are involved.[78,79]

At necropsy, patients with HVZ arteritis may show inflamed necrotic arteries, granulomatous changes,[74] or occluded arteries, with scant inflammation. Doyle and colleagues were able to demonstrate virions that were characteristic of HVZ in the nuclei and cytoplasm of smooth-muscle cells in the involved arteries.[76] Presumably, the virus spreads from the infected gasserian ganglion through trigeminovascular connections to the proximal portions of the ipsilateral MCA and ACA.[79,80] Trigeminovascular projections also go from V[1] to the SCA, and the upper cervical ganglia probably project to the VAs, the basilar artery, and to the AICA and SCA.[80] Spread to the intima could activate the endothelium to release factors promoting thrombosis. As in other virus diseases, inflammation is not always visible under the microscope.

Arteritis

Systemic Vasculitides, Including Collagen Vascular Diseases

The systemic vasculitis syndromes can be conveniently divided into polyarteritis nodosa, allergic angiitis and granulomatosis (Churg-Strauss syndrome), hypersensitivity vasculitis, Wegener's granulomatosis, and overlap syndromes sharing features of the other subtypes.[73,81–84] All have in common multisystem involvement.

Polyarteritis nodosa (PAN) affects small- and medium-sized arteries, especially at branch points.[73,83] Infiltration of polymorphonuclear leukocytes and monocytes is followed by intimal proliferation, fibrinoid necrosis, and thrombosis of arteries.[73] Probably the most common neurological signs relate to mononeuritis multiplex. CNS involvement occurs in 20 to 40 percent of patients, and the onset is usually after systemic symptoms and signs and neuropathy.[73] Some patients have a diffuse encephalopathy, and others have focal or multifocal abnormalities. Occasionally, hemispheral, spinal cord, and cerebellar and brainstem strokes occur. When strokes occur, it is usually late in the illness. Hypertension is very common in patients with PAN and is responsible for many of the ischemic infarcts and hemorrhages. I have not personally seen or known of a report of PAN presenting initially as a stroke syndrome.

Patients with the *Churg-Strauss syndrome* invariably have pulmonary involvement and eosinophilia.[85–87] There is usually also a history of previous allergic disorders. The lesions tend to involve smaller vessels, especially capillaries and venules.[73,87] Encephalopathy and peripheral neuritis are common, but strokes are extremely rare.

The *hypersensitivity vasculitides* are a group of disorders in which the cause is usually known and a major finding is a rash, often with palpable purpuric skin lesions, especially on the legs. Some are drug induced, postinfectious, or related to known foreign antigens (e.g., serum sickness). Mixed cryoglobulinemia and Henoch-Schönlein purpura are other forms of hypersensitivity vasculitis. Neurological involvement is not prominent in patients with the various hypersensitivity vasculitis syndromes, and when it occurs, neuropathies, plexopathies, and encephalopathies predominate.[73] Strokes do not occur, except occasionally due to bleeding related to systemic purpura.

Wegener's granulomatosis is a necrotizing, often fatal, granulomatous vasculitis that involves chiefly the lungs, sinuses, and upper respiratory tract, and the kidneys.[88] Orbital involvement, palsies of extraocular muscles, and ischemic changes in the retina and optic nerve are often reported.[89-91] The diagnosis can be made by biopsy and detection of anti-neutrophilic cytoplasmic antibody and is treatable with cyclophosphamide and other immune suppressants.[92] The findings can closely mimic temporal arteritis,[91] but strokes rarely—if ever—occur.

Nervous-system findings are quite common in patients with *systemic lupus erythematosus* (SLE). Headaches (often sharing features with migraine), seizures, psychosis with decreased cognition, chorea, and mono- and polyneuropathies are important features of SLE.[93] The usual assumption has been that vasculitis underlies these diverse neurological syndromes, but necropsy and clinical studies indicate that true arteritis is not a common cause of the CNS findings.[94,95] In a necropsy study, Johnson and Richardson found very scant evidence of inflammation of brain arteries.[94] However, sudden-onset neurological signs do occur in patients with SLE and can be a prominent clinical feature. MRI now often shows discrete focal lesions in patients with SLE, usually in the absence of a clinical history of stroke.[96] The infarcts are of diverse causes. Small-vessel vasculopathy with small deep infarcts and hemorrhages are usually due to hypertension, which accompanies the renal disease of SLE. Large-artery infarcts are most often due to abnormalities of coagulation and cardiac-origin embolism. Angiography often shows occlusion of intracranial artery branches.[97]

Hematological disorders are extremely common in SLE. The presence of lupus anticoagulant (LA) often correlates with clinical hypercoagulability, characterized by miscarriages, recurrent thrombophlebitis, and strokes.[98] Thrombocytopenia and other platelet abnormalities are also common, as is reduced prostacyclin activity.[99] In a 1988 clinicopathological study of 50 patients dying with SLE, a syndrome clinically resembling thrombotic thrombocytopenic purpura (TTP) developed in 14 (28%).[95] Seven of these 14 had, at necropsy, platelet-thrombi occluding their capillaries and arteries, segmental subendothelial hyalin deposits, and arteriolar microaneurysms—findings typical for TTP.[95] In this same study, vasculitis was not seen in the brain or spinal cord in any of the 50 patients.

Echocardiography in patients with SLE now shows a high incidence of valvular disease, especially Libman-Sacks endocarditis.[100] Other heart lesions are also common. Devinsky et al., in their clinicopathological study, found that 25 of the 50 patients had cardiac lesions that were potentially embolic.[95] These included Libman-Sacks vegetations (8), acute and chronic mitral valvulitis (12), marantic endocarditis (2), bacterial endocarditis (1), and 2 patients had mural thrombi—1 in the left atrium and 1 in the left ventricle.[95] Myocarditis is also a feature of SLE. Evaluation of patients with SLE who have focal neurological signs or focal lesions on MRI should include careful hematological and cardiac evaluation.

TTP is characterized clinically by fever, renal failure, thrombocytopenia, and microangiopathic hemolytic anemia.[101,102] Transient focal neurological signs, which improve quickly, and a more diffuse encephalopathy are common features.[101-103] Occasional reports document persistent neurological deficits, and even occlusion of medium-sized arteries (the PCA) has been documented.[104] Modern neuroimaging will probably show in the future that strokes are rather common in TTP but are usually minor and nondisabling. Plasma exchange can be an effective treatment, so this condition is important to recognize.[105] I have also seen intracranial bleeding in the form of small ICHs and SAHs in patients with TTP.

Severe *rheumatoid arthritis* (RA) can be complicated by neuropathies, meningitis, and rheumatoid dural nodules. True arteritis with fibrinoid necrosis is occasionally seen and can cause an encephalopathy or multifocal small infarcts.[106-108] In active RA, levels of fibrinogen, fibrinogen turnover, and fibrin degradation products are increased.[106-109] Also, very high titers of circulating rheumatoid factor can cause a hyperviscosity syndrome.[110] Undoubtedly, these serological changes contribute to brain infarcts in patients with RA.

Patients with *Sjögren syndrome* have a high incidence of neuropathy, especially involving the trigeminal nerves.[111] They also often have cognitive and behavioral changes.[112,113] In a recent neuroimaging study of 38 patients with the Sjögren syndrome, 8 patients had focal neurological deficits—most often hemiparesis, aphasia, and ataxia, as well as other cognitive and behavioral abnormalities.[113] MRI, in this study, showed CNS abnormalities in 75 percent of patients, most often in the white matter, but occasionally, discrete cortical lesions were seen, which looked like infarcts.[113] Vasculitis has been found at necropsy in patients with Sjögren syndrome, but many of the lesions clinically and on MRI resemble multiple sclerosis.[113,114]

Headache is common in patients with *systemic sclerosis (scleroderma)*, and occasionally brain infarcts and SAH are reported.[115,116] Hypertension is very common in scleroderma, and some of the vascular symptoms are probably due to high blood pressure and reversible vasoconstriction.

Sarcoidosis

Sarcoidosis does cause a cerebral vasculitis; almost invariably accompanying CSF pleocytosis, and retinal inflammatory changes are present.[117-120] The cerebrovascular changes probably represent spread from the meninges through Virchow-Robin spaces to the smaller pial vessels. Veins are predominantly affected, so the vascular lesion is probably most accurately classified as a phlebitis or venulitis.[121] Periphlebitis can be noted on ophthalmoscopic examination of the fundus. The lesions are characterized by a yellowish white focal or diffuse sheathing of retinal veins. Hard exudates, sometimes termed *taches de bougie* because of their resemblance to candle-wax drippings, are often related to the periphlebitis and can leave white choreoretinal scars.[118,122] TIAs, strokes, and evidence of meningeal, hypothalamic, and pituitary dysfunction are the clinical features of *angiitic neurosarcoidosis,* a disorder that can also affect the spinal cord, peripheral nervous system, and muscle. The periphlebitis and meningitis often respond to corticosteroids when given in substantial doses and over long periods (60 mg of prednisone daily for 3 to 6 months or more).

Temporal arteritis

This very important inflammatory disorder usually affects elderly men and women. Although the branches of the ECA, especially the superficial temporal and occipital arteries, are most frequently involved, the ICA, VA, subclavian, coronary, femoral, and even intracranial arteries can be affected.[123,124] Blindness is due to granulomatous arteritis in the arteries supplying the optic nerve and retina (Figure 9.4B). The lesions most often causing strokes are located in the distal extracranial ICA, just as it enters the carotid siphon, and in the distal extracranial VAs.[125] Rare patients have been described with encephalopathy and multifocal neurological signs who have the findings of temporal arteritis in pial and brain arteries.[126]

Temporal arteritis usually presents as a systemic illness. Patients often develop headache different from past headaches they might have had. The headache is not pulsatile and is accompanied by aching in the proximal muscles, low-grade fever, weight loss, malaise, fatigue, and jaw claudication. Jaw claudication results from ischemia of the masseter muscles supplied by branches of the ECAs. The superficial temporal arteries may be tender, cordlike, and nonpulsatile, and the scalp may be diffusely tender. The best-known and most feared complication is visual loss. An ischemic optic neuropathy results from occlusion of the posterior ciliary arteries. Additionally, occlusion of the central retinal artery can lead to an ischemic retina. If visual loss occurs, it is usually severe. Involvement of one eye is often followed by involvement of the other.

Laboratory findings that may be of help are an elevated erythrocyte sedimentation rate, mild anemia, and an elevated leukocyte count. Temporal arteritis may be present, with a normal erythrocyte sedimentation rate. Biopsy of the temporal artery is the most secure manner of making the diagnosis. Angiography with opacification of the ECA branches and the intracranial circulation can be suggestive. If possible, I choose to biopsy a smaller scalp branch of the superficial temporal artery. A long segment of the artery is taken, to avoid possible skip lesions, but the major portion of this artery is preserved. I feel that it is important to look for the general features of temporal arteritis in all elderly patients with stroke. Stroke, however, is rarely the first manifestation of temporal arteritis.

Treatment with prednisone, 60 to 80 mg/day, is undertaken prior to biopsy in patients with probable temporal arteritis. In such cases, there is usually rapid relief of headache and other systemic symptoms. The steroids are tapered by titrating the dose against the erythrocyte sedimentation rate.

Treatment will not reverse established central or ocular ischemia but will help prevent further involvement of blood vessels.

Isolated Central-Nervous-System Angiitis

In some patients, arteritis is limited to the CNS and can be difficult to diagnose. Any age can be affected (mean age about 49 years), and there is a male predominance (nearly 2/1).[127] The disorder (usually "granulomatous angiitis") can be acute, with symptoms developing within a few weeks, or it can evolve during a period of months to years.[127,128] Usually, the clinical picture is that of a diffuse or multifocal encephalopathy.[73,127–129] Cognitive and behavioral changes are found in more than 60 percent of patients, and headache, asymmetric motor signs, somnolence, and seizures are common findings.[127–129] Occasionally, TIAs or sudden strokes are described.[127–130] A myelopathy may also be present.[127,128] Focal signs may occur at onset, but more often, steplike worsenings punctuate the course of a progressive multifocal encephalopathy. The erythrocyte sedimentation rate is elevated in about two thirds of patients, but other serological and systemic tests are not helpful.[127] The CSF usually has a slight to moderate pleocytosis and the CSF protein is usually high (80%), often over 100 mg/dl.[127] CT or MRI may show small or large focal lesions, usually infarcts, but frank small hematomas and hemorrhage infarcts have also been noted.[127] In about half of the patients, angiography is abnormal and shows segmental narrowing and sausage-shaped dilation of arteries ("beading");[127] in many patients, however, angiography is completely normal.

Biopsy or necropsy shows a segmental, necrotizing granulomatous vasculitis affecting mostly the leptomeningeal and cortical and spinal vessels. Any size of artery or vein can be involved, but usually vessels < 500 μm in diameter are most affected. In some patients, the granulomatous changes have been predominantly venular.[127,128] The intima and adventitia of arteries are infiltrated with lymphocytes, giant cells, and granulomas. Granulomas can extend into the adjacent brain parenchyma. Specific diagnosis is very important because treatment with prednisone and immunosuppressant agents such as cyclophosphamide may allow recovery from a disease that is nearly always fatal when untreated.[73,84,127,129] Biopsy should be pursued in patients with multifocal lesions and encephalopathy, especially if they have a CSF pleocytosis and a high protein content. Moore urges biopsy of the nondominant hemisphere, especially the tip of the temporal lobe, choosing tissue that contains a longitudinally oriented surface vessel.[129]

Takayasu's Arteritis

Often called "pulseless disease," Takayasu's arteritis was originally described in young Japanese females.[131] Now the disorder is well known in other countries but is still uncommon in North America.[132] Some patients have a prodromal phase of malaise, fever, and night sweats, and laboratory analysis reveals anemia and an increased sedimentation rate. Later, severe occlusive disease of the aortic arch and its branches develops, often leading to absent neck and limb pulses.[133,134] Surprisingly, strokes or focal neurological signs are not the predominant feature. Headache, dizziness, syncope, and visual blurring are more common. In some patients, neurological function is well preserved despite striking radiological signs of occlusion of vessels at their origin from the arch.[135] Occlusions, stenosis, luminal irregularities, and ectasia or aneurysm formation are found. The commonest sites of involvement are the midportion of the left CCA, the left and right subclavian arteries, and the middle of the innominate artery.[135-137] The inflammatory process involves the media and adventitia, which are infiltrated with plasma cells, lymphocytes, and histiocytes.[136,137] Arm and leg claudication are commonly related to the subclavian, aortic, and iliofemoral disease.

Hypertension is present in more than half of the patients and may be difficult to control. The chronic proximal occlusive disease often leads to retinal microaneurysms and arteriovenous anastomoses, and visual loss can result from the chronic eye ischemia.[138] The proximal occlusive disease leads to extensive collateral circulation. Hypertension and increased flow through collateral channels can cause SAHs and ICHs similar to the situation in the moyamoya syndrome. Corticosteroids, immunosuppressive therapy, and surgical bypass treatment[139] have all been used. Moore[73] and others[140] are impressed that corticosteroids (prednisone 30 mg/day initially, then tapered to 5–10 mg/day maintenance) may prevent or diminish vascular complications.

Behçet's Disease

Behçet's disease is a relapsing, remitting illness first described by a Turkish dermatologist who recognized the triad of oral ulcers, genital ulcers, and uveitis. The disease is most often found in Turkey, Saudi Arabia, other Mediterranean countries, and Japan but does occur in North America, Europe, and worldwide and is a very important disease for neurologists to recognize. The predominant clinical systemic findings are aphthous ulcers in the mouth and genital tissues, uveitis, synovitis, other skin findings (such as folliculitis and erythema nodosum), ulcerative lesions in the bowel mucosa (especially the colon), and thrombophlebitis.[141-143] The disorder affects mostly young adults in their 20s, and there is a 2/1 to 4/1 male predominance.[141-145] Neurological involvement probably occurs in about 6 to 10 percent of patients. Among a large series containing 323 patients with Behçet's disease followed in a clinic in Turkey, only 46 were referred because of headache and neurological signs, and only 17 (5.3%) had neurological abnormalities.[144]

The most common neurological syndromes are a *meningitic form*, in which headache is the major symptom; an *encephalitic form,* with gradually evolving multifocal signs; *strokes,* characterized by relatively acute-onset focal signs; and *headache,* with papilledema due to dural sinus thrombosis.[144–149] Characteristically, the neurological signs come in attacks with remissions between, a course that closely mimics multiple sclerosis. Recently, CT and MRI show that the most frequent site of involvement is the pons and midbrain, followed by the basal ganglia and thalamus. The lesions most often are small foci that have high signals on T2-weighted MRI images and are iso or hypointense on T1-weighted images.[146,147] Some lesions are larger. The spinal cord is also frequently involved clinically and by MRI. The lesions often contain hemosiderin, and the distribution in gray and white matter separates the lesions from those found in multiple sclerosis. Angiography usually does not show arterial abnormalities.

The CSF is almost always abnormal, including pleocytosis, high protein content, and increased levels of immunoglobulins, which are produced intrathecally.[150] The CSF pressure is sometimes elevated. The levels of oligoclonal bands of IgA and IgM correlate well with neurological disease activity and are useful to follow. At necropsy, there often is a diffuse meningoencephalitis with perivascular lymphocytic cuffing, predominantly around veins, venules, and capillaries, with occasional arterial involvement.[145,147] The dural sinuses and large veins may be occluded.[144,148,149] Thromboses of the leg veins and even the vena cava are important systemic features, and the pathology is predominantly venous. The brain shows areas of necrosis, demyelination, and scarring, especially in the upper brainstem, internal capsule, and basal ganglia, as well as in the spinal cord. The lesions probably represent focal hemorrhagic venous infarcts and areas of encephalitic change. Corticosteroids may suppress the ocular and brain symptoms.[73,141] Moore recommends "early and aggressive treatment of CNS involvement with corticosteroids."[73]

Cogan's Syndrome

Cogan described a syndrome of interstitial keratitis with vestibuloauditory dysfunction.[151] The condition is probably an autoimmune vasculitic disorder that affects young adults. The earliest symptoms are photophobia, reduced vision, and redness of the eyes.[151–153] An interstitial keratitis is found on ophthalmological examination, occasionally with uveitis. Blindness can result from corneal opacification. Tinnitus, reduced hearing, vertigo, and ataxia appear before, during, or after the eye abnormalities. Microscopic study shows a vasculitis of small- and medium-sized arteries. Some patients have fever, and the aortic valve and bowel may be involved.[152] I am not aware of brain infarcts or CNS findings in patients with Cogan's syndrome.

Eales's Disease

Eales described a disorder characterized by abnormal retinal vessels and recurrent vitreous hemorrhages. The disease affects mostly young men and is common in the Middle East and India. The visual symptoms include specks, floaters, cobwebs and curtains, and blurred vision.[154] Ophthalmological examination shows prominent sheathing of veins and arteries, flame-shaped retinal hemorrhages, and vitreous hemorrhages. Although the symptoms usually begin in one eye, both eyes are invariably involved. The macular arteries are relatively spared, so that central vision is often preserved.[154] A vasculitis affecting both retinal arteries and veins causes the eye findings. Sometimes, the uvea is also involved. CNS involvement has been described in the form of meningitis, focal infarcts, and vascular occlusions.[155–158] In one patient, a left cerebral infarct was due to MCA occlusion.[155] Spinal-cord involvement is also common.[157] Usually, there are no systemic symptoms or characteristic laboratory abnormalities, although the CSF may show a pleocytosis.[155] The diagnosis is made on the basis of the characteristic ophthalmoscopic abnormalities.

Vascular Occlusive Lesions of Unknown Cause (Possibly Vasculitic)

Microangiopathy of the brain, ear, and retina

An unusual, but I believe distinct, occlusive vascular disorder was called "microangiopathy of the brain and retina" by Susac and colleagues.[159] Although this condition resembles granulomatous angiitis in some ways, there are important differences. In microangiopathy of the brain and retina, there is always obliteration of large retinal arteries, causing gradual severe bilateral visual loss.[159–162] The retinal vascular changes are easily observed through the ophthalmoscope. Some retinal arteries are amputated, while others are severely narrowed or attenuated, and light streaking characterizes their thickened arterial walls. Tinnitus and hearing loss are also prominent. The most important clinical signs are dementia, bilateral motor weakness with pyramidal signs, and cerebellar dysfunction. The disorder affects mostly young women in their second to fourth decade and progresses stepwise or gradually. The CSF protein is very high, sometimes more than 1 gm/dl, but usually there is no major pleocytosis. Brain biopsy has shown obliteration of small arteries without prominent inflammation or granulomas, as well as multiple microinfarcts.[157,160] Some patients with this condition have improved at least temporarily after corticosteroids and immunosuppressive therapy.[162]

Sneddon's syndrome

Sneddon's syndrome is characterized by livedo reticularis and recurrent strokes often in young patients without risk factors for stroke.[163–165] The most important and diagnostic clinical feature is livedo reticularis, a grayish pale mottling of the skin that usually involves the trunk and all limbs. The cutaneous findings are obvious by simply looking at the skin with the patient undressed. I have now seen a number of patients with Sneddon's syndrome who had undergone multiple invasive tests but apparently had never been examined without clothes. Usually, the hands and feet are cold and peripheral pulses are reduced. Hand angiography shows dramatic occlusions of digital arteries with areas of narrowing and dilation.[165] The neurologic findings are multiple acute onset strokes. Cerebral angiography often shows occlusion of large- or medium-sized intracranial arteries. At times, the disorder is familial. Some patients with Sneddon's syndrome have antiphospholipid antibodies.[166]

Kohlmeier-Degos Syndrome

This disorder, also called "malignant atrophic papulosis," is another vascular occlusive disorder with characteristic skin changes. The skin lesions begin as small yellow-pink raised lesions, usually on the trunk and arms.[167,168] The central part of the skin lesions comes to appear atrophic and looks porcelain-white, flat, and depressed, and each lesion is surrounded by a raised pink zone, often with telangiectasis.[167] Small- and medium-sized arteries in the skin undergo a progressive fibrosis, with infarcts of the skin.[168] Biopsy shows fibrous proliferation between the intima and the internal elastica, with rare inflammatory changes.[167,168] The bowel is also involved, causing ulcers, decreased motility, bowel dilation, and often perforation.[168] Although the vessels in other visceral organs are often involved at necropsy, systemic symptoms are usually limited to the skin and gut. CNS symptoms occur in about one fifth of patients with Kohlmeier-Degos syndrome.[167] Strokes do occur, and angiography may show occlusion and beading of distal branches of intracranial arteries.[167] Neuropathological examination shows hyalinization or fibrous proliferation between the endothelium and internal elastic membrane, often with superimposed thrombosis.[167] Occasionally, SAH and dural sinus thrombosis are present.[167] At times, the strokes precede skin and bowel involvement.

Vasculopathy in Drug Abusers

Unfortunately, drug abuse has become an important cause of stroke in adolescents and young adults. ICH due to drugs is considered in Chapter 13 and is most often due to amphetamines and cocaine. Ischemic stroke usually relates to one of five different situations: (1) heroin addiction, (2) amphetamine abuse, (3) abuse of drugs synthesized for oral use, (4) infection as a complication of an addictive life-style, and (5) cocaine use.

Heroin Addiction

In *heroin addicts,* strokes are invariably ischemic and may be cerebral or spinal. Stroke frequently follows the reintroduction of IV heroin after a period of abstention.[169–172] Cerebral ischemia may directly follow the injection but is more often delayed by 6 to 24 hours. Heroin addicts also have a number of well-documented serological and systemic abnormalities, including eosinophilia, elevated immune and gamma globulins, false-positive serology, Coombs-positive hemolysis, and lymph-node hypertrophy.[171] Increased binding of serum globulins by morphine has been found in rabbits with implanted morphine pellets, and in some narcotic addicts, morphine also binds gamma globulins.[173] Illicitly available heroin is frequently adulterated with a host of fillers and foreign substances. These data make it likely that *immune-complex deposition or other hyperimmune mechanisms underlie the strokes in patients who are chronically exposed to many recurrently introduced antigens.*[171] Unfortunately, definitive immunological or pathological studies of strokes in heroin addicts are wanting.

Amphetamine Abuse

In *amphetamine abuse,* necrotizing angiitis has been demonstrated pathologically. The lesions resemble polyarteritis nodosa and can affect the brain and other viscera.[174] In experimental animals[175] and humans[176] who have taken amphetamines orally or intravenously, angiography shows segmental changes in intracerebral vessels, with prominent beading. The commonest clinical syndrome is ICH, usually beginning shortly after amphetamine exposure, but ischemic infarcts have been found at necropsy.

Abuse of Drugs Synthesized for Oral Use

A different pattern of disease affects patients who inject intravenously drugs that have been synthesized for oral use; *methylphenidate* (Ritalin) and *pentazocine* (Talwin) with pyribenzamine are the best-documented drugs. These compounds contain talc, microcrystalline cellulose, and other fillers designed to maintain the chemicals in pill form. Addicts mash the pills, dissolve them in tap water, and inject them intravenously, or occasionally even directly into the carotid artery.[177] Particles of drugs and fillers still remain and are trapped by the lung arterioles and small arteries, causing an obliterative arteritis.[177,178] Pulmonary arteriovenous shunts develop and are probably responsible for crystals reaching the brain and eyes of addicts.[176–179] Strokes and seizures usually follow quickly after IV injection, and deep small cerebral arteries such as the lenticulostriate[177] and anterior spinal arteries are affected.[180]

Infection as a Complication of an Addictive Life-Style

Drug abusers seldom follow strict sterile precautions. Hepatitis, AIDS, infective endocarditis, and fungal infections are common complications of their *habit and life-style*. Endocarditis can cause embolic strokes. Fungal infections, especially with *Nocardia* and *Aspergillus*, can cause focal necrotic infarcts or brain abscesses.[71,72]

Cocaine Use

Cocaine use has become the most common cause of drug-related strokes. Unfortunately, cocaine use has become rampant. In a 1990 study, among 214 patients ages 15 to 44 years, admitted to the San Francisco General Hospital during a 10-year period, 34 percent were drug users, and cocaine was the predominant drug used.[181] Cocaine can be snorted or injected as cocaine hydrochloride or can be smoked as the free-base alkaloidal form usually called "crack cocaine."[182–184] Crack cocaine is made by mixing aqueous cocaine hydrochloride with ammonia and sometimes baking soda. The free-base cocaine is usually smoked after the cocaine has become alkalinized and precipitated. Crack cocaine produces a more rapid high than does snorted or injected cocaine hydrochloride, and its use is associated with a higher frequency of brain infarcts.[185] The strokes usually begin shortly after cocaine use, irrespective of the portal of entry (snorted, inhaled, or injected). These strokes have a predilection for the brainstem.[186] The mechanism of ischemia is unknown. Bowel and myocardial ischemia and an eosinophilic myocarditis are also found after cocaine abuse.[187] Vasoconstriction, increased platelet aggregation, and apparent vasculitis are posited as potential causes of stroke in cocaine users.

   Cocaine use is also associated with both SAHs and ICHs. For unclear reasons, there is a higher incidence of aneurysms and vascular malformations in cocaine-related hemorrhages than in hemorrhages after amphetamine use. Angiography should be performed unless the cocaine-related hemorrhage is in a characteristic location for hypertensive ICH.

Migraine and Vasoconstriction

Vascular headaches are among the most common disorders treated by physicians and neurologists. Migraine is prevalent at all ages, including young children and the elderly. During migraine attacks, angiography, CBF studies, and TCD have clearly documented changes in intracranial vessel diameter, flow velocities, and CBF. During the past decades, reversible vasoconstriction has been shown to be a very important cause of ischemia, especially in the coronary circulation, and in the brain after subarachnoid bleeding. Migraine is a clinical diagnosis usually applied when there is a past history and family history of pulsating, usually unilateral headaches, with or without characteristic visual, somatosensory, or other migraine accompaniments, and followed by nausea and vomiting. Although vasoconstriction and vasodilation have been shown to occur during migraine attacks, not all vasoconstriction is usually equated with migraine.

Neuroimaging in patients with migraine shows a more-frequent-than-expected incidence of infarcts. Migraine-related strokes have also been reported recently more often than in the past.[188-190] Infarction can be due to prolonged intense vasoconstriction, causing permanent ischemia or thrombosis of arteries. Intense vasoconstriction can impede flow, promoting thrombosis; platelets are activated during migraine, and the vasoconstrictive process itself may stimulate the endothelium to release factors that promote thrombosis. My own investigations on stroke within the PCA[191] and basilar-artery territories in patients with migraine[190] show that many have thrombi within the basilar artery and the PCA.

Migrainous accompaniments can precede, accompany, or follow headache and can occur in the absence of headache. Transient vasoconstriction accounts for many examples of temporary spells of neurological dysfunction in the elderly,[192,193] including transient global amnesia (TGA).[194,195] Fisher[192,193] and I have tried to separate migraine accompaniments from atherosclerotic ischemia by analyzing the clinical features of each (Table 9.1). To complicate matters, atherosclerotic lesions in the coronary arteries of humans—and in the extracranial and retinal arteries of experimental animals—seem to predispose them to superimposed vasoconstriction. Thus, vasoconstriction can complicate atherostenosis. TCD shows promise in identification of vasoconstriction by showing high velocities that change with time and with various pharmacological treatments.

Call and colleagues called attention to a syndrome that they called "reversible cerebral segmental vasoconstriction."[196] The syndrome most often affects young women, especially during the puerperium, but is found at all ages. Some patients have developed this syndrome after carotid endarterectomy. Vasoconstriction involves many large-, medium-, and small-sized cerebral arteries. The clinical findings include severe headache, decreased alertness, seizures, and changing multifocal neurological signs. Brain edema and death can occur. Angiography shows sausage-shaped focal regions of vasodilation and multifocal regions of vascular narrowing. TCD shows high velocities in many intracranial arteries. CT and MRI may show brain edema and small areas of infarction and hemorrhage. Corticosteroids, calcium-channel blockers, anticonvulsants, and treatments for increased ICP have all been used to treat this disorder. Many of the patients have had migraine in the past.

More recently, ICH has been shown to occasionally complicate a

TABLE 9.1
Migraine Accompaniments versus Atherosclerotic Ischemia

Migraine	*Atherosclerosis*
1. Sensory modalities involved sequentially—e.g., vision → tactile → speech	Modalities involved together—e.g., visual, somatosensory, and aphasic abnormalities noted at same time
2. Within each modality, first symptoms are "positive"—e.g., visual brightness, shining; somatosensory paresthesias	Usually negative symptoms—loss of vision, numbness
3. Symptoms gradually progress within each modality; visual loss gradually affects field; paresthesias move from one finger to hand to body—often takes 20 minutes to travel fully	Visual field or body involved at once
4. Within each modality, positive followed by negative—e.g., brightness leaves scotoma in its wake; paresthesias followed by numbness	Usually negative effects only
5. One modality clears before the next is involved	Modalities are involved simultaneously
6. Headache most often followed after neurological symptoms have cleared	Headache accompanies persistent deficits or is absent
7. Attacks usually last 15–30 minutes (average 20 minutes)	Usually 1–2 minutes; often <5 minutes
8. Different attacks involve different sides and different vascular territories	Usually always the same vascular territory
9. Spells may occur over years	Usually self-limited to days, weeks, months
10. Stroke risk factors often absent	Risk factors present
11. Women predominate over men	Men predominate over women

severe migraine attack.[197] Intense vasoconstriction leads to ischemia of a local brain region, with edema and ischemia of the small vessels perfused by the constricted artery. Then, when vasoconstriction abates, blood flow to the region is augmented, and the reperfusion can cause hemorrhage from the damaged arteries and arterioles.[198] The mechanism is the same as found in hemorrhage after carotid endarterectomy, and in reperfusion after brain embolization.

I believe that vasoconstriction accounts for many more strokes than is currently recognized or appreciated. Surveys of strokes in the young now attribute many infarcts to migraine. I take very seriously the risk of stroke in patients with prolonged classic migraine attacks, especially if the deficits last for hours or more after the attack. In these patients and in those with migraine-related infarcts, I use prophylactic agents (most often phenytoin, calcium-channel blockers, cyproheptadine, or methysergide), along with agents that modify platelet function and coagulation. Aspirin is used most often, but I sometimes use warfarin in patients with prior infarcts.

Moyamoya Syndrome

Moyamoya, although sometimes referred to as a disease, is probably better thought of as a syndrome, defined by a characteristic angiographic appearance. The intracranial ICAs undergo progressive tapering and progressive occlusion at their intracranial bifurcations (the so-called T portion of the ICAs). Basal penetrating branches of the ICAs, ACAs, and MCAs enlarge, so that they can provide collateral circulation. These vessels form large prominent anastomosing channels—basal telangiectasias—which angiographically appear as a cloud of smoke; these arteries appear especially prominent because of the paucity of MCA sylvian branches. The appearance of these basal telangiectasias led to the Japanese clinicians' use of the term *moyamoya*, which means "something hazy like a puff of cigarette smoke drifting in the air."[199,200] Although first described in Japan,[200] the disease has been reported worldwide.[199,201]

Necropsy studies, although few, have shown severe vascular occlusive changes characterized by endothelial hyperplasia and fibrosis with intimal thickening and abnormalities of the internal elastic lamina.[202] In contrast, the intracerebral perforating arteries show microaneurysm formation, focal fibrin deposition and thinning of the elastic laminas and arterial walls. These changes in the perforating arteries are probably the result of greatly increased flow through these small vessels.[199,200] Inflammatory changes have universally been absent. In 1991, Ikeda studied at necropsy the extracranial arteries of 13 Japanese patients with spontaneous occlusions of the circle of Willis, who met the research definition of moyamoya syndrome.[203] The extracranial arteries showed the same intimal lesions as the intracranial arteries. Characteristically, the proximal pulmonary arteries had fibrous nodular intimal thickening without inflammatory abnormalities.[203] Moyamoya changes have been found in a variety of situations, including sickle-cell disease, neurofibromatosis, young women (especially those who smoke cigarettes and take oral contraceptives),[202] and fibromuscular dysplasia. A variety of different conditions can probably cause intimal changes, which lead to fibrosis and luminal narrowing.

Clinically, the disorder has an interesting bimodal distribution, occurring often in children under age 15 years and in adults in their third to fifth decades of life. Children usually present with transient episodes of hemiparesis or other focal neurological signs, often precipitated by physical exercise or hyperventilation. Others have sudden-onset deficits such as hemiplegia or the gradual development of intellectual deterioration. Headaches and seizures are common.[199,200] These symptoms are often accompanied by CT evidence of infarction and CBF studies that reveal regions of hypoperfusion.

Adults, in contrast, usually present with brain hemorrhages—usually in the thalamus, basal ganglia, or deep white matter. These hemorrhages are the result of the degenerative changes (aneurysmal dilation and thinning) in the anastomotic basal vessels, which are overtaxed and cannot accommodate the volume of blood needed for perfusion. At times, the hemorrhages are subarachnoid and intraventricular. Angiography shows progressive changes that may be asymmetrical initially but always involve the intracranial ICAs bilaterally and usually also involve the MCA and ACA branches. As the intracranial arteries narrow, collaterals develop, involving the basal penetrating arteries, the orbital vessels (so-called ethmoidal moyamoya), and vessels over the vault derived from transdural anastomoses from the meningeal and superficial temporal arteries.[199] Later, the telangiectasias may regress and become less prominent. Suzuki and others have staged the severity of disease by the angiographic findings.[199,200]

Some patients with moyamoya stabilize clinically, often after they have developed disabilities. The best treatment is not known. A variety of different surgical revascularization procedures have been used, but whether they improve the outcome is not yet certain.

Hematological Disorders, Including Abnormalities of Coagulation, Viscosity, and Serum Constituents

In the 1980s and 1990s, the knowledge of blood constituents and their function in the coagulation process has dramatically advanced. Brain ischemia and hemorrhage often result from these hematological disorders, rather than from primary diseases of the blood vessels. The endothelia, blood vessels, and circulating blood are so intricately interwoven that it is often difficult to be sure of which changes are primary and thereby cause the disorder and which are a result of the etiology. For example, sickle-cell disease causes intimal fibrovascular changes, and occlusive diseases of all varieties activate coagulation factors, leading to readily detectable changes in the blood. I have already discussed most of the conditions in Chapters 4 and 5, regarding laboratory diagnosis and treatment, so the scope of this book permits only a brief cataloging of these disorders here.

Cellular Abnormalities

Changes in the *formed cellular constituents of the blood* may be *quantitative* or *qualitative*. Polycythemia has long been known to increase blood viscosity, decrease CBF, and increase thrombosis. Sickle-cell disease and sickle-cell–hemoglobin-C disease are examples of qualitative RBC abnormalities that affect blood flow. Sickle-cell disease is associated with occlusive changes in large intracranial arteries and small penetrating vessels.[204,205] Subcortical, cortical, and border-zone infarcts are often found on CT and MRI;[205] angiography has shown intracranial occlusions of the major basal arteries. TCD now offers a noninvasive method for detecting velocity changes related to IC narrowing and allows monitoring of patients with sickle-cell disease.

Increased platelet counts, especially those over 1 million, are also associated with hypercoagulability. The thrombocytosis can be primary, so-called essential thrombocythemia, can be associated with other myeloproliferation, or less often, can be secondary to systemic disease. Essential thrombocythemia is associated with strokes and digital occlusions.[206–208] The lack of correlation between the platelet count and the thrombotic complications has led to the assumption that there are also qualitative abnormalities of platelet function.[206–209] In some patients, increased coagulability has been attributed to *increased adhesion* and *aggregation of platelets* (so-called sticky platelets) in the absence of thrombocytosis.[210,211] Unfortunately, platelet function in vitro may not reflect true in vivo activity and function.

Leukemia is complicated occasionally by brain hemorrhages and microinfarcts. When the WBC count is very high (increased leukocrit), the WBCs can pack capillaries, leading to microinfarcts and vascular rupture with small hemorrhages in the brain. Larger intraparenchymatous hemorrhages and SAHs are most often related to thrombocytopenia, due to replacement of the bone marrow with leukocyte precursors.

Serological Abnormalities

Normally, *natural inhibitors of coagulation* circulate to discourage spontaneous blood clotting. The best known of these inhibitors—*antithrombin III* and *proteins C and S*—can be deficient on a hereditary basis or can be reduced by disease. Congenital deficiency of antithrombin III may be quantitative or qualitative and is most often an autosomal-dominant condition.[209,212] Reduced synthesis of antithrombin III, as in patients with liver disease, or renal loss in the nephrotic syndrome can lead to acquired deficiencies. Inherited deficiencies of protein C[213] and protein S can also contribute to or cause increased coagulability.[209] Most often, clotting is venous, but arterial occlusions have also been described.

Systemic and inherited conditions can *alter the levels of the serine protease coagulation factors*. The best known of these disorders is *hemophilia*, which causes bleeding into the joints, skin, and cranium. In 1989, my colleagues and I measured Factor VIII levels in a large number of patients with brain ischemia.[214] Some patients have chronically increased concentrations, with frequent episodes of thrombophlebitis, spontaneous abortion, and strokes.[215] In others, Factor VIII levels are high, probably as an epiphenomenon to the initial thromboembolic event. Some patients with infectious and inflammatory diseases, such as Crohn's disease and ulcerative colitis, have increased Factor VIII levels as a result of serological changes induced by the primary disease.[216,217] Venous dural sinus occlusions, thrombophlebitis, and arterial occlusions may result. Hematological changes in inflammatory bowel disease are complex because elevated levels of Factors V and VIII, reduced levels of antithrombin III, and quantitative and qualitative platelet abnormalities have all been described.[217]

Cancers are also often associated with hypercoagulability.[218,219] In 1989, my colleagues and I studied patients with mucinous adenocarcinomas, who had venous occlusions, large-artery thrombi, and multiple small-artery occlusions.[220] Mucin was seen inside and directly outside of small vessels, presumably contributing to the hypercoagulability evident clinically. In some situations (e.g., during pregnancy, the puerperium, or use of oral contraceptives), the mechanism of the hypercoagulability is not fully known.

The advent of thrombolytic and fibrinolytic treatment, especially with rtPA has led to more detailed study of the body's normal fibrinolytic activity and abnormalities of the fibrinolytic system.[221,222] Plasminogen deficiencies, dysfibrinogenemias, and abnormalities of tPA and its inhibitors can all cause an increased tendency toward thrombosis.[209,223] Thrombin and fibrinolytic activity can be monitored during acute stroke by measuring a number of substances:[224,225] For example, the levels of fibrinopeptide A correlate with thrombin activity, and the levels of cross-linked D-dimer, a breakdown product of fibrin polymer, are a useful index of fibrinolytic activity.[224,225]

Immunological Abnormalities

Recently, attention has been drawn to the presence of circulating antibodies that react to various hematological and vascular components. The best known of these disorders are the so-called *lupus anticoagulant* (LA) and *anticardiolipin antibodies*. These substances both react against phospholipids, and the presence of LA or anticardiolipins has been referred to as the *antiphospholipid antibody* (APLA) syndrome. The LA (a misnomer because it is associated with increased coagulability, not bleeding) is a phospholipid antibody that interferes with the formation of the prothrombin activator.[226,227] In the laboratory, there is a prolonged activated partial thromboplastin time (aPTT) that does not correct when normal plasmin is added, indicating the presence of an inhibitor of clotting rather than a deficiency of a needed component.[226–228] Some patients with LA have SLE, but most do not. When antiphospholipids of the IgG, IgM, or IgA classes are found in the absence of a known systemic illness, the disorder is now referred to as a primary APLA syndrome.[227–232] Clinically, these patients have an increased incidence of spontaneous abortions, thrombophlebitis, pulmonary embolism, and large- and small-artery occlusions. In addition to the presence of LA and/or anticardiolipins, laboratory abnormalities include positive VDRL, thrombocytopenia, and antinuclear antibodies. Some patients have mitral and aortic valve abnormalities and ocular ischemia.[227,231,232] The mechanism of increased coagulability and valvular changes is not known, but these probably relate to immune-related endothelial and valve-surface injuries.

Disseminated intravascular coagulation (DIC) is a disorder that affects both cellular and serological factors. When a primary disorder leads to local or diffuse clotting, the coagulation cascade may be activated, with generation of excess intravascular thrombin. The coagulation system then is activated further, fibrin is deposited into the microcirculation, hemostatic elements have a shortened survival, and the fibrinolytic system is activated.[233] The most common disorders inciting DIC are infections, obstetric and vascular emergencies, and cancer.[234,235] Head trauma, SAH, brain tumors, and vascular malformation can also cause DIC.[234,236] The laboratory findings usually include thrombocytopenia, reduced fibrinogen levels, prolongation of PT and PTT, and increased levels of fibrin split products. DIC can be associated with nonbacterial thrombotic endocarditis, especially in patients with cancer.[220,234,236] Neurological findings are frequent and include an encephalopathy with multifocal signs and frank thrombotic and embolic infarcts. Bleeding can also occur.

Blood flow, especially in the brain microcirculation, depends heavily on the *viscosity of the blood*, while blood viscosity is affected most by the *erythrocyte content* of the blood and the serum fibrinogen level.[237,238] Polycythemia and hyperfibrinogenemia can each increase whole-blood viscosity and can decrease CBF, especially in patients with cerebrovascular disease. Less often, increased viscosity is caused by high levels of globulins (e.g., in Waldenström's macroglobulinemia or in other disorders with abnormal proteins or cryoglobulins, such as multiple myeloma).[239] Rarely, very high levels of serum lipids cause significant hyperviscosity.[240]

Clinically, patients with hyperviscosity syndromes have an encephalopathy characterized by somnolence, stupor, headache, seizures, ataxia, and decreased vision.[239] A clue to the presence of hyperviscosity is the ophthalmoscopic appearance of the retina. Retinal veins are very dilated and tortuous and may show segmentations in the blood columns within the retinal vessels. Serum viscosity is measured relative to water; the average normal level is about 1.8. Serum viscosity of 5 or 6 is usually associated with encephalopathy, but lower levels may be very important in patients with hypertensive microvasculopathy and atherosclerotic disease.

Cerebral Venous Thrombosis

The advent of CT and later MRI have led to increased recognition of occlusions of dural sinuses and to improved knowledge of the causes, clinical findings, and possible treatment of this potentially serious condition.[241-243] The etiologies are diverse. Local infectious processes—such as otitis media, mastoiditis, and sinusitis—can lead to thrombosis of adjacent dural sinuses. Cancer, meningitis, dehydration (especially in children), and Behçet's disease are other well-known causes.[241,244] Since 1980, coagulopathies related to systemic diseases such as SLE, primary APLA syndrome, and ulcerative colitis[245] have been recognized as causes of dural-sinus occlusion. Some patients with congenital coagulation disorders—such as antithrombin III, protein C, and plasminogen deficiencies—develop this complication.[246] In some patients, congenital anomalies of a sinus, such as a congenitally bifurcated sagittal sinus, can promote occlusion.[247]

Of special importance is the frequency of dural-sinus occlusions, especially of the sagittal sinus, in young women. Pregnancy, the postpartum period, and the use of oral contraceptives seem to convey additional risks for developing this disorder. In one series, among 20 young women of childbearing age who had intracranial venous thrombosis, 13 developed thrombosis during the postpartum period, and 6 did so while taking oral contraceptives.[248] In India, venous dural sinus thrombosis is one of the most common types of stroke in young adults, especially during pregnancy and the puerperium.[249] In these patients, there is sometimes laboratory evidence of hypercoagulability.[248]

The clinical picture varies. Some patients present with a pseudotumor cerebri syndrome, characterized by headache and papilledema, with increased CSF pressure. These findings are due to decreased absorption of CSF because of the increased cranial venous pressure. In others, spread of thromboses from the sagittal sinus leads to venous infarction. The infarcts are most often bilateral, posterior parietal, and hemorrhagic. Frank hematomas may develop. Seizures, hemiplegia, and focal signs dominate the clinical picture in patients with infarcts.[241] Brain edema and increased ICP can be fatal. At times, the deep cerebral venous system is involved. Occlusion of the vein of Galen and the straight sinus can lead to infarction in the midbrain and thalamus, which has usually been discovered at necropsy in the past.[250,251] Hypersomnolence and abulia with headache and increased ICP are found clinically. Some patients with deep venous thrombosis do survive.[252]

CT may show nonspecific signs, such as small ventricles and brain edema or bilateral hemorrhagic infarcts. The occluded sinus may be hyperdense, without contrast, or may show a filling defect (delta sign). MRI has proven much more effective in showing venous sinus occlusions. MRA and other newer techniques usually show the occlusion in its full extent, as well as venous collaterals.[242,243,253] MRA has virtually eliminated the need for standard angiography to diagnose venous occlusive disease.

Treatment of patients with dural-sinus occlusions remains controversial. The sinus occlusions can extend into the internal jugular veins and can cause pulmonary embolization. Anticoagulation with heparin and warfarin theoretically might prevent extension of thrombosis and embolization, but clinicians feared that hemorrhagic infarctions and frank hematomas would develop or worsen in anticoagulated patients. A retrospective review of outcome in patients with dural-sinus occlusion indicated that those on anticoagulants fared better than those not given heparin or warfarin.[254] A preliminary study of heparin in 20 patients with venous thrombosis showed a clear benefit of heparin.[255] Among 10 heparin-treated patients, after 3 months, 8 had a complete recovery, and 2 had slight deficits; among the placebo-treated group, 3 died, 6 had deficits, and only 1 recovered completely.[255] A retrospective review by the same authors showed that heparin did not increase the risk of bleeding, even in patients with ICH before treatment.[255] In another study, 5 patients treated with both heparin and urokinase recovered completely.[256] Instillation of thrombolytic agents through catheters threaded into the dural sinuses is a possible effective treatment for the future, but insufficient data are now available on efficacy and risks.

Neoplastic Conditions

Neoplastic angioendotheliosis is a rare disorder in which tumor cells proliferate within the brain's blood vessels. Biopsy or autopsy usually shows endothelial proliferation and the presence of irregular crowding of pleomorphic cells with mitotic figures and multiple nuclei.[257] The cells occlude small arteries, leading to multiple microinfarcts. The disorder can be systemic, producing erythematous skin plaques and patches, subcutaneous nodules, high sedimentation rates, fever, and renal failure.[258,259] The cells are probably of lymphomatous origin. The disorder can affect the spinal cord.[260]

    Lymphomatoid granulomatosis is another disorder, probably related to lymphoma, in which granulomatous nodules can involve brain arteries and veins and can produce strokelike deficits.[261,262] *Hodgkin's disease in the meninges* often causes occlusions of meningeal arteries and veins, with hemorrhagic infarction in the underlying cerebral cortex. I have already commented on *leukemic blockage* of small arteries and on the *coagulopathies associated with cancer*, especially of the mucinous adenocarcinoma type.

Some Genetic Disorders That Cause Strokes

Many of the conditions already discussed in this chapter—for example, hereditary disorders of connective tissue and familial CAA—are known to be genetically determined. Many others are probably influenced by genetic predispositions. Dyslipoproteinemias, hemoglobinopathies, diabetes, hypertension, and atherosclerosis are all strongly governed by genetic factors. I close this chapter by briefly discussing a few other disorders with Mendelian etiologies. Knowledge of the genetic factors in stroke is still primitive but is growing rapidly.[263]

The *MELAS syndrome* (mitochondrial myopathy, encephalopathy, lactic acidosis, and strokelike episodes) is one form of mitochondrial encephalomyopathy.[264] Seizures, headaches, and intellectual deterioration are most prominent clinically.[265,266] Affected patients often have abrupt episodes of visual deterioration, hemiparesis, and ataxia, often with seizures. Lactic and pyruvic acid levels in the blood are often high, and muscle biopsy may show ragged red fibers.[265] CT and MRI show discrete multifocal infarcts that are mostly parieto-occipital and cerebellar.[266,267] These infarcts affect the cortex and underlying white matter. Basal-ganglia calcifications are also prominent. The cause of the strokes is unknown.

Strokes, renal failure, painful dysesthesias, and cutaneous angiokeratomas characterize *Fabry's disease*. The disorder is a sex-linked lysosomal storage disease, with most clinical cases being homozygous men; occasionally, heterozygous women are affected.[268,269] The diagnosis is suggested by finding the characteristic small, dark-red papules that are located predominantly along the inner thighs, perineum, and near the umbilicus. Because of a deficiency of a lysosomal enzyme (α-galactosidase), trihexosyl ceramide (a sphingolipid) accumulates and causes a diffuse vasculopathy.[270,271] Multiple vascular occlusions and strokes are common. Renal transplantation may delay vascular complications and may improve the prognosis.[271]

Homocystinuria is probably the most common genetic disease that affects the brain vasculature and leads to premature atherosclerosis and strokes.[272] An enzyme deficiency that is transmitted recessively and autosomally limits the body's ability to convert homocysteine to methionine;[272] homocysteine can cause injury to the vascular endothelium, making vessels susceptible to thrombus formation.[273,274] Homozygous individuals with homocystinuria often have a Marfanlike habitus, both myopia and dislocated lenses, osteoporosis, and mental slowness, as well as multiple venous and arterial occlusions.[272] The diagnosis is made by a positive nitroprusside test on the urine and elevated blood levels of homocysteine. Somewhat more controversial is whether heterozygotes are also susceptible to premature vascular occlusions.[275] A 1985 study showed an unusually high frequency of elevated blood levels of homocysteine after methionine loading challenges in patients under 50 years of age who had occlusive cerebrovascular and peripheral arterial occlusive disease.[272] Dietary therapy and pyridoxine may prevent some of the vascular occlusive complications of the disease.[272]

The scope of this book does not permit full discussion of other disorders occasionally complicated by strokes. Neurofibromatosis, Menkes's kinky-hair syndrome, various hemoglobinopathies and coagulation and platelet disorders, and other rare metabolic disorders clearly can predispose to stroke.[263] Hypercalcemia can cause stroke by its tendency to cause hypertension, vasoconstriction, and platelet activation.[276] Because of the limitations of this discussion, I have heavily referenced this chapter, grouping the references under the heading of each condition. These references should be explored for more details.

References

Arterial Dissection

1. Ojemann RG, Fisher CM, Rich JC. Spontaneous dissecting aneurysms of the internal carotid artery. Stroke 1972;3:434–400.
2. Fisher CM, Ojemann RG, Roberson GH. Spontaneous dissection of cervicocerebral arteries. Can J Neurol Sci 1978;5:9–19.
3. Caplan LR, Zarins C, Hemmatti M. Spontaneous dissection of the extracranial vertebral artery. Stroke 1985;16:1030–1038.
4. Caplan LR, Tettenborn B. Vertebrobasilar occlusive disease: review of selected aspects: I. spontaneous dissection of extracranial and intracranial posterior circulation arteries. Cerebrovasc Dis 1992;2:256–265.
5. Ehrenfeld WK, Wylie EG. Spontaneous dissection of the internal carotid artery. Arch Surg 1976;111:294–330.
6. Hart RG, Easton JD. Dissection of cervical and cerebral arteries. In: Barnett HJM, ed. Neurologic clinics: vol 1. cerebrovascular disease. Philadelphia: Saunders, 1983:155–182.
7. Ehrenfeld WK, Wylie EG. Spontaneous dissection of the internal carotid artery. Arch Surg 1976;111:294–330.
8. Friedman WA, Day AL, Quisling RG, et al. Cervical carotid dissecting aneurysms. Neurosurgery 1980;7:207–214.
9. Mokri B, Houser OW, Sandok BA, Piepgras DG. Spontaneous dissection of the vertebral arteries. Neurology 1988;38:880–885.
10. Bogousslavsky J, Despland PA, Regli F. Spontaneous carotid dissection with acute stroke. Arch Neurol 1987;44:137–140.
11. Pozzali E, Giuliani G, Poppi M, Faenza A. Blunt traumatic carotid dissection with delayed symptoms. Stroke 1989;20:412–416.
12. Sturzenegger M. Ultrasound findings in spontaneous carotid artery dissection: the value of duplex sonography. Arch Neurol 1991;48:1057–1063.
13. Hennerici M, Steinke W, Rautenberg W. High-resistance Doppler flow pattern in extracranial ICA dissection. Arch Neurol 1989;46:670–672.
14. Touboul PJ, Mas JL, Bousser MG, Laplane D. Duplex scanning in extracranial vertebral artery dissection. Stroke 1987;18:116–121.
15. Krueger BR, Okazaki H. Vertebral–basilar distribution infarction following chiropractic cervical manipulation. Mayo Clin Proc 1980;55:322–332.
16. Sherman DG, Hart RG, Easton JD. Abrupt change in head position and cerebral infarction. Stroke 1981;12:2–6.
17. Cook JW, Sanstead JK. Wallenberg's syndrome following self-induced manipulation. Neurology 1991;41:1695–1696.
18. Rothrock JF, Hesselink JR, Teacher TM. Vertebral artery occlusion and stroke from cervical self-manipulation. Neurology 1991;41:1696–1697.
19. Tramo MJ, Hainline B, Petito F, et al. Vertebral artery injury and cerebellar stroke while swimming: case report. Stroke 1985;16:1039–1042.

20. Hope EE, Bodensteiner JB, Barnes P. Cerebral infarction related to neck position in an adolescent. Pediat 1983;72:335–337.
21. Bostrom K, Liliequist B. Primary dissecting aneurysm of the extracranial part of the internal carotid and vertebral arteries. Neurology 1967;17:179–186.
22. Grossman FI, Davis KR. Positional occlusion of the vertebral artery: a rare cause of embolic stroke. Neuroradiology 1982;23:227–230.
23. Yonas H, Agamanolis D, Takaoka Y, White RJ. Dissecting intracranial aneurysms. Surg Neurol 1977;8:407–415.
24. Caplan LR, Baquis G, Pessin MS, et al. Dissection of the intracranial vertebral artery. Neurology 1988;38:868–879.
25. Anson J, Crowell RM. Cervicocranial arterial dissection. Neurosurg 1991; 29:89–96.
26. O'Connell B, Towfighi J, Brennan R, et al. Dissecting aneurysms of head and neck. Neurology 1985;35:993–997.

Fibromuscular Dysplasia

27. So EL, Toole JF, Dalal P, et al. Cephalic fibromuscular dysplasia in 32 patients. Arch Neurol 1981;38:619–622.
28. Corrin LS, Sandok BA, Houser OW. Cerebral ischemic events in patients with carotid artery fibromuscular dysplasia. Arch Neurol 1981;38:616–618.
29. Sandok BA. Fibromuscular dysplasia of the internal carotid artery. In: Barnett HJM, ed. Neurologic clinics: vol 1. Cerebrovascular disease. Philadelphia: Saunders, 1983:17–26.
30. Luscher TF, Lie JT, Stanson AW, et al. Arterial fibromuscular dysplasia. Mayo Clin Proc 1987;62:931–952.
31. Mettinger K, Ericson K. Fibromuscular dysplasia and the brain. Stroke 1982;13:46–52.

Heritable Disorders of Connective Tissue

32. Lebwohl MG, Distefano D, Prioleau PG, et al. Pseudoxanthoma elasticum and mitral-valve prolapse. N Engl J Med 1982;307:228–231.
33. Strole WE, Margolis R. Case records of the Massachusetts General Hospital: Case 10—1983. N Engl J Med 1983;308:579–585.
34. Altman LK, Fialkow PJ, Parker F, et al. Pseudoxanthoma elasticum: an under-diagnosed genetically heterogenous disorder with protein manifestations. Arch Intern Med 1974;134:1048–1054.
35. Rios-Montenegro E, Behrens MM, Hoyt WF. Pseudoxanthoma elasticum: association with bilateral carotid rete mirabile and unilateral carotid-cavernous sinus fistula. Arch Neurol 1972;26:151–155.
36. Leier CV, Call TD, Fulkerson PK, Wooley CF. The spectrum of cardiac defects in the Ehlers-Danlos syndrome types I and III. Ann Intern Med 1980;92: 171–178.
37. Pretorius ME, Butler IJ. Neurologic manifestations of Ehlers-Danlos syndrome. Neurology 1983;33:1087–1089.
38. Lach B, Nair SG, Russell NA, Benoit BG. Spontaneous carotid-cavernous fistula and multiple arterial dissections in type IV Ehlers-Danlos syndrome. J Neurosurg 1987;66:462–467.

39. Pyeritz RE, McKusick VA. The Marfan syndrome: diagnosis and management. N Engl J Med 1979;300:772–777.

Dilatative Arteriopathy

40. Read D, Esiri MM. Fusiform basilar artery aneurysm in a child. Neurology 1979;29:1045–1049.
41. Hirsch CS, Roessmann U. Arterial dysplasia with ruptured basilar artery aneurysm: report of a case. Hum Pathol 1975;6:749–758.
42. Makos MM, McComb RD, Hart MN, Bennett DR. Alpha-glucosidase deficiency and basilar artery aneurysm: report of a sibship. Ann Neurol 1987;22: 629–633.
43. Pessin MS, Chimowitz MI, Levine SR, et al. Stroke in patients with fusiform vertebrobasilar aneurysms. Neurology 1989;39:16–21.
44. Moseley IF, Holland IM. Ectasia of the basilar artery: the breadth of the clinical spectrum and the diagnostic value of computed tomography. Neuroradiology 1979;18:83–91.
45. Little JR, St Louis P, Weinstein M, et al. Giant fusiform aneurysms of the cerebral arteries. Stroke 1981;12:183–188.
46. Echiverri HC, Rubino FA, Gupta SR, Gujrati M. Fusiform aneurysm of the vertebrobasilar arterial system. Stroke 1989;20:1741–1747.
47. Nishizaki T, Tamaki N, Takeda N, et al. Dolichoectatic basilar artery: a review of 23 cases. Stroke 1986;17:1277–1281.
48. Shokunbi MT, Vinters HV, Kaufmann JC. Fusiform intracranial aneurysms: clinicopathologic features. Surg Neurol 1988;29:263–270.
49. Cohen MM, Hemalatha CP, D'Addario RT, Goldman HW. Embolism from a fusiform middle cerebral artery aneurysm. Stroke 1980;11:158–161.
50. Hennerici M, Rautenberg W, Schwartz A. Transcranial Doppler ultrasound for the assessment of intracranial arterial flow velocity: II. evaluation of intracranial arterial disease. Surg Neurol 1987;27:523–532.

Cerebral Amyloid Angiopathy

51. Vinters HV. Cerebral amyloid angiopathy: a critical review. Stroke 1987;18:311–324.
52. Vinters HV, Gilbert JJ. Cerebral amyloid angiopathy: incidence and complications in the aging brain: II. the distribution of amyloid vascular changes. Stroke 1983;14:924–928.
53. Okazaki H, Reagan TJ, Campbell RJ. Clinicopathological studies of primary cerebral amyloid angiopathy. Mayo Clin Proc 1979;54:22–31.
54. Cosgrove G, Leblanc R, Meagher-Villemure K, et al. Cerebral amyloid angiopathy. Neurology 1985;34:625–631.
55. Gilbert JJ, Vinters HV. Cerebral amyloid angiopathy: incidence and complications in the aging brain: I. cerebral hemorrhage. Stroke 1983;14:915–923.
56. Smith DB, Hitchcock M, Philpott PJ. Cerebral amyloid angiopathy presenting as transient ischemic attacks: case report. J Neurosurg 1985;63:963–964.
57. Gray F, Dubas F, Roullet E, Escourolle R. Leukoencephalopathy in diffuse hemorrhagic cerebral amyloid angiopathy. Ann Neurol 1985;18:54–59.
58. Loes DJ, Biller J, Yuh WTC, et al. Leukoencephalopathy in cerebral amyloid

angiopathy: MR imaging in four cases. AJNR 1990;11:485–488.

59. DeWitt LD, Louis DN. Case records of the Massachusetts General Hospital: Case 27—1991. N Engl J Med 1991;325:42–54.

60. Grubb A, Jensson O, Gudmundsson G, et al. Abnormal metabolism of Y-trace alkaline microprotein: the basic defect in hereditary cerebral hemorrhage with amyloidosis. N Engl J Med 1984;311:1547–1549.

61. Stefansson K, Antel JP, Ojer J, et al. Autosomal dominant cerebrovascular amyloidosis: properties of peripheral blood lymphocytes. Ann Neurol 1980;7:436–440.

62. Greene GM, Godersky JC, Biller J, et al. Surgical experience with intracerebral hemorrhage secondary to cerebral amyloid angiopathy. Stroke 1990;21:170.

Vasculitis

Listeria monocytogenes

63. Weinstein AJ, Schianone WA, Furlan AJ. Listeria rhomboencephalitis. Arch Neurol 1982;39:514–516.

64. Brown RH, Sobel RA. Case records of the Massachusetts General Hospital. New Engl J Med 1989;321:739–750.

65. Frayne J, Gates P. Listeria rhomboencephalitis. Clin Exp Neurol 1987;24: 175–179.

Lyme Disease

66. Rahn DW, Malawista SE. Lyme disease: recommendations for diagnosis and treatment. Ann Intern Med 1991;114:472–481.

67. Halperin JJ, Luft BJ, Anand AK, et al. Lyme neuroboreliosis: central nervous system manifestations. Neurology 1989;39:753–759.

68. Pachner AR, Duray P, Steere AC. Cerebral nervous system manifestations of Lyme disease. Arch Neurol 1989;46:790–795.

69. Uldry PA, Regli F, Bogousslavsky J. Cerebral angiopathy and recurrent strokes following *Borrelia burgdorferi* infection. J Neurol Neurosurg Psychiatry 1987;50:1703–1704.

Fungal Infections

70. Kobayashi RM, Coil M, Niwayama G, Trauner D. Cerebral vasculitis in coccidioidal meningitis. Ann Neurol 1977;1:281–284.

71. Walsh TJ, Hier DB, Caplan LR. Fungal infection of the central nervous system: comparative analysis of the risk factors and clinical signs in 57 patients. Neurology 1985;35:1654–1657.

72. Walsh TJ, Hier DB, Caplan LR. Aspergillosis of the central nervous system: clinicopathological analysis of 17 patients. Ann Neurol 1985;18:574–582.

Virus-Related Vasculitis

73. Moore PM, Cupps TR. Neurologic complications of vasculitis. Ann Neurol 1983;14:155–167.

74. Bourdette DN, Rosenberg NL, Yatsu FM. Herpes zoster ophthalmicus and delayed ipsilateral cerebral infarction. Neurology 1983;33:1428–1432.

75. Hilt DC, Buchholz D, Krumholz A, et al. Herpes zoster ophthalmicus and delayed contralateral hemiparesis caused by cerebral angiitis: diagnosis and management approaches. Ann Neurol 1983;14:543–553.

76. Doyle PW, Gibson G, Dolman C. Herpes zoster ophthalmicus with contralateral hemiplegia: identification of cause. Ann Neurol 1983;14:84–85.

77. Powers JM. Herpes zoster maxillaris with delayed occipital infarction. J Clin Neuroophthalmol 1986;2:113–115.

78. Snow BJ, Simcock JP. Brainstem infarction following cervical herpes zoster. Neurology 1988;38:1331.

79. Ross MH, Abend WK, Schwartz RB, Samuels MA. A case of C2 herpes zoster with delayed bilateral pontine infarction. Neurology 1991;41:1685–1686.

80. Saito K, Moskowitz MA. Contributions from the upper cervical dorsal roots and trigeminal ganglia to the feline circle of Willis. Stroke 1989;20:524–526.

Systemic Arteritis

73. Moore PM, Cupps TR. Neurologic complications of vasculitis. Ann Neurol 1983;14:155–167.

81. Fauci AS, Haynes BF, Katz P. The spectrum of vasculitis: clinical, pathologic, immunologic and therapeutic considerations. Ann Intern Med 1978;89:660–676.

82. Scott DG. Classification and treatment of systemic vasculitis. Br J Rheumatol 1988;27:251–257.

83. Moore PM, Fauci AS. Neurologic manifestations of systemic vasculitis: a retrospective and prospective study of the clinico-pathologic features and responses to therapy in 25 patients. Am J Med 1981;71:517–524.

84. Kissel JT, Rammohan KW. Pathology and therapy of nervous system vasculitis. Clin Neuropharm 1991;14:28–48.

85. Churg J, Strauss L. Allergic granulomatosis, allergic angiitis, and periarteritis nodosa. Am J Pathol 1951;27:277–301.

86. Chumbley LC, Harrison EG, DeRemee RA. Allergic granulomatosis and angiitis (Churg-Strauss syndrome): report and analysis of 30 cases. Mayo Clin Proc 1977;52:477–484.

87. Hauser SL, Shahani B, Hedley-White ET. Case records of the Massachusetts General Hospital: Case 38—1990. N Engl J Med 1990;323:812–822.

Wegener's Granulomatosis

88. Fauci AS, Haynes BF, Katz P, Wolff SM. Wegener's granulomatosis: prospective clinical and therapeutic experience with 85 patients for 21 years. Ann Intern Med 1983;98:76–85.

89. Haynes BF, Fishman ML, Fauci AS, Wolff SM. The ocular manifestations of Wegener's granulomatosis: fifteen years' experience and review of the literature. Am J Med 1977;63:131–141.

90. Lapresle J, Lasjaunias P. Cranial nerve ischemic arterial syndromes. Brain 1985;109:207–215.

91. Palaic M, Yeadon C, Moore S, Cashman N. Wegener's granulomatosis mimicking temporal arteritis. Neurology 1991;41:1694–1695.

92. Nölle B, Specks U, Lüdemann J, et al. Anticytoplasmic autoantibodies: their immunodiagnostic value in Wegener's granulomatosis. Ann Intern Med 1989;111:28–40.

Systemic Lupus Erythematosus (SLE)

93. Feinglass EJ, Arnett SC, Dorsch CA, et al. Neuropsychiatric manifestations of systemic lupus erythematosus: diagnosis, clinical spectrum, and relationship to other features of the disease. Medicine 1976;55:323–339.
94. Johnson RT, Richardson EP. The neurological manifestations of systemic lupus erythematosus: a clinical–pathological study of 24 cases and review of the literature. Medicine 1968;47:337–369.
95. Devinsky O, Petito C, Alonso D. Clinical and neuropathological findings in systemic lupus erythematosus: the role of vasculitis, heart emboli, and thrombotic thrombocytopenic purpura. Ann Neurol 1988;23:380–384.
96. Alsen AM, Gabrulsen TO, McCune WJ. MR imaging of systemic lupus erythematosus involving the brain. AJNR 1985;6:197–201.
97. Trevor RF, Sondheimer FK, Fessel WJ, et al. Angiographic demonstration of major cerebral vessel occlusion in systemic lupus erythematosus. Neuroradiology 1972;4:202–207.
98. Hart R, Miller V, Coull B, et al. Cerebral infarction associated with lupus anticoagulants: preliminary report. Stroke 1984;15:114–118.
99. McVerry BA, Machin SJ, Parry H, et al. Reduced prostacycline activity in systemic lupus erythematosus. Ann Rheum Dis 1980;39:524–525.
100. Galve E, Candell-Riera J, Pigrau C, et al. Prevalence, morphological types, and evaluation of cardiac valvular disease in systemic lupus erythematosus. N Engl J Med 1988;319:817–823.

Thrombotic Thrombocytopenic Purpura (TTP)

101. Petitt RM. Thrombotic thrombocytopenic purpura: a thirty year review. Semin Thromb Hemost 1980;6:350–355.
102. Kwaan HC. Clinicopathological features of thrombotic thrombocytopenic purpura. Semin Hematol 1987;24:71–81.
103. Silverstein A. Thrombotic thrombocytopenic purpura: the initial neurological manifestations. Arch Neurol 1968;18:358–362.
104. Rinkel G, Wijdicks E, Hené R. Stroke in relapsing thrombotic thrombocytopenic purpura. Stroke 1991;22:1087–1088.
105. Shepard KV, Bukowski RM. The treatment of thrombotic thrombocytopenic purpura with exchange transfusions, plasma infusions and plasma exchange. Semin Hematol 1987;24:178–193.

Rheumatoid Arthritis

106. Ramos M, Mandybur TI. Cerebral vasculitis in rheumatoid arthritis. Arch Neurol 1975;32:271–275.
107. Watson P. Intracranial hemorrhage with vasculitis in rheumatoid arthritis. Arch Neurol 1979;36:58.
108. Watson P, Fekete J, Dick J. Central nervous system vasculitis in rheumatoid arthritis. Can J Neurol Sci 1977;4:269–271.

109. Takeda Y. Studies of the metabolism and distribution of fibrinogen in patients with rheumatoid arthritis. J Lab Clin Med 1967;69:624–633.
110. Jasin HE, LoSpalluto J, Ziff M. Rheumatoid hyperviscosity syndrome. Am J Med 1970;49:484–493.

Sjögren Syndrome

111. Alexander EL, Provost TT, Stevens MB, Alexander GE. Neurologic complications of primary Sjögren's syndrome. Medicine 1982;61:247–257.
112. Alexander GE, Provost TT, Stevens MB, Alexander EL. Sjögren syndrome: central nervous system manifestations. Neurology 1981;31:1391–1396.
113. Alexander EL, Beall S, Gordon B, et al. Magnetic resonance imaging of cerebral lesions in patients with the Sjögren syndrome. Ann Intern Med 1988;108: 815–823.
114. Alexander EL, Malinow K, Lijewski JE, et al. Primary Sjögren syndrome with central nervous system disease mimicking multiple sclerosis. Ann Intern Med 1986;104:323–330.

Scleroderma

115. Estey E, Lieberman A, Pinto R, et al. Cerebral arteritis in scleroderma. Stroke 1979;10:595–597.
116. Pathak R, Gabor AJ. Scleroderma and central nervous system vasculitis. Stroke 1991;22:410–413.

Sarcoidosis

117. Stern BJ, Krumholz A, Johns C, et al. Sarcoidosis and its neurological manifestations. Arch Neurol 1985;42:909–917.
118. Caplan LR, Corbett J, Goodwin J, et al. Neuro-ophthalmological signs in the angiitic form of neurosarcoidosis. Neurology 1983;33:1130–1135.
119. Meyer J, Foley J, Campagna-Pinto D. Granulomatous angiitis of the meninges in sarcoidosis. Arch Neurol Psychiatry 1953;69:587–600.
120. Alajouanime T, Bertrand J, Degos R, et al. Sarcoidose ganglionaire, cutanée et oculaire, avec atteinte secondaire diffuse, periphérique et centrale du système nerveux. Rev Neurol (Paris) 1958;99:421–447.
121. Urich H. Some outstanding problems in sarcoidosis of the central nervous system. In: Iwai K, Hosoda Y, eds. Proceedings of the Sixth International Conference on Sarcoidosis. Baltimore: University Park Press, 1974:338–339.
122. Karmi A. Ophthalmic changes in sarcoidosis. Acta Ophthalmol (Suppl) 1979;141:1–94.

Temporal Arteritis and Granulomatous Angiitis

123. Goodwin J. Temporal arteritis. In: Vinken P, Bruyn G, eds. Handbook of clinical neurology: vol 39, pt 2. neurological manifestations of systemic diseases. Amsterdam: North Holland, 1980:313–342.
124. Klein RG, Hunder GG, Stanson AW, et al. Large artery involvement in giant cell arteritis. Ann Intern Med 1975;83:806–812.
125. Wilkinson I, Russel R. Arteries of the head and neck in giant cell arteritis. Arch Neurol 1972;27:378–391.

126. Enzmann D, Scott WR. Intracranial involvement of giant-cell arteritis. Neurology 1977;27:794–797.

Granulomatous Angiitis Limited to CNS

127. Hankey GJ. Isolated angiitis/angiopathy of the central nervous system. Cerebrovasc Dis 1991;1:2–15.
128. Kolodny EH, Rebeiz JJ, Caviness VS, Richardson EP. Granulomatous angiitis of the central nervous system. Arch Neurol 1968;19:510–524.
129. Moore PM. Diagnosis and management of isolated angiitis of the central nervous system. Neurology 1989;39:167–173.
130. Burger PC, Burch JG, Vogel FS. Granulomatous angiitis: an unusual etiology of stroke. Stroke 1977;8:29–35.

Takayasu's Arteritis

131. Shimizuki K, Sano K. Pulseless disease. J Neuropathol Clin Neurol 1951;1: 37–47.
132. Ask-Upmark E. On the pulseless disease outside of Japan. Acta Med Scand 1954;149:161–178.
133. Lupi-Herrera E, Sanchez-Torres G, Marcushamer J, et al. Takayasu's arteritis: clinical study of 107 cases. Am Heart J 1977;93:94–103.
134. Ishikawa K. Natural history and classification of occlusive thromboaortopathy (Takayasu's disease). Circulation 1978;57:27–35.
135. Sano K, Alga T, Saito I. Angiography in pulseless disease. Radiology 1970; 94:69–74.
136. Hall S, Barr W, Lee JT, et al. Takayasu arteritis: a study of 32 North American patients. Medicine 1985;54:89–99.
137. Hargraves RW, Spetzler RF. Takayasu's arteritis: case report. Barrow Neurological Institute Quarterly 1991;7:20–23.
138. Ishikawa K, Uyama M, Asayama K. Occlusive thromboaortopathy (Takayasu's disease): cervical occlusive stenosis, retinal artery pressure, retinal micro-aneurysms and prognosis. Stroke 1983;14:730–735.
139. Takagi A, Tada Y, Sato O, et al. Surgical treatment for Takayasu's arteritis: a long-term follow-up study. J Cardiovasc Surg 1989;30:553–558.
140. Fraga A, Mintz G, Valle L, Flores-Izquierdo G. Takayasu's arteritis: frequency of systemic manifestations (study of 22 patients) and favorable response to maintenance steroid therapy with adrenocorticosteroids (12 patients). Arthritis Rheum 1972;15:617–624.

Behçet's Disease

141. Chajek T, Fainaro M. Behçet's disease: report of 41 cases and a review of the literature. Medicine 1975;54:179–195.
142. Shimizu T, Ehrlich GE, Inaba G, et al. Behçet's disease (Behçet's syndrome). Semin Arthritis Rheum 1979;8:223–260.
143. Wechsler B, Davatchi F, Mizushima Y, et al. Criteria for diagnosis of Behçet's disease. Lancet 1990;335:1078–1080.
144. Serdaroglu P, Yazici H, Ozdemir C, et al. Neurologic involvement in Behçet's syndrome: a prospective study. Arch Neurol 1989;46:265–269.

145. Herskovitz S, Lipton RB, Lantos G. Neuro-Behçet's disease: CT and clinical correlates. Neurology 1988;38:1714–1720.
146. Al Kawi MZ, Bohlega S, Banna M. MRI findings in neuro-Behçet's disease. Neurology 1991;41:405–408.
147. Banna M, El-Ramahi K. Neurologic involvement in Behçet disease: imaging findings in 16 patients. AJNR 1991;12:791–796.
148. Pamir MN, Kansu T, Erbengi A, Zileli T. Papilledema in Behçet's syndrome. Arch Neurol 1981;38:643–645.
149. Bousser MG, Chiras J, Bories J, Castaigne P. Cerebral venous thrombosis—a review of 38 cases. Stroke 1985;16:199–213.
150. Sharief MK, Hentges R, Thomas E. Significance of CSF immunoglobulins in monitoring neurologic disease in Behçet's disease. Neurology 1991;41:1398–1401.

Cogan's Syndrome

151. Cogan DG. Syndrome of nonsyphilitic interstitial keratitis and vestibulo-auditory symptoms. Arch Ophthal 1945;33:144–149.
152. Cheson BD, Bluming AZ, Alroy J. Cogan's syndrome: a systemic vasculitis. Am J Med 1976;60:549–555.
153. Peeters GJ, Pinckers AJ, Cremers CW, Hoefnagels WH. Atypical Cogan's syndrome: an autoimmune disease. Ann Otol Rhinol Laryngol 1986;95:173–175.

Eales's Disease

154. Miller NR. Walsh and Hoyt's clinical neurophthalmology: vol 4, ch 60. vasculitis. 4th ed. Baltimore: Williams and Wilkins, 1991:2575–2729.
155. Gordon MF, Coyle PK, Golub B. Eales disease presenting as stroke in the young adult. Ann Neurol 1988;24:264–266.
156. Herson RN, Squier M. Retinal perivasculitis with neurological involvement. J Neurol Sci 1978;36:111–117.
157. Singhal BS, Dastur DK. Eales disease with neurological involvement. J Neurol Sci 1976;27:312–321,323–345.
158. White RH. The etiology and neurological complications of retinal vasculitis. Brain 1961;84:262–273.

Microangiopathy of the Brain, Ear, and Retina

159. Susac J, Hardman J, Selhorst J. Microangiopathy of the brain and retina. Neurology 1979;29:313–316.
160. Coppeto J, Currie J, Monteiro M, et al. A syndrome of arterial-occlusive retinopathy and encephalopathy. Am J Ophthalmol 1984;98:189–202.
161. Swanson R, Mario L, Monteiro M, et al. A microangiopathic syndrome of encephalopathy, hearing loss and retinal artery occlusion. Neurology 1985;35(Suppl 1):145.
162. Bogousslavsky J, Gaio JM, Caplan LR, et al. Encephalopathy, deafness, and blindness in young women: a distinct retino-cochleo-cerebral arteriolopathy. J Neurol Neurosurg Psychiatry 1989;52:43–46.

Sneddon's Syndrome

163. Sneddon B. Cerebro-vascular lesions and livedo reticularis. Brit J Derm 1965;77:180–185.
164. Thomas DJ, Kirby JD, Britton KE, Galton DJ. Livedo reticularis and neurological lesions. Brit J Derm 1982;106:711–712.
165. Rebollo M, Val JF, Garijo F, et al. Livedo reticularis and cerebrovascular lesions (Sneddon's syndrome). Brain 1983;106:965–979.
166. Levine SR, Langer SL, Albers JW, Welch KMA. Sneddon's syndrome: an anti-phospholipid antibody syndrome? Neurology 1988;38:798–800.

Kohlmeier-Degos Syndrome

167. Petit WA, Soso MJ, Higman H. Degos disease: neurologic complications and cerebral angiography. Neurology 1982;32:1305–1309.
168. Strole WE, Clark WH, Isselbacher KJ. Progressive arterial occlusive disease (Kohlmeier-Degos). N Engl J Med 1967;276:195–201.

Strokes and Vasculopathy in Drug Abusers

169. Brust J, Richter R. Stroke associated with addiction to heroin. J Neurol Neurosurg Psychiatry 1978;39:194–199.
170. Woods B, Strewler G. Hemiparesis occurring six hours after intravenous heroin injection. Neurology 1972;22:863–866.
171. Caplan LR, Hier DB, Banks G. Stroke and drug abuse. Curr Concepts Cerebrovasc Dis (Stroke) 1982;27:9–13.
172. Brust JC. Stroke and drugs. In: Vinker P, Bruyn G, Klawans H, eds. Handbook of clinical neurology: vol 11, pt 3, ch 55. vascular diseases. Amsterdam: Elsevier Science, 1989:517–531.
173. Pearson J, Richter R. Addiction to opiates: neurologic aspects. In: Vinken P, Bruyn G, eds. Handbook of clinical neurology: vol 37, pt 2. intoxications of the nervous system. Amsterdam: North Holland, 1979:365–400.
174. Citron B, Halpern M, McCarron M, et al. Necrotizing angiitis associated with drug abuse. N Engl J Med 1970;283:1003–1011.
175. Rumbaugh C, Bergeron R, Gang H, et al. Cerebral vascular changes secondary to amphetamine abuse in the experimental animal. Radiology 1971;101:345–351.
176. Rumbaugh C, Bergeron R, Gang H, et al. Cerebral angiographic changes in the drug abuse patient. Radiology 1971;101:335–344.
177. Caplan LR, Thomas C, Banks G. Central nervous system complications of "T's and blues" addiction. Neurology 1982;32:623–628.
178. Szwed JJ. Pulmonary angiothrombosis caused by "blue velvet" addiction. Ann Intern Med 1970;73:771–774.
179. Atlee W. Talc and cornstarch emboli in the eyes of drug abusers. JAMA 1972;219:49–51.
180. Mizutami T, Lewis R, Gonatas N. Medial medullary syndrome in a drug abuser. Arch Neurol 1980;37:425–428.
181. Kaku D, Lowenstein DH. Emergence of recreational drug abuse as a major risk factor for stroke in young adults. Ann Intern Med 1990;133:821–827.

182. Levine SR, Welch KM. Cocaine and stroke: current concepts of cardiovascular disease. Stroke 1988;19:779–783.
183. Daras M, Tuchman AJ, Marks S. Central nervous system infarction related to cocaine abuse. Stroke 1991;22:1320–1325.
184. Levine SR, Washington JM, Jefferson MF, et al. "Crack" cocaine associated stroke. Neurology 1987;37:1849–1853.
185. Levine SR, Brust JC, Futrell N, et al. A comparative study of the cerebrovascular complications of cocaine—alkaloidal versus hydrochloride—a review. Neurology 1991;41:1173–1177.
186. Rowley HA, Lowenstein DH, Rowbotham MC, Simon RP. Thalamomesencephalic strokes after cocaine abuse. Neurology 1989;39:428–430.
187. Isner JM, Estes NA, Thompson PD, et al. Acute cardiac events temporally related to cocaine. N Engl J Med 1986;315:1438–1443.

Migraine

188. Rothrock JF, Walicke P, Swendon M, et al. Migrainous stroke. Arch Neurol 1988;45:63–67.
189. Bogousslavsky J, Regli F, Van Melle G, et al. Migraine stroke. Neurology 1988;38:223–227.
190. Caplan LR. Migraine and vertebrobasilar ischemia. Neurology 1991;41:55–61.
191. Pessin MS, Lathi ES, Cohen MB, et al. Clinical features and mechanisms of occipital infarction in the posterior cerebral artery territory. Ann Neurol 1987;21:290–299.
192. Fisher CM. Late-life migraine accompaniments as a cause of unexplained transient ischemic attacks. Can J Neurol Sci 1980;7:9–17.
193. Fisher CM. Late-life migraine accompaniments: further experience. Stroke 1986;17:1033–1042.
194. Caplan LR, Chedru F, Lhermitte F, Mayman C. Transient global amnesia and migraine. Neurology 1981;31:1167–1170.
195. Caplan LR. Transient global amnesia: characteristic features and overview. In: Markowitsch HJ, ed. Transient global amnesia and related disorders. Toronto: Hogrife and Huber, 1990:15–27.
196. Call GK, Fleming MC, Sealfon S, et al. Reversible cerebral segmental vasoconstriction. Stroke 1988;19:1159–1170.
197. Cole AJ, Aube M. Migraine with vasospasm and delayed intracerebral hemorrhage. Arch Neurol 1990;47:53–56.
198. Caplan LR. Intracerebral hemorrhage revisited. Neurology 1988;38:624–627.

Moyamoya Syndrome

199. Suzuki J, Kodama N. Moyamoya disease—a review. Stroke 1983;14:104–109.
200. Suzuki J. Moyamoya disease. Berlin: Springer-Verlag, 1986.
201. Taveras JM. Multiple progressive intracranial arterial occlusions: a syndrome of children and young adults. Am J Roentgenol 1969;106:235–268.
202. Bruno A, Adams HOP, Bilbe J, et al. Cerebral infarction due to moyamoya disease in young adults. Stroke 1988;19:826–833.
203. Ikeda E. Systemic vascular changes in spontaneous occlusion of the circle of Willis. Stroke 1991;22:1358–1362.

Sickle-Cell Disease

204. Rothman SM, Fulling KH, Nelson JS. Sickle cell anemia and central nervous system infarction: a neuropathological study. Ann Neurol 1986;20:684–690.
205. Adams RJ, Nichols FT, McKie V, et al. Cerebral infarction in sickle cell anemia: mechanisms based on CT and MRI. Neurology 1988;38:1012–1017.

Thrombocytosis and Other Platelet Disorders

206. Murphy S, Iland H, Rosenthal D, Laszlo J. Essential thrombocythemia: an interim report from the polycythemia vera study group. Semin Hematol 1986;23:177–182.
207. Jabaily J, Iland HJ, Laszlo J, et al. Neurologic manifestations of essential thrombocythemia. Ann Intern Med 1983;99:513–518.
208. Hehlmann R, Jahn M, Baumann B, Kopcke W. Essential thrombocythemia. Clinical characteristics and course of 61 cases. Cancer 1988;61:2487–2496.
209. Hart RG, Kanter MC. Hematologic disorders and ischemic stroke: a selective review. Stroke 1990;21:1111–1121.
210. Al-Mefty O, Marano G, Rajaraman S, et al. Transient ischemic attacks due to increased platelet aggregation and adhesiveness. J Neurosurg 1979;50:449–453.
211. Trip MD, Cats VM, van Capelle FJL, Vreeken J. Platelet hyperreactivity and prognosis in survivors of myocardial infarction. N Engl J Med 1990;322:1549–1554.

Coagulopathies

212. Thaler E, Lechner K. Antithrombin III deficiency and thromboembolism. Clin Haematol 1981;10:369–390.
213. Camerlingo M, Finazzi G, Casto L, et al. Inherited protein C deficiency and nonhemorrhagic arterial stroke in young adults. Neurology 1991;41:1371–1373.
214. Estol C, Pessin MS, DeWitt LD, Caplan LR. Stroke and increased factor VIII activity. Neurology 1989;39(Suppl 1):1159.
215. Kosik KS, Furie B. Thrombotic stroke associated with elevated factor VIII. Arch Neurol 1980;8:435–437.
216. Talbot RW, Heppell J, Dozois RR, Beart RW. Vascular complications of inflammatory bowel disease. Mayo Clin Proc 1986;61:140–145.
217. Johns DR. Cerebrovascular complications of inflammatory bowel disease. Am J Gastroenter 1991;86:367–370.
218. Sack GH, Levin J, Bell WR. Trousseau's syndrome and other manifestations of chronic disseminated coagulopathy in patients with neoplasms. Medicine 1977;56:1–37.
219. Graus F, Rodgers LR, Posner JB. Cerebrovascular complications in patients with cancer. Medicine 1985;64:16–35.
220. Amico L, Caplan LR, Thomas C. Cerebrovascular complications of mucinous cancers. Neurology 1989;39:523–526.
221. Sloane MA. Thrombolysis and stroke—past and future. Arch Neurol 1986;44:748–768.
222. Del Zoppo GH, Zeumer H, Harker LA. Thrombolytic therapy in stroke: possibilities and hazards. Stroke 1986;17:595–607.

223. Francis RB. Clinical disorders of fibrinolysis. Blut 1989;59:1–14.
224. Hunt FA, Rylatt DB, Hart R, Bundesen PG. Serum cross-linked fibrin (XDP) and fibrinogen/fibrin degradation products (FDP) in disorders associated with activation of the coagulation or fibrinolytic systems. Br J Haematol 1985;60:715–722.
225. Feinberg WM, Bruck DC, Ring ME, Corrigan JJ. Hemostatic markers in acute stroke. Stroke 1989;20:582–587.

Lupus Anticoagulant and Antiphospholipid Antibodies

226. Levine SR, Welch KMA. Cerebrovascular ischemia associated with lupus anti-coagulant. Stroke 1987;18:257–263.
227. DeWitt LD, Caplan LR. Antiphospholipid antibodies and stroke. ANJR 1991;12:454–456.
228. Coull BM, Goodnight SH. Antiphospholipid antibodies, prethrombotic states, and stroke. Stroke 1990;21:1370–1374.
229. Levine SR, Kim S, Deegan MJ, Welch KMA. Ischemic stroke associated with anticardiolipin antibodies. Stroke 1987;18:1101–1106.
230. Montalban J, Codina A, Ordi J, et al. Antiphospholipid antibodies in cerebral ischemia. Stroke 1991;22:750–753.
231. Pope JM, Canny CL, Bell DA. Cerebral ischemic events associated with endo-carditis, retinal vascular disease, and lupus anticoagulant. Am J Med 1991; 90:299–309.
232. The Antiphospholipid Antibodies in Stroke Study (APASS) Group. Clinical and laboratory findings in patients with antiphospholipid antibodies and cerebral ischemia. Stroke 1990;21:1268–1273.

Disseminated Intravascular Coagulation

233. Bick RL. Disseminated intravascular coagulation and related syndromes: a clinical review. Semin Thromb Hemost 1988;14:299–338.
234. Wen PY, Sobel RA. Case records of the Massachusetts General Hospital: Case 36—1991. N Engl J Med 1991;325:714–726.
235. Colman RW, Rubin RN. Disseminated intravascular coagulation due to malignancy. Semin Oncol 1990;17:172–186.
236. Schwartzman RJ, Hill JB. Neurologic complications of disseminated intra-vascular coagulation. Neurology 1982;32:791–797.

Hyperviscosity

237. Grotta J, Ackerman R, Correia J, et al. Whole blood viscosity parameters and cerebral blood flow. Stroke 1982;13:296–301.
238. Coull BM, Beamer N, de Garmo P, et al. Chronic blood hyperviscosity in sub-jects with acute stroke, transient ischemic attack, and risk factors for stroke. Stroke 1991;22:162–168.
239. Fahey JL, Barth WF, Solomon A. Serum hyperviscosity syndrome. JAMA 1965;192:464–467.
240. Rosenson RS, Baker AL, Chow M, Hay R. Hyperviscosity syndrome in a hyper-cholesterolemic patient with primary biliary cirrhosis. Gastroenterology 1990;98:1351–1357.

Venous Occlusive Disease

241. Bousser MG, Chiras J, Bories J, Castaigne P. Cerebral venous thrombosis—a review of 38 cases. Stroke 1985;16:199–213.
242. Hulcelle RJ, Dooms GC, Mathurin P, Cornelis G. MRI assessment of unsuspected dural sinus thrombosis. Neuroradiology 1989;31:217–221.
243. Mas J-L, Meder JF, Meary E, Bousser MG. Magnetic resonance imaging in lateral sinus hypoplasia and thrombosis. Stroke 1990;21:1350–1356.
244. Hickey WF, Garnick MB, Henderson IC, Dawson D. Primary cerebral venous thrombosis in patients with cancer—a rarely diagnosed paraneoplastic syndrome. Am J Med 1982;73:746–750.
245. Yerby MS, Bailey GM. Superior sagittal sinus thrombosis 10 years after surgery for ulcerative colitis. Stroke 1980;11:294–296.
246. Schutta HS, Williams EC, Baranski BG, Sutula TP. Cerebral venous thrombosis with plasminogen deficiency. Stroke 1991;22:401–405.
247. Hosley MA, Fisher M, Lingley JF. Thrombosis in a congenitally bifurcated superior sagittal sinus. Stroke 1991;22:396–400.
248. Estanol B, Rodriguez A, Conte G, et al. Intracranial venous thrombosis in young women. Stroke 1979;10:680–684.
249. Srinivasan K. Ischemic cerebrovascular disease in the young: two common causes in India. Stroke 1984;15:733–735.
250. Krayenbuhl HA. Cerebral venous and sinus thrombosis. Clin Neurosurg 1967;14:1–24.
251. Bots GAM. Thrombosis of the Galenic system veins in the adult. Acta Neuropathol 1971;17:227–233.
252. Haley EC, Brashear R, Barth J, et al. Deep cerebral venous thrombosis: clinical, neuroradiological and neuropsychological correlates. Arch Neurol 1989;46:337–340.
253. Sze G, Simmons B, Krol G, et al. Dural sinus thrombosis: verification with spin echo techniques. AJNR 1988;9:679–686.
254. Levine SR, Twyman RE, Gilman S. The role of anticoagulation in cavernous sinus thrombosis. Neurology 1988;38:517–522.
255. Einhaupl KM, Mehracin S, Haberl RL, et al. Heparin treatment in sinus venous thrombosis. Lancet 1991;338:597–600.
256. DiRocco C, Ianelli A, Leone G, et al. Heparin–urokinase treatment in aseptic dural sinus thrombosis. Arch Neurol 1981;38:431–435.

Neoplastic Conditions

257. Petito CK, Gottlieb GJ, Dougherty JH, Petito FA. Neoplastic angioendotheliosis: ultrastructural study and review of the literature. Ann Neurol 1978;3:393–399.
258. Beal MF, Fisher CM. Neoplastic angioendotheliosis. J Neurol Sci 1982;53:359–375.
259. LeWitt PA, Forno LS, Brant-Zawadzki M. Neoplastic angioendotheliosis: a case with spontaneous regression and radiographic appearance of cerebral arteritis. Neurology 1983;33:39–44.
260. Hamada K, Hamada T, Satoh M, et al. Two cases of neoplastic angioendotheliomatosis presenting with myelopathy. Neurology 1991;41:1139–1140.

261. Fauci A, Haynes BF, Costa J, et al. Lymphatoid granulomatosis: prospective clinical and therapeutic experience over 10 years. N Engl J Med 1982;306: 68–74.
262. Hogan PJ, Greenberg MK, McCarty GE. Neurologic complications of lymphomatoid granulomatosis. Neurology 1981;31:619–620.

"Genetic" Disorders

263. Natowicz M, Kelley RI. Mendelian etiologies of stroke. Ann Neurol 1987; 22:175–192.

MELAS Syndrome

264. Pavlakis SG, Phillips PC, DiMauro S, et al. Mitochondrial myopathy, encephalopathy, lactic acidosis, and stroke-like episodes: a distinctive clinical syndrome. Ann Neurol 1984;16:481–488.
265. Kuriyama M, Umezaki H, Fukuda Y, et al. Mitochondrial encephalomyopathy with lactate-pyruvate elevation and brain infarctions. Neurology 1984;34: 72–77.
266. Allard JC, Tilak C, Carter AP. CT and MR of MELAS syndrome. AJNR 1988;9:1234–1238.
267. Matthews PM, Tampieri D, Berkovic SF, et al. Magnetic resonance imaging shows specific abnormalities in the MELAS syndrome. Neurology 1991;41: 1043–1046.

Fabry's Disease

268. Brady RO, Gal AE, Bradley RM, et al. Enzymatic defect in Fabry's disease: ceramide trihexosidase deficiency. N Engl J Med 1967;276:1163–1167.
269. Dawson DM, Miller DC. Case records of the Massachusetts General Hospital: Case 2—1984. N Engl J Med 1984;310:106–114.
270. Kint JA. Fabry's disease: α galactosidase deficiency. Science 1970;167: 1268–1269.
271. Philippart M, Franklin SS, Gordon A. Reversal of an inborn sphingolipidosis (Fabry's disease) by kidney transplantation. Ann Int Med 1972;77:195–200.

Homocystinuria

272. Boers GH, Smals AG, Trijbels FJ, et al. Heterozygosity for homocystinuria in premature peripheral and cerebral occlusive disease. N Engl J Med 1985;313: 709–715.
273. Harker LA, Slichter SJ, Scott CR, Ross R. Homocystinemia: vascular injury and arterial thrombosis. N Engl J Med 1974;291:537–543.
274. Wall RT, Harlan JM, Harker LA, Striker GE. Homocysteine-induced endothelial cell injury in vitro: a model for the study of vascular injury. Thromb Res 1980;18:113–121.
275. Brattstrom LE, Hardebo JE, Hultberg BJ. Moderate homocysteinemia—a possible risk factor for arteriosclerotic vascular disease. Stroke 1984;15:1012–1016.

Hypercalcemia

276. Gorelick PB, Caplan LR. Calcium, hypercalcemia, and stroke. Curr Concepts Cerebrovasc Dis (Stroke) 1985;20:13–17.

CHAPTER 10

Brain Embolism

Cardiac-origin embolism was once considered a rare and unusual stroke mechanism. Aring and Merritt[1] and Whisnant et al.[2] classified only 3 and 8 percent of strokes in their respective series as cardiac-origin embolism. In recent years, with improvement in technologies available to investigate stroke mechanisms, the incidence of embolic stroke has been estimated as high as 30 percent.[3] Emboli usually arise from three major sources: the heart, the large arteries, and the venous circulation.

Clinical and Laboratory Findings

Regardless of source, emboli travel distally until they lodge in an extra-cranial or intracranial artery. The recipient vessel, of course, cannot distinguish the source of the embolic material, nor do the clinical neurological findings differ among emboli of cardiac, intra-arterial, or venous origin. The size of the embolic material will determine where it lodges, and the type of material also differs among the three sources. A variety of different particles with different physical properties can arise from the heart, arteries, or circulation.[4] Table 10.1 enumerates these different particles from cardiac and intra-arterial sources. Unlike thrombi formed locally at sites of prior atherosclerotic narrowing, emboli are only loosely adherent to vessel walls. They can and do readily fragment, dislodge, and move to more distal arteries. When arteriography is performed more than 48 hours after the first symptoms of an embolic stroke, emboli frequently have passed and cannot be seen.[3] Even at necropsy, emboli are frequently no longer visible in arteries supplying hemorrhagic infarcts.[5,6] Fisher and Perlman called attention to the nonsudden embolus, which they explained in terms of an embolus leaving its original lodging place and moving distally.[7] Dalal et al. reported 9 patients that had emboli that were seen on initial angiography but later disappeared.[8] Others have documented disappearance or movement of emboli.[9]

Emboli have a predilection for arterial bifurcations, particularly the MCA branches, the upper and lower trunks of the MCAs, the distal basilar

TABLE 10.1
Types of Embolic Materials

Cardiac Origin	Intra-arterial
1. So-called red thrombi	1. So-called red thrombi
2. White platelet–fibrin aggregates	2. White platelet–fibrin aggregates
3. Marantic endocarditis vegetations	3. Cholesterol crystals
4. Bacteria from endocarditis vegetations	4. Atheromatous plaque debris
5. Calcium (valves and mitral annulus calcification [MAC])	5. Calcium from vascular calcification
6. Myxoma and fibroelastoma fragments	6. Air
	7. Fat
	8. Tumor cells and tumor mucin
	9. Talc or microcrystalline cellulose from injected drugs

Modified with permission from Caplan LR. Of birds and nests and brain emboli. Rev Neurol 1991;147:265–273.

artery, and the PCAs. They also lodge at sites of narrowing in the ICA, VAs, and basilar arteries. In experimental models of carotid-circulation embolization, which used balloon catheters, emboli most often reached the MCA or one of its branches.[10] The ACA was a rare destination. Emboli usually reach the PCAs by way of the VAs and basilar artery but occasionally enter a PCA that originates from the ICA.

Embolic infarcts may be pale, spotted with small petechial hemorrhages, or frankly hemorrhagic. Hemorrhage is thought to result when ischemic tissues are reperfused.[5] Capillaries and arterioles are injured by ischemia. When an embolus passes distally into a previously ischemic zone, reperfusion into regions that contain incompetent, damaged vessels causes blood to leak into the infarcted brain tissue.

Embolic strokes most often begin suddenly, the clinical signs evolving during seconds or a few minutes. The deficit may begin during physical activity but more often than not occurs during rest or activities of daily life.[3,11] Traditionally, the neurological deficit in patients with embolic stroke is described as maximal at onset. A focal brain region, suddenly deprived of its oxygen and fuel supply, quickly loses its function. When the embolus arises from the heart or venous system, there are no preceding TIAs referable to the same arterial supply territory, but there may be a history of TIA or stroke in another arterial bed. Preceding TIAs in the same vascular territory favor a proximal intra-arterial source of embolism. In patients with cardiac-origin embolism, there is often a history of valvular heart disease, congestive heart failure, myocardial infarction (MI), or arrhythmias. Patients with intra-arterial embolism frequently have a history of atherosclerotic coronary or peripheral vascular disease.

Experience with acute angiography since the late 1980s has shown a high rate of demonstration of intracranial emboli in patients with cardiac-origin sources and extracranial occlusive disease.[12] My own experience with patients evaluated for a trial of rtPA also shows that early angiography very often shows intracranial blockage. Recently, TCD ultrasound insonation of patients with sudden-onset hemispheric strokes shows frequent MCA occlusion; sequential TCD shows opening of the blocked arteries.[12,13] Fluctuations and worsening of deficits can be noted when emboli move distally and were present in 21 percent of emboli in the Harvard Stroke Registry (HSR)[3] and 19 percent of Michael Reese Stroke Registry (MRSR) embolic strokes.[8] Passage of emboli can also lead to rapid improvement in the neurological deficit.

The nature of the clinical neurological signs will depend on the location of the occluded vessel and will be similar to those described in Chapters 6 and 7 on large-artery thrombosis. An occluded ACA will cause leg weakness, abulia, and left-arm apraxia. When the occluded vessel is the upper trunk of the left MCA, Broca's aphasia and weakness of the right face, hand, and arm will result. An occluded left MCA inferior trunk causes Wernicke's aphasia and a right homonymous hemianopia. An occluded PCA will cause a homonymous hemianopia, while an embolus at the top of the basilar artery can cause blindness, lethargy or agitation, and abnormal eye movements. At times, emboli may be large enough to occlude a normal or an already stenotic ICA, MCA stem, VA, or basilar artery, producing more severe neurological deficits.

Neuroimaging with CT and MRI can suggest brain embolism. Because emboli most often lodge in distal arteries that supply cortical zones, embolic infarcts are often V-shaped and abut on the superficial cortical surface. Multiple cortical infarcts in various vascular supply regions suggest cardiac-origin embolism. In 1989, Ringelstein and colleagues analyzed the CT pattern of infarction among 60 patients with cardiogenic embolism. Most were large, cortically based infarcts (41 lesions). Some patients had small, cortical, subcortical, and insular infarcts, and a few patients had deep infarcts in the striatocapsular region.[14] In Chapter 6, I commented on the mechanism of these deep infarcts: namely, blockage of the MCA before the lenticulostriate branches, with preservation of collateral flow to the convexity. At times, on noncontrast CT, acute emboli are imaged as hyperdense arteries. Most often, the hyperdensity takes the course and shape of the MCA.[15,16] Occasionally, calcific fragments can also be seen within arteries on noncontrast CT scans.

MRA and standard catheter angiography, especially if performed within 48 hours of stroke onset, may allow visualization of the embolus. A sudden sharp, abrupt termination of a distal or medium-sized vessel, without visible atherosclerosis, or a filling defect in the lumen of an artery suggests embolization. Disappearance of the obstruction in subsequent films or on later angiograms substantiates the diagnosis but is seldom practical. Sequential TCD examinations that show clearing of an obstruction suggest embolism. Detection of a potential embologenic cardiac source of embolism is also helpful. Echocardiography, cardiac nuclide scanning, Holter rhythm monitoring, and platelet scintigraphy can document cardiac abnormalities. However, because cardiac disease and atherosclerotic occlusive cerebrovascular disease often coexist, the presence of a potential cardiac embolic source does not mean that the cerebral infarct is necessarily embolic. Noninvasive tests of the extracranial and intracranial arteries and angiography can also reveal potential intra-arterial sources of embolization.

A 31-year-old carpenter, TL, was evaluated after the sudden onset of confusion and right-hand weakness. The symptoms began suddenly at work. Three years earlier, he had had what he called a minor stroke, characterized by numbness and weakness of the left arm and leg. Cerebral angiography was normal, but he was given warfarin during the 2 years following this event. He gave no history of cardiac or vascular disease, and examination of the heart and vessels was normal, except for a slight tachycardia. Blood pressure was 130/60. On neurological examination, his speech was fluent but contained many paraphasic errors. He had difficulty repeating spoken language, and he read, wrote, and spelled poorly. His right arm was weak, and he could not recognize objects placed in his right hand.

This young man had a lesion clinically localized to the left central and parietal region. The prior lesion was probably in the right cerebral hemisphere. The lesions were each of sudden onset and were in very different vascular territories. The differential diagnostic considerations included cardiac-origin embolism, coagulopathy, or an unusual multifocal vascular disease. There were no positive features from the history or physical examination that strongly favored any of these diagnoses.

The CT in TL showed a small region of lucency involving the left angular and postcentral gyri. There were also small old infarcts in the right frontal lobe and left cerebellum. Hematological, serological, and coagulation studies were normal. Angiography on the third hospital day revealed a sharp cutoff of the left angular artery. The proximal vessels were all normal. Cardiac echocardiography showed an enlarged heart with a reduced ejection fraction, suggestive of a cardiomyopathy. Myocardial biopsy later revealed cardiac sarcoidosis. During the next year, he had no further brain emboli while taking warfarin.

In this case, the negative hematological studies, absence of risk factors for atherosclerosis, and normal proximal extracranial and intracranial arteries suggested cerebral embolism despite the absence of known cardiac disease. Cardiac evaluation finally clarified the diagnosis. I have seen similar patients with multiple cerebral infarcts and negative hematological and vascular studies, in whom cardiac investigations failed to identify a definite cardiogenic source of embolism. Embologenic sources are often too small to be visualized, and thrombi sometimes form transiently and have disappeared by the time of the investigations.[4]

Cardiac Sources of Emboli

Many different types of cardiac lesions can give rise to cerebral emboli (Table 10.2). Cardiomyopathies, valvular and endocardial disease, rhythm disturbances, cardiac tumors, and ischemic lesions are all potential sources of emboli. Congestive heart failure alone increases the risk of stroke, often from an embolic mechanism.[17] Thrombi can often be found in the cardiac apex and trabeculae carneae in the hearts of patients who have died with congestive heart failure.[18] In young people with recurrent strokes, intensive cardiac evaluation—including cardiac catheterization—may be necessary to uncover the nature of the cardiac diseases.

Myocardial Infarction

Cardiac-muscle dysfunction after MI can be a source of embolic stroke. In small infarcts, the endothelium of the heart muscle may be damaged, allowing deposition of platelet and fibrin material and, later, thrombus, which can subsequently embolize. A greater risk of embolic stroke exists in patients with large transmural MIs. In such cases, the heart muscle may be severely damaged, producing stagnant nonfunctioning heart muscle, such as akinetic segments or ventricular aneurysms. Mural thrombi form within akinetic regions. Such clots can be so small that they are beyond the resolution of either echocardiography or cardiac angiography, yet be large enough to obstruct significant brain blood vessels.[4,19] Formation and embolization of clots are dynamic processes. When a clot fragments or dislodges, it sometimes leaves no detectable clues to its former presence.[4] With time, a new mural clot forms. If the patient is imaged or even studied at necropsy after the embolus has dislodged, it will escape detection. Emboli are probably most frequent in the first 3 months after MIs[17,18] but can arise later if there is a persistent mural clot or aneurysm.

> A 68-year-old man, CA, was admitted to the coronary care unit with a large MI. The creatine kinase peaked at 1200 IU/l. On the tenth day, while straining at stool, he became confused. Examination at that time showed a normal heart rhythm, Wernicke's aphasia, and a right superior quadrantanopia. Echocardiography showed an akinetic ventricular segment. The patient was treated with heparin and subsequently switched to warfarin, which was continued for the next 6 months.

The diagnosis of cardiac-origin embolism was more obvious in CA than in the previous patient. CT confirmed an infarct in the left temporal lobe in the distribution of the lower trunk of the MCA, a frequent site of embolism. Although embolism is a well-recognized complication of acute MI, the incidence is relatively low. Most observers do not recommend routine anticoagulation of all patients with cardiac infarcts. Only those with high risk of embolization and venous occlusion or those already known to have either

TABLE 10.2
Some Cardiac Sources of Emboli

Coronary artery disease
  Mural thrombi
  Ventricular aneurysms
  Hypokinetic zones
Arrhythmias
  Atrial fibrillation
  Sick-sinus syndrome
Valvular disease
  Mitral stenosis, rheumatic
  Aortic stenosis, rheumatic
  Bicuspid aortic valve
  Mitral annulus calcification (MAC)
  Calcific aortic stenosis
  Mitral valve prolapse (MVP)
  Bacterial endocarditis
  Nonbacterial thrombotic endocarditis
Cardiomyopathies or endocardiopathies
  Endocardial fibroelastosis
  Alcoholic cardiomyopathy
  Cocaine cardiomyopathy
  Myocarditis
  Sarcoidosis
  Amyloidosis
Intracardiac lesions
  Myxomas
  Fibroelastomas
  Malignant cardiac tumors
  Metastatic tumors
  Ball-valve thrombi
Septal abnormalities or paradoxical emboli
  Atrial septal defects
  Patent foramen ovale
  Atrial septal aneurysms

of these complications are treated. Wright et al. reported the results of anticoagulant treatment in a randomized series of patients with MI.[20] Among the 589 patients treated with anticoagulants, approximately 0.7 percent had clinically recognizable cerebral emboli, compared with 4.9 percent among the 442 patients in the control group.[20] In three other large studies, there were also definite, but small, differences in the rate of embolic complications of MI, favoring anticoagulant therapy.[21-23] These studies all antedated the introduction of newer cardiac diagnostic techniques, and the anticoagulation intensity was more than is customarily used today.

Rhythm Disturbances

Abnormal cardiac rhythms are also a cause of embolic stroke. The most embologenic rhythms are chronic atrial fibrillation, intermittent atrial fibrillation, and the so-called sick-sinus syndrome. In 1951, Daley and colleagues recognized atrial fibrillation in the setting of rheumatic heart disease as a source of systemic emboli.[24] Hinton et al. examined at necropsy the hearts of 333 patients known to have atrial fibrillation.[25] As expected, the percentage of patients with symptomatic systemic arterial embolism was high in those with atrial fibrillation and rheumatic mitral stenosis (41%), ischemic heart disease (35%), and combined rheumatic and ischemic heart disease (35%). Even those with no recognized heart disease or other miscellaneous cardiopathies with atrial fibrillation had a high rate of systemic embolism (17%).[25] A control group of 66 patients with ischemic heart disease but no known history of atrial fibrillation had, in contrast, only a 7 percent incidence of embolism.[25] In this and other series, the majority of symptomatic arterial emboli were cerebral.[3,8,25] Seventy-three percent of patients with emboli had involvement of the brain.[25] Data from the Framingham study[26,27] and from a review of patients with atrial fibrillation studied at the Massachusetts General Hospital[28] corroborate the relatively high risk of stroke in patients with this arrhythmia. Now, all agree that the presence of atrial fibrillation is an important risk factor for cardiogenic embolism. The Cerebral Embolism Task Force, in their first report, concluded, "Nonrheumatic nonvalvular atrial fibrillation is the most common cardiac condition associated with presumed embolic stroke, accounting for almost half of cardiogenic embolic strokes in recent clinical series."[29]

The origin of the embolic material in patients with atrial fibrillation is probably in the left atrium or left atrial appendage. In postmortem studies, these areas were far more likely to contain clot in patients with cerebral emboli than in those without emboli.[25] The presence of rheumatic heart disease;[25,30] the onset of atrial fibrillation within the preceding 3 months;[31] an enlarged left atrium, as measured by echocardiography;[32,33] and left ventricular dysfunction[33] all place patients with atrial fibrillation at increased risk for embolization.

Paroxysmal atrial fibrillation is also embologenic, with thrombi thought to form during the arrhythmia. Chronic atrial fibrillation is often preceded by paroxysmal atrial fibrillation. Kannel et al., in an epidemiological study, found that cerebral embolism commonly preceded the onset of chronic atrial fibrillation.[27] Brain emboli presumably occur during a paroxysm of atrial fibrillation. Wolf and colleagues supported this hypothesis by confirming that emboli most often occur soon after the onset of atrial fibrillation.[31] My own experience also includes patients who have had brain embolism at the time of cardioversion of their atrial fibrillation.

Brain embolism also occurs in the setting of sinoatrial pacemaker disturbances (sick-sinus syndrome).[34,35] In the series by Fairfax and colleagues, systemic embolism occurred in 16 of 100 patients with sick-sinus syndrome, 13 of which were brain emboli.[35] Patients with sick-sinus syndrome, in addition to having periods of unexplained sinus bradycardia or sinoatrial arrests, have attacks of atrial tachycardia, atrial fibrillation, and atrial flutter. Rubenstein and colleagues speculated that emboli might be related to paroxysms of atrial fibrillation.[34] Fairfax and colleagues found emboli more commonly in patients with evidence of prolonged atrial asystoles.[35] In atrial asystole, as in atrial fibrillation, the atria are mechanically inactive, increasing the risk of thrombus formation and subsequent embolization. Patients with sinoatrial disease at greatest risk for embolization have the brady–tachycardia syndrome.[36] These patients are at greater risk than either patients with sinoatrial disease but no tachycardia or patients with atrioventricular block.[36]

Valvular Disease

Abnormalities of the heart valves provide another source of embolism. The high rate of embolism with rheumatic valvular disease is well known. Noninfected calcific stenotic valves, particularly the mitral but also the aortic valve, may serve as a template for deposition of platelet and fibrin clots, which can embolize. Three other relatively common abnormalities—mitral valve prolapse (MVP), mitral annulus calcification (MAC), and bicuspid aortic valves[37–44]—have also been suspected of having embologenic potential. The association between MVP and cerebral infarction has been clearly demonstrated.[38–40] Some necropsy specimens have shown fibrin, platelets, and thrombi on prolapsed mitral valves, which also showed thickening and myxomatous degeneration.[40] MVP is a common finding in young patients with otherwise unexplained stroke. Hart and Easton estimated that if one third of all strokes in young adults were due to MVP (a very high estimate), the risk of stroke in an individual young adult with MVP would be 1 per 6000 young adults per year.[41] The association of MVP with strokes in older patients is more difficult to determine, as strokes from other mechanisms in this age group are much more common. The mechanisms of stroke in patients with MVP remain undefined. Speculations include thrombus formation on the atrial side of the prolapsing valve, in areas of stagnant flow;[42] clot formation secondary to a hypercoagulable state;[42] or myxomatous change in the valve, which allows endothelial tears, platelet adhesion, and agglutination, followed by fibrin deposition and embolization.[43]

Calcification of the mitral valve annulus (MAC) has also been reported more commonly in patients with embolic stroke than in age-matched controls.[44] In an early clinicopathological review of this entity, 4 of 14 patients described had suffered cerebral infarction, 1 of whom was not in atrial fibrillation.[45] Because MAC is commonly found in elderly patients, other stroke mechanisms must be investigated before MAC can be implicated as the cause of the stroke. Stroke in patients with MAC may occur secondary to extrusion of calcific material or embolization of platelet–fibrin material deposited in the region of the mitral valve annulus. In the MRSR, 7 patients were found with MAC as the only recognized source of stroke among 127 patients who were believed clinically to have had brain emboli.[8]

Infected heart valves are also a source of embolic material. In a large series of patients with infective endocarditis, 33 percent with infection of natural valves and 50 percent of those with prosthetic valve infection had brain emboli.[46] In natural-valve infections, cerebral emboli were most likely to occur if the aortic valve was infected; Group D streptococcus and *Staphylococcus aureus* were the most common organisms. In prosthetic valve endocarditis, aspergillosis was the most common infection causing early cerebral emboli, while *Streptococcus viridans* was the most common late cause.[46] In another series, neurological complications occurred more often with *Staphylococcus aureus* infection (67%) than with *Streptococcus viridans* (22%).[47]

Myxomatous mitral valves with prolapse can also become infected and can lead to bacterial endocarditis and even marantic nonbacterial endocarditis.[48] Brain emboli occur prior to, during, or after the diagnosis and treatment of infective endocarditis. Vegetations sterilized by antibiotic therapy can still embolize. Additional diagnostic features include constitutional symptoms, intermittent fevers, and emboli to other organs (lungs, spleen, kidneys, and peripheral vessels). Patients with infective endocarditis may also develop an encephalopathy characterized by restlessness, sleepiness, and confusion, without prominent focal neurological signs. Encephalopathy is more common in patients with virulent organisms, older age, and uncontrolled infection, and it is probably due to infective microemboli.[47] Brain abscess formation is rare.

Emboli from infected valves also embolize to the adventitia of blood vessels, producing mycotic aneurysms. Mycotic aneurysms are typically located in sites unusual for berry aneurysms, far beyond the circle of Willis. SAH and hemorrhagic infarction can also result from pyogenic arteritis, which causes vascular necrosis and bleeding.[47,49,50] Echocardiography, especially transesophageal, occasionally visualizes valvular vegetations, but a normal echocardiogram does not exclude endocarditis as a cause of stroke.

Nonbacterial thrombotic endocarditis is another cause of embolic stroke. This syndrome is usually associated with cancer, particularly with malignant melanoma and carcinoma of the pancreas, lung, or prostate. It has also been seen in patients with other debilitating diseases, such as SLE, pneumonia, inflammatory bowel disease, congestive heart failure, chronic renal failure, and perforated duodenal ulcer.[51] The mitral valve is more commonly affected than is the aortic valve; tricuspid and pulmonic valve lesions are rare. Bivalvular lesions are common. The vegetations, which consist of bland fibrin–platelet thrombi, are usually very small—less than 5 mm—making their identification during life by echocardiography and cardiac catheterization difficult. Heart murmurs are present in about one half of patients with nonbacterial thrombotic endocarditis but are usually hemodynamic and are often not caused by the vegetations.[51]

Stroke is common, occurring in more than one half of patients with nonbacterial thrombotic endocarditis. Stroke may be characterized by single or multiple large-vessel occlusions, with focal neurological signs; by multiple small micro-occlusions of leptomeningeal arteries producing multifocal and diffuse dysfunction; or by both small- and large-vessel occlusions. Systemic arterial thromboses are also common. The coexistence of nonbacterial thrombotic endocarditis with disseminated intravascular coagulation and multiple small-vessel occlusions suggests an associated primary clotting disorder.[52] Stroke due to nonbacterial thrombotic (also called marantic) endocarditis can be the initial manifestation of cancer, especially mucinous adenocarcinomas.[53,54]

Diagnosis is often difficult antemortem and must be based on high clinical suspicion. Suggestive findings include an underlying disease process that predisposes to nonbacterial thrombotic endocarditis; single or multiple sudden-onset strokes; heart murmur; infarction of multiple organs, including the brain, spleen, kidney, and heart; and absence of bacterial endocarditis or other embologenic cardiac diseases. Though a full cardiac evaluation may not reveal the source of emboli, arteriography may show evidence of multiple small arterial occlusions.

Prosthetic and even porcine heart valves can be sites of deposition of fibrin, platelet, or thrombin nidi that can suddenly embolize. Initial studies with Starr-Edwards valves demonstrated the embologenic nature of prosthetic valves.[55] The incidence of emboli is probably related to valve type, with the degree of thrombogenicity declining from non-cloth-covered prosthetic valves to cloth-covered prosthetic valves to tissue valves. Special substances are used to coat the valve surfaces to inhibit thrombus formation.

The incidence of stroke in patients with mechanical heart valves, even on anticoagulation, is about 2 to 5 percent a year, with mitral-valve prostheses more frequent offenders than aortic prostheses.[56] Tissue valves, without anticoagulation, have a similar rate of thromboembolism,[56] although some reports have noted embolic complications in 12 to 23 percent of such patients.[57] The high frequency of embolism in patients with mitral-valve replacement may be related to the frequent association of atrial fibrillation with mitral-valve disease. In prosthetic valves, thrombus formation is most likely to occur at the component-tissue interface or in areas of relative stenosis. In one postmortem study, up to 30 percent of valves were so affected.[58] The patients at greatest risk for embolization have been those who also had atrial fibrillation, left atrial enlargement, and stenotic valves.[57] The neurological stroke syndromes can vary from a mild transient deficit to severe permanent impairment. The size of the infarction will depend on the size of the embolus, the recipient artery, the stability of the embolus, and the variability of the collateral circulation. Strokes may occur either early or late after surgery, with early stroke often related to foreign-body embolization. Echocardiography is useful in evaluating dysfunction of prosthetic valves and in excluding large residual thrombi.

Cardiac Tumors

Atrial myxomas, although rare, are important and treatable causes of embolic infarction. These tumors arise from either side of the atrial septum, in the region of the fossa ovalis. Cardiac myxomas more frequently arise in the left atrium but have been known to originate in the left ventricle and simultaneously in both atria.[59] The tumors may be firmly attached to the atrial wall or may be attached to a stalk that allows movement about the atrial cavity, at times obstructing the cardiac valves. Grossly, the tumors are gelatinous, round, or polypoid masses that may be caked with platelet–fibrin clots. Emboli take the form of thrombi or tumor fragments.

In one series, 27 percent of atrial myxomas presented with cerebral ischemia, but in most cases, cardiac and constitutional symptoms predominate.[60] These symptoms include fainting due to change in cardiac output, heart murmurs, congestive heart failure, polyarthralgias, fever, and weight loss.[59] The erythrocyte sedimentation rate is often increased, and anemia is common. Heart murmurs may vary with position. Cardiac arrhythmias occur and vary from time to time. Myxomatous emboli frequently go to the vasa vasorum and produce multiple aneurysmal vascular dilations similar to the mycotic aneurysms found in bacterial endocarditis.[60,61]

Cardiac papillary fibroelastomas are rare tumors that also tend to embolize.[62] The tumor consists of frondlike papillary growths, which most often attach to valves but can appear over the papillary muscles, chordae tendineae, ventricular septum, and surface of the endocardium.[62] Metastatic tumors also are occasionally found in the heart. Myxomas and other intracardiac tumors are usually easily identified by echocardiography. Occasionally, echocardiography will be negative in the presence of a myxoma.[63] Atrial thrombi can be difficult to distinguish from tumors. Surgical removal of the myxomas relieves both the source of emboli and constitutional symptoms. Follow-up of patients with surgically removed myxomas indicates that myxomatous material in brain vessels or in the brain seldom grows.[60]

Cardiomyopathies and Endocardiopathies

Nonischemic diseases of the myocardium are also commonly complicated by embolism.[29,64] Although the major target of these disorders is the heart muscle—hence, the terms *myocarditis* and *cardiomyopathy*—the adjacent endocardium is also involved. Fibrin–platelet or thrombin can deposit on endocardial surfaces and embolize. Stasis within the heart cavities—due to poor myocardial function, congestive heart failure, and arrhythmias—also potentiate formation of thrombi. Mural thrombi are quite common in series of patients with alcoholic and other cardiomyopathies.[65–68] Mural thrombi have been found in as many as 53 percent of necropsies in patients with dilated cardiomyopathies.[68] Brain embolism has been estimated to occur in about 15 percent of patients with cardiomyopathy;[66] dilated and restrictive types of cardiomyopathies have a higher frequency of embolism than does hypertrophic subaortic stenosis.[67]

Elderly patients with cardiac amyloidosis are also prone to embolism. I have seen a patient with sarcoid myocardiopathy who presented with behavioral disturbances secondary to multiple cerebral emboli.[69] Even idiopathic hypertrophic subaortic stenosis (IHSS), a focal disorder of the muscle of the ventricular septum, is occasionally complicated by embolism, particularly if atrial fibrillation and left atrial enlargement are present.[70,71] Cocaine use can cause cardiac ischemia and a myocarditis with infiltration of eosinophils.[72] Recurrent brain embolism has been reported to originate from myocarditis associated with chronic cocaine use.[73,74] Echocardiography is especially helpful in detecting cardiac-muscle diseases and separating them into dilated, restrictive, and infiltrative types.

Artery-to-Artery Emboli

Intra-arterial embolism is a frequent presentation of most arterial diseases. Clots or fibrin–platelet clumps are formed after large-vessel occlusion in areas of tight stenosis and in vessels with ulcerated plaques. The idea of intra-arterial emboli is not new, but rather has been rediscovered since the early 1970s. Chiari, in the early 1900s, observed this phenomenon and reported a relatively high frequency (7 in 400 autopsies) of carotid thrombus and subsequent cerebral embolization.[75] Intra-arterial embolism occurs during three different time periods (immediate, early, and late) after large-vessel occlusion. In the immediate group, embolic phenomena are present shortly after occlusive thrombosis. These patients have a stroke of sudden onset, without prior episodes of transient neurological dysfunction.[76] Angiography in these patients shows tandem lesions, consisting of a proximal large-vessel occlusion and a more distal intracranial embolic occlusion.[12,76,77] In general, outcome in these patients is not as favorable as in patients without embolization. Fresh clot that is poorly adherent—usually in the ICA, VA, or basilar artery—breaks loose into the more distal circulation. Strokes may also occur in the early period—that is, within the first 1 to 2 weeks after the occlusion—probably due to emboli originating from the tail of occlusive thrombi.[76]

Embolic strokes can also occasionally occur late (more than 2 weeks) after large-vessel occlusions.[78] In some patients, these new strokes occur during rehabilitation and recovery from the original stroke. The mechanism of these delayed strokes is controversial. Barnett and colleagues have drawn attention to the carotid stump as a possible embolic source.[79] Within the stump, there are atheromatous ulcers on which thrombi develop. The turbulence of flow in this area produces conditions further conducive to both platelet–fibrin aggregation and embolization of formed thrombus. The embolic material is then carried through the collateral circulation to cause ipsilateral cerebral or retinal ischemia. Arteriography in these patients usually shows thrombus in the stump or an atheromatous ulcer protruding into the stump. The likelihood that the stump is a nidus for embolic material is probably related to stump length: Stumps longer than 5 mm are more often associated with ischemic events. Other potential mechanisms for delayed stroke after large-vessel occlusion include emboli from the contralateral or external carotid circulation, which traverse into the territory of the occluded vessel; hemodynamic factors causing low distal perfusion; and new occlusive disease distal to the prior occlusion.[78,80] Ischemia due to low perfusion is usually transient, positionally sensitive, and often precipitated by overzealous blood-pressure reduction.

Emboli from atherosclerotic plaques are composed of two types of material: platelet–fibrin clumps and atheromatous cholesterol debris. Atherosclerotic plaques are a common finding at postmortem examination. Most plaques are asymptomatic. What makes a plaque symptomatic is not clearly understood and may include multiple processes. I suspect that nonstenosing, nonulcerative plaques are an infrequent cause of major strokes. A review of the pathology of 44 cases of carotid plaques surgically removed from sites appropriate to focal cerebral symptoms revealed no cases of isolated simple plaques.[81] The stenotic plaque, however, is a frequent cause of intra-arterial embolism. I judge stenosis not by the percentage of luminal narrowing, but rather by the residual lumen size. Lumens less than 2 mm in diameter are significantly stenotic, even if this represents only a 50 percent reduction in an already congenitally small vessel.[82] Pessin et al., in their series of acute carotid-territory strokes, described a group of patients with embolic stroke, in whom the ICA lumen was less than 2 mm.[76] These stenotic vessels thrombose because of reduction in flow or altered thromboxane/prostacyclin balance. A study of carotid endarterectomy specimens shows that severe stenosis is often associated with ulceration, crevices, adherence of platelet–fibrin aggregates, and attached red fibrin-dependent thrombi.[83]

Cholesterol crystals lie within clefts of atherosclerotic plaques and sometimes discharge into the circulation, reaching the eye and brain. Hollenhorst described cholesterol material at bifurcations of retinal arteries, which was visible as bright refractile, light-refringent particles that moved distally with time.[84] Among Hollenhorst's 24 patients with cholesterol crystals in the optic fundus, 8 had repeated episodes of transient monocular blindness, but 16 had no symptoms.[84] Because single crystals are quite small, they do not impede blood flow, an observation corroborated by experimental data.[85] Nonetheless, groups of cholesterol crystals, especially if accompanied by other debris or fibrin–platelet clumps, can and do block small arteries. In past reports[86,87] and my own experience, showers of emboli often cause TIAs and accompanying prominent symptoms and signs of extremity, retinal, and renal ischemia. Patients who have these showers seldom have large strokes. Careful repeated ophthalmoscopic examinations and skin, renal, and muscle biopsy are often diagnostic. Some have suggested that anticoagulants have an adverse effect on cholesterol embolism.[86] At times, cholesterol embolism has followed cardiac or aortic surgery or radiography. When the source of the emboli has been an aortic aneurysm, surgery can be curative. Necropsy studies and the results of transesophageal echocardiography (TEE) now document the aorta, especially any protruding aortic atheromas, as frequent sources of cholesterol and other emboli.[88] No definitive data are available on the effects of various proposed medical therapies, such as agents that reduce serum lipids or platelet-antiaggglutinating agents, in patients with cholesterol-crystal emboli.

Embolization from the aorta may account for an important number of strokes after open-heart surgery.[89,90] Aortic plaques are often layered, broad-based, and immobile, but they may also be pedunculated and may protrude into the lumen.[91] Mobile plaques jutting into the lumen are more apt to be associated with embolism.[91] In a 1991 study, TEE showed that 38 of 556 (7%) patients studied had intra-aortic atherosclerotic debris, and 36 of these patients had an embolic event.[91] Cholesterol-crystal embolization from the aorta seems to occur in periodic flurries and can be precipitated by aortography or aortic clamping.

Thrombi can occasionally form within large arteries—such as the ICA or the VA—even in the absence of atherosclerosis. Among a series of nine patients with carotid luminal thrombi, three had underlying serious medical disease, such as cancer, rheumatoid arthritis, and chronic pulmonary insufficiency.[92] Figure 10.1 shows a luminal thrombus from this series of patients. Cancer can predispose to arterial, as well as venous, occlusion. One mechanism of hypercoagulability is the release of *mucin*, a substance that promotes thrombosis, into the circulation.[54] In other patients, various coagulopathies can promote intravascular clotting. These large intracarotid clots can be seen at angiography and are perhaps best treated with anticoagulants.[93]

Aneurysms are another infrequent but important source of distal embolism.[94] Large berry or fusiform aneurysms often harbor clots that can block orifices directly or occasionally can embolize to the more distal territories of the vessel harboring the aneurysm. Dolichoectatic aneurysms often harbor large or small pancakelike clots, especially in regions of outpouching and altered flow.[95] The evaluation of some patients with TIAs shows an unsuspected aneurysm as the only explanation for the attacks.[96] Dissecting aneurysms are even more likely to provide an embolic source near the time of the dissection.[94] Blood dissects within the wall of the artery and can reenter the lumen as a loosely adherent clot. In addition, the lumen may be so compromised by the expanded vascular wall that blood flow is reduced, and the slow-flowing intraluminal blood may thrombose. The association of embolization with ICA or VA dissection[97] has led many to recommend heparin and short-term anticoagulation therapy, beginning as soon as a dissection is recognized.

Paradoxical Emboli

In addition to the heart and the arterial circulation, the venous circulation is also a source of emboli. Thrombi most often form in the legs or pelvic

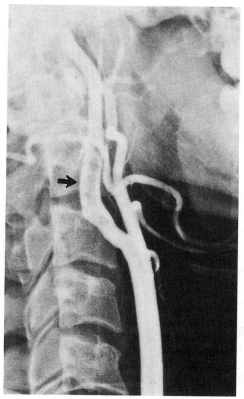

FIGURE 10.1 Carotid arteriogram, lateral view: Dark filling defects within the artery (black arrow) represent luminal clots.

veins and pass through an intra-atrial septal defect or a probe-patent foramen ovale to enter the systemic circulation. Perhaps as many as 35 percent of patients have a probe-patent foramen ovale at necropsy.[98] Another source of paradoxical embolism involves pulmonary arteriovenous fistulas, lesions especially common in patients with hereditary hemorrhagic telangiectasia.[99,100] Embolic material goes directly into pulmonary veins and then into the left heart chambers and systemic arterial circulation. When the pulmonary particles are infected, brain abscesses occur. Pulmonary shunts are also the likely mechanism by which foreign particles injected intravenously by drug users reach the eye and brain.[101] In patients with atrial septal defects, there is usually some shunting of blood from the right to the left side of the heart. During the Valsalva maneuver and straining, right-heart pressure rises and can promote paradoxical embolization.

In my experience, some patients with paradoxical emboli have no prior history of heart disease, no obvious right ventricular hypertrophy, and no

history of thrombophlebitis.[102] Atrial septal aneurysms are often fenes-
trated and show minor degrees of right-to-left shunting detectable by contrast echocardiography during Valsalva maneuver.[64] Other atrial septal
aneurysms are accompanied by larger septal defects.[103,104] These aneurysms
usually represent localized bulging in the region of the fossa ovalis; most protrude alternately into the left and right atria, as pressure gradients shift, but
some remain in the right atrium.[64] Stenosis and altered flow within the
aneurysms can also lead to thrombosis and embolization to the lungs, brain,
or systemic organs. These lesions are now better detected with TEE.

Newer technology using saline injection and Doppler probes at the
time of echocardiography improves diagnosis. TEE has been a great advance
because it shows the septum so well.[105] TCD has also been a helpful advance. Introduction of agitated saline while monitoring with a TCD probe
over the MCA, reveals short bursts of high voltage shortly after injection in
patients with cardiac shunts.[106] TCD has also been effectively used to
detect emboli during carotid endarterectomy[107] and heart surgery[108] and in
experimental animals.[109]

Conditions that predispose to venous thrombosis—for example, prolonged bed rest, anovulatory drugs, cancer, and obesity—are often present in
young adults with paradoxical embolism to the brain.[102,110] Anticoagulation, vena cava plication, and surgical repair of atrial septal defects have all
been effective in controlling embolization.[103] More recently, small
muscular ventricular septal defects in children have been closed percutaneously.[111] Figure 10.2 depicts the common mechanisms of paradoxical
embolization.

Differential Diagnosis

In Part I of this book, I discussed the differential diagnosis between ischemia
distal to an occlusive lesion in a large artery (called "thrombus") and
ischemia due to embolism. Separation of these two mechanisms is often difficult, sometimes impossible. In the case of thrombotic occlusion of large extracranial arteries, both mechanisms—that is, distal hypoperfusion and
embolism—are often operative. Table 10.3 lists points of distinction, but
none of these guidelines is absolute.[3] In practice, when it is clear that the
lesion is ischemic, but distinction of the mechanism cannot be made from
the available clinical data, both mechanisms should be fully explored. A
search for both cardiac and arterial lesions is appropriate. In some patients,
even after a full evaluation that includes CT, ultrasound, angiography, and
cardiac evaluation, the stroke mechanism is still uncertain. Treatment for
each remaining possible mechanism should, in that circumstance, be
considered.

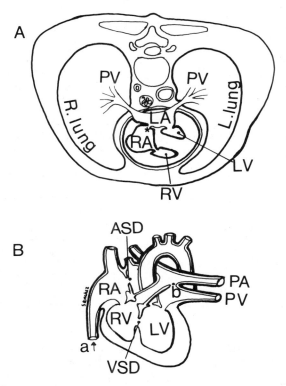

FIGURE 10.2 Common routes of paradoxical embolism. (A) Cross-section through the thorax showing patent foramen ovale (asterisk). (B) Right-to-left shunts; atrial septal defect (ASD), ventricular septal defect (VSD), and fistula between the pulmonary artery and pulmonary vein (b). Clot from the leg vein ascends via the interior vena cava (a). RA = right atrium; LA = left atrium; RV = right ventricle; LV = left ventricle; PA = pulmonary artery; PV = pulmonary vein.

Treatment

Several alternative strategies are applicable, depending on the source of emboli, the severity of the neurological deficit, and the general medical condition of the patient.

Removal or Repair of the Source

Cardiac surgery to repair ventricular aneurysms, replace a sclerotic or rheumatic valve, or close an intra-atrial septal defect have proven effective. In one patient, surgical removal of a protruding aortic atheromatous plaque removed the source of multiple cholesterol emboli.[112] Pharmacological or

TABLE 10.3
Differentiating Signs of Thrombosis and Embolism

Thrombosis	Embolism
1. Preceding brief, frequent shotgun-like TIAs	1. Single or infrequent but longer-lasting TIAs or strokes
2. TIAs all in same vascular territory	2. Deficits maximal at onset
3. Onset of stroke after sleep	3. Onset during activity or sudden strain, cough, or sneeze
4. Postural sensitivity of the symptoms	4. Infarcts in multiple vascular territories
5. Occlusion or severe stenosis of a large artery, shown by ultrasound or angiography	5. Presence of distal intraarterial embolus by angiography or TCD
6. Absence of distal embolus by angiography	6. Hemorrhagic cerebral infarct on CT or MRI
7. Infarct on CT or MRI near border zone of affected artery	7. Infarct on CT or MRI in heart of vascular territory, wedge-shaped and abutting on cortical surface
8. Presence of risk factors for atherosclerosis: hypertension, hypercholesterolemia, angina, etc.	8. Presence of known cardiac, arterial, or venous source of embolus

electrical control of arrhythmias and antibiotics for bacterial endocarditis are other examples of treatment aimed at the cardiac source. Clipping of large arterial aneurysms and endarterectomy to remove plaques causing severe luminal compromise are other examples of surgical correction of embolic sources. In most instances, however, either the source is uncertain or the lesion is not operable.

Anticoagulant and Anti-Platelet-Agglutinating Agents

Anticoagulants have long been used to prevent embolism in patients with acute MI and rheumatic heart disease. Three large, controlled trials, individually and together, showed reduced risk of strokes in patients with acute MIs who were anticoagulated.[29,113–115] Anticoagulants have also been shown to reduce the rate of embolism in patients with rheumatic heart disease, especially mitral stenosis with atrial fibrillation.[116] These studies were mostly performed when the intensity of anticoagulation was greater than the amount that is used now. Bleeding complications did occur, especially during long-term therapy.

Since the first edition of this book, there have been a number of randomized, controlled trials of anticoagulation in patients with atrial fibrillation who did not have valve disease. Once atrial fibrillation had been shown to be an important risk factor for brain embolism, clinicians rightly questioned whether the risk of anticoagulant-related hemorrhage in the multitude of individuals with atrial fibrillation, many of whom were elderly and frail, would outweigh the benefit of stroke reduction.

Three recent trials have now shown conclusively that warfarin is effective in preventing brain emboli in patients with atrial fibrillation.[117–121] In the Danish AFASAK study, 1007 patients with atrial fibrillation were randomly assigned to warfarin (at an INR of 2.8 to 4.2), aspirin (75 mg/day), or placebo.[117] Warfarin, but not aspirin, was effective in preventing severe thromboembolic events.[117] In the Boston area anticoagulation trial for atrial fibrillation, warfarin (target PT of 1.2 to 1.5 times the control) was compared with best other medical therapy (which could include aspirin) in preventing stroke and death among 420 atrial fibrillation patients.[119] Warfarin proved very effective in preventing both stroke and death, but there were insufficient data to judge the effect of aspirin.[119]

The stroke prevention in atrial fibrillation (SPAF) study was larger (1244 patients), and the study design was more complex than in the other trials.[118,120,121] In atrial fibrillation patients eligible for warfarin prophylaxis, the effect of warfarin (INR 1.7 to 4.6), aspirin (325 mg/day), and placebo were compared; in patients not eligible for warfarin, placebo and aspirin were compared.[118] Both warfarin and aspirin were more effective than placebo, so that the placebo trials were discontinued, and now aspirin and warfarin effectiveness are being compared.[118–120] Only the SPAF study showed a superiority of aspirin over placebo in preventing stroke in atrial fibrillation patients.[122] The stroke and systemic embolism rate was 3.2 percent per year in 517 patients given aspirin, compared to 6.3 percent in 528 patients treated with placebo, a nearly 50 percent risk-reduction rate in favor of aspirin.[118,122] All studies showed a very low rate of bleeding complications. Clearly, anticoagulants are indicated for patients with atrial fibrillation, but the timing and intensity of treatment are not settled.

The timing of anticoagulation has been controversial. Clinicians want to prevent the next embolus but do not want to transform the acute infarct into a hematoma. Recent studies have shown that most often, anticoagulants can be given immediately after a brain embolism, with a very low incidence of hemorrhagic complications. Furlan et al. studied 54 consecutive patients with nonseptic cardiogenic cerebral emboli treated with anticoagulants; 25 received anticoagulants within 24 hours.[123] Seven patients, all inadequately anticoagulated, had recurrent emboli within the first week, and no patient had evidence of brain hemorrhage.

Koller[124] and Hart et al.[125] emphasized the frequency of early recurrent embolism within 10 days of the initial embolus. In Koller's experience, there were no adverse effects from therapeutic levels of anticoagulation within the first 48 hours.[124] The timing of anticoagulation was studied in a randomized prospective trial that admitted 45 patients studied within 48 hours of a cardiac-origin cerebral embolism, who had no CT evidence of hemorrhage.[126] The group was randomized to receive immediate heparinization (average time 32 hours post-onset) or no anticoagulation until after 14 days.

There were four adverse events, all in the nonanticoagulant treatment group: 2 patients had recurrent embolism, and 2 had delayed-onset hemorrhagic infarction.[126] No adverse effects of immediate anticoagulation were noted.

Others have reported isolated anecdotal examples of cerebral hemorrhage or hemorrhagic infarction complicating anticoagulant therapy for cerebral embolism.[127-130] Bleeding is probably most common in patients with large infarcts,[129,130] with hypertension, and with coagulation parameters indicating excess anticoagulation. Bolus heparin therapy also may yield a higher risk than continuous heparin infusion.[130] Patients with bacterial endocarditis, prosthetic valves, and rheumatic heart disease[127] may also have higher risks of bleeding.

Another factor to consider is the nature of the cardiac lesion. Some lesions carry a higher risk of reembolism. Paroxysmal atrial fibrillation, recent MI, and rheumatic mitral stenosis with atrial fibrillation are high-risk conditions, while MVP, MAC, and long-standing atrial fibrillation with normal-sized atria are less risky, with regard to imminent recurrence. The duration of anticoagulation will depend on the chronicity or reversibility of the cardiac lesion. Acute conditions such as thyrotoxic atrial fibrillation, cardioversion of atrial fibrillation, or acute MI without ventricular aneurysm might warrant short-term treatment, while a permanent irreversible lesion might warrant indefinite prophylaxis.

Clinicians have usually not started anticoagulants or stopped their use if hemorrhagic infarction is found on CT. My colleagues and I recently reported a series of patients who were continued on anticoagulants after hemorrhagic changes were seen.[131,132] None developed worsening clinically or by CT. Physicians are accustomed to giving heparin immediately to individuals with pulmonary embolism even if they have hemoptysis and with the knowledge that pulmonary embolic infarcts are often beefy red.

If the patient with acute embolism has a large or hemorrhagic infarct, I delay heparinization. In any case, I avoid bolus heparin. If the cardiac lesion is such that the risk of reembolism is high and the infarct is not large or hemorrhagic, I advise immediate heparinization. If the risk of reembolization is low, then I delay anticoagulant use for at least 48 to 72 hours.

The role of aspirin treatment in patients with cardiac embolization is unclear. The results cited in the trials of atrial fibrillation prophylaxis are suggestive, but not conclusive, that aspirin may have some role to play. Some studies have reported low embolism rates in patients with bioprosthetic valves and atrial fibrillation treated with platelet antiaggregants.[133,134] Addition of dipyridamole (400 mg per day) decreased embolic events in patients with prosthetic aortic valves who were on warfarin.[135]

Treatment of intra-arterial embolism from proximal atherosclerotic lesions has been discussed elsewhere. I suggest using aspirin for irregular, nonstenotic disease, and warfarin for tight stenotic and occlusive thrombi. When occlusive thrombosis has occurred, I continue to prescribe warfarin for 2 to 3 months only, and then I prescribe aspirin.

References

1. Aring CD, Merritt H. Differential diagnosis between cerebral infarction and cerebral hemorrhage. Arch Intern Med 1935;56:435–456.
2. Whisnant JP, Fitzgibbon JP, Kurland LT, et al. Natural history of stroke in Rochester, Minnesota, 1945–1954. Stroke 1971;2:11–22.
3. Mohr JP, Caplan LR, Melski JW, et al. The Harvard Cooperative Stroke Registry: a prospective registry. Neurology 1978;29:754–762.
4. Caplan LR. Of birds and nests and brain emboli. Rev Neurol 1991;147:265–273.
5. Fisher CM, Adams R. Observations on brain embolism with special reference to the mechanism of hemorrhagic infarction. J Neuropathol Exp Neurol 1951;10:92–93.
6. Fisher CM, Adams RD. Observations on brain embolism with special reference to hemorrhagic infarction. In: Furlan AJ, ed. The heart and stroke. London: Springer-Verlag, 1987:17–36.
7. Fisher CM, Perlman A. The nonsudden onset of cerebral embolism. Neurology 1967;17:1025–1032.
8. Dalal P, Shah P, Sheth S, et al. Cerebral embolism: angiographic observations on spontaneous clot lysis. Lancet 1965;1:61–64.
9. Liebeskind A, Chinichian A, Schechter M. The moving embolus seen during cerebral angiography. Stroke 1971;2:440–443.
10. Gacs G, Merel MD, Bodosi M. Balloon catheter as a model of cerebral emboli in humans. Stroke 1982;13:39–42.
11. Caplan LR, Hier DB, D'Cruz I. Cerebral embolism in the Michael Reese Stroke Registry. Stroke 1983;14:530–536.
12. Fieschi C, Argentino C, Lenzi G, et al. Clinical and instrumental evaluation of patients with ischemic stroke within the first six hours. J Neurol Sci 1989;91:311–322.
13. Kushner MJ, Zanette EM, Bastianello S, et al. Transcranial Doppler in acute hemisphere brain infarction. Neurology 1991;41:109–113.
14. Ringelstein EB, Koschorke S, Holling A, et al. Computed tomographic patterns of proven embolic brain infarctions. Ann Neurol 1989;26:759–765.
15. Gacs G, Fox AJ, Barnett HJ, Vinuela F. CT visualization of intracranial arterial thromboembolism. Stroke 1983;14:756–763.
16. Tomsick T, Brott T, Barsan W, et al. Thrombus localization with emergency cerebral computed tomography. Stroke 1990;21:180.
17. Wolf PA, Dawber TR, Kannel WB. Heart disease as a precursor of stroke. In: Schoenberg BS, ed. Advances in neurology: vol. 19. New York: Raven Press, 1978:567–577.
18. Bean WB. Infarction of the heart: III. clinical concern and morphological findings. Ann Intern Med 1958;12:71–94.
19. Kase C, White R, Vinson T, et al. Shotgun pellet embolus to the middle cerebral artery. Neurology 1981;31:458–461.
20. Wright IS, Marple CD, Beck DF. Myocardial infarction: its clinical manifestations and treatment with anticoagulants—a study of 1031 cases. New York: Grune & Stratton, 1954.
21. Drapkin A, Mersky C. Anticoagulant therapy after myocardial infarction: relation of therapeutic benefit to patient's age, sex, and severity of infarction. JAMA 1972;222:541–549.

22. Medical Research Council. Assessment of short-term anticoagulant administration after cardiac infarction. Br Med J 1969;1:335–342.
23. Veteran's Administration Cooperative Study. Anticoagulants in acute myocardial infarction: results of a cooperative trial. JAMA 1973;225:724–729.
24. Daley R, Mattingly TW, Holt CL, et al. Systemic arterial embolism in rheumatic heart disease. Am Heart J 1951;42:566–581.
25. Hinton RC, Kistler JP, Fallon JT, et al. Influence of etiology of atrial fibrillation on incidence of systemic embolism. Am J Cardiol 1977;40:509–515.
26. Wolf PA, Dawber TR, Thomas HE, et al. Epidemiologic features of chronic atrial fibrillation and risk of stroke: the Framingham study. Neurology 1978;28:975–977.
27. Kannel WB, Abbott RD, Savage DP, et al. Epidemiologic features of chronic atrial fibrillation: the Framingham study. N Engl J Med 1982;306:1018–1022.
28. Fisher CM. Reducing risks of cerebral embolism. Geriatrics 1979;34:59–66.
29. Cerebral Embolism Task Force. Cardiogenic brain embolism. Arch Neurol 1986;43:71–84.
30. Selzer A. Atrial fibrillation revisited. N Engl J Med 1982;306:1044–1045.
31. Wolf P, Kannel W, McGee D, et al. Duration of atrial fibrillation and imminence of stroke: the Framingham study. Stroke 1983;14:664–667.
32. Caplan LR, D'Cruz I, Hier DB, et al. Atrial size, atrial fibrillation, and stroke. Ann Neurol 1986;19:158–161.
33. The Stroke Prevention in Atrial Fibrillation Investigators. Predictors of thromboembolism in atrial fibrillation: II. echocardiographic features of patients at risk. Ann Intern Med 1992;116:6–12.
34. Rubenstein JJ, Schulman LL, Yurchak PM, et al. Clinical spectrum of the sick sinus syndrome. Circulation 1972;46:5–13.
35. Fairfax AJ, Lambert CD, Leatham A. Systemic embolism in chronic sinoatrial disorder. N Engl J Med 1976;295:190–193.
36. Bathen J, Sparr S, Rokseth R. Embolism in sinoatrial disease. Acta Med Scand 1978;203:7–11.
37. Pleet A, Massey E, Vengrowe M. TIA, stroke, and the bicuspid aortic valve. Neurology 1981;31:1540–1542.
38. Barnett HJM, Boughner DR, Taylor DW, et al. Further evidence relating mitral valve prolapse to cerebral ischemic events. N Engl J Med 1980;302:139–144.
39. Scharf RE, Hennerici M, Bluschke V, et al. Cerebral ischemia in young patients: is it associated with mitral valve prolapse and abnormal platelet activity in vivo? Stroke 1982;13:454–458.
40. Lauzier S, Barnett HJM. Cerebral ischemia with mitral valve prolapse and mitral annulus calcification. In: Furlan AJ, ed. The heart and stroke. London: Springer-Verlag, 1987:63–100.
41. Hart RG, Easton JD. Mitral valve prolapse and cerebral infarction. Stroke 1982;13:429–430.
42. Kostuk WJ, Boughner DR, Barnett HJM, et al. Strokes: a complication of mitral-leaflet prolapse? Lancet 1977;2:313.
43. Rice GPA, Boughner DR, Stiller C, et al. Familial stroke syndrome associated with mitral valve prolapse. Ann Neurol 1980;7:130–134.
44. De Bono DP, Warlow CP. Mitral-annular calcification and cerebral or retinal ischemia. Lancet 1979;2:383–385.
45. Korn D, DeSanctis RW, Sell S. Massive calcification of the mitral annulus. N Engl J Med 1962;267:900–909.

46. Garvey GT, Neu HC. Infective endocarditis: an evolving disease. Medicine 1978;57:105–127.
47. Kanter MC, Hart RG. Neurologic complications of infective endocarditis. Neurology 1991;41:1015–1020.
48. Geyer JJ, Franzini DA. Myxomatous degeneration of the mitral valve complicated by nonbacterial thrombotic endocarditis with systemic embolization. Am J Clin Pathol 1979;72:489–492.
49. Hart RG, Kagan-Hallet K, Jocens SE. Mechanisms of intracranial hemorrhage in infective endocarditis. Stroke 1987;18:1048–1054.
50. Hart RG, Foster JW, Luther MF, Kanter MC. Stroke and infective endocarditis. Stroke 1990;21:695–700.
51. Deppisch L, Fayem A. Nonbacterial thrombotic endocarditis. Am Heart J 1976;92:723–729.
52. Reagan TJ, Okazaki H. The thrombotic syndrome associated with carcinoma. Arch Neurol 1974;31:390–395.
53. Kooiker JC, McLean JM, Sumi SM. Cerebral embolism, marantic endocarditis, and cancer. Arch Neurol 1976;33:260–264.
54. Amico L, Caplan LR. Thomas C. Cerebrovascular complications of mucinous cancer. Neurology 1989;39:522–526.
55. Akbarian M, Austen G, Yurchak PM, et al. Thromboembolic complications of prosthetic cardiac valves. Circulation 1968;37:826–831.
56. Kloster FE. Complications of artificial heart valves. JAMA 1979;241:2201–2203.
57. Edmiston WA, Harrison EC, Diuck GF, et al. Thromboembolism in mitral porcine valve recipients. Am J Cardiol 1978;41:508–511.
58. Silver MD. Late complications of prosthetic heart valves. Arch Pathol Lab Med 1978;102:281–284.
59. Schwartz GA, Schwartzman RJ, Joyner CR. Atrial myxoma. Neurology 1972;22:1112–1121.
60. Sandok BA, Van Estorff I, Giuliani ER. Central nervous system embolism due to atrial myxoma. Arch Neurol 1980;37:485–488.
61. Roeltapen DR, Weiner GR, Patterson LD. Delayed neurologic complications of left atrial myxoma. Neurology 1981;31:8–13.
62. Kasarskis E, O'Connor W, Earle G. Embolic stroke from cardiac papillary fibroelastomas. Stroke 1988;19:1171–1173.
63. Thompson J, Kapor W, Wechsler LR. Multiple strokes due to atrial myxoma with a negative echocardiogram. Stroke 1988;19:1570–1571.
64. Cerebral Embolism Task Force. Cardiogenic brain embolism: the second report of the Cerebral Embolism Task Force. Arch Neurol 1989;46:727–743.
65. Vost A, Wolochow D, Howell D. Incidence of infarcts of the brain in heart disease. J Pathol Bacteriol 1964;88:463–470.
66. Demakis J, Proskey A, Rahimtoola S, et al. The natural course of alcoholic cardiomyopathy. Ann Intern Med 1974;80:293–297.
67. Salgado ED, Furlan AJ, Conomy JP. Cardioembolic sources of stroke. In: Furlan AJ, ed. The heart and stroke. London: Springer-Verlag, 1987:47–61.
68. Roberts WC, Ferrans VJ. Pathological aspects of certain cardiomyopathies. Circulation Res 1974;4/35(suppl):128–144.
69. Harthorne J. Case records of the Massachusetts General Hospital (Case 46—1975). N Engl J Med 1975;293:1138–1145.
70. Glancy D, O'Brien K, Gold H, et al. Atrial fibrillation in patients with

idiopathic hypertrophic subaortic stenosis. Br Heart J 1970;32:652–659.
71. Russell JW, Biller J, Hajduczok Z, et al. Ischemic cerebrovascular complications and risk factors in idiopathic hypertrophic subaortic stenoses. Stroke 1991;22:1143–1147.
72. Isner JM, Estes NAM, Thompson PD, et al. Acute cardiac events temporally related to cocaine abuse. N Engl J Med 1986;315:1438–1443.
73. Petty GW, Brust JC, Tatemichi TK, Barr ML. Embolic stroke after smoking "crack" cocaine. Stroke 1990;21:1632–1635.
74. Sauer CM. Recurrent embolic stroke and cocaine-related cardiomyopathy. Stroke 1991;22:1203–1205.
75. Chiari H. Über das verhalten des teilungs winkels der carotis communis bei der endarteritis chronica deformans. Verh Dtsch Ges Pathol 1905;9:326–330.
76. Pessin MS, Hinton RL, Davis KE, et al. Mechanism of acute carotid stroke. Ann Neurol 1979;6:245–252.
77. Ringelstein E, Zeumer H, Angelou D. The pathogenesis of strokes from internal carotid artery occlusion: diagnostic and therapeutic implications. Stroke 1983;14:867–875.
78. Barnett HJM. Delayed cerebral ischemic episode distal to occlusion of major cerebral arteries. Neurology 1978;28:769–774.
79. Barnett HJM, Peerless SJ, Kaufman JCE. Stump of internal carotid artery: a source for further cerebral embolic ischemia. Stroke 1978;9:448–456.
80. Finkelstein S, Kleinman GM, Cuneo R, et al. Delayed stroke following carotid occlusion. Neurology 1980;30:84–88.
81. Imparato AM, Riles TS, Gorstein F. The carotid bifurcation plaque: pathologic findings associated with cerebral ischemia. Stroke 1979;10:238–245.
82. Caplan LR, Baker R. Extracranial occlusive vascular disease: does size matter? Stroke 1980;11:63–66.
83. Fisher CM, Ojemann RG. A clinico-pathologic study of carotid endarterectomy plaques. Rev Neurol 1986;142:573–589.
84. Hollenhorst RW. Significance of bright plaque in the retinal arterioles. JAMA 1961;178:125–129.
85. Steiner TJ, Rail DL, Rose F. Cholesterol crystal embolization in rat brain: a model for atheroembolic cerebral infarction. Stroke 1980;11:184–189.
86. Beal MD, Williams RS, Richardson EP, et al. Cholesterol embolism as a cause of transient ischemic attacks and cerebral infarction. Neurology 1981;31:860–865.
87. McDonald WI. Recurrent cholesterol embolism as a cause of fluctuating cerebral symptoms. J Neurol Neurosurg Psychiatry 1967;30:489–496.
88. Ammenco P, Duyckaerts C, Tzourio C, et al. The prevalence of ulcerated plaques in the aortic arch in patients with stroke. N Engl J Med 1992;326:221–225.
89. Marshall WG, Barzilai B, Kouchoukos NT, Saffitz J. Intraoperative ultrasonic imaging of the ascending aorta. Ann Thorac Surg 1989;48:339–344.
90. Gardner TJ, Horneffer PJ, Manolio TA, et al. Stroke following coronary artery bypass grafting: a ten-year study. Ann Thorac Surg 1985;40:574–581.
91. Karalis DG, Chandrasekaran K, Victor MF, et al. Recognition and embolic potential of intra-aortic atherosclerotic debris. J Am Coll Cardiol 1991;17:73–78.

92. Caplan LR, Stein R, Patel D, et al. Intraluminal clot of the carotid artery detected radiographically. Neurology 1984;34:1175–1181.

93. Gates P, Buchan A, Barnett HMJ. Luminal thrombus in the cerebral circulation. Stroke 1985;16:140.

94. Duncan A, Rumbaugh C, Caplan LR. Cerebral embolic disease: a complication of carotid aneurysms. Cardiology 1979;133:379–384.

95. Pessin MS, Chimowitz MI, Levine SR, et al. Stroke in patients with fusiform vertebrobasilar aneurysms. Neurol 1989;39:16–21.

96. Fisher M, Davidson R, Marcus E. Transient focal cortical ischemia as a presenting manifestation of unruptured cerebral aneurysms. Ann Neurol 1980;8: 367–372.

97. Caplan LR, Zarins C, Hemmatti M. Spontaneous dissection of the extracranial vertebral artery. Stroke 1985;16:1030–1038.

98. Thompson T, Evans W. Paradoxical embolism. Q J Med 1930;23:135–150.

99. Roman G, Fisher M, Peil D, et al. Neurological manifestations of hereditary hemorrhagic telangiectasis (Rendu-Osler-Weber disease): report of 2 cases and review of the literature. Ann Neurol 1978;4:130–144.

100. Regeura JM, Colmenero JD, Guerrero M, et al. Paradoxical cerebral embolism secondary to pulmonary arteriovenous fistula. Stroke 1990;21:504–505.

101. Caplan LR, Banks G, Thomas C. Central nervous system complications of addiction to "T's and blues." Neurology 1982;32:623–628.

102. Jones HR, Caplan LR, Come PC, et al. Cerebral emboli of paradoxical origin. Ann Neurol 1983;13:314–319.

103. Shenoy MM, Vijaykumer PM, Friedman SA, Greef E. Atrial septal aneurysm associated with systemic embolism and interatrial right-to-left shunt. Arch Intern Med 1987;147:605–606.

104. Belkin RN, Hurwitz BJ, Kisslo KB. Atrial septal aneurysm: association with cerebrovascular and peripheral embolic events. Stroke 1987;18:856–862.

105. Tegeler CH, Downes TR. Cardiac imaging in stroke. Stroke 1991;22:1206–1211.

106. Chimowitz M, Nemec JJ, Marwick TH, et al. Transcranial Doppler ultrasound identifies patients with right to left cardiac or pulmonary shunts. Neurology 1991;41:1902–1904.

107. Spencer MP, Thomas GI, Nicholls SC, et al. Detection of middle cerebral artery emboli during carotid endarterectomy using transcranial Doppler ultrasonography. Stroke 1990;21:415–423.

108. Harrison MJ, Pugsley W, Neuman S, et al. Detection of middle cerebral emboli during coronary artery bypass surgery using transcranial Doppler sonography. Stroke 1990;21:1512.

109. Russell D, Madden KP, Clark WM, et al. Detection of arterial emboli using Doppler ultrasound in rabbits. Stroke 1991;22:253–258.

110. Loscalo J. Paradoxical embolism: clinical presentation, diagnostic strategies and therapeutic options. Am Heart J 1986;112:141–145.

111. Bridges ND, Perry SB, Keane JF, et al. Preoperative transcatheter closure of congenital muscular ventricular septal defects. N Engl J Med 1991;324:1312–1317.

112. Tunick PA, Culliford AT, Lamperello PJ, Kronzon I. Atheromatosis of the aortic arch as an occult source of multiple systemic emboli. Ann Intern Med 1991;114:391–392.

113. Drapkin A, Mersky C. Anticoagulant therapy after acute myocardial infarction. Relation of therapeutic benefit to patient's age, sex and severity of infarction. JAMA 1972;222:541–549.
114. Medical Research Council. Assessment of short-term anticoagulant administration after myocardial infarction. Br Med J 1969;1:335–342.
115. Veteran's Administration Cooperative Study. Anticoagulants in acute myocardial infarction: results of a cooperative trial. JAMA 1973;225:724–729.
116. DeWar HA, Weightman D. A study of embolism in mitral valve disease and atrial fibrillation. Br Heart J 1983;49:133–140.
117. Peterson P, Boysen G, Godtfresen J, et al. Placebo controlled randomized trial of warfarin and aspirin for prevention of thromboembolic complications in chronic atrial fibrillation: The Copenhagen AFASAK Study. Lancet 1989; 1:175–179.
118. Stroke Prevention in Atrial Fibrillation Study Group Investigators. Preliminary report of the stroke prevention in atrial fibrillation study. N Engl J Med 1990;322:863–868.
119. The Boston Area Anticoagulation Trial for Atrial Fibrillation Investigators. The effect of low-dose warfarin on the risk of stroke in patients with nonrheumatic atrial fibrillation. N Engl J Med 1990;323:1505–1511.
120. Cheesbro JH, Fuster V, Halperin J. Atrial fibrillation—risk marker for stroke. N Engl J Med 1990;323:1556–1558.
121. Albers G, Sherman DG, Gress DR, et al. Stroke prevention in nonvalvular atrial fibrillation: a review of prospective randomized trials. Ann Neurol 1991;30:511–518.
122. Stroke Prevention in Atrial Fibrillation Investigators. Stroke prevention in atrial fibrillation study—final results. Circulation 1991;84:527–539.
123. Furlan A, Cavalier S, Hobbs R, et al. Hemorrhage and anticoagulation after nonseptic embolic brain infarction. Neurology 1982;32:280–282.
124. Koller R. Recurrent embolic cerebral infarction and anticoagulation. Neurology 1982;32:283–285.
125. Hart RG, Coull BM, Hart PD. Early recurrent embolism associated with nonvalvular atrial fibrillation. Stroke 1983;14:688–693.
126. Cerebral Embolism Study Group. Immediate anticoagulation of embolic stroke: a randomized trial. Stroke 1983;14:668–676.
127. Calandre L, Ortega J, Bermejo F. Anticoagulation and hemorrhagic infarction in cerebral embolism secondary to rheumatic heart disease. Arch Neurol 1984;41:1152–1154.
128. Drake M, Shin C. Conversion of ischemic to hemorrhagic infarction by anticoagulant administration. Arch Neurol 1983;40:44–46.
129. Shields R, Laureno R, Lachman T, et al. Anticoagulant related hemorrhage in acute cerebral embolism. Stroke 1984;15:426–437.
130. Cerebral Embolism Study Group. Immediate anticoagulation of embolic stroke: brain hemorrhage and management options. Stroke 1984;15:779–789.
131. Pessin MS, Estol CJ, Lafranchise EF, Caplan LR. Safety of anticoagulation in hemorrhagic infarction. Neurology 1991;41:263.
132. Pessin MS, Teal PA, Caplan LR. Hemorrhage infarction: guilt by association? AJNR 1991;12:1123–1126.
133. Nunoz L, Aguado G, Larrea JL, et al. Prevention of thromboembolism using aspirin after mitral valve replacement with porcine bioprosthesis. Ann Thorac Surg 1984;37:84–87.

134. Gonzalaz-Laven L, Tandon AP, Chi S, et al. The risk of thromboembolism and hemorrhage following mitral valve replacement. J Thorac Cerebrovasc Surg 1984;87:340–351.
135. Sullivan J, Harkin D, Gorlin R. Pharmacologic control of thromboembolic complications of aortic valve replacement. N Engl J Med 1971;284:1391–1394.

CHAPTER 11

Hypoxic–Ischemic Encephalopathy

The brain is particularly vulnerable to any decrease in its blood, oxygen, or fuel supply. Patients with hypotension or hypoxia often present to their physicians or the emergency room because of cerebral dysfunction. Most often, decreased cerebral perfusion is due to cardiac disease, either arrhythmia or pump failure, often caused by an acute MI. Because circulatory failure usually leads to hypoventilation, and hypoxia soon causes diminished cardiac function, hypoxia and hypoperfusion are usually combined. The general term *hypoxic–ischemic encephalopathy* reflects the dual nature of the CNS stress. Pulmonary embolism is another acute disorder that causes hypotension and diminished blood oxygenation. In some patients, decreased cerebral perfusion is due to acute blood loss or hypovolemia.

Clinical Findings

A general decrease in perfusion causes generalized nonfocal brain dysfunction. Dizziness, light-headedness, confusion, and difficulty in concentrating are common. Focal symptoms and signs such as hemiplegia, hemianopia, and aphasia are rarely caused by circulatory failure but are the rule in the other categories of ischemic stroke. At times, prior strokes or vascular occlusions do lead to asymmetries on neurological examination. Examination of the patient with globally decreased cerebral perfusion usually reveals an ill-appearing person with sweating, tachycardia, hypotension (especially postural), and signs of cardiac dysfunction upon physical or electrocardiographic examination. There are two common circumstances in which neurologists might see patients with cerebral hypoperfusion due to systemic causes: (1) acute CNS symptoms in the absence of a known incident of circulatory failure, and (2) after known cardiac arrest, hypotension, or cardiac surgery. In the first circumstance, the major problem is diagnosis. When there is a known cardiac arrest, the consulting physician usually asks the neurologist about the prognosis of the brain injury.

Patient 1

A 63-year-old white man, LB, suddenly became agitated and restless and seemed confused. He had entered the hospital 2 days before for abdominal pain, had had no neurological symptoms or abnormalities, and was having routine gastrointestinal x-rays. A psychiatrist who was called to examine and calm the patient requested neurological consultation because of concern about an organic cause for the behavioral change. Neurological examination showed a very agitated, restless man. He did not know his whereabouts, nor could he give any account of the previous few days. He recalled none of three objects told to him 3 minutes before and could not even remember that he had been given objects to recall. He spoke normally and could repeat and understand spoken language. He could write but not read. He also could not identify by sight objects in his environment and saw only parts of pictures shown to him. When the same objects were placed in his hands, he correctly named them. There were no abnormalities of motor, reflex, or somatosensory function. Gait was normal, but he held his hands outstretched as if feeling for the walls.

This patient had abnormalities in three major spheres—memory, vision, and behavior. These findings indicate bilateral dysfunction of the posterior portions of the cerebral hemispheres. Embolization to the rostral basilar artery causing bilateral temporo-occipital-lobe infarcts in the PCA territory could cause these findings. Alternatively, an unrecognized episode of prolonged hypotension might have led to hypoperfusion in the posterior border zone between the MCA and PCA territories. Distal-field infarction most often affects the posterior hemispheres, possibly because they are the regions farthest from the heart.[1]

Lesions in the posterior watershed (between the MCA and the PCA) often disconnect the preserved calcarine visual cortex in the occipital lobe from the more anterior centers that control eye movement. A visual problem first described by an ophthalmologist, called Balint's syndrome, often results.[1-4] Patients act as if they cannot see but surprisingly sometimes notice very small objects. The features of Balint's syndrome are

1. *Asimultagnosia*—Patients see things piecemeal; they do not see all the objects in their field of vision at one time and may notice only parts of objects. To test for this problem, ask patients to count the number of people or objects in a picture or on a table; ask patients to read a paragraph aloud, to determine whether they omit words or phrases; and show patients multiple objects held up together, for verbal identification.

2. *Optical ataxia*—Patients cannot coordinate hand and eye movements and point erratically at objects. Test by asking patients to touch the

noses of people in a picture or to touch the crossing point of several Xs on a page. Ask patients to trace, first with one hand and then the other, a complex drawing constructed by the examiner.

3. *Apraxia of gaze*—Patients are unable to gaze directly where desired. Ask patients to look at an object held to the side, then to look at the examiner's nose, and then to repeat the same task. Notice how patients explore a picture.

The visual abnormalities can be more severe in either the left or the right visual field. Balint's original cases probably were caused by systemic hypoperfusion, the commonest mechanism of the bilateral parieto-occipital damage. PCA infarction can also lead to Balint's syndrome. Occasional patients with Alzheimer's or Creutzfeldt-Jakob disease can have features of Balint's syndrome, but the findings develop gradually and insidiously rather than abruptly. Memory dysfunction and agitation can also be caused by bilateral PCA-territory infarcts or border-zone ischemia. (See the discussion in Chapter 7 on the PCA.)

When hypotension is more severe, lesions can spread to the anterior border zones between the ACA and the MCA and may extend like a triangle toward the ventricle (Figure 11.1).[5,6] The area of the motor homunculus most affected is usually the shoulder and arm. The face territory in the central portion of the MCA territory and the foot region in the center of the ACA supply are spared. The distribution of weakness has been likened by Mohr to a "man in a barrel."[1,7]

Among a prospective series of 34 patients with coma presumably due to an episode of systemic hypotension, 11 had the man-in-the-barrel syndrome.[7] They moved neither arm but moved both legs either spontaneously or in response to pain. The frontal eye fields are also affected, so that roving eye movements and hyperactive doll's-eye reflexes result. At times, perhaps because of previously asymmetrical occlusive disease of extracranial and intracranial arteries, the signs can be quite asymmetrical, with unilateral or asymmetric arm paralysis and conjugate-eye deviation toward the side of the larger lesion. Stupor results from extensive bilateral border-zone ischemia.

LB was sedated and a CT scan ordered. The scan showed small but definite, roughly symmetric hypodensities in the posterior parietal regions, with sparing of the medial calcarine cortex and temporal lobes. An ECG showed evidence of acute MI and multifocal frequent premature ventricular contractions.

CT confirmed that the lesions were between the PCA and the MCA territories, supporting the diagnosis of border-zone infarction. This led to more cardiac testing, which showed an unsuspected MI and potentially serious arrhythmia. In retrospect, after further questioning by the patient's physician, the acute abdominal pain was probably due to coronary disease. The

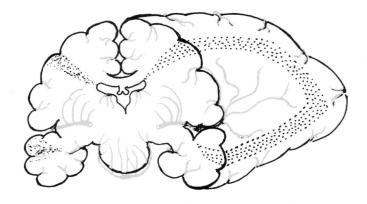

A

FIGURE 11.1   Coronal brain section showing distribution of border zone infarction. Pattern of infarct in "watershed" ischema: watershed areas seen are between the anterior and middle cerebral arteries and between the posterior and middle cerebral arteries and the left hemisphere.

diagnosis of border-zone ischemia leads to a different array of diagnostic tests than those that apply to infarction in the center of a vascular territory. I have also occasionally seen demented patients whose neurological examination and CT scans indicated border-zone infarcts due to repeated unrecognized episodes of hypotension or globally decreased cerebral perfusion.

LB had a relatively slight insult and recuperated well with time. The nature of the insult and its reversibility should be emphasized. In general, it is unwise to push the patient back to work too quickly, or self-confidence may be lost. Many patients are not restored mentally for weeks after cardiac surgery but gradually regain their usual intellectual vigor. Time and reassurance are needed.

Patient 2

A 45-year-old previously well man, AR, collapsed at work, clutching his chest in pain. Paramedics found him pulseless minutes later and administered cardiopulmonary resuscitation (CPR) on the way to the hospital. Pulse and blood pressure were restored, but the patient lay comatose. A neurologist examined the patient the next morning, 18 hours after the arrest. The patient was very sleepy but could be momentarily aroused by shouting or pinching. He would appropriately flick off painful stimuli but did not speak or obey oral commands or answer queries. There were spontaneous restless limb movements. Blinking, swallowing, and tongue-protrusion movements were seen. Pupillary, corneal, and doll's-eye reflexes were normal. Plantar responses were extensor, but there was no abnormal limb posturing.

In this patient, the consulting physician knew that the abnormal neurological state was due to cardiac arrest. Was the CNS insult likely to be lethal? What would be the quality of survival? Should orders not to resuscitate be given? This scenario is frequent in hospital practice today. Successful CPR, once rare, has now become commonplace. Advances in technique, widespread teaching of medical, paramedical, and lay volunteer personnel, and the availability of special mobile equipment and facilities in some communities have saved many lives.[8,9] The heart is often able to recover from ischemia, but unfortunately, the brain has often been irreversibly damaged by the ischemic–anoxic insult of circulatory failure. New technology can prolong life indefinitely in a vegetative state, at great cost to the community and to the family. Physicians involved with CPR must be familiar with prognostic indicators for cerebral recovery after cardiac arrest and should consider their own ethical and moral values in applying this knowledge.

Pathology and Prognosis

The signs of brain dysfunction secondary to hypoxic–ischemic insults can best be remembered by visualizing the brain regions most vulnerable to circulatory failure and their pathology. The location and severity of the pathology depends on the patient's age, the completeness of the circulatory arrest, serological factors such as the blood sugar and pH, and the relative admixture of hypoxia and ischemia.

Severe prolonged hypoxic–ischemic insults cause necrosis of the cerebral and cerebellar cortex, cerebral edema, and injury to brainstem nuclei. Patients with severe injury usually remain deeply comatose after resuscitation and do not awaken later. Brainstem reflex functions are lost (no corneal, pupillary, oculocephalic, or oculovestibular response). Pupils are dilated, and spontaneous respirations are absent. This state, if persistent, is incompatible with independent survival.

Patients with less severe cerebral injury usually show some signs of reaction to the environment shortly after resuscitation. Restless limb motions and eye opening develop. When the eyelids are passively opened by the examiner, the eyes are seen to rove from side to side and may temporarily fixate on an object. Noise, a light shined in the eye, or painful stimuli evoke alerting or withdrawal responses other than obligatory decorticate or decerebrate posturing. Spontaneous blinking, swallowing, yawning, and licking movements with the tongue are noted if patients are observed closely.[10] In some patients, the mouth lies constantly open, with the tongue protruding. When a tongue blade is inserted, patients may bite down hard on the blade, preventing the examiner from removing it.

As stupor lightens, agitation, restlessness, confusion, and even delirium supervene. After awakening, examination often uncovers features of Balint's syndrome, as described in the first patient. Other patients have a selective difficulty with memory and are unable to recall recent happenings or to make new lasting memories. This amnesic state clinically resembles Korsakoff's syndrome and is due to selective vulnerability of the hippocampus and adjacent medial temporal structures to hypoxic–ischemic insults.[11-14] *Active memory testing* is required to identify and quantify the memory loss. Give patients a 10-fact story, three objects, or three pictures, emphasizing that you will later ask about the material they will be expected to recall. Ask them to repeat the information to be certain that it has registered. Later, ask the patients to recite the things to be recalled, grading the performance—for example, as three out of five objects after 5 minutes. *Passive memory testing*—for example, asking patients what happened that morning or what they ate at their last meal—is less useful and reliable than is active testing.

The cerebral cortex often undergoes selective damage to the middle lamina that relatively spares both the deeper and the more superficial cortical layers.[15-17] This laminar necrosis frequently causes seizures. Seizures may follow severe or moderate laminar injury and may take the form of multifocal myoclonic jerks, twitches, or frank grand mal seizures. Myoclonic jerks are often exaggerated or provoked by moving or stimulating a limb. Seizures caused by diffuse hypoxic–ischemic injury are relatively resistant to treatment. Care should be taken to avoid overdosing with anticonvulsants, thus compounding the patient's stupor. If seizures create respiratory compromise or cause myoglobinuria or release of high levels of muscle enzymes, curarization and mechanical ventilation may be necessary. Repetitive generalized myoclonus lasting more than 30 minutes carries a very poor prognosis in patients who have survived a cardiac arrest.[18] In one series of 11 such patients, none regained consciousness after resuscitation, and all remained comatose until death.[18] Each of these patients had extensive anoxic-ischemic damage to the cerebral cortex, especially the hippocampus and calcarine cortices. The basal ganglia, thalamus, cerebellum, and brainstem nuclei were all severely damaged.[18]

Severe laminar necrosis can be associated with extensive loss of cortical functions so that the patient survives in a persistent vegetative state, with little meaningful response to the environment but preserved brainstem function. These patients appear awake. They have sleep–wake cycles with eyes open but make no response to stimulation or to the environment.[16,19] Necropsy examinations of 10 patients with the persistent vegetative state showed extensive cortical necrosis, often laminar in distribution, and multiple microinfarcts.[16]

Prolonged partial ischemia, especially in the young, can cause damage to the basal ganglia, particularly the globus pallidus and the thalamus. Strangulation and carbon monoxide poisoning produce a similar insult,[20] in which hypoxia antedates and overshadows circulatory compromise. Rigidity, decorticate posturing, and flexion of all limbs result. Although the eyes are open and fixate, patients are often mute and usually do not respond to environmental stimuli. Patients with mutism and rigidity after cardiac arrest have a very poor prognosis for recovery.

In some patients, especially youths, sudden and severe circulatory arrest may lead to necrosis of the brainstem and its nuclei, with relative preservation of cerebral and basal-ganglionic structures.[21,22] This pattern of selective injury to brainstem nuclei is also found in the experimental animal.[23] Brainstem reflexes are absent, but patients frequently retain the ability to control respiration. Despite the absence of brainstem function, the EEG may show preserved cerebral activity. This state mimics pontine hemorrhage or basilar-artery occlusion and carries a dire prognosis unless there is rapid improvement. Necropsy reveals necrosis of many brainstem nuclei.

Although ischemic–anoxic cerebellar damage is commonly found at necropsy, clinical signs of cerebellar dysfunction are rare and usually are overshadowed by cerebral abnormalities. Some patients, after cardiac arrest, have spontaneous arrhythmic fine or coarse muscle jerking, markedly exaggerated when the limbs are used. This disorder of movements, usually called "action myoclonus" or the "Lance-Adams syndrome," after the physicians who originally described it,[24] is often accompanied by gait ataxia. The movement disorder can progress even without further ischemic stress. Some patients, especially those with preexisting occlusive disease of the VAs, may have prominent ataxia due to border-zone cerebellar infarcts, mostly between the main supply of the three major circumferential cerebellar arteries.

Plum and colleagues described progressive deterioration after a single hypoxic insult.[25] Delayed deterioration is common after carbon-monoxide intoxication and has been described after strangulation.[20] Progressive worsening is rare after cardiac arrest, though it has been described. The mechanism of progressive loss of function after single self-limited insults is uncertain.

The most reliable way of judging prognosis is to perform careful repeated neurological examinations within the first hours and days after the insult. The level of consciousness is very important. If patients are alert or arousable during the first hours after the hypoxic–ischemic insult, the prognosis is good for excellent recovery of brain functions. Most patients who will eventually recover awaken within 72 hours. In one series of 63 patients, 90 percent of patients who did recover alertness did so within the first 3 days.[26] Especially important is assessment of brainstem reflexes; most often, prolonged brainstem dysfunction means a very severe insult to the nervous system and to the cerebral cortex. Dilated, nonreactive pupils at 12 hours after arrest carries a poor prognosis. Corneal reflex, oculocephalic responses to passive horizontal and vertical movement of the head (doll's eyes) and oculovestibular reflexes (movement of the eyes when cold water is instilled in the ear canals) are also excellent indices of the function of the brainstem tegmentum.[10] When these reflexes are absent hours after CPR, the prognosis is grave.[27–29] In one series, among 63 patients, no survivor had absent pupillary responses to light and absent corneal reflexes at 6 hours after cardiopulmonary arrest.[29] In survivors, all brainstem reflex responses returned to normal within 48 hours.[29] Absence of spontaneous respiration and prolonged low blood pressure are also poor prognostic signs. Snout, pharyngeal, and cough reflexes, and jaw jerks have less correlation with survival and outcome.

Willoughby and Leach divided cardiac-arrest patients into two groups, depending on their responses to pain when tested 1 hour after arrest.[30] Eighteen patients had either no response to pain (5) or decorticate (9) or decerebrate posturing (4). Ten of these patients died, and the remaining 8 had significant intellectual impairment and did not improve while in the hospital. All survivors who responded to pain at 1 hour without obligatory posturing had preserved intellectual function.[30] Plum and Caronna used the patient's response to deep supraorbital ridge or interphalangeal pain to assess prognosis.[31] They watched for eye opening or a verbal or motor response to pain. Patients who did not respond to pain within 24 hours died or were left in a persistent vegetative state.[31] In a larger series, among 133 patients who were comatose after cardiac arrest, only 15 survived without neurological deficit, while all survivors among 151 patients who were not comatose after arrest left the hospital without neurological deficit.[32] The appearance of roving eye movements or purposeful face or limb movements by 12 to 24 hours bodes well. At 48 hours, the return of intelligible speech and response to commands is a good prognostic sign.[33] The use of multiple variables helps improve prognostication.[34]

The following criteria are often used as indications of *brain death*, an irreversible state in which there is no precedent for meaningful survival:[35,36]

1. coma with loss of cerebral reactivity
2. absence of spontaneous respiration
3. loss of brainstem reflexes (pupillary, corneal, oculovestibular, and oculocephalic)
4. electrocerebral silence (a so-called flat EEG) for greater than 12 hours (in the absence of hypothermia or sedative drugs)

Physicians can declare death if criteria for brain death are met, despite persistence of cardiac function.

In AR, blood sugar was 150 mg/dl on admission. The pH was 7.32 one hour after arrest. CT was normal. EEG showed diffuse delta and theta slowing, but the background changed when the patient was pinched or light was shown in the face. By day 3, he had awakened and spoke normally but had a severe amnesic syndrome.

The level of blood sugar at the time of arrest may be one factor that affects recovery. Myers and Yamaguchi demonstrated that young monkeys given infusions of glucose before induced cardiac arrest had more cerebral damage than similarly studied animals infused with saline.[37] Others have corroborated these findings in adult animals and have shown that more severe damage also results when glucose is given after the ischemic insult.[38]

The damage may be caused by production of lactate, which can injure brain tissue.[38,39] Systemic lactic acidosis can clearly compound the cerebral damage. Poor neurological recovery after cardiac arrest was linked to higher blood-sugar levels (greater than 300 mg/dl) in one human study.[40] Theoretically, high blood calcium levels could also have a deleterious effect.[41–43]

EEGs of patients in coma after cardiac arrest are usually very abnormal and contain diffuse slowing in the theta and delta ranges, as well as periodic phenomena and epileptiform discharges. In the most severe injuries, the EEG may be flat—electrocerebral silence. Severe slowing or low amplitude of the background activity has a very bad prognosis, especially if documented in EEGs 12 or 24 hours apart.

Some patients in deep coma from hypoxic–ischemic injury have preserved alpha activity. *Alpha coma activity* differs from normal rhythms, as follows:[44–46]

1. It is usually faster (9–12 cycles/second), as compared to the usual (8–10 cycles/second) alpha.
2. It is more frontal, central, and parietal, as compared with the usual occipital location.
3. It is usually temporary.
4. It does not respond to auditory, photic, or tactile stimuli.

Evoked-response testing may also help determine the degree of cerebral injury. Regional cerebral blood flow (rCBF) studies using SPECT invariably show hypoperfusion in patients with prolonged cardiac arrests.[47] Usually the decreased perfusion is most severe frontally.

The brains of patients who were considered brain dead before death was pronounced are usually soft and necrotic. Angiography before death reveals an absence of intracranial circulation. Brain swelling is so extensive as to block antegrade flow of blood into the cranium. Obviously, absence of blood flow into the intracranial vessels is not compatible with survival. Korein and colleagues introduced a test that uses a bolus injection of radioisotope, with subsequent cranial recording, to test CBF.[48,49] Absence of the appearance of the isotope in the head correlates with no flow in angiography and other criteria for brain death. TCD also has been used since the early 1990s to evaluate patients for the determination of brain death.[50–52]

Treatment

Little is known about optimal treatment of patients to minimize cerebral damage after cardiac arrest, although many experimental and clinical studies deal with this problem. Certainly, it is important to maintain good cardiac output and ventilation and to prevent complications of the stuporous state, such as aspiration, pneumonia, and urosepsis. Theoretical advantages can be cited for

1. hemodilution
2. artificially induced hypertension to augment CBF
3. hypothermia
4. barbiturate anesthesia to reduce cerebral metabolism
5. lowering of blood sugar
6. use of corticosteroids
7. use of G_{M1} gangliosides
8. use of calcium-channel blockers
9. use of free-radical scavengers

When many of these treatments are combined in the experimental animal, brain damage is reduced, although evidence that any single treatment is effective is scanty.[53] Much more work is needed to answer the important question of how to treat patients with brain dysfunction after cardiac arrest.

References

1. Mohr JP. Neurological complications of cardiac valvular disease and cardiac surgery including systemic hypotension. In: Vinken P, Bruyn G, eds. Handbook of clinical neurology: vol 38. neurological manifestations of systemic disease, pt I. Amsterdam: North Holland Publishing, 1979:143–171.
2. Balint R. Seelenlahmung des Schauens, optische Ataxie, raumliche Storung der Aufmerksamheit. Z Psychiatr Neurol 1909;25:51–81.
3. Tyler HR. Cerebral disturbance of vision in Neuro-ophthalmology: vol 4. St. Louis: Mosby, 1968:266–281.
4. Hecaen H, Ajuriaguerra J. Balint's syndrome and its minor forms. Brain 1954; 77:373–400.
5. Zulch K. On the circulatory disturbances in the borderline zones of the cerebral and spinal vessels. In: Proceedings of the Second International Congress on Neuropathology: vol 8. Amsterdam: Excerpta Medica, 1955:894–895.
6. Romanul F, Abramowicz A. Changes in brain and pial vessels in arterial border zones. Arch Neurol 1974;11:40–65.
7. Sage JI, Van Uitest RL. Man-in-the-barrel syndrome. Neurology 1986;36: 1102–1103.
8. Copley D, Mantel J, Rogers W, et al. Improved outcome for prehospital cardio-pulmonary collapse with resuscitation by bystanders. Circulation 1977;56: 901–905.
9. Lund I, Skulberg A. Cardiopulmonary resuscitation by lay people. Lancet 1975;2:702–704.
10. Fisher CM. The neurological examination of the comatose patient. Acta Neurol Scand 1969;45(Suppl 36):5–56.
11. Caronna J, Finkelstein S. Neurologic syndrome after cardiac arrest. Stroke 1978;9:517–520.
12. Volpe B, Hirst W. The characterization of an amnesic syndrome following hypoxic–ischemic injury. Arch Neurol 1983;40:436–440.
13. Cummings J, Tomiyasu U, Reed S, et al. Amnesia with hippocampal lesion after cardiopulmonary arrest. Neurology 1984;34:679–681.

14. Petito C, Feldmann E, Pulsinelli W, Plum F. Delayed hippocampal damage in humans following cardiorespiratory arrest. Neurology 1987;37:1281–1286.

15. Brierley JB, Adams JH, Graham D, et al. Neocortical death after cardiac arrest: a clinical, neurophysiological, and neuropathological report of two cases. Lancet 1971;2:560–565.

16. Dougherty J, Rawlinson D, Levy D, et al. Hypoxic–ischemic brain injury and the vegetative state: clinical and neuropathologic correlation. Neurology 1981; 31:991–997.

17. Adams JH, Brierley JB, Connor RCR, Treip CS. The effects of systemic hypotension upon the human brain: clinical and neuropathological observations in 11 cases. Brain 1966;89:235–268.

18. Young GB, Gilbert JJ, Zochodne DW. The significance of myoclonic status epilepticus in postanoxic coma. Neurology 1990;40:1843–1848.

19. Jennett B, Plum F. Persistent vegetative state after brain damage: a syndrome in search of a name. Lancet 1972;1:734–737.

20. Dooling E, Richardson E. Delayed encephalopathy after strangling. Arch Neurol 1976;33:196–199.

21. Gilles F. Hypotensive brainstem necrosis. Arch Pathol 1969;88:32–41.

22. Boisen E, Siemkowicz E. Six cases of cerebromedullospinal disconnection after cardiac arrest. Lancet 1976;1:1381–1383.

23. Miller J, Myers R. Neuropathology of systemic circulatory arrest in adult monkeys. Neurology 1972;22:888–904.

24. Lance J, Adams R. The syndrome of intention and action myoclonus as a sequel to hypoxic encephalopathy. Brain 1963;86:111–133.

25. Plum F, Posner JB, Hain R. Delayed neurologic deterioration after anoxia. Arch Intern Med 1962;110:56–67.

26. Snyder BD, Loewenson RB, Gumnit RJ, et al. Neurologic prognosis after cardiopulmonary arrest: II. level of consciousness. Neurology 1980;30:52–58.

27. Allen N. Life or death after cardiac arrest. Neurology 1977;27:805–806.

28. Snyder B, Ramirez-Lassepas M, Lippert D. Neurologic status and prognosis after cardiopulmonary arrest. Neurology 1974;24:582–588.

29. Synder BD, Gumnit RJ, Leppik IE, et al. Neurologic prognosis after cardiopulmonary arrest: IV. brainstem reflexes. Neurology 1981;31:1092–1093.

30. Willoughby J, Leach B. Relation of neurological findings after cardiac arrest to outcome. Br Med J 1974;33:437–439.

31. Plum F, Caronna J. Can one predict outcome of medical coma? In: Outcome of severe damage to the central nervous system: a Ciba Foundation symposium. New York: Elsevier, 1975:121–139.

32. Bell J, Hodgson H. Coma after cardiac arrest. Brain 1974;97:361–372.

33. Finkelstein S, Caronna J. Outcome of coma following cardiac arrest. Neurology 1977;27:367–368.

34. Longstreth W, Diehr P, Inui T. Prediction of awakening after out-of-hospital cardiac arrest. N Engl J Med 1983;308:1378–1382.

35. A definition of irreversible coma. Report of the Ad Hoc Committee of the Harvard Medical School to examine the definition of brain death. JAMA 1968; 205:337–340.

36. Walker A, et al. An appraisal of the criteria of cerebral death. JAMA 1977;237: 982–986.

37. Myers C, Yamaguchi S. Nervous system effects of cardiac arrest in monkeys. Arch Neurol 1977;34:65–74.
38. Plum F. What causes infarction in ischemic brain? Neurology 1983;33:222–233.
39. Myers R. A unitary theory of causation of anoxic and hypoxic brain pathology. In: Fahn S, Davis J, Rowland L, eds. Advances in neurology: vol 26. cerebral hypoxia and its consequences. New York: Raven Press, 1979:195–213.
40. Longstreth W, Inui T. High blood glucose level on hospital admission and poor neurological recovery after cardiac arrest. Ann Neurol 1984;15:59–63.
41. Hass W. Beyond cerebral blood flow, metabolism, and ischemic thresholds: an examination of the role of calcium in the initiation of cerebral infarction. In: Meyer J, Lechner H, Reivich M, et al., eds. Cerebral vascular disease: proceedings of the Tenth International Salzburg Conference: vol 3. Amsterdam: Excerpta Medica, 1981:3–17.
42. Siesjo BK, Bengtsson F. Calcium fluxes, calcium antagonists, and calcium-related pathology in brain ischemia, hypoglycemia, and spreading depression. J Cereb Blood Flow Metab 1989;9:127–140.
43. Cheung JY, Bonventre JV, Malis CD, Leaf A. Calcium and ischemic injury. N Engl J Med 1986;314:1670–1676.
44. Caplan LR. Neurology of the acute cardiac. In: Donoso E, Cohen S, eds. Critical cardiac care. New York: Stratton International Medical Books, 1979:183–197.
45. Westmoreland B, Klass D, Sharbrough F, et al. Alpha coma. Arch Neurol 1975;32:713–718.
46. Chokroverty S. "Alpha-like" rhythms in electroencephalograms in coma after cardiac arrest. Neurology 1975;25:655–663.
47. Roine RO, Launes J, Nikkinen P, et al. Regional cerebral blood flow after human cardiac arrest. Arch Neurol 1991;48:625–629.
48. Korein J, Braunstein P, George A, et al. Brain death: I. angiographic correlation with the radioisotopic bolus technique for evaluation of critical deficit of cerebral blood flow. Ann Neurol 1973;2:195–205.
49. Perrson J, Korein J, Harris J, et al. Brain death: II. neurological correlation with the radioisotope bolus technique for evaluation of critical deficit of cerebral blood flow. Ann Neurol 1977;2:206–210.
50. Caplan LR, Brass LM, DeWitt LD, et al. Transcranial Doppler ultrasound: present status. Neurology 1990;40:696–700.
51. Kirkham F, Levin S, Padayachee T, et al. Transcranial pulsed Doppler ultrasound findings in brainstem death. J Neurol Neurosurg Psychiatry 1987;50:1504–1513.
52. Ropper A, Kehne S, Wechsler L. Transcranial Doppler in brain death. Neurology 1987;37:1733–1735.
53. Giswold S, Safar P, Rao G, et al. Multifaceted therapy after global brain ischemia in monkeys. Stroke 1984;15:803–812.

CHAPTER 12

Subarachnoid Hemorrhage

Intracranial hemorrhage involves the brain parenchyma, the subarachnoid space, or both. Twenty percent of strokes are hemorrhagic, with subarachnoid hemorrhage (SAH) and ICH each accounting for 10 percent. *SAH* occurs when a blood vessel near the brain surface leaks, causing extravasation of blood into the subarachnoid space. SAH is most often caused by rupture of a saccular aneurysm or by an arteriovenous malformation (AVM). Less common causes are head injury, the use of illicit drugs—especially amphetamines and cocaine—venous-sinus thrombosis, and bleeding disorders. Blood in the subarachnoid space acts as a meningeal irritant and incites a typical clinical response regardless of etiology. Patients with SAH characteristically complain of headache, photophobia, and stiff neck, and they may also vomit. Confusion, restlessness, and transient or persistent decreased levels of consciousness are also common.

Saccular Aneurysms

Incidence and Importance

Ruptured saccular aneurysms are a common and very serious medical problem. Approximately 6 percent of the population harbor aneurysms.[1] In a necropsy series of adult patients (20 years of age or older), about 10 percent in each decade have had saccular aneurysms. Fortunately, the annual incidence of rupture of saccular aneurysms is less, approximately 10 to 12 per 100,000.[2,3] Overall, ruptured aneurysms are more common in women: Although men dominate the age group below 40 years, women prevail after age 40.[4,5]

   Despite the low incidence of rupture, the high prevalence of aneurysms and the poor prognosis of patients with SAH make the social and economic consequences of this disease tremendous. Among 100 typical patients with SAH caused by ruptured aneurysms, it is estimated that 33 will die before reaching medical attention. Another 20 will die while in the hospital or will remain incapacitated from the original hemorrhage. Seventeen patients who survive the initial hemorrhage will deteriorate later, with 8 recovering and 9 suffering severe neurological sequelae.[6] Only 30 of the original 100 patients will do well, surviving without major disability. If the ruptured aneurysm remains surgically untreated, and the patient does not have recurrent hemorrhage during the first 6 months, about 3 percent of the remaining patients will rebleed each year.[7] Even among patients admitted to the hospital in good condition, the prognosis is poor. In one series, 29 percent of these patients died, and only 55 percent made a good recovery at 90 days.[8] Unfortunately, there is often a delay in referring patients with SAH to neurological and neurosurgical centers for treatment. In one series, among 150 consecutive patients with aneurysmal SAH, only 36 percent were referred within 48 hours, and the median time to referral was 3.6 days.[9] Tragically, delayed diagnosis by physicians and both logistic and policy issues accounted for more than 70 percent of the delays.[9]

Pathogenesis

Saccular aneurysms typically form at arterial bifurcations (see Figure 2.15). Common sites in the anterior circulation are the junction between the anterior communicating artery and the anterior cerebral artery (ACA); the bifurcation of the middle cerebral artery (MCA); and the ICA junction with the ophthalmic artery, posterior communicating artery, anterior choroidal artery (AChA), and MCAs. In the posterior circulation, the apex of the basilar artery and the origins of the posterior inferior cerebellar artery (PICA) and the superior cerebellar artery (SCA) from the basilar artery are common sites. About 25 percent of patients with aneurysms have more than one.[1] Saccular aneurysms are more common in patients with polycystic kidney disease, coarctation of the aorta, fibromuscular dysplasia, pseudoxanthoma elasticum (PXE), and Marfan's syndrome.

At present, there is no completely satisfactory explanation of the origin, growth, and rupture of saccular aneurysms. Intracerebral arteries are normally composed of an outer collagenous adventitia, a prominent muscular media, an internal elastic lamina, and an intima lined by endothelial cells. There is no external elastic lamina. Intracranial arteries are more susceptible than extracranial vessels to aneurysm formation because, intracranially, the arterial walls are thin, there is less elastin, there is no external elastic lamina, and vessels lying in the subarachnoid space lack surrounding supporting tissue. Various theories cite congenital and genetic abnormalities causing defects in the arterial media, hypertensive and atherosclerotic degenerative changes in the vessel walls, inflammatory proliferative arteritis, and focal degeneration of the internal elastic lamina. Some investigators emphasize that aneurysms form because of congenital defects in the media of arteries. These medial defects are focally absent muscular media, often located at arterial bifurcations.

A plausible and inclusive hypothesis was proposed by Ferguson,[10] who suggested that cerebral aneurysms result from mechanically induced degeneration of arteries. There is maximal hemodynamic stress at the apices and bifurcations of vessels. Imbalance between the strength of a vessel at a particular bifurcation and the hemodynamic stresses applied to it lead to degeneration of the internal elastic lamina and aneurysmal outpouching. Turbulent flow in and around aneurysms produces vibration in vessel walls, further weakening the vessel's structural integrity and allowing aneurysm growth.[10] The observation that aneurysms may form either at sites of increased flow feeding AVMs or in vessels providing collateral blood flow supports the contention that increased pressure and flow contributes to aneurysm formation. Vessel-wall stress increases as aneurysms become thinner, the radius of the aneurysm enlarges, or the intra-aneurysmal pressure increases because of elevated blood pressure. When the wall stress exceeds the wall strength, aneurysms rupture.

Aneurysms may rupture at any time, but especially when blood pressure or blood flow are increased. Rupture often occurs during strenuous activity, such as weight lifting, exercise, coition, defecation, and heavy work. However, many aneurysms leak during relatively inactive periods. One third of the aneurysms in the Cooperative Study of Intracranial Aneurysms and SAH[5,6] ruptured while patients were asleep, and another third occurred during ordinary daily activities.[11] Size also plays a major role; up to a point, the larger the aneurysm, the more likely it is to rupture. In different autopsy series, the critical size for rupture has varied from 4 to 10 mm.[12–15]

Aneurysms greater than 2.5 cm in size are usually referred to as "giant aneurysms." The notion that they rarely rupture and produce SAH is erroneous. Drake reported that 33 percent of giant aneurysms present with bleeding, and another 10 percent have a history of remote hemorrhage.[16] Giant aneurysms often have intra-aneurysmal thrombi.

Once an intracranial aneurysm has ruptured, the course is often stormy and the outcome poor. It is estimated that of the 28,000 victims of ruptured aneurysms each year in the United States and Canada, 7,000 are misdiagnosed, never referred, or referred too late for definitive therapy.[9,17] The greatest impact in improving morbidity and mortality from SAH will not be through the efforts of neurologists or neurosurgeons, but rather through early recognition of SAH by primary-care physicians. Diagnosed early, these patients can be referred, while still relatively intact, to centers with appropriate neurological, neurosurgical, neuroradiological, and neuroanesthetic capabilities. Neurological intensive care units (ICUs) are also important for definitive treatment of ruptured aneurysms and their complications.

Clinical Findings

A 32-year-old woman, PN, came to the emergency ward because of a headache that had been unremitting for 48 hours. She had had migraine headaches as an adolescent. One month ago, she awakened at night with moderately severe headache and vomiting. After that headache had persisted for 3 days, she consulted her physician, who diagnosed "the flu." Although she had no fever, she felt too ill to do her daily chores and stayed in bed for 1 week, after which the headache gradually cleared. Two days ago, she developed a severe headache that came on very suddenly. She had been taking heavy trash cans out for garbage collection when the pain struck her in the right temple and top of the head and quickly radiated to the neck and back. Her knees buckled with the pain and she vomited. She stumbled into the house and was in bed and rather sleepy when her husband returned from work and insisted she go to the hospital.

Headache

Intracranial saccular aneurysms often present with a warning leak or socalled *sentinel hemorrhage*—a minute rent in the aneurysm leaks for only seconds, spilling blood into the subarachnoid space under high pressure. The patient has sudden severe headache, often occipital or nuchal in location, and constant. The headache generally resolves in 48 hours but can last longer. It is best distinguished from migraine by its rapidity of onset and longer duration. Only seconds elapse before it reaches maximum intensity. Migraine headaches, on the other hand, are usually more throbbing and build in intensity over minutes. Sentinel headaches usually last from days to a week, during which time patients are seldom able to continue normal activities. Unfortunately, sentinel hemorrhages are often misdiagnosed as migraine, flu, hypertensive encephalopathy, aseptic meningitis, cervical neck strain, or even gastroenteritis.[18]

In the patient PN, the headache 1 month earlier was probably a warning leak. The duration was too long for migraine, and inability to carry out daily activities should have alerted the physician to study her further. In the MRSR and the University of Illinois stroke registry, 31 percent of patients with SAH had sentinel headaches.[19] In the Danish Aneurysm Study, a warning leak was present in 166 of 1076 patients (15.4%).[20] In 99 of the 166 (54%) patients with warning leaks, the headache episode was evaluated by a doctor but was misdiagnosed.[20] Ostergaard emphasized that as many as 50 to 60 percent of patients with SAH have headache or other warning signs before presenting with major bleeds.[21] In patients with headaches of acute onset, the index of suspicion for SAH should be high and the threshold for lumbar puncture (LP) low. In patients with sudden severe headache without focal neurological signs, the only absolute contraindications to LP are no back and no needle. I feel that if series of LPs for headache contain only taps positive for blood, then too few LPs are being performed and sentinel hemorrhages are being missed.

PN's headache that began 2 days earlier was typical of that found in SAH. Sudden onset with rapid radiation, especially to the neck and back or sciatic region, suggests meningeal irritation. Often, the headache is accompanied by sudden loss of posture or alertness. Vomiting is common at outset. In migraine, vomiting more often comes later. The focal asymmetric headache is a fairly reliable sign that the bleeding lesion was on the right—that is, the side of the head pain.

Neurological Symptoms

Examination of PN showed a restless but sleepy woman with a stiff neck. The right eyelid was droopy, and when the lid was lifted, the right eye rested down and out. The right pupil was dilated and unreactive to light. Plantar responses were bilaterally extensor.

Aneurysms may present by compressing adjacent brain tissue or cranial nerves. Giant aneurysms are particularly noted for their tendency to cause focal symptoms and signs related to mass effect. Giant MCA aneurysms can cause seizures, hemiparesis, or dysphasia. The third nerve can be compressed by aneurysms of the ICA and posterior communicating artery junction or by SCA aneurysms. A giant SCA aneurysm can cause contralateral hemiplegia (Weber's syndrome) by compressing the pyramidal tracts in the midbrain. An isolated sixth-nerve paresis can be caused by mass effect. In the cavernous sinus, an aneurysm may compress the sixth, fourth, or third cranial nerves, producing ophthalmoplegia. Basilar bifurcation aneurysms that point forward can mimic pituitary tumors and can cause visual-field defects and hypopituitarism. Basilar bifurcation aneurysms that point vertically can cause an amnesic syndrome combined with third-nerve paresis, bulbar signs, and quadriparesis.[22] In this patient, the right third-nerve palsy suggested a right posterior communicating artery localization.

Rarely, aneurysms present with transient neurological deficits. These TIAs may be secondary to ischemia or seizures. Stewart et al. reported short, recurrent, stereotyped episodes in three patients with ischemia and in a fourth with transient spells secondary to partial complex seizures.[23] CT of the brain, LP, and EEG were all normal. No cardiac source of embolism could be identified. Cerebral arteriography showed aneurysms in appropriate locations to explain the symptoms in all cases. Clots may form within aneurysms, dislodge, and then embolize distally, causing stroke. Sutherland et al. have confirmed this hypothesis, showing deposition of platelets within giant aneurysms.[24] In three of the six patients in their series with active platelet deposition, episodes of recurrent transient neurological dysfunction occurred. Identification of aneurysms presenting in this manner is another indication for performing arteriography in patients with recurrent transient neurological deficits, particularly those in whom no cardiac source has been identified and those under 45 years of age. MRI scans now also often show heterogeneous signals, indicating thrombi within aneurysms (Figures 12.1 and 12.2).

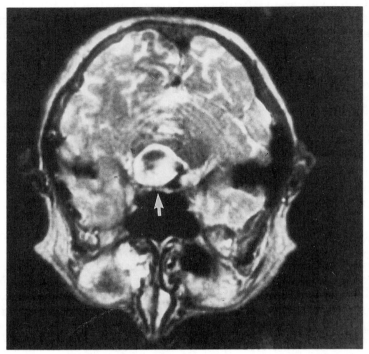

FIGURE 12.1   MRI, T2-weighted: White arrow points to large basilar artery aneurism containing heterogeneous signals representing thrombus formation.

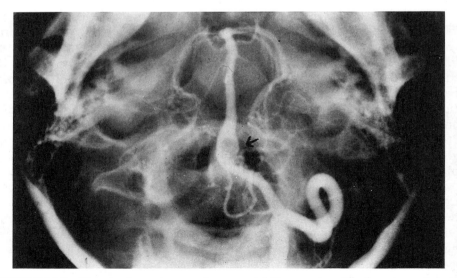

FIGURE 12.2   Vertebral arteriogram, intracranial Towns view: Black arrow points to a filling defect in a VA aneurysm, representing thrombus.

Patients with SAH usually report sudden-onset, constant headache that reaches maximal intensity within seconds. Nausea, vomiting, stiff neck, and transient loss of consciousness are common accompaniments. The patient is often quite agitated and restless. The headache is of such note that the patient is sometimes later able to describe in minute detail the circumstances surrounding the episode. SAH is rarely present without headache. Occasionally, I have cared for patients in whom the initial manifestation of the subarachnoid bleed was neck pain or backache, with sciatic radiation. Patients may not report headache if they have confusion, lethargy, aphasia, or amnesia for the event. Transient loss of consciousness is caused by the sudden increase of ICP that occurs as arterial blood suddenly enters the subarachnoid space. The increased ICP, dissection of blood into the optic-nerve sheath, and increased pressure in central retinal veins can cause retinal hemorrhages, usually subhyloid in location. These hemorrhages appear as large red masses of blood spreading outward from the optic disc into the retina. Papilledema may develop later. Unilateral or bilateral sixth-nerve paresis is also common and is a reflection of increased ICP. Some focal signs that suggest the sites of aneurysmal rupture have been previously discussed. Additional signs include

1. leg weakness, confusion, and bilateral Babinski signs in anterior communicating artery aneurysms[25]
2. homonymous hemianopia in PCA aneurysms
3. aphasia, hemiparesis, and anosognosia in MCA aneurysms
4. monocular visual disturbances in ophthalmic-artery aneurysms

Because aneurysms that have previously bled may become adherent to the adjacent brain, recurrent rupture often is characterized by both intracerebral and subarachnoid bleeding, so-called meningocerebral hemorrhage.

The patient's clinical state can be graded according to the scale of Hunt and Hess (Table 12.1),[26] which is useful for predicting short- and long-term prognosis.[27] In general, the higher the grade, the worse the prognosis. I classified patient PN as Hunt and Hess Grade II.

Laboratory Findings

Cranial CT in PN was suboptimal because of motion. There was diffuse opacification of the cortical gyri, and blood was visible in the basal cisterns. LP revealed bloody fluid, with an opening pressure of 420 torr. She was placed at bed rest and observed carefully.

Computed tomography

CT of the brain is the first diagnostic step in the evaluation of patients with suspected SAH. CT often verifies the presence of blood in the subarachnoid space and demonstrates associated intraparenchymal blood. The location of the blood may suggest the site of rupture.[25,28,29] A temporal-lobe hematoma or a collection of blood in the sylvian fissure suggests an MCA aneurysm. In

TABLE 12.1
Hunt and Hess Classification of Subarachnoid Hemorrhage

Classification	Symptoms
Grade I	Asymptomatic or minimal headache and slight nuchal rigidity
Grade II	Moderate to severe headache, nuchal rigidity, no neurological deficit other than cranial-nerve palsy
Grade III	Drowsiness, confusion, or mild focal deficit
Grade IV	Stupor, moderate to severe hemiparesis, possible early decerebrate rigidity and vegetative disturbance
Grade V	Deep coma, decerebrate rigidity, moribund appearance

Reprinted by permission from Hunt W, Hess R. Surgical risk as related to time of intervention in the repair of intracranial aneurysms. J Neurosurg 1968;28:14–20.

anterior communicating artery aneurysms, blood fills the subfrontal region, anterior intrahemispheric fissure, pericallosal cistern, and septum.[25] Large aneurysms greater than 10 mm in size are occasionally also demonstrated. In an infused CT scan, aneurysms appear as small, round densities on the circle of Willis. Giant aneurysms may also be shown as contrast-enhancing masses.[30,31] CT is not very good at detecting asymptomatic aneurysms; in one series, 14 of 85 aneurysms (16%) were seen on CT,[32] but in another series, none was detected.[33] The amount of blood helps predict the likelihood of subsequent vasospasm. CT may show a dilated ventricular system with hydrocephalus due to disturbance of CSF dynamics by blood clogging the basal cisterns and the pacchionian granulations. A normal CT scan does not rule out SAH; a normal scan occurs if the hemorrhage is small, especially if the scan is delayed 24 to 72 hours. In PN, SAH was confirmed by the CT; the amount of blood was moderate, but no local aneurysm or asymmetry of distribution was noted.

Magnetic resonance imaging

MRI is probably less sensitive than CT in showing acute subarachnoid blood.[34] However, AVMs—especially cavernous angiomas—are well seen on MRI as very well circumscribed structures with heterogeneous signals. MRA, a relatively new technique with rapidly developing improvements in technology, is a very promising noninvasive method of studying aneurysms. In one series, aneurysms as small as 3 to 4 mm were usually reliably detected by MRA, but some lesions (3 among 21 aneurysms) were missed.[35] Some vessels and aneurysms were not well imaged, and details were often insufficient for surgeons to define the neck and the extent of the aneurysms. At present, MRA is best used as a screening test for asymptomatic or large aneurysms but not as a definitive test in patients with SAH.

Lumbar puncture

I advocate LP as the next diagnostic step, especially if the CT is normal and clinical suspicion of SAH is still present.[36] The spinal fluid usually shows

1.   large numbers of RBCs without clearing of cells between the first and last tubes
2.   faint pink color of the supernatant fluid if examined within 4 to 5 hours of hemorrhage
3.   deep yellow (xanthochromic) color in the centrifuged supernatant fluid, secondary to breakdown of heme pigments; hemoglobin is first formed and later is transformed to bilirubin
4.   elevated protein
5.   pleocytosis, usually mononuclear
6.   increased pressure
7.   normal glucose

Spinal fluid obtained after 72 hours may show only an elevated pressure, xanthochromia, and increased protein. Spectrophotometry, by quantifying the amounts of hemoglobin and bilirubin, gives information about the age of the hemorrhage.[36]

Controversy exists as to the advisability of LP in confirmed SAH. Some argue that sudden lowering of pressure may provoke bleeding. I advocate LP even in CT-confirmed SAH. The initial LP gives a baseline pressure and quantification of the number of RBCs. This information may be useful later if the patient deteriorates and a second bleed is suspected. The level of CSF pressure is an important parameter to follow. Spinal tap also helps remove blood and CSF and, by lowering the CSF pressure, often relieves headache. Subsequent taps help to document the pressure and blood contents. Surgical complications are more common when the CSF pressure is over 180 torr at the time of operation.

Angiography

PN gradually became more alert, and her headache waned. By the third hospital day (5 days after onset of SAH), the plantar responses were flexor. Angiography showed a 7-mm irregular aneurysm at the junction of the right ICA and posterior communicating artery. There was no important focal or generalized vascular narrowing. On the next day, repeat LP showed an opening pressure of 160 torr and no fresh blood. Surgical clipping of the aneurysm was accomplished on the following day.

Cerebral angiography remains the definitive method of demonstrating intracranial aneurysms. Arterial digital subtraction angiography (DSA) is now the preferred technique, allowing excellent arterial opacification and rapid filming, with less dye. In patients with confirmed SAH, I delay angiography until the patient is considered operable. If the diagnosis is uncertain, however, I often pursue early angiography. Some physicians always obtain immediate arteriograms to define the bleeding aneurysm. If the patient is quite sick, definitive angiography is often difficult early, so I prefer to wait.

Vasospasm may also be potentiated by angiography, making complete studies difficult. In patient PN, I waited to perform angiography until she could be classified as Grade I. Because aneurysms may be multiple, all four intracranial arteries should be studied, with anteroposterior, lateral, and oblique views, if needed. If multiple aneurysms are identified, the bleeding aneurysm is usually

1.   the largest aneurysm
2.   the most irregularly shaped aneurysm
3.   the aneurysm with the most associated focal spasm, as discussed later in this chapter
4.   the aneurysm in the vascular territory explaining the focal signs
5.   the aneurysm that best explains the collection of blood on CT

At times, despite well-documented SAH, no aneurysm is identified angiographically. In general, the prognosis of these patients is better than when an aneurysm is demonstrated.[37]

Other diagnostic techniques

TCD is a very useful technology for detecting AVMs[38–41] and for monitoring the intracranial circulation for vasospasm.[38,42–45] Serial TCD measurements of flow velocities in the basal arteries after modest and large volume SAH often show an increase in velocities during days 3 to 10 and maximum velocities between days 11 and 20. Time-averaged maximum velocities in the MCA over 140 cm per second accurately predict vascular narrowing at angiography, and velocities over 200 cm per second predict severe vasospasm.[38] Doppler-measured velocities in the MCA have an inverse relationship with vascular diameter.

SPECT is also a useful test for monitoring for the presence of vasospasm. Regional hypoperfusion correlates well with vasospasm and delayed brain infarcts in patients with SAH.[46]

Differential Diagnosis

Van Gijn and colleagues noted that a high proportion of patients with SAH that is located predominantly in the perimesencephalic cisterns by CT, have normal angiography.[47,48] The clinical course in patients with perimesencephalic hemorrhage is also different from aneurysmal SAH because few patients die, rebleed acutely, or develop delayed cerebral infarction or hydrocephalus.[48] The outcome is much more benign than in patients with aneurysms shown by angiography.[49] As yet, the etiology of perimesencephalic hemorrhage is unknown.

Patients with SAH and normal angiography probably have a variety of different etiologies. I have seen a number of patients who had hemorrhage into the caudate nucleus, with extension into the ventricular system, simulating SAH.[50] AVMs also may involve the subependymal region and may bleed directly into the ventricles and the CSF. Before the era of CT scans, these and other intraventricular hemorrhages may have accounted for some examples of SAH with normal arteriography. Other explanations include

1. subarachnoid hemorrhage secondary to trauma
2. blood dyscrasias
3. a nonvisualizing angioma
4. an unseen small aneurysm
5. thrombosis of an aneurysm at or near the time of rupture
6. leakage from a small nonaneurysmal artery on the brain surface[51]
7. spinal AVMs

The possibility of an erroneous diagnosis of SAH must also be entertained; other conditions—such as cerebral venous thrombosis, tumor, infection, or traumatic LP—can mimic SAH. If the clinical picture is characterized by back pain, radicular signs, or myelopathic signs, I order a spinal MRI and prone and supine myelograms, looking for a spinal AVM. In situations where vasospasm is prominent but no aneurysm is seen, I repeat angiography after the clinical state improves, to better visualize the intracranial arteries.

Complications of Aneurysmal Subarachnoid Hemorrhage and Their Management

Rebleeding

Management of patients with SAH can be one of the most difficult problems in clinical medicine today. The complications are myriad, and management trends change almost yearly. Table 12.2 lists common complications of SAH, during both the acute and the later period. The most feared complication in patients with SAH is recurrent aneurysmal rupture. Rebleeding is heralded by sudden abrupt severe headache, meningismus, focal signs associated with intraparenchymal hemorrhage, and rapid development of coma. Among aneurysms that rebleed, about 20 percent will do so in the first 2 weeks, 30 percent by the end of the first month, and 40 percent by the end of 6 months. Beyond 6 months, rerupture occurs at a rate of 3 percent per year.[2,5] Rebleeding is associated with 40 percent mortality.[5] No infallible rules predict which patients will have recurrent hemorrhage.

Efforts are directed to reducing those factors that may promote rebleeding. Patients are placed at bed rest, with minimal stimuli. Pain is controlled with analgesics. Sedatives are used. Patients are kept from straining at stool, by regular use of laxatives and stool softeners. These measures are attempts to avoid elevations in blood pressure, which could increase intra-aneurysmal pressure and so increase the risk of rebleeding.

TABLE 12.2
Complications of Subarachnoid Hemorrhage (The Nine H's)

Early
  Hypertension (intracranial)
  Hypertension (systemic)
  Heart failure and arrhythmia
  Hematoma
Delayed
  Hemorrhage (rebleed)
  Hypoperfusion (vasospasm)
  Hydrocephalus
  Hypovolemia
  Hyponatremia

Blood pressure control

Care must be taken in managing blood pressure. Elevated ICP causes an increase in venous pressure inside the cranium. In order to perfuse the brain, an arteriovenous pressure gradient must be maintained so that systemic blood pressure rises. Ordinarily, if the blood pressure is not excessively high, I do not routinely lower it, especially if vasospasm is present. If the blood pressure is excessive (for example, above 160/100 torr), I do attempt to reduce it while carefully monitoring the patient's level of alertness and neurological signs, to ensure that hypoperfusion does not develop as the pressure is lowered. If blood pressure remains excessive, I prescribe hydrochlorothiazide, low doses of propranolol, nifedepine, angiotensin-converting-enzyme inhibitors such as captopril or enalapril, or sodium nitroprusside. I prefer sodium nitroprusside because of its rapid and easily titratable effects.[52] There are no absolute levels of blood pressure to aim for; rather, the patient's clinical state should be observed to ensure that there is adequate blood flow and cerebral perfusion.

Antifibrinolytic agents

Antifibrinolytic agents have been used in patients with SAH, to prevent rebleeding.[53,54] The commonest antifibrinolytic drug used is Amicar (epsilon aminocaproic acid), which is usually given in a dose of 24 gm/day intravenously for 3 days, followed by oral administration for 3 weeks or until surgery. Antifibrinolytic agents inhibit plasmin by partially blocking the conversion of plasminogen to plasmin and by binding with the receptor protein on the portion of the plasmin that binds fibrin.[53] Inhibition of plasmin activity prevents lysis of the clot that covers the rent in the aneurysm, allowing endothelial repair and development of fibrous tissue to replace the clot.

Hypothetically, antifibrinolytic therapy might predispose to clotting or hypercoagulability. Phlebothrombosis is already a very significant problem in patients with SAH on prolonged bed rest; antifibrinolytic agents could exaggerate this hazard. Kassell and colleagues reviewed the experience of the Cooperative Study of Intracranial Aneurysms and SAH,[5,6] with respect to antifibrinolytic drugs.[55] Although Amicar decreased the rate of rebleeding, it did not improve morbidity or mortality. Vasospasm, thrombophlebitis with pulmonary embolism, and hydrocephalus were all more common in patients given antifibrinolytic agents.[55] Though they may be useful in selected patients with high potential for rebleeding, antifibrinolytic agents have too many adverse effects to be recommended for general use in patients with SAH.

Delayed cerebral ischemia (vasospasm)

Second only to rebleeding as a cause of significant morbidity and mortality is vasoconstriction. *Vasoconstriction* is defined as abnormal narrowing of intracranial arteries. Vasoconstriction has customarily been called "vasospasm." Purists argue that the *constriction* may be structural, while *spasm* usually refers to functional reversible changes. I use the term *vasospasm* here but am cognizant of the dispute over names. The pathogenesis of vasospasm is unknown but is probably related to the release of substances into the CSF from the subarachnoid blood and to the interaction of these substances within the arteries in the subarachnoid space. The most likely putative substance is oxyhemoglobin, which affects the function of platelet-derived growth factor (PDGF), released from platelets adherent to the arterial wall; endothelial factors, especially endothelial-derived relaxing factor (EDRF); components of the coagulation cascade, especially thrombin, plasmin, and fibrinogen.[56-58] There is either an abnormal contraction or failure of relaxation of the arterial smooth muscle. Patients who die from SAH with vasospasm less than 3 weeks after the initial hemorrhage show necrosis of the media, while patients who live longer than 3 weeks show marked concentric intimal thickening, subendothelial fibrosis, and medial atrophy.[59-61] In experimental animals subjected to SAH, intracranial arteries show severe subintimal proliferation, fibrosis of medial smooth muscle, and interruption of the internal elastic membrane.[62]

SAH probably induces vasospasm, which is then followed by arterial wall necrosis. Vasospasm usually has its onset 3 to 5 days after the hemorrhage. The peak timing for vasospasm is 5 to 9 days, with most vasospasm resolving after the second to fifth week.[56,63,64] Vasoconstriction also occurs postoperatively, probably because of the handling of arteries and at times is due to intraoperative bleeding. Vasospasm has been detected arteriographically in 30 to 70 percent of SAH patients.[65] Angiographic diagnosis is based on the narrowed appearance of the intracranial arteries.[66] Severe vasospasm is associated with a lumen size of less than 0.5 mm, with delayed forward flow, and with evidence of collateral flow from anastomotic circulation. Some vessels are diffusely narrowed, whereas others show focal constrictions. Fortunately, only about half of the patients with arteriographically demonstrable vasospasm are symptomatic.

Early signs of spasm include tachycardia, hypertension, electrocardiographic changes, and decreased level of consciousness. Many patients, especially those with diffuse vasospasm, develop signs of diffuse brain dysfunction, including headache, stupor, and confusion. Focal signs often accompany these global signs and depend on the vessel involved. Most often, the severest vasospasm is in the vessel harboring the aneurysm or lying within the surrounding blood clot. Occasionally, maximal spasm occurs at a distance from the aneurysm. Patients with MCA vasospasm develop hemiparesis, hemisensory loss, aphasia, anosognosia, and confusion. With ACA vasospasm, there may be weakness in one or both lower extremities, abulia, and apraxia. PCA territory ischemia causes hemianopia and hemisensory loss. CT scan of the brain provides confirmatory data, ruling out intraparenchymal hemorrhage and hydrocephalus as a cause of the delayed deterioration. Focal hypodensity, representing infarction, is often seen.

The following findings correlate with the development of significant vasospasm:

1. thick blood clots localized in the subarachnoid cisterns[67] and the amount of subarachnoid blood[67,68]
2. lumen size less than 0.5 mm, with low distal perfusion[66]
3. aneurysms located on the circle of Willis[69]
4. decreased level of consciousness[68]
5. intraventricular blood[68]
6. treatment with antifibrinolytic agents (treatment increases likelihood of vasospasm)[68]

The ideal treatment of vasospasm is prevention. Prevention to date has taken three directions: early surgery, volume expansion, and prophylactic drug regimens.[70,71] Blood can be washed from the subarachnoid space during early surgery, and some authors report a low incidence of symptomatic vasospasm in those patients in whom postoperative CT scanning showed removal of blood.[71-73] The only nonsurgical therapy that has been proven effective in preventing delayed cerebral ischemia is expansion of intravascular volume.[56,70,74,75] Blood and serum volumes are often low in patients with SAH.[76] Patients with normal blood volumes seldom have symptomatic ischemia, despite angiographically shown vasoconstriction.[76] Aggressive volume expansion, either given prophylactically to all patients with SAH or only to those with demonstrated vasospasm, is effective in decreasing the incidence of infarction.[75] Volume expansion has no known effect on the vascular narrowing but maintains CBF above ischemic thresholds by increasing cardiac output and improving blood rheology.[75-77]

Since 1980, interest has centered around the use of calcium-channel blocking agents, especially nimodipine. A preliminary trial by Allen and colleagues, reported in 1983, suggested the possibility that nimodipine might decrease the incidence and severity of vasospasm and could improve outcome.[78] A prospective randomized trial conducted in British neurosurgical units showed some benefit from nimodipine use.[79] In this study, 60 mg of nimodipine, given orally every 4 hours, was started on admission and was continued for 21 days. In patients treated with nimodipine, there were fewer episodes of delayed ischemia and infarction, and fewer treated patients had poor outcomes.[79] Subsequent experience with nimodipine, nicardipine, and other calcium-channel blocking agents showed that these drugs can cause decreased blood pressure and decreased renal function, especially when given intravenously. Although these drugs may diminish vasoconstriction, they do not seem to improve outcome when volume expansion is used liberally. Thus, enthusiasm for treatment of SAH patients with nimodipine has waned considerably.

Since 1989, patients with vasoconstriction that was demonstrated angiographically, who have related neurological symptoms, have been treated by interventional radiologists with transluminal angioplasty, using various catheter devices.[80,81] The technology is quite new and changes almost daily. Unfortunately, at present, only a few physicians are trained and experienced in these intravascular interventions. Clearly, this treatment shows great promise for the future.

At present, it seems prudent to prevent hypovolemia by the liberal use of fluids orally and intravenously in all patients with SAH. In those with vasoconstriction shown angiographically, vigorous volume expansion and maintenance of blood pressure should be pursued. This is best supervised in an ICU, and usually, measurement of pulmonary wedge pressures are needed during aggressive volume expansion. ICP monitoring is also helpful, to follow the effects of osmotic diuretics, steroids, and fluid removal on ICP and on CBF. TCD and SPECT are also useful in monitoring blood-flow velocities in the basal arteries and hemispheric blood flow. Surgery should be performed as early as possible when patients are in good condition.[82] I do not routinely give nimodipine but do believe that further studies using calcium-channel blockers are warranted.

Hydrocephalus

In addition to rebleeding and vasospasm, other complications can lead to deterioration of patients with ruptured aneurysms. Acute hydrocephalus is caused by alteration in normal CSF dynamics. CSF flow is blocked by blood in the cisterns around the brainstem, and reabsorption is impaired when blood attaches to the pacchionian granulations. The syndrome can be recognized by increasing headache, lethargy, incontinence, and decreased spontaneity. Diagnosis can be readily confirmed by noncontrast CT scans. In a very large study of the timing of aneurysm surgery, the authors analyzed factors that predicted hydrocephalus among 3521 patients with SAH, who were admitted within 3 days of bleeding.[83] The factors that increased the likelihood of hydrocephalus were older age, hypertension (by history, admission blood pressure, and postoperative measures), thick local or diffuse blood on CT, intraventricular hemorrhage, use of antifibrinolytic drugs, and reduced level of consciousness.[83] Often, repeat LPs are adequate to treat ventricular enlargement, which often becomes obvious early after SAH. A few patients will need ventricular drainage shunts. In the months to years that follow SAH, normal-pressure hydrocephalus may develop, as the arachnoid becomes fibrotic, and adhesions prevent normal CSF flow.

Cardiac complications

Cardiopulmonary complications often occur in patients with SAH. Careful surveillance for cardiac rhythm disturbances, heart failure, and MI is required. I monitor cardiac rhythm, obtain baseline and follow-up ECGs and cardiac enzymes, and carefully watch for clinical signs of congestive heart failure. Severe SAHs can be accompanied by both ECG changes and enzyme elevations mimicking MI.[84-86] Most common are so-called waterfall T waves, which are seen across the endocardium. Subendocardial hemorrhages and myofibrillary degeneration have been noted at necropsy.[87,88] Cardiac muscle cells die in a hypercontracted state. Early calcium entry with calcifications are seen in regions of myocytolysis. ECG changes include alterations in QRS configuration, Q–T interval prolongation, T-wave abnormalities, and S–T segment elevation or depression.[89-91]

In a prospective study of cardiac-rhythm disturbances in 15 patients who had no known underlying cardiac disease, hypoxemia, or electrolyte abnormalities, all had transient cardiac arrhythmias.[90] Most patients with arrhythmia had no clinical hemodynamic symptoms. The commonest arrhythmias were sinus bradycardia, sinus tachycardia, and the tachy–bradycardia syndrome. Four patients showed more severe life-threatening arrhythmias: 3 patients had ventricular tachycardias, and 1 had atrioventricular dissociation. A prolonged Q–T interval was a frequent harbinger of subsequent ventricular arrhythmias. Ventricular arrhythmias often occurred in patients who subsequently died.

Elevated circulating serum catecholamines or sympathetic discharges originating from the hypothalamus and affecting the myocardium may be responsible for these changes.[89,91] The cardiac lesions probably represent excitotoxin-induced injury. Although ECG changes are common, MI is rare.[86]

Cardiac abnormalities are occasionally accompanied by both clinical and necropsy evidence of pulmonary edema. In one series of 178 fatal SAHs, 71 percent had necropsy evidence of pulmonary edema, recognized clinically in only 31 percent.[92] Pulmonary edema is neurogenic in origin. It is characterized by rapid onset, high protein in the edema fluid, and acutely elevated ICP. Weir suggested that pulmonary edema is caused by an acute rise in ICP, which triggers a massive autonomic discharge that results in increased cerebral perfusion but accumulation of fluid within the lungs and hypoxemia.[92] Treatment is directed both at lowering ICP and at eliminating excess fluid. Intubation, controlled ventilation, positive end-expiratory pressure, osmotic and loop diuretics, and drainage of spinal fluid may all be needed.

Fluid and electrolyte abnormalities

Less common, but still an important cause of neurological worsening, are fluid and electrolyte abnormalities. Slight sodium and potassium shifts without clinical consequence occurred among 25 percent in one series of aneurysm patients.[93] Sodium levels were in the range of 130 to 135 meq/l, and potassium levels were in the range of 4.5 to 5 meq/l. In another 14 percent of patients, more severe abnormalities included 5 cases of diabetes insipidus, 2 disturbances of thirst regulation, 1 instance of inappropriate secretion of antidiuretic hormone, and 9 cases of serious sodium and potassium shifts.[93] In these cases, the serum sodium was less than 130 meq/l, and the potassium was greater than 5 meq/l. Hyponatremia is associated with a poor prognosis. Water and electrolyte disturbances are most frequent with aneurysms of the anterior communicating artery. In postmortem studies, severe fluid and electrolyte abnormalities are associated with hemorrhage or ischemic changes in the hypothalamus.[94] In the past, hyponatremia has been attributed to inappropriate secretion of antidiuretic hormone, but in 1991, it was shown that the plasma concentration of atrial natriuretic factor is elevated and is higher in those patients with suprasellar and intraventricular blood.[95] Peerless identified 30 additional less common causes of neurological deterioration after SAH, including enlargement of the aneurysm, seizures, pulmonary emboli, infection, medication side effects, renal failure, and hepatic failure.[96]

Surgery

The definitive treatment of an aneurysm is surgical obliteration. The patient is anesthetized using hypotensive anesthesia. The brain is made slack by using dehydrating agents and controlled removal of CSF, and the neurosurgeon uses a dissecting microscope to approach the aneurysm. Ideally, the aneurysm is clipped at its origin from the parent artery, at its neck. If this is not possible, the aneurysm may be trapped between two clips, wrapped in supportive material, or the feeding vessels may be obliterated. During operations to obliterate aneurysms, rebleeding and ischemic infarction may occur. Infarction is secondary to vessel injury during retraction of the brain or from injury to penetrating vessels as aneurysms are approached and treated. Amnesic syndromes are common after surgery for anterior-communicating-artery aneurysms, particularly if the aneurysms are trapped rather than ligated at their neck.[97,98] Trapping leads to disruption of the perforators that originate from the anterior communicating artery, with resultant ischemia in the area of the anterior wall of the third ventricle and the orbital frontal lobes and basal forebrain nuclei.[97,98]

There is little doubt that patients with surgical obliteration of aneurysms, if they survive surgery, do better in the long term than those who are treated only medically. The best timing for surgery remains controversial. Proponents of late surgery suggest that operations should be delayed until at least 10 to 14 days after the hemorrhage. The patient's medical condition should be optimal after medical complications have been treated. This technically difficult surgery will be easier to perform as the brain edema resolves and the clot and blood in the subarachnoid space are diminished. Rebleeding at the time of surgery will also be minimized, as the clot in the aneurysm will be better organized.

In contrast, proponents of early surgery suggest operation during the first 72 hours.[71,80] They argue that the surgery may be technically more difficult, but early operation affords two advantages. First, if the aneurysm is successfully clipped, the possibility of rebleeding is eliminated. Second, early surgery may also afford a better outcome with regard to vasospasm. If clot can be removed from the subarachnoid space at the time of surgery, vasospasm may be less likely to occur. If it does occur, because the aneurysm has been clipped, more aggressive medical treatment can be given.

I favor early surgery in Grade I or II patients. For these individuals, I order an early arteriogram, followed by prompt mobilization of the surgical team. For patients in higher grades, I favor the later time frame. I monitor the clinical signs, blood pressure, spinal fluid pressure, and blood-flow velocities, as shown with TCD. Surgery is performed when the patient becomes alert and in Hunt and Hess Grade I or II, when spinal fluid pressure is below 180 torr on spinal puncture, and when blood-flow velocities do not indicate severe vasoconstriction.

Unruptured Aneurysms

Management of patients with unruptured aneurysms presents a challenging problem in risk-factor analysis. An unruptured aneurysm may be discovered as part of the evaluation of another ruptured aneurysm, during investigation of a mass lesion, or during evaluation of another neurological problem, such as ischemic vascular disease. Unruptured aneurysms that are not compressing neural structures are thought to bleed at a rate of 2 to 3 percent per year.[99] Aneurysms that cause neurological symptoms rupture at a higher rate, with 15 percent bleeding within 6 months of onset of symptoms.[15] The operative mortality in patients with ruptured aneurysms and normal neurological function is 1.6 percent or less.[100] Therefore, surgical therapy can be recommended. However, the rate of aneurysm rupture is probably related to size. I concur with Kassell and Drake that the data support the idea that aneurysms 5 to 10 mm in size more often bleed than do smaller lesions.[17] I also agree that aneurysms larger than 5 mm should be surgically treated, if possible, in good-risk patients, while lesions smaller than 5 mm should be followed with arteriography. If these smaller aneurysms show growth, then surgical therapy can be undertaken. MRA may facilitate recognition of unruptured aneurysms because patients can be studied noninvasively as outpatients.

Once a cerebral aneurysm has ruptured, the course is stormy, and the prognosis may be grim, even in the best of hands. In order to make a major impact on the morbidity and mortality of cerebral aneurysms, there must be early recognition of this serious disease, so that appropriate therapy can be undertaken while the patient is still in good condition. I stress the need for a high index of suspicion of SAH and for a low threshold for use of LP in suspected cases.

Arteriovenous Malformations

AVMs are the second most common cause of nontraumatic SAH. AVMs are one tenth as common as aneurysms; an estimated 1000 new cases are identified each year in the United States.[101] Cerebral aneurysms have a peak incidence of rupture beyond the age of 30 years; AVMs, however, rupture more commonly in the second and third decades of life.[102] Hemorrhage from an AVM is not strictly limited to the subarachnoid space. Often, there is a large parenchymatous component.

Classification and Distribution

McCormick classified AVMs into five subtypes, based on the predominant vasculature.[103] Most common are *venous angiomas*, which are composed of anomalous veins; there is no direct arterial input. The next most common vascular abnormality is *telangiectasia*, usually found deep within the brain, particularly the brainstem; telangiectases are composed of vessels morphologically resembling capillaries but slightly larger; this vascular abnormality is often merely a curiosity found at the time of necropsy. Another less common vascular abnormality, which also rarely causes symptoms, is the *varix*, which is simply a dilated vein. The two most common symptomatic angiomas are *arteriovenous angiomas* and *cavernous angiomas*.

AVMs are clusters of abnormal vessels composed of arteries and veins of varying size, without intervening capillaries. The arteries within the cluster are large, thin-walled vessels with poorly developed internal elastic lamina and media, while the arteries feeding this abnormality have hypertrophic media and endothelial thickening.[103] The hypertrophic media and endothelial thickening sometimes lead to thrombosis of feeding vessels. Some studies have shown stenosis of afferent arteries feeding AVMs.[104]

Some patients with AVMs have more diffuse occlusive arterial disease despite the fact that they have no atherosclerotic risk factors.[105] Blood circulates rapidly through the central core of AVMs and is quickly shunted into the large dilated draining veins. The substance of cavernous angiomas is composed of vessels of a sinusoidal variety. Often, they have no large feeding artery and are termed *occult* because they are not opacified by catheter angiography and are therefore obscured from view.[106] Cavernous angiomas are often multiple and can be familial.[106–108]

Any part of the brain and spinal cord can harbor an angioma. Angiomas vary in size from microscopic to large. The cavernous malformations and AVMs are often larger than the other types and more commonly cause symptoms. Telangiectases are usually asymptomatic but can be a source of repeated small bleeds. Some very extensive malformations extend from the cortical surface to abut on the ventricular surface. Angiomas may be limited to the brain, the subarachnoid space, or the dura, or they may involve more than one of these regions. Angiomas are most common in the cerebral hemispheres (75%) and basal ganglia (18%); posterior-fossa angiomas (6%) are much less frequent.[109] In the posterior fossa, the pons is by far the most common location.[110] Angiomas that abut on either the ventricular or the meningeal surface may leak solely into the CSF, so that those patients present with symptoms and signs of SAH. The blood supply of large AVMs is usually extensive, originating from the anterior and posterior intracranial circulations, as well as from extracranial components. AVMs are believed to arise in early fetal life, as a result of the failure of primitive vessels to differentiate into normal arteries, veins, and capillaries. Despite their congenital origin, angiomas rarely produce symptoms during the first decade of life. The asymptomatic nature of lesions in early life is probably related to their small size and the inherent plasticity of the developing brain, which allows the function of one area of the brain to be assumed by another. Angiomas enlarge as individuals age. There is growth of the feeding arteries and draining veins and recruitment of additional vasculature. Malformations may enlarge for multiple reasons. Hook suggested that undifferentiated arteries and veins might not tolerate arterial pressure well and therefore would enlarge.[111] Small recurrent ICHs cause loss of brain substance, as clot and necrotic brain are reabsorbed. The decrease in supporting tissue around malformations might allow growth of the vascular anomaly.[112] Decreased strength of supporting tissue may also be caused by pulsation of arteries, which can damage the surrounding brain.

Clinical Symptoms and Signs

As malformations enlarge, symptoms are related to a number of mechanisms. Consider the following patient:

At 15 years, AG began to have spells in which she saw sparkling lights off to her left. Some spells were followed by loss of consciousness and a generalized seizure. By age 21, she noted progressive loss of vision toward her left. Four years later, during the first trimester of her first pregnancy, while shopping, she fell to the ground with a severe headache, nausea, vomiting, and a stiff neck. Examination showed a left homonymous hemianopia.

The most frequent and dramatic presentation of angiomas is bleeding. Fifty percent of symptomatic angiomas present in this manner,[111] as in the patient described. The immediate cause of the rupture is unknown but probably relates to fragility of the abnormal vessels. Vessels on the cortical or ventricular surfaces are more prone to rupture because they lack the support offered by the surrounding brain parenchyma. The angiomas that most frequently rupture are the arteriovenous type.[108] Symptoms and signs depend on the location of the hemorrhage. With CSF extension of blood, there are signs of meningeal irritation similar to those accompanying aneurysmal rupture. Not all ruptures are symptomatic. Frequently, patients with no clinical history of hemorrhage will show evidence of bleeding at surgery or necropsy. In one surgical series, 6 of 55 patients with angiomas had evidence of hemorrhage without recognized symptoms.[101]

In the years before the hemorrhage, AG had partial seizures with secondary generalization and progressive neurological signs. An estimated 46 percent of patients with angiomas present with epilepsy, and 21 percent have progressive neurological deficits.[113] Progressive symptoms are probably caused by two mechanisms: First, large volumes of blood may be shunted or stolen through the malformation to the venous circulation; this shunt could deprive adjacent brain tissue of blood, causing relative ischemia. Second, the ischemic process is aggravated by the pulsatile nature of the malformation; the pulsating blood vessels compress adjacent brain tissue and can lead to local atrophy. Also, partially ischemic tissue is prone to electrical instability and seizures.

Chronic headaches are also a frequent complaint in patients with vascular malformations. The headaches are often migrainous in nature, sometimes closely mimicking classic migraine. Unfortunately, there are no good rules to distinguish migrainous headaches related to vascular malformations. Migraine accompaniments that are always stereotyped and occur on the same side, or headaches always localized to the same side, should lead doctors to suspect AVM. Even patients with unruptured AVMs can have increased ICP and papilledema.[114] The increased pressure may contribute to headaches.

In the brainstem, angiomas may present with serious bleeding or gradually progressive neurological deficits. Depending on location, there may be cranial nerve, cerebellar, pyramidal, or sensory dysfunction. Some have a fluctuating course of neurological dysfunction, which may simulate multiple sclerosis.[115,116] Distinction between these two processes is possible. With angiomas, the neurological dysfunction can be localized to one site. CT or MRI shows hemorrhage or cystic changes at the site of prior bleeding. In demyelinating disease, confirmatory laboratory findings—such as the presence of oligoclonal bands, abnormal visual evoked responses, enhancing periventricular plaques, or other cerebral abnormalities on MRI—are helpful.

Rarely, angiomas present with hydrocephalus. In such cases, the mass of blood vessels can compress the ventricular system, disrupting the normal flow of CSF. Aneurysms of the vein of Galen are the most common cause of this rare presentation. Prior small bleeds can also block absorption of CSF, leading to hydrocephalus. Rarely, patients with large AVMs can present because of a bruit that is audible either to the patient or to the doctor. In children, large AVMs can produce enough shunting of blood to cause high-output congestive heart failure.

In the spinal cord, vascular malformations typically present with back pain, myelopathic symptoms, and root dysfunction. However, because headache so often accompanies spinal AVM rupture, cerebral sources of hemorrhage will often be sought, and the spinal origin can be missed. In one series, 80 percent of patients with spinal malformations had intracranial symptoms, including headache, mental status changes, loss of consciousness, papilledema, decreased vision, nystagmus, diplopia, seizures, sixth nerve paresis, and oculomotor paresis.[117]

Laboratory Findings

The diagnosis of vascular malformations can be suspected clinically. Typical features include

1. prior history of a seizure disorder or progressive neurological deficit
2. a patient in the second or third decade of life
3. SAH in a pregnant woman (Pregnancy is said to be a particularly hazardous time for women with AVMs; peak time for hemorrhages is when the cardiac output is increased, particularly early in pregnancy and during labor and delivery)[118]
4. clinical signs and symptoms of intraparenchymal and subarachnoid blood
5. cranial bruit

CT scan of the brain may be able to confirm the diagnosis. Serpiginous channels sometimes can be seen on plain CT and can be enhanced after IV contrast administration.[119,120] There is some debate over the optimal dose and timing of contrast-enhanced CT in order to best image AVMs. Hayman and colleagues studied the usefulness of various contrast doses and timings in some patients with small AVMs.[121] Delayed high-dose contrast documented one cryptic lesion not seen on plain or early contrast scans and demonstrated zones of encapsulated hemorrhage or infarction not seen in early studies. However, two venous angiomas seen on immediate scans were not visibly opacified on delayed studies. Moreover, in half of the patients, larger blood vessels faded on delayed scans, making the late scan less diagnostic than the early one.[121] Probably a combination of early and delayed scans is most helpful. In addition to the malformation, there may be both atrophy of brain and dilation of ventricles adjacent to the malformation. Small calcifications may be seen within malformations. Sometimes, frank cysts are also found adjacent to AVMs.[122] If there has been a recent hemorrhage, these recent findings may be obscured by the intraparenchymal, subarachnoid, and intraventricular blood. Rapid immediate radionuclide brain scans also successfully image large AVMs. MRI has definitely improved the diagnosis of AVMs and of cavernous angiomas. The latter usually appear as well-circumscribed, well-defined lesions, with a central core of mixed heterogenous signal intensity surrounded by a rim of signal void.[123-126] MRI can also be helpful by showing hemosiderin resulting from old hemorrhage, both in the lesion and in the adjacent meninges. MRA may help noninvasively to identify large AVM feeding arteries and veins.

TCD is also helpful in diagnosing and following AVMs.[38-41] The increased flow to the AVMs is associated with increased flow velocities in arteries feeding the malformations. At times, musical-type murmurs can be heard and unusual unmodulated high- or middle-frequency bands are seen on the Doppler spectrum.[40] Abnormal collateralization and steal effects can be found with reduction of mean and peak flow velocities in some arteries.[40] Changes in velocities can be monitored during therapeutic embolization and after surgical or radiation therapy.[41]

A detailed angiogram is needed to identify all possible arterial feeders. Angiographic features typical of vascular malformations are

1. large feeding arteries
2. a central tangle of vessels
3. enlarged, tortuous draining veins
4. rapid arterial-to-venous shunting of blood

Some angiographic findings—such as large size, presence of multiple feeding arteries, and drainage into peripheral cortical veins—correlate with the development of progressive neurological signs that have been attributed by some to stealing of blood from normal vessels to the malformations.[127] Four circumstances may arise in which the clinical syndrome appears to be an SAH secondary to a vascular malformation, but arteriography is normal: (1) There may have been spontaneous thrombosis of the malformation; this represents a self-cure. (2) With rupture, there may have been obliteration of the malformation, representing another cure. (3) Alternatively, the malformation may be a cavernous angioma, without a direct arterial feeder and therefore not visualized on angiography. (4) Finally, when a malformation or aneurysm is not found during the investigation of an SAH, a spinal malformation must be considered; the history and physical examination should be repeated, looking closely for a history of back pain and myelopathic or radicular symptoms and signs.

Prognosis

In the short term, the prognosis of ruptured AVMs and cavernous angiomas is better than that of aneurysms. The rebleeding rate is low during the first months. Only 6 percent rebleed during the first year,[128] and vascular spasm occurs only rarely. Mortality from the first hemorrhage is low, only about 10 percent. However, in the long term, the prognosis of vascular malformations is not as good. Estimates of recurrent hemorrhage during subsequent years vary from 1 percent in four to seven years[113] to 2 percent per year after the first year.[128] With subsequent hemorrhages, the mortality rate is higher, about 20 percent.[128]

With each recurrence, the chances of additional hemorrhages increase.[113] In one large series of 137 patients with AVMs treated conservatively between 1942 and 1967, 10 percent died of their AVMs, 24 percent were disabled, and only 40 percent were well at the time of the 1970 report;[128] by 7 years later, only 19 percent of the initial group were well.[129,130] Because AVMs tend to occur in younger patients, the probability that recurrent hemorrhage with severe disability or death will occur is substantial. Almost 50 percent of patients with recurrent hemorrhage will have some deterioration in working capacity or will become an invalid during the 20 to 40 years following the first hemorrhage.[131] There are no clear rules to predict which patients will have recurrent hemorrhage. Parietal, central, and infratentorial malformations may be more likely to bleed than frontal, temporal, or occipital malformations.[130] This poor prognosis necessitates an aggressive approach to the treatment of patients who present with hemorrhage from AVMs.

Patients who present with seizures alone have a better prognosis: there is only a 25 percent chance of a clinically symptomatic hemorrhage in 15 years.[131] In one long-term series of patients with seizures, there was only a 12 percent mortality and an additional 16 percent overall disability.[130] A more conservative approach, prescribing only anticonvulsant therapy for patients with seizures alone, is reasonable. Seizures can be well controlled by anticonvulsants, and surgical removal of malformations often does not improve seizure control.[132] Patients presenting with progressive neurological deficits have a poor prognosis, but these patients also often have the largest malformations, which are difficult to treat.[127]

Data are not available regarding long-term prognosis in patients with asymptomatic vascular malformations. These are usually discovered during the evaluation of other problems. With the advent of CT and MRI, it is now possible to collect information regarding the fate of these malformations and the outcome of patients who harbor them. Aminoff has argued convincingly for conservative management of most unruptured malformations.[132]

Treatment of Vascular Malformations

A 33-year-old, right-handed school teacher, BC, had occasional left-sided throbbing headaches while in college. At age 27 years, he had his first epileptic seizure, which began with a warm feeling in his right lip and tongue. The feeling rapidly spread to his hand, and then he lost consciousness. At age 33, while shoveling snow, he developed a severe diffuse headache and vomited. On examination, he was restless and complained of headache but had no abnormal neurological signs except a right extensor plantar response. LP showed blood-tinged CSF at a pressure of 210 torr. CT showed a thin layer of subarachnoid blood, and contrast injection opacified a very large sylvian group of tortuous veins. Angiography revealed a large parasylvian central AVM fed primarily from the left MCA.

How should this patient be treated? In this case, the diagnosis of AVM is certain. The prodromal history of headaches and seizures was typical. The present bleed was subarachnoid, arising from the surface of the lesion. There was no intraparenchymatous hematoma, either clinically or by CT. In this patient, surgery or embolization carries the risk of aphasia or right hemiparesis, each possibly disabling. Because there were no important neurological signs, I chose to watch the patient during the next years to see the natural history of the lesion. If he had presented with an intracerebral hematoma and had had aphasia and right hemiplegia, the situation would have been quite different, and surgery might have been indicated.

There are four therapeutic options available that can be used in combination or alone to treat AVMs: (1) surgery, (2) interventional radiology including embolization, (3) radiotherapy, and (4) a strictly medical approach.

Surgery

A surgical approach is the oldest. Initially, neurosurgeons ligated the major feeding vessels to the malformation. This method of treatment has been largely abandoned because of its failure to obliterate the lesion and the hazards inherent in the procedure. Stroke often occurred as blood flow to normal brain was interrupted. The malformations continued to draw blood from the nonligated, deep inaccessible vessels.

Direct surgical excision of lesions has been improved with the use of the operating microscope. Lesions are meticulously approached, avoiding critical cerebral vessels and vital neurological structures. Operations may be performed using local anesthesia and with evoked response control, so that the exact location of vital areas can be accurately determined. Dissection is done, if possible, in the gliotic plane that surrounds the tangle of vessels, so that malformations can be removed en bloc. Surgical excision can be carried out in appropriate patients with a low morbidity and mortality.[101,129,130]

The major complications of surgical excision are loss of normal brain tissue, with additional loss of neurological function, and the so-called *breakthrough phenomenon*.[133] This term is used to describe massive brain swelling and ICH occurring postoperatively, which is caused by redirection of the large volume of blood that previously flowed into the malformation into the small vessels surrounding the malformation. These vessels are unable to handle the large volume of blood, and cerebral edema or hemorrhage results.[133]

Interventional radiology approaches, including embolization

Embolization of AVMs can be used alone, prior to surgery, or at the time of surgery. Initially, small pellets were used to fill the abnormal vessels within the central nidus. Because flow to malformations is increased, pellets released into feeding arteries tend to travel to the malformations. There, they occlude the lumens of vessels, it is hoped, in sufficient quantity to thrombose the vascular malformation. However, the particle embolization technique has many problems. Emboli rarely enter arteries with acute or right angles. Furthermore, as vessels within malformations become occluded, flow to the malformations equals the flow to the normal brain, and particles stray into the normal circulation, causing ischemia. Advances reported in 1991 have greatly improved the embolization technique.[134]

Since the early 1980s, calibrated-leak balloon catheters have been advanced into feeding arteries, close to the malformation. Next, a rapidly setting tissue adhesive such as isobutyl-2-cyanoacrylate is released.[135] It forms a clot in the segment of the lesion irrigated predominantly by that artery. Several feeding arteries are then injected. This technique often reduced the size of the lesion but rarely totally obliterated the abnormality.

Embolization can also be done at the time of surgery, when the material can be injected into cannulized blood vessels. Complications of this technique, in addition to postembolization hemorrhage related to altered blood flow, include hemorrhage or ischemic stroke, induced by the balloon catheter; gluing of the balloon catheter complex in place by the tissue adhesive; or occlusion of normal arteries by the plastic material. Also, buccylate is toxic to tissues and causes angionecrosis and does escape into the extravascular spaces.[136]

Endovascular techniques are especially important in treating lesions that are not very surgically accessible and as an adjunct to surgical removal. Newer imaging technology has clearly facilitated the use of various interventional techniques.

Radiotherapy

Attempts have been made to use radiotherapy to obliterate AVMs. High energy from conventional x-rays, gamma rays, or protons induces subendothelial deposition of collagen and hyaline substances, which narrow the lumen of small vessels and shrink the nidus of the malformation by progressive occlusion of vessels during the months after treatment.[137] Newer techniques focus the radiation beam on small regions. An example is the so-called *gamma knife,* a system that uses a cobalt source to generate highly collimated gamma rays that converge on a focal point. Modified linear accelerators can now deliver radiation to a defined volume of tissue with very good accuracy. Radiation necrosis occurs in about 9 percent of patients.[138] About 40 percent of AVMs are obliterated in 1 year, 84 percent after 2 years, and 97 percent after 3 years.[138] Bleeding has occurred after treatment, especially during the period of obliteration. Recent reports on the use of Bragg-peak proton-beam radiotherapy[137] and stereotactic helium-ion Bragg-peak radiation[139] have been very encouraging. Complications include radionecrosis of normal brain; hydrocephalus; immediate post-therapy seizures; loss of body temperature regulation; and possibly long-term cognitive-function deficits. Further data will be needed before the frequency of these complications and the therapeutic utility of focused radiotherapy may be known. At present, focused radiotherapy is probably best reserved for rather small deep lesions not easily amenable to surgery that have bled.

Medical approach

The most conservative therapeutic option for AVMs is a medical approach. Blood pressure is strictly controlled within the normal range. Anticoagulants and platelet-antiaggregant drugs are avoided. Because the rate of hemorrhage in pregnant women with AVMs is relatively high, I discuss the risk of pregnancy in fertile women and suggest appropriate contraception if desired.

Vascular malformations, if left untreated, are hazardous, but as yet, no one therapeutic option is entirely successful or without risk. Treatment of the vascular lesion is often complicated by numerous feeding arteries, extensive size, or location within the brain parenchyma in areas vital to normal neurological function. Decisions regarding therapy must consider these factors. Of additional importance is the age of the patient and the mode of presentation. These two factors are major determinants of the natural history of the disease.

For the most common mode of presentation, ICH, I recommend an aggressive approach, including surgery or surgery combined with embolization if the following criteria are met:

1. The patient is relatively young (less than 55 years and has a life expectancy of greater than 15 years).

2.   Recovery of neurological function after the hemorrhage is moderately good, so that a reasonable life-style can be anticipated.
3.   The malformation is superficial in location and does not extensively involve vital neurological structures—so-called eloquent brain.

Because the rate of early rebleeding is very low, I wait until the patient is in good medical condition before suggesting surgery. The presence of a remaining neurological deficit related to the bleeding is a factor favoring surgery, while postbleed return to complete normality would argue against surgery.

I adopt a more conservative approach utilizing embolization, radiotherapy if available, or strictly medical management if the following criteria are met:

1.   The patient is older than 55 or 60, and life expectancy is less than 10 years.
2.   The deficit from the initial hemorrhage is severe.
3.   The malformation is extensive, deep within the dominant hemisphere, in the brainstem, or in other vital eloquent areas.

I use these same criteria for patients who present with progressive neurological deficits.

I treat patients who present with seizures medically. Anticonvulsants are given to control the spells, blood pressure is regulated, and anticoagulants and platelet antiaggregating drugs are avoided. If seizures remain intractable despite medical therapy, a more aggressive plan utilizing surgical excision might be considered.

In asymptomatic patients (including those with only headache), I follow a conservative medical approach. Because the natural history of asymptomatic lesions is unknown, it is unreasonable to undertake therapy that may be more hazardous than the lesion itself. Furthermore, initial hemorrhages are rarely fatal; if a hemorrhage does occur, the opportunity for more aggressive therapy will be available.

References

1.   McCormick WF. The natural history of intracranial saccular aneurysms. Neurol Neurosurg (Weekly Update) 1978;1(3):2.
2.   Parkarinen S. Incidence, etiology, and prognosis of primary subarachnoid hemorrhage: a study based on 589 cases diagnosed in a defined urban population during a defined period. Acta Neurol Scand 1967;43(Suppl 29):1–128.
3.   Phillips LH, Whisnant JP, O'Fallan W, et al. The unchanging pattern of subarachnoid hemorrhage in a community. Neurology 1980;30:1034–1040.

4. Garraway WM, Whisnant JP, Furlan AJ, et al. The declining incidence of stroke. N Engl J Med 1979;300:449–452.

5. Locksley HB. Report of the Cooperative Study of Intracranial Aneurysms and Subarachnoid Hemorrhage: sec V, pt I. natural history of subarachnoid hemorrhage, intracranial aneurysms, and arteriovenous malformation—based on 6,368 cases in the cooperative study. J Neurosurg 1966;25:219–239.

6. Locksley HB. Report of the Cooperative Study of Intracranial Aneurysms and Subarachnoid Hemorrhage: sec V, pt II. natural history of subarachnoid hemorrhage, intracranial aneurysms, and arteriovenous malformation. J Neurosurg 1966;25:321–368.

7. Heros RC, Kistler JP. Intracranial arterial aneurysms, an update: current concepts of cerebrovascular disease. Stroke 1983;14:628–631.

8. Winn WR, Richardson AE, Jane JA. The long-term prognosis in untreated cerebral aneurysms: I. the incidence of late hemorrhage in cerebral aneurysms—a ten year evaluation of 364 patients. Ann Neurol 1977;1:358–370.

9. Kassell NF, Kongable GL, Torner JC, et al. Delay in referral of patients with ruptured aneurysms to neurosurgical attention. Stroke 1985;16:587–590.

10. Ferguson GG. Physical factors in the initiation, growth, and rupture of human intracranial saccular aneurysms. J Neurosurg 1972;37:666–677.

11. Adams HP, Kassell N, Torner JC, et al. Early management of aneurysmal subarachnoid hemorrhage. J Neurosurg 1981;54:141–145.

12. Locksley HB. Natural history of subarachnoid hemorrhage, intracranial aneurysms and arteriovenous malformation. In: Sahs A, Perret G, Locksley H, Nishioke H, eds. Intracranial aneurysms and subarachnoid hemorrhage: a cooperative study. Philadelphia: Lippincott, 1969:37–108.

13. Crompton MR. Mechanism of growth and rupture in cerebral berry aneurysms. Br Med J 1966;1:1138–1142.

14. McCormick WF, Acosta-Rua GJ. The size of intracranial saccular aneurysms: an autopsy study. J Neurosurg 1970;33:422–427.

15. Wiebers DO, Whisnant JP, O'Fallon WM. The natural history of unruptured intracranial aneurysms. N Engl J Med 1981;304:696–698.

16. Drake CG. Giant intracranial aneurysm: experience with surgical treatment in 174 patients. In: Carmel PW, ed. Clinical neurosurgery. Baltimore: Williams & Wilkins, 1979:12–95.

17. Kassell N, Drake CG. Review of the management of saccular aneurysms. In: Barnett HJM, ed. Neurological clinics: vol 1. cerebrovascular disease. Philadelphia: Saunders, 1983:73–86.

18. Adams HP, Jergenson DD, Kassell NF, Sahs AL. Pitfalls in the recognition of subarachnoid hemorrhage. JAMA 1980;244:794–796.

19. Gorelick PB, Hier DB, Caplan LR, Langenberg P. Headache in acute cerebrovascular disease. Neurology 1986;36:1445–1450.

20. Hauerberg J, Andersen BB, Eskesen V, et al. Importance of the recognition of a warning leak as a sign of a ruptured intracranial aneurysm. Acta Neurol Scand 1971;83:61–64.

21. Ostergaard JR. Warning leak in subarachnoid haemorrhage. Brit Med J 1990;301:190–191.

22. Drake CG. The treatment of aneurysms of the posterior circulation. In Carmel PW, ed. Clinical neurosurgery. Baltimore: Williams & Wilkins, 1979:96–144.

23. Stewart RM, Samsom D, Diehl J, et al. Unruptured cerebral aneurysms presenting as recurrent transient neurological deficits. Neurology 1980;30:47–51.

24. Sutherland GR, King ME, Peerless SJ, et al. Platelet interaction within giant intracranial aneurysms. J Neurosurg 1982;56:53–61.

25. Weisberg LA. Ruptured aneurysms of anterior cerebral or anterior communicating arteries. Neurology 1985;35:1562–1566.

26. Hunt WE, Hess RM. Surgical risk as related to time of intervention in the repair of intracranial aneurysms. J Neurosurg 1968;28:14–20.

27. Alvord EC, Loeser JD, Bailey WL, et al. Subarachnoid hemorrhage due to ruptured aneurysm: a simple method of estimating prognosis. Arch Neurol 1972;27:273–284.

28. Weisberg L. Computed tomography in aneurysmal subarachnoid hemorrhage. Neurology 1979;29:802–808.

29. Liliequist B, Lindquist M. Computer tomography in the evaluation of subarachnoid hemorrhage. Acta Radiol (Diag) 1980;21:327–331.

30. Schubiger O, Valvanis A, Hayek J. Computed tomography in cerebral aneurysms with special emphasis on giant intracranial aneurysms. J. Comput Assist Tomogr 1980;4:24–32.

31. Golding R, Peatfield R, Shawdon H, et al. Computed tomographic features of giant intracranial aneurysms. Clin Radiol 1980;31:41–45.

32. Atkinson JLD, Sundt TM, Houser OW, Whisnant JP. Angiographic frequency of anterior circulation intracranial aneurysms. J Neurosurg 1989;70:551–555.

33. Asari S, Satoh T, Sakurai M, et al. Delineation of unruptured cerebral aneurysms by CT angiotomography. J Neurosurg 1982;57:527–534.

34. DeLaPaz RL, New PF, Buonano FS, et al. NMR imaging of intracranial hemorrhage. J Comput Assist Tomogr 1984;8:599.

35. Ross J, Masaryk T, Modic M, et al. Intracranial aneurysms: evaluation by MR angiography. AJNR 1990;11:449–456.

36. Caplan LR, Flamm ES, Mohr JP, et al. Lumbar puncture and stroke. Stroke 1987;18:540A–544A.

37. Hayward RS. Subarachnoid hemorrhage of unknown etiology. J Neurol Neurosurg Psychiatry 1977;40:926–931.

38. Caplan LR, Brass LM, DeWitt LD, et al. Transcranial Doppler ultrasound: present status. Neurology 1990;40:696–700.

39. Lindegaard K, Grolemund P, Aaslid R, Normes H. Evaluation of cerebral AVMs using transcranial Doppler ultrasound. J Neurosurg 1986;65:335–344.

40. Schwartz A, Hennerici M. Noninvasive transcranial Doppler ultrasound in intracranial angiomas. Neurology 1986;36:626–635.

41. Petty GW, Massaro AR, Tatemichi TK, et al. Transcranial Doppler ultrasonographic changes after treatment for arteriovenous malformations. Stroke 1990;21:260–266.

42. Aaslid R, Huber P, Nornes H. Evaluation of cerebrovascular spasm with transcranial Doppler ultrasound. J Neurosurg 1984;60:37–41.

43. Harders AG, Gilsbach JM. Time course of blood velocity changes related to vasospasm in the circle of Willis measured by transcranial Doppler ultrasound. J Neurosurg 1987;66:718–728.

44. Sloan MA, Haley EC, Kassell NF, et al. Sensitivity and specificity of transcranial Doppler ultrasonography in the diagnosis of vasospasm following subarachnoid hemorrhage. Neurology 1989;391:1514–1518.

45. Sekhar L, Wechsler L, Yonas H, et al. Value of transcranial Doppler examination in the diagnosis of cerebral vasospasm after subarachnoid hemorrhage. Neurosurgery 1988;22:813–821.

46. Davis S, Andrews J, Lichtenstein M, et al. A single-photon emission computed tomography study of hyperperfusion after subarachnoid hemorrhage. Stroke 1990;21:252–259.

47. Van Gijn J, van Dongen KJ, Vermeulan M, et al. Perimesencephalic hemorrhage: a nonaneurysmal and benign form of subarachnoid hemorrhage. Neurology 1985;35:483–487.

48. Rinkel GJ, Wijdicks E, Vermeulen M, et al. The clinical course of perimesencephalic nonaneurysmal subarachnoid hemorrhage. Ann Neurol 1991;29:463–468.

49. Rinkel GJ, Wijdicks E, Vermeulen M, et al. Outcome in perimesencephalic (nonaneurysmal) subarachnoid hemorrhage: a follow-up study in 37 patients. Neurology 1990;40:1130–1132.

50. Stein RW, Kase CS, Hier DB, et al. Caudate hemorrhage. Neurology 1984;34:1549–1554.

51. Hochberg F, Fisher CM, Roberson G. Subarachnoid hemorrhage caused by rupture of a small superficial artery. Neurology 1974;24:309–311.

52. Calhoun DA, Oparil S. Treatment of hypertensive crises. N Engl J Med 1990;323:1177–1183.

53. Adams HP. Current status of antifibrinolytic therapy for treatment of patients with aneurysmal subarachnoid hemorrhage. Stroke 1982;13:256–259.

54. Ramirez-Laseppas M. Antifibrinolytic therapy in subarachnoid hemorrhage caused by ruptured intracranial aneurysm. Neurology 1981;31:316–322.

55. Kassell N, Torner D, Adams H. Antifibrinolytic therapy in the acute period following aneurysmal subarachnoid hemorrhage. J Neurosurg 1984;61:225–230.

56. Kassell NF, Sasaki T, Colohan AR, Nazar G. Cerebral vasospasm following aneurysmal subarachnoid hemorrhage. Stroke 1985;16:562–572.

57. White RP, Robertson JT. Role of plasmin, thrombin, and antithrombin as etiological factors in delayed cerebral vasospasm. Neurosurg 1985;16:27–35.

58. Macdonald RL, Weir B. A review of hemoglobin and the pathogenesis of cerebral vasospasm. Stroke 1991;22:971–982.

59. Hughes JT, Schianchi PM. Cerebral artery spasm: a histological study at necropsy of the blood vessels in cases of subarachnoid hemorrhage. J Neurosurg 1978;48:515–525.

60. Conway LW, McDonald LW. Structural changes of the intradural arteries following subarachnoid hemorrhage. J Neurosurg 1972;37:715–723.

61. Wellum GR, Peterson JW, Zervas NT. The relevance of in vivo smooth muscle experiments to cerebral vasospasm. Stroke 1985;16:573–581.

62. Clower BR, Smith RR, Haining JL, Lockard J. Constrictive endarteropathy following experimental subarachnoid hemorrhage. Stroke 1981;12:501–508.

63. Kwak R, Niizuma H, Ohi J, et al. Angiography study of cerebral vasospasm following rupture of intracranial aneurysms: I. time of the appearance. Surg Neurol 1979;11:257–262.

64. Weir B, Grace M, Hansen J, et al. Time course of vasospasm in man. J Neurosurg 1978;48:173–178.

65. Heros RC, Zervas NT, Varsos V. Cerebral vasospasm after subarachnoid hemorrhage: an update. Ann Neurol 1983;14:599–608.

66. Fisher CM, Roberson GH, Ojemann RG. Cerebral vasospasm with ruptured saccular aneurysm: the clinical manifestations. Neurosurgery 1977;1:245–248.

67. Fisher CM, Kistler JP, Davis JM. Relation of cerebral vasospasm to subarachnoid hemorrhage visualized by computed tomographic scanning. Neurosurgery 1980;6:1–9.

68. Hijdra A, van Gijn J, Nagelkerke NJ, et al. Prediction of delayed cerebral ischemia, rebleeding, and outcome after aneurysmal subarachnoid hemorrhage. Stroke 1988;19:1250–1256.

69. Graf CJ, Nibbelink DW. Cooperative Study of Intracranial Aneurysms and Subarachnoid Hemorrhage: report on randomized treatment study: III. intracranial surgery. Stroke 1974;5:559–601.

70. Wilkins RH. Attempts at prevention or treatment of intracranial arterial spasm: an update. Neurosurgery 1986;18:808–825.

71. Auer LM. Acute operation and preventive nimodipine improve outcome in patients with ruptured cerebral aneurysms. Neurosurgery 1984;15:57–66.

72. Mizukami M, Kawase T, Usami T, et al. Prevention of vasospasm by early operation with removal of subarachnoid blood. Neurosurgery 1982;10:301–307.

73. Taneda M. Effect of early operation for ruptured aneurysm in prevention of delayed ischemic symptoms. J Neurosurg 1982;5:622–628.

74. Kassell NF, Peerless SJ, Durward QJ, et al. Treatment of ischemic deficits from vasospasm with hypervolemia and induced arterial hypertension. Neurosurgery 1982;11:337–343.

75. Solomon RA, Fink ME, Lennihan L. Prophylactic volume expansion therapy for the prevention of delayed cerebral ischemia after early aneurysm surgery. Arch Neurol 1988;45:325–332.

76. Solomon RA, Post KD, McMurty JG. Depression of circulating blood volume in patients after subarachnoid hemorrhage: implications for the management of symptomatic vasospasm. Neurosurgery 1984;15:354–361.

77. Wood JH, Simeone FA, Kron RE, et al. Rheological aspects of experimental hypervolemic hemodilution with low molecular weight dextran. Neurosurgery 1982;11:739–753.

78. Allen GS. Cerebral arterial spasm: a controlled trial of nimodipine in subarachnoid hemorrhage patients—the nimodipine cerebral arterial spasm study group. Stroke 1983;14:122.

79. Pickard JD, Murray GD, Illingworth R, et al. Effect of oral nimodipine in cerebral infarction and outcome after subarachnoid hemorrhage: British aneurysm nimodipine trial. Br Med J 1981;298:636–642.

80. Higashida RT, Halbach VV, Cahan LD, et al. Transluminal angioplasty for treatment of intracranial arterial vasospasm. J Neurosurg 1989;71:648–653.

81. Newell DW, Eskridge JM, Mayberg M, et al. Angioplasty for the treatment of symptomatic vasospasm following subarachnoid hemorrhage. J Neurosurg 1989;91:654–660.

82. Auer LM. Unfavorable outcome following early surgical repair of ruptured cerebral aneurysms: a critical review of 238 patients. Surg Neurol 1991;35:152–158.

83. Graff-Radford NR, Torner J, Adams HP, Kassell NF. Factors associated with hydrocephalus after subarachnoid hemorrhage. Arch Neurol 1989;46:744–752.

84. Hammermeister KE, Reichenbach DD. QRS changes, pulmonary edema, and myocardial necrosis associated with subarachnoid hemorrhage. Am Heart J 1969;78:94–100.

85. Hunt D, McRae C, Zupf P. Electrocardiographic and serum enzyme changes in subarachnoid hemorrhage. Am Heart J 1969;77:479–488.

86. Brouwers PJ, Wijdicks EF, Hasan D, et al. Serial electrocardiographic recording in aneurysmal subarachnoid hemorrhage. Stroke 1989;20:1162–1167.

87. Greenhoot JH, Reichenbach DD. Cardiac injury and subarachnoid hemorrhage: a clinical, pathological, and physiological correlation. J Neurosurg 1969;30: 521–531.

88. Koskela P, Punsar S, Sipila W. Subendocardial hemorrhage and ECG change in intracranial bleeding. Br Med J 1964;1:1479–1480.

89. Weintraub BM, McHenry LC. Cardiac abnormalities in subarachnoid hemorrhage: a resume. Stroke 1974;5:384–392.

90. Vidal BE, Dergal EB, Cesarman E, et al. Cardiac arrhythmias associated with subarachnoid hemorrhage: prospective study. Neurosurgery 1979;5:675–680.

91. Samuels MA. Electrocardiographic manifestations of neurologic disease. Seminars in Neurology 1984;4:453–460.

92. Weir BK. Pulmonary edema following fatal aneurysm rupture. J Neurosurg 1978;49:502–507.

93. Landolt AM, Yasargil MG, Krayenbuhl H. Disturbances of the serum electrolytes after surgery of intracranial arterial aneurysm. J Neurosurg 1972;37: 210–218.

94. Takaku A, Shindo K, Tanaki S, et al. Fluid and electrolyte disturbances in patients with intracranial aneurysms. Surg Neurol 1979;11:349–356.

95. Diringer MN, Lim JS, Kirsch JR, Hawley DF. Suprasellar and intraventricular blood predict elevated plasma atrial natriuretic factor in subarachnoid hemorrhage. Stroke 1991;22:572–581.

96. Peerless SJ. Pre- and postoperative management of cerebral aneurysm. Clin Neurosurg 1979;26:209–231.

97. Garde A. Amnesia after operations on aneurysms of the anterior communicating artery. Surg Neurol 1982;18:46–49.

98. Damasio AR, Graff-Radford N, Eslinger P, et al. Amnesia following basal forebrain lesions. Arch Neurol 1985;42:263–271.

99. Winn HR, Berga SL, Richardson AE, et al. Long-term evaluation of patients with cerebral aneurysms. Ann Neurol 1981;10:106.

100. Sundt TM, Whisnant JP. Subarachnoid hemorrhage from intracranial aneurysm. N Engl J Med 1978:299:116–122.

101. Stein BM, Wolpert SM. Arteriovenous malformations of the brain: I. current concepts and treatment. Arch Neurol 1980:37:1–5.

102. Tonnis W, Schiefer W, Walter W. Signs and symptoms of supratentorial arteriovenous aneurysms. J Neurosurg 1953;15:471–480.

103. McCormick WF. The pathology of vascular ("arteriovenous") malformations. J Neurosurg 1966;27:807–816.

104. Omojola M, Fox A, Vinuela F, Debrun G. Stenosis of afferent vessels of intracranial arteriovenous malformations. AJNR 1985;6:791–793.

105. Mawad ME, Hilal SK, Michelson J, et al. Occlusive vascular disease associated with cerebral arteriovenous malformations. Radiology 1984;153:401–408.

106. Rigamonti D, Hadley MN, Drayer BP, et al. Cerebral cavernous malformations: incidence and familial occurrence. N Engl J Med 1988; 319:343–347.

107. Savoiardo M, Strada L, Passerini A. Intracranial cavernous hemangiomas: neuroradiologic review of 36 operated cases. AJNR 1983;4:945–950.
108. Mason I, Aase JM, Orrison WW, et al. Familial cavernous angiomas of the brain in an Hispanic family. Neurology 1988;38:324–326.
109. Newton TH, Troost BT. Arteriovenous malformations and fistulas. In: Newton TH, Potts DG, eds. Radiology of the skull and brain: vol. 2. angiography. St. Louis: Mosby, 1974:2490–2565.
110. McCormick WF, Hardman JM, Boulter TR. Vascular malformations ("angiomas") of the brain, with special reference to those occurring in the posterior fossa. J Neurosurg 1968;28:241–254.
111. Hook C, Johanson C. Intracranial arteriovenous aneurysms: a follow-up study with particular attention to their growth. Arch Neurol Psych 1958;80:39–54.
112. Patterson JH, McKissock W. A clinical survey of intracranial angiomas with special reference to their mode of progression and surgical treatment: a report of 110 cases. Brain 1965;79:233–266.
113. Svien J, McRae JA. Arteriovenous anomalies of the brain. J Neurosurg 1965;23:23–28.
114. Chimowitz MI, Little JR, Awad IA, et al. Intracranial hypertension associated with unruptured cerebral arteriovenous malformations. Ann Neurol 1990;27:474–479.
115. DeJong RN, Hicks SP. Vascular malformation of the brainstem: report of a case with long duration and fluctuating course. Neurology 1980;30:995–997.
116. Stahl SM, Johnson KP, Malamud N. The clinical and pathological spectrum of brainstem vascular malformations. Arch Neurol 1980;37:25–29.
117. Caroscio JT, Brannan T, Budabin M, et al. Subarachnoid hemorrhage secondary to spinal arteriovenous malformation and aneurysm. Arch Neurol 1980;37:101–103.
118. Robinson JC, Hall CS, Sedzimir CB. Arteriovenous malformations, aneurysms, and pregnancy. J Neurosurg 1974;41:63–70.
119. Jensen H, Klinge H, Lemke J, et al. Computerized tomography in vascular malformations of the brain. Neurosurg Rev 1980;3:119–127.
120. Caplan LR. Computed tomography and stroke. In: McDowell F, Caplan LR, eds. Cerebrovascular surgery report for the National Institute of Neurological and Communicative Disorders and Stroke (NINCDS). Washington, DC: NINCDS, rev. 1985:61–74.
121. Hayman L, Fox A, Evans R. Effectiveness of contrast regimens in CT detection of vascular malformations of the brain. AJR 1981;2:421–425.
122. Daniels D, Houghton V, Williams A, et al. Arteriovenous malformation simulating a cyst on computed tomography. Radiology 1979;133:393–394.
123. Rigamonti D, Drayer B, Johnson PC, et al. The MRI appearance of cavernous malformations (angiomas). J Neurosurg 1987;67:518–524.
124. Gomori JM, Grossman RI, Hackney DB, et al. Variable appearances of subacute intracranial hematomas on high-field spin–echo MR. AJR 1988;150:171–178.
125. Farmer J-P, Cosgrove GR, Villemure FG, et al. Intracerebral cavernous angiomas. Neurology 1988;38:1699–1704.
126. Requena I, Arias M, Lopez-Iber L. Cavernomas of the cerebral nervous system in clinical and neuroimaging manifestations in 47 patients. J Neurol Neurosurg Psychiatry 1991;54:590–594.

127. Marks M, Lane B, Steinberg G, Chang P. Vascular characteristics of intracerebral arteriovenous malformations in patients with clinical steal. AJNR 1991; 12:489–496.
128. Drake CG. Arteriovenous malformations of the brain: the options for management. N Engl J Med 1983;309:308–310.
129. Heros RC, Tu Y-K. Is surgical therapy needed for unruptured arteriovenous malformations? Neurology 1987;37:279–286.
130. Drake CG. Cerebral arteriovenous malformations: considerations for and experience with surgical treatment in 166 cases. Clin Neurosurg 1979;26:145–208.
131. Forster DMC, Steiner L, Hakanson S. Arteriovenous malformations of the brain: a long-term clinical study. J Neurosurg 1972;37:562–570.
132. Aminoff MJ. Treatment of unruptured cerebral arteriovenous malformations. Neurology 1987;37:815–819.
133. Spetzler RF, Wilson CB, Weinstein P, et al. Normal perfusion pressure breakthrough theory. Clin Neurosurg 1978;25:651–672.
134. Fournier D, TerBrugge KG, Willinsky R, et al. Endovascular treatment of intracerebral arteriovenous malformations: experience in 49 cases. J Neurosurg 1991;75:228–233.
135. Vinuela F, Fox AJ, Debrun G, et al. Progressive thrombosis of brain arteriovenous malformations after embolization with isobutyl-2-cyanoacrylate. AJNR 1983;4:959–966.
136. Vinters HV, Lundie MJ, Kaufmann JC. Long-term pathological follow-up of cerebral arteriovenous malformations treated by embolization with buccylate. N Engl J Med 1986;314:477–483.
137. Kjellberg RN, Hanamura T, Davis KR, et al. Bragg-peak proton beam therapy for arteriovenous malformations of the brain. N Engl J Med 1983;309:269–274.
138. Heros R, Korosue K. Radiation treatment of cerebral arteriovenous malformations. N Engl J Med 1990;323:127–129.
139. Steinberg G, Fabrikant J, Marks MP, et al. Stereotactic heavy-charged-particle Bragg-peak radiation for intracerebral arteriovenous malformations. N Engl J Med 1990;323:96–101.

CHAPTER 13

Intracerebral Hemorrhage

Bleeding into the substance of the brain was recognized as a cause of stroke by Morgagni in 1761.[1] Cheyne wrote a treatise on apoplexy and coma in 1812, in which he included examples of ICH.[2] Clinicians of the nineteenth and twentieth centuries considered ICH invariably lethal. Postmortem examples were usually studied, because the tests available could not identify ICH during life. Clinicians correlated the clinical signs and features with the size and location of the hemorrhages found in brains at necropsy. Gowers[3] and Osler,[4] writing at the turn of the twentieth century, included in their respective textbooks long and detailed chapters on the usual locations of ICH and the nature of accompanying clinical signs and symptoms. Aring and Merritt,[5] in 1935, correlated the clinical and pathological findings in 245 patients with stroke who came to necropsy at the Boston City Hospital and emphasized the features that separated hemorrhage from infarction. The major teachings emanating from these works can be summarized in a few general rules:

1. ICH occurred at a younger age than brain infarction.
2. The major cause of ICH was hypertension, often of an extreme nature.
3. Symptoms of ICH began abruptly.
4. Loss of consciousness was a nearly constant feature.
5. Headache always accompanied ICH and was usually severe.
6. The commonest locations for ICH were the putamen, internal capsule, thalamus, pons, and cerebellum.
7. ICH was invariably fatal or devastating, with few, if any, intact survivors.

However, this work was B.C.—that is, before CT scanning. These teachings evolved from correlation with fatal cases. There had been no way to diagnose less severe hemorrhages during life, especially if the lesions did not communicate with the CSF. CT now allows for accurate localization of small- and medium-sized hemorrhages. CT not only shows clinicians whether a lesion is a hemorrhage, but also accurately shows them the location, size, spread within the brain, drainage into the ventricles and spaces around the brain, and presence of edema and mass effect. MRI, by its capability of showing the presence of hemosiderin, can help define whether lesions are old hemorrhages. Old infarcts and old hemorrhages can look similar on CT. When the subject of ICH is reviewed in light of results with newer imaging techniques, the old rules are found to apply to only a small fraction of ICHs—the larger hemorrhages. I begin this chapter by reviewing the general rules and findings applicable to ICH at any site, and then I review the findings in hemorrhages at their common locations in the brain.

Incidence and Epidemiology

Approximately 10 percent of strokes are due to ICH. The pilot Stroke Data Bank (SDB),[6] the Michael Reese Stroke Registry (MRSR),[7] and the Harvard Stroke Registry (HSR)[8] all found that about 1 stroke in 10 was caused by parenchymatous brain hemorrhage; the same figure was reached in studies of stroke at the Mayo Clinic in Rochester, Minnesota.[9,10] There is a higher incidence of ICH in populations that have a high frequency of hypertension, such as African-Americans and individuals of Chinese, Japanese, and Thai ancestry. ICH affects a very wide age range, with many examples in the seventh, eighth, and ninth decades of life. Figure 13.1 displays the age and sex distribution of ICH in the HSR,[11] and Figure 13.2 is a graph of age distribution in the combined MRSR and SDB. Though it is probably accurate to say that a higher percentage of strokes in patients under age 40 years are hemorrhagic, ICH is certainly not rare during the later years of life.

Clinical Course and Accompanying Symptoms

JT, a 44-year-old black school teacher had rushed to arrive at a very important job interview for which he was 10 minutes late. While being stressfully interrogated, he noted tingling in his left hand, which gradually spread to his arm. He excused himself to go to the washroom and then noted a similar feeling in the left leg. As he washed his hands, he realized his left hand and arm were clumsy and weak. He tripped on his left foot as he walked back. The interviewer was alarmed by slurring of words and a droop of the left face that he noticed when the teacher returned. An ambulance was called. JT began to feel a headache over his right scalp. When the emergency team arrived in 10 minutes, JT could no longer move his left arm and leg but seemed unaware and unconcerned with his handicap. He complained of a severe headache and was now sleepy. While being placed on a stretcher, he began to vomit. He had no history of hypertension or drug use. Blood pressure was 175/110 torr when he was first examined by the emergency personnel.

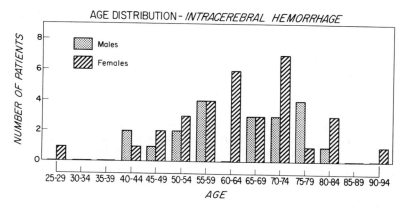

FIGURE 13.1 Age distribution in patients with intracerebral hemorrhage (from the Harvard Stroke Registry). Reprinted with permission from Caplan LR, Mohr JP. Intracerebral hemorrhage: an update. Geriatrics 1978;33:42–52.

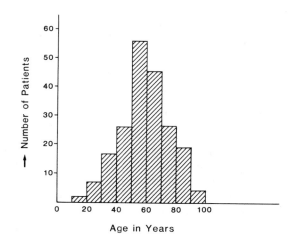

FIGURE 13.2 Age distribution by decade of 111 patients with intracerebral hemorrhage from the Michael Reese Stroke Registry and the Stroke Data Bank.

The course of illness in this patient was the gradual accumulation of focal neurological signs during a period of about 20 minutes. As the symptoms and disability worsened, headache, decreased alertness, and vomiting developed.

ICH develops gradually. Bleeding into the brain tissues from small, deep penetrating vessels is usually under arteriolar or capillary pressure. This contrasts with the situation in SAH, in which arteries on the brain surface leak blood under systemic arterial pressure. Symptoms in patients with

SAH begin instantaneously and consist of headache, loss of concentration, and vomiting. These symptoms are caused by sudden increase in ICP due to blood rapidly disseminating through the CSF around the brain substance. In ICH, hemorrhage develops gradually during minutes or sometimes hours. Fisher examined serial sections of ICH studied at necropsy.[12] At the center of the lesions was a large mass of blood. At the periphery were many of what he called "fibrin globes," representing little caps of fibrinous material that plugged small vessels, which had broken and leaked during life. As ICH develops, pressure within the central core increases and compresses small vessels at the periphery of the hematoma. These peripheral arteries in turn break, and blood escapes, enlarging the lesion. The hematoma grows like a snowball rolling downhill and accumulating more snow on its outer circumference as it rolls. ICP rises as the lesion enlarges, and tissue pressure around the lesion also mounts. Eventually, an equilibrium is reached, and bleeding stops. If the hematoma reaches the ventricle or brain surface, it may communicate with the CSF and discharge part of its contents at the same time.

Visualizing the pathology of the lesion and its development helps predict the pace of the symptoms. Bleeding is directly into the brain parenchyma, rather than into the CSF, as it is in SAH. The brain itself is devoid of pain fibers, so the initial release of blood does not cause headache. Instead, blood disrupts the function of that particular local brain region. If the hematoma began in the left putamen, the patient might note weakness of the right limbs. As the hemorrhage grows during the next few minutes, the weakness would become more severe, and sensory symptoms, loss of speech, and conjugate eye deviation to the side of the hemorrhage might ensue. In JT, the combination of sensory (tingling) and motor symptoms in the left face, arm, and leg suggests a process in the deep structures of the right cerebral hemisphere affecting the internal capsule region. If the hemorrhage then grew to a size that increased ICP and distorted adjacent meningeal structures, the patient would develop headache, vomiting, and reduced alertness. In JT, headaches, sleepiness, and vomiting started and evolved *after* he became hemiplegic and his lesion had expanded. If the hematoma continued to grow, coma and death would result from compression of vital brainstem centers.

Sometimes, clinical symptoms and signs evolve over a period of days rather than minutes or hours. Herbstein and Schaumburg studied a group of patients with ICH, to determine whether progressive clinical decline was due to continued bleeding or edema around the lesion.[13] They tagged RBCs with chromium 51 and injected these erythrocytes into the circulation 1 to 5 hours after their initial examination. Counts of radioactivity were made from the hematoma cavities at necropsies performed from 1 to 15 days later. There was no increase in radioactivity within the hematomas, but patients who developed secondary (Düret lesion) brainstem hemorrhages after the injection had increased activity within the brainstem lesions but not within the primary hemorrhages. Hematomas were often surrounded by edema.[13] Although this study suggests that in most cases, hematomas do not expand after the initial hours, studies in the 1980s show that sometimes, hematomas do expand dramatically.[14,15] Repeat CT may show dramatic enlargement of hematoma mass and ventricular drainage, developing within hours after the first CT scan.[15] Invariably, clinical worsening was also present and initiated the request for repeat scanning. Patients with ICH who have a bleeding diathesis are especially prone to have hematomas, which expand gradually and enlarge over periods of days.[16]

Analysis of the course of illness in 54 well-documented patients with ICH studied in the HSR showed that 37 had gradual development of symptoms during a period of minutes or a few hours.[11] In the 17 other patients, there seemed to be no progression of symptoms after the patients were first found by others. In many of this latter group, an accurate account of the earliest development of symptoms was not available because of aphasia, lack of awareness of the deficit, or stupor. A smooth, gradual worsening of function over minutes, followed by headache and vomiting, was the rule in larger lesions. Some patients who had stabilized during the first 24 to 48 hours later developed progressively decreased alertness and increased focal signs within 48 to 72 hours, probably due to edema around the hematoma.

I find an early description of the gradual evolution of symptoms in a fatal case of ICH very dramatic and memorable.[17] This patient, seen in 1937, developed and evolved his hematoma while entirely under observation. He was sent to the hospital because of "malignant hypertension." While his history was being taken, he noted weakness and dizziness.

He stated that he had noted numbness and tingling of the hands just before he left the station at which his heart had been examined. As the taking of the history continued he became extremely restless and apprehensive. He complained of inability to hear, difficulty in swallowing and dyspnea. The patient was placed on the examining table and the blood pressure was found to be 245 systolic and 170 diastolic. Under the eyes of several examiners complete bilateral palsy of the sixth nerve developed; both pupils dilated, and the corneal reflexes disappeared. The patient was still able to talk, but with a typical bulbar speech, and he seemed almost totally deaf. The left leg now became paretic, rapid clonic movements being observed. The Babinski sign was present bilaterally. By 4:15 the patient was completely stuporous and the blood pressure had risen to 280 systolic and 170 diastolic. This rapidly progressive chain of events was most unpleasant to witness and produced a depressing effect on the nurses and physicians.

I had a similar experience during my first week as a medical intern at the Boston City Hospital:

An elderly hypertensive Chinese man had come to the emergency room with slight weakness of his right limbs. He spoke normally. He was placed on the danger list and I and a porter pushed his stretcher through the underground hospital tunnels toward the ward. As we went, his right limbs became weaker, and he stopped talking. Soon his eyes and head deviated to the left and we could not arouse him. By the time we reached the ward, he was comatose and decerebrate. He died within hours.

Like Kornyey and his colleagues, I felt desperately helpless watching brain function inexorably vanish.

Headache

Headache was not an invariable symptom in the 60 HSR patients with ICH and was described in only 17 patients (28%) near the outset of their neurological symptoms.[11] Another 7 patients (12%) noted headache later. Twenty-four patients (40%) had no headache at any time during their ICH. The 12 (20%) stuporous or comatose patients could not provide data regarding headache.[11] Headache was much more frequent with larger lesions and was often absent or minimal in patients with small lesions.

Loss of Consciousness

Loss of consciousness accompanied only the larger hematomas, and those in the brainstem. Diminished alertness in patients with ICH is due to mass effect and increased ICP or to direct involvement of the brainstem reticular activating system. In the HSR, 30 of 60 patients were alert when first seen, 14 (23%) were lethargic, and 16 (27%) were stuporous or comatose.[11] In the SDB patients with ICH, decreased level of consciousness was the most important adverse prognostic sign, as it has been in nearly all studies of prognosis in ICH.[18] All patients with severely reduced levels of consciousness died. Early reduction of consciousness is not an invariable accompaniment of ICH, but when it occurs, it has an ominous prognosis. The sleepiness that developed in JT was a serious finding and should have triggered urgent evaluation and treatment when he arrived at the hospital.

Vomiting

JT had started to vomit as he was being taken to the hospital and continued to vomit in the emergency room. This is an especially important sign in patients with ICH. In both ICH and SAH, vomiting is usually caused by increased ICP or local distortion of the fourth ventricle. Few patients with ischemic lesions within the cerebral hemispheres vomit, but nearly half of the patients with hemispheral hemorrhages vomit. In the posterior circulation, vomiting usually reflects dysfunction of the vestibular nuclei, or the so-called vomiting center in the floor of the fourth ventricle.[19] Vomiting occurs in about one third of patients with occlusive posterior-circulation disease and in more than one half of patients with posterior-circulation

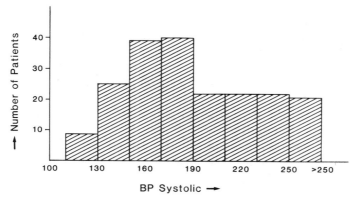

FIGURE 13.3   Systolic blood pressure distribution in 110 patients with intracerebral hemorrhage in the Michael Reese Stroke Registry and the Stroke Data Bank.

hemorrhages. Patients with cerebellar hemorrhage almost always vomit early in the course of the lesion.

Seizures

Seizures are not common during the acute phase of a stroke but are slightly more frequent in ICH than in the other stroke types except embolism.[8] Among two recent series of patients with spontaneous nontraumatic ICH, 12.5 percent and 17 percent of patients had seizures during their early course.[20,21] Lobar hemorrhages, slitlike hemorrhages situated near the gray–white junction of the cortex, and putaminal hemorrhages that undercut the cortex are especially epileptogenic. Neck stiffness is uncommon in putaminal hemorrhage[22] but is often found in patients with thalamic or cerebellar hemorrhages.[23] Subhyaloid retinal hemorrhages, common in SAH, are rare in ICH unless the hematoma has developed rapidly and is large.[24]

Etiologies

Hypertension

The commonest cause of ICH is hypertension, but the blood pressure need not be elevated to malignant ranges. Figure 13.3 shows the distribution of blood pressure in the MRSR and the SDB. Many patients present to the hospital with ICH and have no prior history of hypertension but have high blood pressure on admission. In that circumstance, it is difficult to know how much, if any, of the blood pressure elevation is secondary to raised ICP (the Cushing response) or what the level of blood pressure was prior to the bleed.

When hypertension first develops, the small arteries and capillaries are exposed to a high head of pressure and could leak. This situation is comparable to early left atrial failure in patients with rheumatic mitral stenosis when the pulmonary capillaries are exposed to high pressure, then break and cause hemoptysis. Later, small arteries and arterioles hypertrophy, protecting the capillary bed from the high central pressure. Hemoptysis and brain hemorrhage become less frequent when arterioles hypertrophy, but the heart bears the brunt of the increased peripheral arterial resistance. Later in the course of hypertension, degenerative changes in the form of lipohyalinosis and miliary Charcot–Bouchard aneurysms develop because of the long-standing pressure elevations. ICH occurs when these lesions rupture. The occurrence of ICH is biphasic, patients presenting both at the onset of hypertension and later, after experiencing considerable wear and tear on penetrating blood vessels.[25]

Some hypertensive hemorrhages arise from degenerative changes, such as fibrinoid degeneration and microaneurysms that develop in patients with hypertension. Cole and Yates examined the brains of 100 hypertensive patients and 100 normotensive controls.[26] All 13 patients with ICH had microaneurysms and were hypertensive. Among 63 patients with microaneurysms, 46 had hypertension recognized during life. The age distribution of microaneurysms was also extremely interesting. Among 21 hypertensive patients under age 50 years, only 2 had microaneurysms, whereas 71 percent of hypertensives in the 65- to 69-year age range had microaneurysms.[26]

Rosenblum analyzed the morphology of aneurysms and their parent vessels.[27] Some arteries bore early aneurysmal dilations, while others had sclerosed aneurysms with flask-shaped collections of collagen joined to a small artery by a narrow neck. Microaneurysms are often surrounded by hemosiderin-laden macrophages, indicating previous leakage. The lesions are most common in penetrating vessels that supply the basal ganglia, thalamus, pons and cerebellum, and arteries supplying the gray–white-matter cortical junctions of the hemispheres. The same vessels that bear microaneurysms also contain foci of lipohyalinosis and fibrinoid degeneration, which explains the dictum that ischemic lacunes have the same relative distribution as hypertensive ICH.

Fisher described the results from examination of serial sections of patients with ICH. *Fibrin globes*, meshes of platelets encircled by a thin layer of fibrin, protruded from ruptured sites and clearly marked vessels that had bled.[12] There is a relationship between iris aneurysms and cerebral microaneurysms because rabbits with experimentally induced hypertension develop iris aneurysms roughly proportional to their development of cerebral microaneurysms.[28] Recent studies from Japan of surgical specimens of acute ICH show that penetrating arteries frequently break but often not in relation to microaneurysms.[29,30] Degenerative lipohyalinotic changes were present in the broken and adjacent arteries. Clearly degenerative changes caused by aging and hypertension can predispose to ICH, but it is not certain that microaneurysms represent the bleeding lesion.[29–31]

Considerable evidence has recently accumulated showing that acute changes in blood pressure and blood flow can precipitate rupture of penetrating arteries in the absence of prior hypertension.[25] A large necropsy study of patients who died of ICH used heart weights to estimate the frequency of hypertension; only 46 percent of fatal cases of spontaneous ICH had moderate to severe chronic hypertension.[32] Brott and colleagues reviewed the records of 154 patients with spontaneous ICH in Cincinnati, Ohio, during 1 year, to determine the frequency of hypertension.[33] Only 45 percent had a history of hypertension; another 12 percent without a history of hypertension had left ventricular hypertrophy. The authors judged that about 50 percent of cases were not attributable to chronic hypertension.[33]

In these two series, the location of the hemorrhages, increased blood pressure on admission, and absence of other etiologies makes it highly probable that these hematomas were, in fact, satisfactorily classified as hypertensive ICH. Probably, hypertension was acute and led to bleeding from unprotected capillaries and arterioles. My own observations and those of others have recently documented ICH in situations in which blood pressure probably changed abruptly.[25,31]

My first experience was with patients who developed ICH after exposure to severe *cold weather*.[34] While outdoors in temperatures below −10° F, three patients developed putaminal, thalamic, and cerebellar hematomas, respectively. One was in the midst of alcohol withdrawal, one was removing ice from his car window, and one patient was waiting in line to pay rent. All had increased blood pressure on admission, but their pressures normalized soon thereafter. Immersion in cold is known to be a very strong sympathetic nervous system stimulus. Formerly, the cold-pressure test[35] (immersion of hands in ice water) was used clinically to induce transient hypertension, a phenomenon said to be more common in patients with essential hypertension. Sympathetic stimulation due to alcohol withdrawal and also stress may have added to the effects of cold exposure in these patients.

Dental procedures[36] and surgery or stimulation of the trigeminal nerve[25,37] have also been associated with ICH. In one patient known to have been previously normotensive, dental pain after irrigation of the mouth was followed immediately by a fatal temporal-lobe hemorrhage.[36] Blood pressure was elevated acutely. Necropsy showed no evidence of hypertensive vascular damage in any organ and no other cause for brain hemorrhage. In a series of patients operated on intracranially for trigeminal neuralgia, hematomas developed at locations typical for hypertensive ICH.[37] Other procedures involving manipulation of the trigeminal nerve for treatment of trigeminal neuralgia have also been complicated by ICH.[25,36] Monitoring of blood pressure and heart rate during trigeminal stimulation often shows important fluctuations in blood pressure and pulse. The blood vessels of the brains of animals and humans have very important trigeminal innervation.[38,39]

ICH has now been frequently associated with the use of illicit drugs known to have sympatheticomimetic effects. I discuss drug-induced ICH in more detail later in this chapter because of its growing frequency as an important cause of stroke and ICH. Patients have also developed ICH after sudden augmentation of CBF, either locally to one hemisphere, as in the circumstance of ICH after carotid endarterectomy;[40-42] or more systemically, after correction of congenital heart defects or cardiac transplantation in the young.[25,43,44] In the early 1990s, ICH has been reported to develop during recovery from migraine.[31,45] Intense vasoconstriction leads to diminished flow and perhaps ischemia to local blood vessels, then reperfusion leads to ICH in the zone of prior vascular damage. A similar mechanism probably underlies most examples of hemorrhagic infarction due to cerebral embolism.[46]

Probably more important than the unusual circumstances just cited are events of everyday life that can raise blood pressure. Wilson was quite aware of this concept and wrote in his neurology text,[47] "emotional experience, joy, anger, fear or apprehension may disturb the action of the heart, trivial though the incident may be—an address at a public meeting, trouble with a cook, and so on."

A patient of mine, LF, presented for me a vivid example of the possible interrelationship between daily activities and stresses and the triggering of ICH. He was a retired university professor who came to ask my opinion about what he called a "strange stroke" he suffered a few years previously. Because he never had high blood pressure before or after the stroke, he was puzzled that his physicians had attributed his condition to a hypertensive ICH. He described the events of that day as follows:

> LF had a very active teaching day, with more than the usual responsibilities. He hurried to finish, so as to be on time for an engagement that night. His wife had arranged symphony tickets. They were to hear Mahler (whom he found tedious) and were to go with a couple (whom he considered to be unpleasant bores). He arrived very late at the restaurant where they were to meet and had a hurried and very unpleasant meal. They literally had to run to the symphony hall nearby to arrive in time to be seated, and they rushed to their seats in front. As he hustled toward his seat, he recalls thinking how wonderful it would have been to have remained at work and not agreed to the ordeal of the evening. He got to his seat in a sweat and then began to notice a left hemiparesis gradually developing.

I reviewed his CT and hospital records. A typical small putaminal hemorrhage was present, and his blood pressure was transiently elevated on admission but soon normalized. Both acute fluctuations in blood pressure and flow and chronic degenerative changes are important in the etiology of so-called hypertensive ICH. In either case, bleeding is into the territories of penetrating arteries. At present, it is not known whether the size, location, and clinical picture in these two types of hypertensive ICH differ.[25]

In the case of JT, he was hypertensive when first examined but had no history of hypertension. Could the stressful interview have contributed to an

TABLE 13.1

Distribution by Site: Hypertensive Intracerebral Hemorrhage in Michael Reese Stroke Registry and South Alabama Cases

Site	Number of Patients	Percentage
Caudate nucleus	17	9.0
Putamen	63	32.5
Thalamic	43	22.0
Lobar	38	19.5
Cerebellar	14	7.0
Pons	20	10.0
Total	194	

acute blood pressure rise, or had he developed hypertension recently? His blood pressure stayed elevated during the hospitalization.

Older patients, often in their 70s or 80s, may present with ICH. Is this because of degenerative changes in their arterial system or because of coexistent amyloid angiopathy, now recognized with increasing frequency when sought in elderly patients with lobar hemorrhages? Older patients seem to develop ICH at relatively lower blood pressures than do younger patients. Probably because of atrophy, symptoms of increased ICP—such as headache, vomiting, or reduced alertness—are less common in older patients, even with sizable lesions. This observation makes differentiation between hemorrhage and infarction more difficult in geriatric patients.

The usual loci of hypertensive ICH are shown in Table 13.1, which represents the actual distribution of lesion sites in a combined series of patients with ICH. Because hemorrhages arise from deep penetrating vessels, they primarily affect the brain regions nurtured by these vessels. In postmortem analyses, an increasing number of patients dying of lobar brain hemorrhages are found to have an unsuspected amyloid angiopathy. Rupture of fragile amyloid-encased arteries could be enhanced by raised arterial pressure.

Bleeding Diathesis

A variety of different coagulopathies can lead to bleeding into the brain substance, sometimes accompanied by systemic bleeding. Unfortunately, anticoagulation with heparin or warfarin accounts for an all-too-high percentage of this type of ICH. Considering the large number of patients treated with anticoagulants, the number that develop ICH is small. Among a series of 1626 patients treated with long-term anticoagulants, 30 had ICH, of which two thirds were fatal.[48] The most consistent risk factor for intracranial or systemic bleeding was prolongation of the prothrombin time (PT) beyond the therapeutic range, but some hemorrhages occur even when the PT is subtherapeutic.[16] As with other etiologies of ICH, hypertension aggravates the tendency to bleed intracranially. Three features characterize anticoagulant-induced ICH, as distinct from other causes:

1.   Hemorrhage often develops gradually and insidiously during many hours or even days (6 of 14 patients with anticoagulant-related ICH had a very insidious clinical course).[16]
2.   The cerebellum and cerebral lobes are involved more frequently than in hypertensive ICH.[16]
3.   There is a very high morbidity and mortality rate (15 of 24 patients died,[16] and only patients with smaller hematomas—that is, under 30 cc volume—had a favorable chance for survival; only 1 of 24 patients with ICH had bleeding elsewhere).

Anticoagulant-related ICH is a particularly difficult situation to treat because many patients are taking warfarin to prevent ischemic stroke. Patients with prosthetic heart valves, rheumatic mitral stenosis, or atrial fibrillation have a high risk for cerebral emboli without warfarin therapy. Especially when the indication for anticoagulants is strong and the early presenting symptoms are slight, treating physicians might be inclined to continue therapy, or at least not to reverse the hypoprothrombinemia with vitamin K or fresh frozen plasma. In my experience, this tactic is a mistake because many anticoagulant-related hemorrhages will insidiously progress. Because of their size and locale in the surgically accessible cerebellum and cerebral lobes, many eventually require lifesaving surgery.

The initial clinical diagnosis may also be difficult in the group on warfarin for stroke prophylaxis because the first reaction to the neurological symptoms is to predict that the patient had an ischemic stroke despite the treatment. I have found two axioms very useful: (1) If a patient on anticoagulants develops neurological symptoms, the cause is anticoagulant-related hemorrhage until proven otherwise. (2) If anticoagulant hemorrhage is verified, immediately give vitamin K and fresh frozen plasma, and pursue all measures aggressively to stem bleeding. Although no formal prospective studies clarify the optimal time for restarting anticoagulants after ICH in patients who require long-term treatment, a retrospective study found that after 10 to 14 days, recurrent ICH did not develop.[49] I believe it safe to restart heparin or warfarin 2 to 3 weeks after ICH, when indicated. When the indication for anticoagulation is relative or questionable, it is probably best to discontinue anticoagulants, perhaps using platelet antiaggregants instead.

Leukemia, hemophilia, thrombocytopenia, and disseminated intravascular coagulation (DIC) are other important causes of ICH, although it is unusual in these disorders to have bleeding confined only to the brain. In a 1992 report, some patients given recombinant tissue plasminogen activator (rtPA) to treat coronary artery thrombosis developed ICH, most often in the cerebral lobes or cerebellum.[50] The incidence is rather small, but the brain hematomas are usually devastating or fatal.[50] ICH also occurs after rtPA infusion to treat occlusive cerebrovascular lesions, but in that circumstance, hematomas usually begin within the region of brain infarction.

Drugs

A variety of commonly abused substances are known to cause ICH.[51,52] Alert clinicians should always think of the possibility of drug-related hemorrhage in young patients, in whom other causes of ICH except trauma and AVM are rare. Perhaps best known are *amphetamine* (or "speed") hemorrhages. Hemorrhage often develops within a few minutes of drug use. The most frequent presenting symptoms are headache, confusion, and seizures.[52] Despite large-volume ICHs, there are often surprisingly few focal signs in such patients. This phenomenon is perhaps explained by the frequent coexistence of brain edema, infarcts, and a diffuse vasculopathy, in addition to the focal ICH. In some patients, acute hypertension follows amphetamine use and can potentiate ICH. When first examined by physicians, most patients with amphetamine hemorrhage do not have signs of sympathetic overactivity, such as hypertension, tachycardia, or fever.[51-53]

Citron et al. studied 14 drug abusers, almost all admitting use of methamphetamine, among other drugs.[54] At necropsy, there was fibrinoid necrosis of the media and intima of small and medium-sized arteries, resembling polyarteritis nodosa.[54] Rumbaugh and colleagues studied the angiographic features of a group of methamphetamine abusers and noted beaded arteries with segmental constriction and dilation of intracranial arteries.[55] In monkeys given IV amphetamines, angiography showed similar changes to the human cases, and necropsy revealed small brain hemorrhages, zones of infarction, microaneurysms, and a vasculitis similar to that described by Citron.[56]

I recently reviewed 30 reported, well-documented examples of intracranial hemorrhage after amphetamine use.[51] Among the 30, 24 were known drug abusers; some patients also had used other drugs, and many also often used alcohol. Amphetamine, methamphetamine ("speed"), and dextroamphetamine were the most often used drugs. Seventeen (57%) took oral amphetamines, 12 (40%) administered their drug intravenously, and 1 person inhaled amphetamine nasally. Amphetamine (14) and methamphetamine were responsible for hemorrhage more often than dextroamphetamine (4) in causing intracranial bleeding. The dose used was often unknown or not stated, but hemorrhage followed as small a dose as 20 mg of oral amphetamine.[53] Age among the 22 men and 8 women ranged from 19 to 51 years, with an average of 25.4 years.[51] In 23, the bleeding was intracerebral and most often lobar. In contrast to the situation with cocaine-related hemorrhage, only 1 of the 30 (3%) had an underlying vascular lesion in the form of an aneurysm or AVM.[57] Amphetamine-related hemorrhage can be very serious; 7 patients with hemorrhage died (23%), and 9 required surgical drainage (30%).[51] Recently, a very potent solid form of D-methamphetamine base that can be smoked has begun to appear in the streets under the name "ice." This form is more potent and more rapid acting. The ice–amphetamine relation is likely to prove similar to the crack–cocaine-hydrochloride relationship in terms of complications and potency.

Angiography has often shown striking abnormalities in chronic amphetamine users and other patients with amphetamine-related ICH. Most common are segmental areas of constriction, irregularity, and occasionally fusiform dilation.[51,53,58,59] The focal vascular abnormalities usually emphasize superficial cortical arterial branches and are often referred to as "beading." At times, the changes disappear on subsequent angiography.[58] Customarily, these arteriographic changes have been attributed to arteritis, and immunological phenomena are common in drug users.[51,52] Amphetamines are known to be potent vasoconstrictors. In 1988, series of patients with segmental vasoconstriction and beading thought to be due to vasospasm (commonly in migraine, migrainelike disorders, or after SAH) were described.[60] Vasoconstriction after SAH can become chronic and can produce chronic morphological changes in the media of involved arteries. Segmental changes and beading in some amphetamine users is probably due to pharmacological effects of the drugs used and does not represent a true arteritis.

Since the early 1980s, *cocaine* has far surpassed the amphetamines as a public health problem and as a cause of stroke and drug-related ICH. Cocaine hydrochloride is usually snorted nasally. During the 1980s, addicts turned to *crack cocaine*, a substance made by mixing aqueous cocaine hydrochloride with ammonia and sometimes baking soda. Crack cocaine is smoked or inhaled after the cocaine is mixed in the alkaline solution and precipitated as alkaloidal cocaine. Crack cocaine is absorbed very quickly, reaching the brain in less than 10 seconds.[61] Cocaine hydrochloride can be taken in a variety of ways (orally, vaginally, rectally, sublingually, nasally, and by subcutaneous, intramuscular, or IV injection). Cardiovascular effects begin immediately after use and consist of an increase in pulse, blood pressure, temperature, and metabolism. The pressor effects of cocaine are similar to those of amphetamine and are probably mediated through a peripheral catecholamine mechanism.[56]

In a 1993 text, I reviewed 45 examples of cocaine-related ICH.[51] The series included 28 men and 17 women with ages ranging from 22 to 57 years (average 33.6). Headache, focal neurological signs, and sudden loss of consciousness were the most frequent symptoms and usually began immediately or shortly after the episode of drug use.[51,62] Concurrent use of alcohol was very common. ICH followed use by any route. Fifteen used crack, 14 snorted cocaine nasally, and 11 injected the drug intravenously. The acute mortality was relatively high (14/45, 31%).[51]

The commonest location of cocaine-related ICH was lobar (57%). In others, the bleeding often involved deep structures known to be frequent sites of hypertensive ICH. These included 1 caudate, 3 thalamic, and 8 putaminal hematomas. Of great interest and importance was the frequent presence of an underlying vascular lesion. Twelve patients had AVMs, 3 had aneurysms, and 1 had a glioma with recurrent hemorrhage.[51] Similarly, among 31 cases of SAH after cocaine use, 15 (48.4%) had aneurysms. Among 29 patients with adequate angiographic and/or necropsy study, 25 (86%) had aneurysms.[51] *Cocaine-related ICH has a high mortality, and a very high frequency of underlying aneurysms and AVMs.* Clearly, cocaine-related intracranial bleeding is an indication for angiography, especially when the bleeding is subarachnoid or lobar. Underlying vascular lesions are less common when the ICH is deep. Most authors have attributed cocaine-related hemorrhage to the sympatheticomimetic effects of the drug. In some reported cases, the blood pressure is very high after admission (240/140, 220/110, 210/120 torr, etc.).[51]

Another drug known to have sympatheticomimetic capabilities is *phencyclidine* (PCP, "angel dust"), which has also been occasionally implicated as a cause of ICH[63,64] and of hypertensive encephalopathy.[65] Lysergic acid diethylamide (LSD) and mescaline—two other hallucinogens—are also known to elevate blood pressure and cause vasoconstriction. To my knowledge, however, no reports document ICH after the use of these drugs.

More controversial is the issue of ICH after the use of amphetamine-like drugs. These agents are usually sold over the counter as diet suppressants or stimulants. The most commonly cited agent is *phenylpropanolamine* (PPA), which is often combined with an antihistamine and caffeine. PPA is primarily a partial alpha-adrenergic agonist and has little if any beta-adrenergic agonist activity.[66] PPA has been used in patients with ICH, but the numbers are relatively small, considering the frequency of use of the drug. Among 19 patients, only 4 were men.[51] Ten of the 19 were under 30 years old. In some, the PPA compounds were taken in very high doses in suicidal attempts. Two had SAH only, and 17 had ICH (2 of which were multiple).[67,68] Twelve PPA-related hematomas were lobar, 7 putaminal-capsular, and 2 thalamic.[51] Blood pressures recorded on initial examination were usually within the normal range, but some were very high (210/130, 160/104, 210/110 torr).

Segmental vascular changes similar to those found after amphetamine use have been described.[69] In one patient, the angiographic changes cleared after abstinence from PPA for 1 month.[69] In four patients, histological analysis of tissue removed at surgical drainage of hematomas was available. Three had no indication of vascular lesion on light microscopy, but the fourth did have a necrotizing vasculitis.[70]

The examples of putative PPA-related hemorrhages are difficult to evaluate. In some cases, the use of diet pills was surely incidental, and in other patients, multiple other drugs and risk factors coexisted.[51] In several patients, ICH occurred a few weeks postpartum, a time of vulnerability for spontaneous vascular complications. Although PPA has been shown to be associated with ICH in experimental animals[71] and humans,[51,66,72] it seems reasonable to conclude that reactions to PPA compounds are often idiosyncratic. It is probably dangerous and carries a risk of ICH to use PPA with higher than suggested dose; prior hypertension; additional use of alcohol, coffee, or caffeine; concomitant use of monoamine oxidase inhibitors; and use during the postpartum period.

Occasionally, ICH can develop after the IV use of drugs that are manufactured for oral consumption, such as pentazocine and pyribenzamine ("T's and blues") or methylphenidate.[51,52,73] Talc, methylcellulose, crystals, and cornstarch obliterate the lung arterioles, allowing the particles to get to the systemic circulation following IV use. The damage to brain arterioles then predisposes users to develop ICH.[73]

Amyloid Angiopathy

Congophilic or cerebral amyloid angiopathy (CAA) was recognized by Zenkevich as a potential cause of ICH,[74] but Jellinger is probably most responsible for bringing this disorder to the attention of the neurological community.[75,76] Awareness of the disorder has led to wider use of special stains and recognition that an ever-increasing percentage of ICH, especially in the elderly, is related to CAA. The disorder usually affects small arteries and arterioles in the leptomeninges and cerebral cortex; involved arteries are thickened by an acellular hyaline material that stains positively with periodic acid-Schiff (PAS) stains and has an apple-green birefringence with polarized Congo red stain.[77] Sometimes, the vessel wall seems to be reduplicated or split. CAA predominantly affects persons over age 65 years and increases in frequency in the eighth and ninth decades;[77] in some series of patients, there has been a striking female predilection.[78,79] At necropsy, most patients have senile plaques, and many patients have been diagnosed clinically as suffering from Alzheimer's disease.

The vascular lesions are most commonly found in the occipital and parietal regions, less often in the other cerebral lobes, and rarely, if ever, in the deep basal gray matter, brainstem, or cerebellum. Hemorrhages may be quite large and are often multiple.[79–81] Some patients have recurrent ICH or SAH in different lobar sites, a finding in an elderly person that is virtually diagnostic of CAA. At necropsy, small scattered cerebral infarcts and Alzheimer-related changes are found, along with evidence of old slitlike lobar hemorrhages. Some patients have a Binswanger-like picture with chronic white-matter gliosis and atrophy. Like anticoagulant-related hemorrhages, CAA-related hemorrhages may develop insidiously. Perhaps because of coexisting atrophy, pressure symptoms such as headache and vomiting are less frequent than in younger patients with hypertensive or AVM hemorrhages.

Arteriovenous Malformations

AVMs are uncommon and presumably congenital lesions that occur with approximately one tenth the frequency of intracranial cerebral aneurysms.[82]

Malformations can be composed of small capillaries ("capillary telangiectases"), dilated sinusoidal channels ("cavernous angiomas"), or veins ("veinous angiomas"), but the majority have both arterial and venous elements. Blood is shunted under arterial pressure into the venous system, almost always with dilation of the feeding arteries and recipient veins. Usually, there are numerous thin-walled vascular channels within AVMs that can break.

The lesions most often become symptomatic within the first three decades of life. There is a male preponderance of AVMs, in some series approaching a 2/1 ratio of men to women. Patients with AVM usually present with headache, seizures, or SAH or ICH. Small lesions are more often deep and are generally silent until they bleed, whereas larger lesions are more often associated with headache and seizures.[83]

AVMs can be located in any part of the nervous system. The pons and the periependymal regions are frequent locations. Small AVMs are responsible for the majority of cases of primary intraventricular hemorrhage in the young. When AVMs reside on the surface of the brain or ventricular system, bleeding is often into the brain and subarachnoid space (meningocerebral). Bleeding may be slow because these lesions often have lower pressures than aneurysms. The clinical findings in patients with SAH due to AVM hemorrhage are described in Chapter 12.

Calcifications are sometimes seen on plain skull x-rays. On CT, recent hematomas are readily visible. Contrast enhancement often displays nearby vascular structures and draining veins. MRI is a particularly good technique for visualizing AVMs. Cavernous angiomas produce heterogeneous signals often with evidence of old bleeding. Cavernous angiomas are often familial and multiple[84,85] and are not opacified on angiography. TCD ultrasound has also proven very helpful in detecting and following AVMs. Musical murmurs and patterns of augmented flow are found and can be followed after ablative treatment. In general, short-term mortality from AVM-related ICH is less than that for aneurysmal SAH, but AVMs have a higher rate of rebleeding. Newer techniques of embolization, radiation, and surgery show promise for better eradication of these lesions.[86,87] In young, normotensive, non-drug-abusing men with seizures and recurrent ICH in the same area, AVM is the most likely diagnosis.

Trauma

Trauma can also cause intracerebral bleeding, which is seldom occult. We have seen several patients who were rendered aphasic or stuporous by head blows delivered by others and who could give no history of the trauma; assailants and others did not volunteer their complicity. A search for superficial head bruises or lacerations is worthwhile. Traumatic ICH is most often accompanied by contusions in the basal frontal and temporal lobes, which may be multiple. Occasionally a "spät hemorrhage" (late or delayed hemorrhage) develops into an area of traumatic brain edema when the local swelling subsides.[88]

Arterial Aneurysms

Arterial aneurysms can rupture into both the brain and the CSF, causing so-called meningocerebral hemorrhage. The clinical picture in that circumstance is usually dominated by the SAH, with sudden headache, vomiting, and loss of concentration, but a focal deficit such as hemiparesis or visual field loss is also found on initial examination. The distribution of the bleeding as seen on CT can often help distinguish an aneurysmal meningocerebral hemorrhage from an ICH that has leaked into the CSF. Blood in the basal frontal lobes and the septum pellucidum suggests an anterior communicating artery aneurysm, and blood within the sylvian fissure and adjacent temporal lobe suggests an MCA aneurysm. Aneurysmal bleeding is discussed in detail in Chapter 12 on SAH. Occasionally, a sudden-onset stroke is caused by hemorrhage into a previously unrecognized brain tumor (e.g., metastatic melanoma, hypernephroma, or glioma).

Signs and Symptoms of ICH at Common Locations

Just as there are physicians who believe that chest x-ray made the stethoscope obsolete, some doctors feel that detailed knowledge of the findings on neurological examination of patients with CNS lesions is no longer necessary since the advent of CT. Because hemorrhages are so well imaged by CT, why bother to learn the physical findings? For one thing, in the foreseeable future, physicians will probably not have an inexpensive pocket or portable CT or MRI to take with them to replace the examination of patients. The prognosis and treatment of ICH often depend on the locale of the hemorrhage. Particular locations—such as the cerebral lobes, right putamen, and cerebellum—are relatively accessible to surgical drainage, while others—such as the thalami and brainstem—are not. Because the pace of ICH is often so rapid, the examining physician may have to decide, depending on clinical localization, whether to seek emergent CT for help. Clinical distinction between ICH and superficial cerebral infarction due to large-vessel occlusive disease or cerebral embolism depends on localization of the lesion to deep (ICH) or superficial (infarct) location. Historically, hemorrhages in the cerebellum, thalami, and caudate were recognized before cerebellar, thalamic, or caudate infarction. Awareness of the clinical syndromes associated with ICH in these locations made it possible to later recognize infarcts in these regions. For these and many other regions, it is still very important for clinicians to know the common clinical syndromes in ICH and to be able to localize clinically the lesion in most patients with intracranial hemorrhages.[89]

Keys to localization of ICH are

1. motor signs—quadriparesis, hemiparesis, or no paresis
2. pupillary function—asymmetry, size, and light reaction

	Pathology	CT scan	Pupils	Eye movements	Motor and sensory deficits	Other
Caudate nucleus (blood in ventricle)	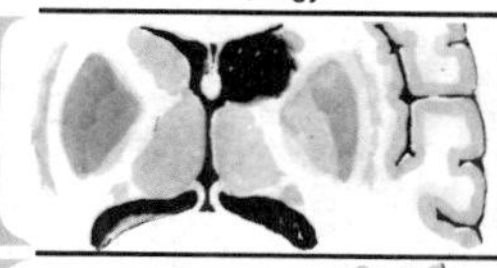	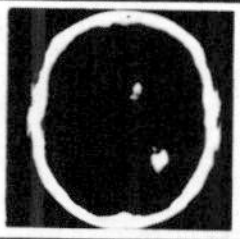	Sometimes ipsilaterally constricted	Conjugate deviation to side of lesion. Slight ptosis	Contralateral hemiparesis, often transient	Headache, confusion
Putamen (small hemorrhage)	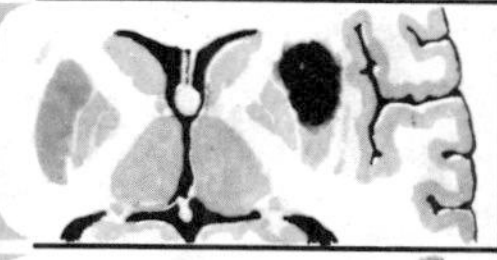	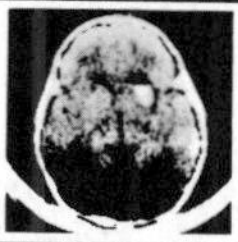	Normal	Conjugate deviation to side of lesion	Contralateral hemiparesis and hemisensory loss	Aphasia (if lesion on left side)
Putamen (large hemorrhage)	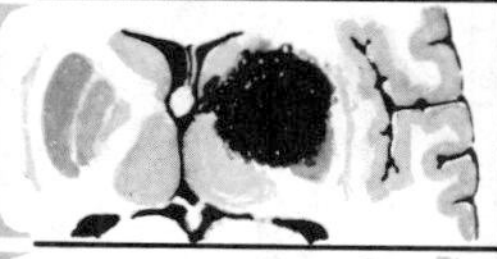	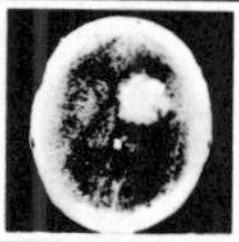	In presence of herniation, pupil dilated on side of lesion	Conjugate deviation to side of lesion	Contralateral hemiparesis and hemisensory loss	Decreased consciousness
Thalamus	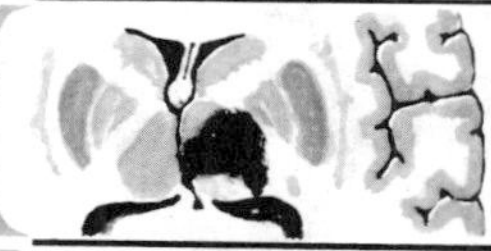	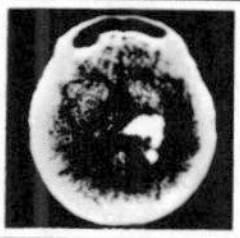	Constricted, poorly reactive to light bilaterally	Both lids retracted. Eyes positioned downward and medially. Cannot look upward	Slight contralateral hemiparesis, but greater hemisensory loss	Aphasia (if lesion on left side)
Occipital lobar white matter	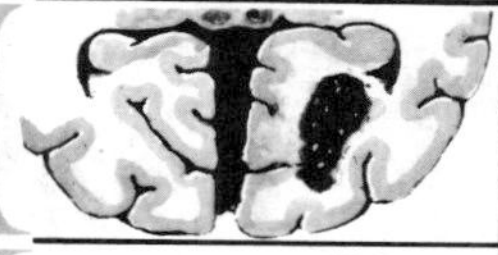	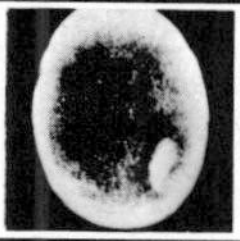	Normal	Normal	Mild, transient hemiparesis	Contralateral hemianopsia
Pons	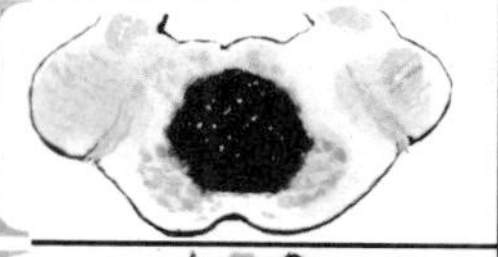	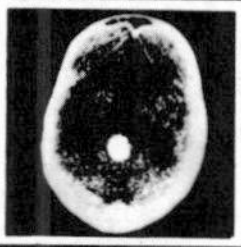	Constricted, reactive to light	No horizontal movements. Vertical movements preserved	Quadriplegia	Coma
Cerebellum	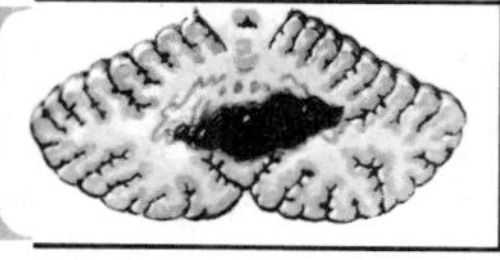	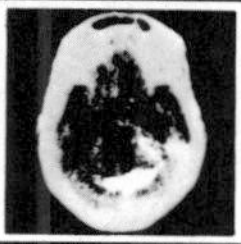	Slight constriction on side of lesion	Slight deviation to opposite side. Movements toward side of lesion impaired, or sixth cranial nerve palsy	Ipsilateral limb ataxia. No hemiparesis	Gait ataxia, vomiting

FIGURE 13.4   Clinical manifestations related to site in intracerebral hemorrhage. (© Copyright 1986 CIBA Pharmaceutical Company, division of CIBA-GEIGY Corporation. Reprinted with permission from The Ciba Collection of Medical Illustrations, illustrated by Frank H. Netter, M.D. All rights reserved.)

3.   extraocular movements—gaze, nuclear, or internuclear palsy
4.   gait abnormalities—especially ataxia

Figure 13.4 and Table 13.2 summarize the usual abnormalities of these functions in patients with hemorrhages at the commonest locations of ICH.

Hemorrhages of the Lateral Basal Ganglia, Putamen, and Internal Capsule

The commonest location of hypertensive ICH is the lateral basal-ganglionic–capsular region. These lesions are usually referred to as *putaminal hemor-*

TABLE 13.2.
Neurologic Findings in Patients with ICH at Common Sites

Locale	Motor Weakness	Sensory Loss	Hemi- anopia	Pupils	Eye Movements	Other
Caudate	Hemiparesis + –	–	–	Normal	– or transient conjugate gaze palsy contralateral	Confusion
Putamen, small	Hemiparesis + +	+	–	Normal	–	–
Putamen, large	Hemiparesis + + + + + +	+ +	+ +	+ – ipsilateral fixed, dilated	Conjugate gaze palsy contralateral	L: aphasia R: left-sided neglect, con- structional apraxia
Thalamus	Hemiparesis +	+ + +	+ –	Small nonreactive	Eyes down, or down and in; vertical gaze palsy; conjugate gaze palsy ipsilateral or contra- lateral; pseudo sixth nerve palsy	Confusion L: aphasia

Lobar					
Frontal	Hemiparesis +	–	Normal	–	Abulic
Parietal	Hemiparesis +	+++	++	Normal	–	L: aphasia; R: left-sided neglect, constructional apraxia
Temporal	–	–	++	Normal	–	L: aphasia, agitation
Occipital	– or transient	– or transient	++++	Normal	–	–
Pontine						
Median	Quadraparesis ++++ ⎤					
Large	Quadraparesis ++++ ⎦	+ –	–	Small reaction	Bilateral horizontal conjugate gaze palsy, bobbing	Hyperventilation
Lateral tegmental	– or transient	Contralateral hemisensory +++	–	Ipsilateral small reaction	1½ syndrome	Limb ataxia
Cerebellar	–	–	–	Small reaction	Ipsilateral sixth nerve palsy or ipsilateral conjugate gaze palsy	Gait ataxia

Note: L = left-sided lesion, R = right-sided lesion.

rhage because they most often begin in the putamen. The usual findings include contralateral hemiparesis, contralateral hemisensory loss, and conjugate deviation of the eyes toward the side of the hematoma. The pupils are generally normal, and gait is hemiparetic. Patients with a left putaminal hemorrhage usually have a nonfluent aphasia with relative preservation of the ability to repeat spoken language. Right-sided lesions are associated with left visual neglect, motor impersistence, and constructional dyspraxia. These abnormalities of higher cortical function are probably due to disconnection and undercutting of cortical zones and are usually more transient than in patients with cortical infarcts of equal size. Some patients develop ipsilateral adventitious movements that the family or observers call "tremor"; these movements are probably due to involvement of ipsilateral descending projections of the extrapyramidal system.

As the lesion enlarges, patients develop increasing stupor; the ipsilateral pupil at first becomes smaller, and later larger than the opposite pupil; the ipsilateral plantar response becomes extensor; and a bilateral horizontal gaze palsy develops. The presence of any of these signs—ipsilateral Babinski sign, abnormal ipsilateral pupil, or ipsilateral gaze paresis—has a very grim prognosis.[11,22] These additional findings are due to midline shift or compression of the rostral brainstem by the expanding hematoma.

The findings described are those found in patients with large hematomas that involve the medial and most anterior portions of the posterior putamen and the anterior two thirds of the posterior limb of the internal capsule.[90,91] This location is the commonest site for putaminal hemorrhage because it is supplied by the largest of the lateral lenticulostriate arteries. Some lesions affect the anterior limb of the internal capsule and anterior putamen and produce a milder, more transient hemiparesis without sensory abnormalities.[90] When hematomas are in the posterior third of the internal capsule and far posterior extreme of the putamen, sensory abnormalities predominate, with little or no hemiparesis. An inferior quadrant anopia or hemianopia may be present. Lesions in the far posterior left putamen may have fluent Wernicke-like aphasia because of undercutting of the temporal lobe or extension of the lesion into the temporal isthmus, giving the hematoma a hockey-stick-like configuration. Figure 13.5 depicts the anatomical distribution of lesions within the lateral basal-ganglionic region on horizontal brain section. The most common and usually the largest lesions affecting the anterior part of the posterior limb of the internal capsule are often referred to as the *middle type*, while the others are termed *anterior* or *posterior types* of putaminal hematomas.[31]

Putaminal hemorrhages vary greatly in size. In one series of 24 patients,[22] the smallest hematoma volume was 20 mm^2, while the largest was 225 mm^2. Patients with small hematomas, as shown in Figure 13.6, have a good outcome. Larger hemorrhages are more likely to rupture into the ventricle and have a much higher mortality than do small putaminal hematomas.[22,92] Most often, the bleeding extends along the anteroposterior

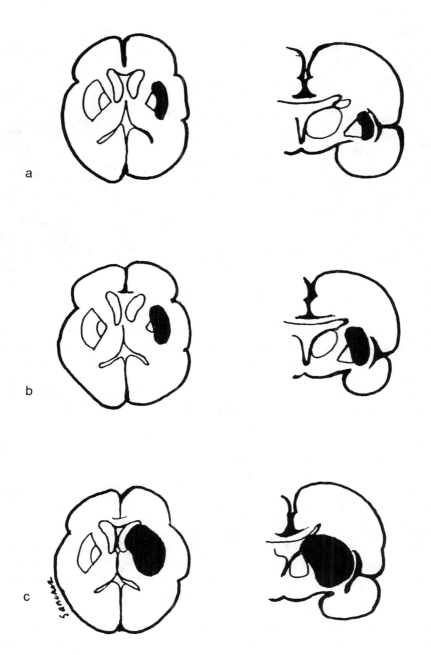

FIGURE 13.5 Examples of putaminal hemorrhage. (a) Hemorrhage within the boundaries of the putamen. (b) Encroachment on the internal capsule. (c) Hematoma progressing into the body of the lateral ventricle.

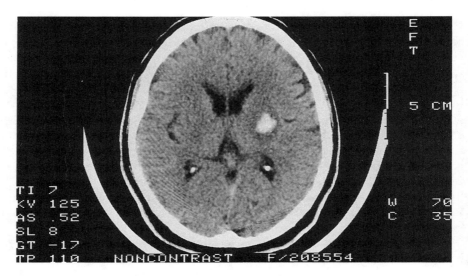

FIGURE 13.6   CT showing a small left putaminal hemorrhage.

axis of the brain, but some lesions are globoid, and others extend laterally toward the cortical surface, along white-matter tracts.[22] Analysis of CT scans at the level of the body of the lateral ventricles can help prognosticate the likelihood of recovery from hemiplegia.[91] When the hematoma occupies CT sections containing the bodies of the lateral ventricles, then the middle type of hematoma is usually present, and hemiplegia is likely to persist. When this region is free of bleeding, hemiparesis is more often absent, slight, or transient.[91]

Cerebral angiography may be helpful in studying patients with putaminal hemorrhage. Mizukami and colleagues studied 60 postmortem specimens from patients with ICH, using microangiography.[93] They identified the source of the bleeding as lateral lenticulostriate arteries, analyzed the postmortem displacement of these vessels, and correlated their findings with the angiographic anatomy in 100 other patients with autopsy or surgically confirmed ICH.[93] In large putaminal hemorrhages, the most lateral lenticulostriate arteries are displaced medially, increasing the distance between the most lateral lenticulostriate arteries and the insular artery. Anterior and posterior lesions have different patterns of displacement of lenticulostriate arteries.[93]

Since the mid-1980s, PET and SPECT have yielded insights into the clinical findings in patients with putaminal hemorrhage.[94] Anterior lesions show depression of frontal-lobe function ipsilaterally, while posterior lesions more often affect the temporal and parietal lobes. The pattern of cortical depression helps predict aphasia type and recovery.[94]

Caudate Hemorrhage

Hemorrhage into the caudate nucleus accounts for approximately 7 percent of ICH.[95] Hematomas at this site frequently discharge quickly into the adjacent lateral ventricle or may spread laterally toward the internal capsule or inferiorly toward the hypothalamus. Early ventricular dilation by blood probably accounts for the most common symptoms of caudate hemorrhage: headache, vomiting, decreased alertness, and stiff neck.[95–97] Some patients also are confused, disoriented, and have poor memory.[95,97] The larger parenchymatous lesions cause a contralateral hemiparesis, conjugate deviation of the eyes to the side of the lesion, conjugate gaze palsy to the opposite side, and an ipsilateral small pupil or Horner's syndrome.[95] Sensory findings are usually absent or minimal. The usual cause of caudate hemorrhage is hypertension, but AVMs are also common, especially in the young. Caudate hematomas have a better prognosis than comparable-sized putaminal hemorrhages.

The symptoms and signs of caudate hemorrhage closely mimic SAH, but the CT appearance of blood in the caudate and lateral ventricles is distinctive.

Thalamic Hemorrhage

Thalamic hematomas are usually posterior to the pyramidal-tract fibers in the internal capsule, so that contralateral sensory abnormalities are usually more prominent than is contralateral hemiparesis. Sometimes, the contralateral limbs are ataxic or have choreic movements. The contralateral hand may rest in a fisted or dystonic posture. The key neurological findings that separate thalamic from caudate or putaminal hemorrhages are the eye signs. Patients with caudate or putaminal hemorrhages have conjugate deviation of the eyes toward the side of the lesion and paresis of conjugate gaze to the opposite side. The commonest oculomotor abnormalities in patients with thalamic hematomas are

1. *paralysis of upward gaze,* often with one or both eyes resting downward
2. *hyperconvergence of one or both eyes,*[23,24,89,98] with a combination of these findings giving patients the appearance of peering downward and inward at the tops of their noses

Other oculomotor signs include:

3. *ocular skewing,* in which one eye rests below the other, with this divergence in vertical eye position remaining constant in gaze in all directions
4. *eyes gazing the wrong way,* resting toward the opposite side.[24]
5. *disconjugate gaze,* with limited abduction of one or both eyes, so-called

pseudo-sixth-nerve paresis;[89,98,99] failure of ocular abduction due to visual fixation by the adducted eye and increased convergence vectors neutralizing abduction—not due to involvement of the sixth nerve[99]

These ocular abnormalities are due to direct extension of the hematoma to the diencephalic–mesencephalic junction or to compression of the quadrigeminal plate region by the thalamic hematoma. In thalamic hemorrhage, the pupils are usually small and react poorly to light because of interruption of the afferent limb of the pupillary reflex arc.

Patients with large left thalamic hemorrhages often have an unusual aphasia.[100–102] After beginning a conversation almost normally, patients may lapse into a remarkable fluent aphasia, with many jargon or nonexistent words and poor communication of ideas. In contrast to patients with Wernicke's aphasia, comprehension of spoken language is good. Patients with thalamic ICH may repeat and duplicate words or syllables at the ends of words in both spoken and written language. Paraphasic errors and poor naming are also common. Patients with right thalamic hematomas often have left visual neglect, anosognosia, and visuospatial abnormalities.[23,103]

Decreased levels of consciousness and alertness and hypersomnolence are extremely common at the onset of thalamic hemorrhage because of involvement of the rostral reticular activating system. The prognosis for recovery from thalamic hemorrhages is not as good as from caudate or putaminal hemorrhages of comparable size, but coma is not as dire a prognostic sign in thalamic lesions as it is in other supratentorial sites. Also, unlike putaminal hemorrhage, both the severity of the deficit and the mortality do not correlate with ventricular extension in thalamic hematomas.[92] Figure 13.7 shows a CT scan from a patient with an anterior thalamic hematoma, which spread into the ventricles. She made an excellent recovery. Thalamic hemorrhages are not accessible surgically unless they extend far laterally. Most studies have not differentiated medial from lateral or posterior thalamic hematomas, although lesions at these various sites yield different clinical syndromes and have different prognoses for recovery.

Since the mid-1980s, using MRI and CT, it has become possible to distinguish syndromes related to small discrete hemorrhages in the thalamus.[104–106] The *posterolateral* type, in the territory of the thalamogeniculate arteries, are the commonest and largest type of thalamic hematoma. These lesions often spill out of the thalamus laterally and cause motor paralysis by involving the internal capsule. Sensorimotor signs predominate, and pupillary and eye-movement abnormalities are slight or absent unless the hematoma is quite large and spreads to or compresses the medial thalamus. *Anterior* or *anterolateral* thalamic hematomas are in the distribution of the tuberothalamic (polar) artery; behavioral abnormalities predominate, especially apathy and abulia. *Medial hematomas* are in the distribution of the thalamic–subthalamic thalamoperforating arteries; abnormalities of consciousness, pupillary function, and vertical gaze

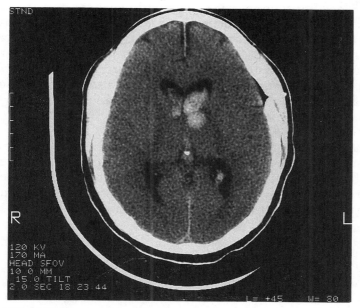

FIGURE 13.7   CT showing a small left anterior thalamic hematoma, which drained into the lateral ventricles; blood casts are seen within the ventricle.

predominate. The hematoma often spreads to the third ventricle and can compress the diencephalic–mesencephalic junction and can obstruct the third ventricle, causing hydrocephalus.[107,108] Far *posterior* lesions predominantly involve the pulvinar in the distribution of the posterior choroidal arteries; slight sensorimotor signs may be found but are usually transient, and aphasia and behavioral abnormalities are common. In patients with hydrocephalus due to third-ventricle obstruction, shunting has resulted in reversal of some of the eye-movement abnormalities.[107,108]

Lobar Hemorrhages

ICH may develop beneath the region of the gray–white junction of the cerebral cortex. These subcortical hemorrhages usually spread in a linear direction along white-matter pathways. When the hematomas absorb, linear cavities remain, giving the lesion the name *slit hemorrhage*. The lesions undercut cortex and often do not obey the strict divisions of cerebral lobes; hence, the term *lobar hemorrhage* actually is inaccurate; nonetheless, I use it here because of its widespread acceptance. Undercutting of the cortex can be epileptogenic, causing repeated focal seizures of limited duration.[109]

Subcortical hemorrhages are important to diagnose because the symptoms and signs are readily misinterpreted as being due to cerebral infarction, and inappropriate therapy might be prescribed. Also, if subcortical hemorrhages are large, they are relatively superficial and are more accessible to surgical drainage than are deeper hematomas. In the past, subcortical hemorrhages were rarely diagnosed antemortem, but CT now has greatly enhanced recognition of these lesions. Many lobar hemorrhages are due to AVMs and CAA, each of which has a predilection for cortical and subcortical regions. Some hypertensive lesions are also subcortical. The parietal and occipital lobes are affected more often than the frontal or parietal regions. Symptoms and signs depend on the lobes affected, as follows:[100,110]

Frontal hematomas—Far anterior lesions usually cause abulia. Patients seem lethargic and have reduced spontaneity, prolonged latency in responding, and short, terse replies. If the lesions extend deeply or toward the precentral gyrus, both conjugate eye deviation toward the side of the hematoma and contralateral hemiparesis are found.

Central hematomas—Lesions near the central sulcus produce contralateral motor and sensory signs, with aphasia if the lesion is in the left hemisphere.

Parietal hemorrhages—These are usually accompanied by contralateral hemisensory loss, with neglect of the contralateral visual field.

Occipital hematomas—These cause a severe contralateral hemianopia, often with slight contralateral hemisensory or motor signs and visual neglect.

Temporal-lobe lesions—These lesions often cause agitation and delirium. Wernicke-type aphasia accompanies left temporal lesions. Temporal-lobe hematomas are particularly likely to swell and may cause herniation without preceding hemiparesis. Brainstem compression may develop insidiously, with deepening stupor and then an ipsilaterally dilated pupil.

Lobar hematomas are in general of smaller volume than are deep lesions, and they have a lower mortality rate.[110] The functional outcome in patients with lobar ICH is also generally better than in other forms of ICH.[109,110] The diagnosis is often quite difficult without CT or MRI. Because of the higher incidence of vascular malformations and other bleeding lesions in patients with lobar hematomas, angiography is often indicated.

Primary Intraventricular Hemorrhages

In some patients, the principal locus of bleeding is into the ventricular cavities. Ventricular bleeding usually arises from small subependymal AVMs or from hemorrhage into the caudate nucleus just adjacent to the ventricles. The clinical syndrome closely mimics SAH—with sudden headache, stiff neck, vomiting, and lethargy. At times, there are bilateral, usually symmetrical hyperreflexia and extensor plantar responses. CT shows blood distending the lateral ventricles and the third ventricle and some blood density within the subarachnoid space. In childhood, the commonest cause is an AVM, which can destroy itself as it ruptures. These small angiomas may arise in the choroid plexus.[111] In adults, most intraventricular hemorrhages are due to ventricular spread of primary hypertensive bleeds into periventricular structures.[112]

Pontine Hemorrhage

Primary brainstem hemorrhages are located most often in the pons. Midbrain and medullary hemorrhages are rare and, when present, are usually caused by blood dyscrasias or AVMs.[113] Raised ICP, especially if it develops quickly, frequently causes secondary lesions, so-called Düret hemorrhages, in the median or paramedian zones of the thalamus, midbrain, and pons, due to stretching of paramedian vascular structures.[114] Pontine hemorrhage usually begins in the center of the pons at the tegmental–basal junction. These hematomas grow quickly and assume a round or oval shape, usually destroying the center of the tegmentum and the base of the pons. The blood may dissect rostrally into the midbrain but rarely extends caudally into the medulla. Hematomas frequently dissect into the fourth ventricle. These large pontine hemorrhages arise from the larger median pontine penetrating vessels that originate from the basilar artery.

The signs accompanying large medial pontine hematomas are quadriparesis, often with limb stiffness and rigidity; coma; absent horizontal eye movements; small but reactive pupils; and rapid or irregular respirations.[89,115-117] Headache and vomiting occasionally occur. Some pontine hemorrhages develop gradually,[17] and early findings may be asymmetrical. Deafness, dysarthria, facial numbness, asymmetric facial or limb weakness, and dizziness occasionally precede the development of coma. Some patients have twitching, shivering, or spasmodic movements of the limbs, usually culminating in decerebrate rigidity. Vertical reflex eye movements are preserved unless the lesion extends into the midbrain. In some patients, the eyes spontaneously and repeatedly bob downward.[113,118] Massive pontine hemorrhages are invariably fatal but not usually instantaneously so. Death usually occurs 24 to 48 hours after onset, but survival for 7 to 10 days is not rare. Some patients with large medial pontine hematomas survive with quadriplegia. Hyperthermia is sometimes noted. CT has now allowed documentation of two other types of pontine hemorrhage: small basal hematomas[119,120] and lateral tegmental pontine hematomas.[117,118] In Silverstein's series of 50 necropsy-proven pontine hemorrhages coming to autopsy at the Philadelphia General Hospital, 28 were massive central hematomas, 11 were located in the lateral basis pontis, and 11 were tegmental.[116] These sites correspond to the usual distribution of penetrating pontine arteries.

Lateral basal hematomas can cause pure motor hemiparesis[119] or ataxic hemiparesis,[120] thus mimicking the findings in lacunar infarction. Lateral basal lesions can spread into the adjacent tegmentum, causing unilateral cranial-nerve signs and contralateral hemiparesis. Lateral tegmental hematomas arise from penetrating vessels that course from lateral to medial after branching from the lateral circumferential pontine arteries. These lesions involve the rostral pons, and the findings on neurological examination are those of a predominantly unilateral tegmental lesion.

Most distinctive and diagnostic are the oculomotor abnormalities, which include ipsilateral conjugate-gaze paresis, ipsilateral internuclear ophthalmoplegia (INO), or a combination of INO and gaze palsy (a "one and one-half syndrome"[24,117]), in which the only preserved eye motion is abduction of the contralateral eye. Because the sensory lemniscus (joining of the medial lemniscus and spinothalamic tracts) is tegmental, accompanying loss of pinprick, temperature, and position sense on the opposite side of the body is common. Limb and truncal ataxia are usually present and may be bilateral or predominantly ipsilateral. Unilateral facial numbness or weakness, ipsilateral miosis, and transient deafness may also be present. When contralateral hemiparesis occurs, it is usually slight and transient. Patients with small pontine hematomas generally survive with slight to moderate clinical neurological deficits.

Cerebellar Hemorrhages

Hemorrhage into the cerebellum probably accounts for about 10 percent of ICH, approximating the relative percentage of weight of the cerebellum in reference to the entire brain. Although the frequency of cerebellar hemorrhage is low, establishing the diagnosis is important because of the potentially serious outcome if not treated and the contrasting good prognosis after surgical treatment. Cerebellar hemorrhage usually originates in the region of the dentate nucleus, arising from distal branches of the SCA and the PICA. Hematomas collect around the dentate and spread into the cerebellar hemispheral white matter, frequently extending into the fourth ventricle. The adjacent brainstem is seldom directly involved but is compressed from above by the lesion.

The most consistent symptom is inability to walk. Some patients even have difficulty remaining in a sitting or standing position, often leaning or tilting toward the side of the hematoma. Patients have been known to crawl, slide, or bump on their bottom to get to the bathroom or to the phone. Vomiting is also very frequent, occurring in 68 (92%) of 72 patients from several series.[113] Headache is also common, usually affecting the occiput or neck or frontal region. Dysarthria, hiccups, and tinnitus occur but are less frequent. Loss of consciousness at onset is distinctly unusual, but by the time these patients reach the hospital, about one third are obtunded.[121–123]

Neurological signs include an ipsilateral abducens or gaze palsy toward the side of the hematoma; small pupils, with the ipsilateral pupil slightly smaller; rebound overshoot of the rapidly elevated ipsilateral arm; and gait ataxia. Hemiparesis probably does not occur in cerebellar hemorrhage, but cerebellar lesions do produce an apparent asthenia or slowness of the affected limbs.[124] Inferior extremity reflexes are usually symmetrically exaggerated, but plantar responses are flexor. Classic cerebellar-type incoordination of the arm on finger-to-nose testing or of the leg on toe-to-object testing and frank intention tremor are uncommon. In my experience with patients with cerebellar infarction and hemorrhage, the single most useful cerebellar sign is elicited when the patient is asked to raise both arms together rapidly, then to brake the ascent quickly. Next, the patient is directed to drop the arms quickly, again braking the descent before the hands hit the bed or table. The arm on the side of the cerebellar lesion lags behind the other arm and overshoots the endpoint.

Patients with larger cerebellar hematomas usually develop brainstem compression. They develop increasing stupor, lateral gaze palsy toward the side of the hematoma, and bilateral extensor plantar responses. Among those patients not comatose on admission in one series, only 20 percent had a smooth, uneventful recovery, but 80 percent deteriorated to coma, 25 percent of these within 3 hours after onset.[121] In the series of Fisher et al.,[122] only 2 of 18 patients had a benign course, and the other 16 developed coma, usually within a few hours. Because the hematoma usually affects the caudal cerebellum, the medulla is the portion of the brainstem compressed, and so vasomotor disturbances and respiratory arrest may develop. Untreated patients with cerebellar hemorrhage who become comatose invariably die of brainstem compression. CT not only documents the size, locale, and position of the hematoma but also yields considerable information about posterior-fossa pressure. An expanding lesion obliterates the cerebellopontine angle and ambient cisterns, and it displaces the fourth ventricle toward the opposite side. Usually, the fourth ventricle compression leads to hydrocephalus, with early distension of the temporal horns of the lateral ventricles.

Occasionally, patients with cerebellar hemorrhage have a more indolent course, presenting with symptoms and signs of hydrocephalus. Abulia, dementia, slow-stepped shuffling gait, and incontinence are the characteristic signs of hydrocephalus. The patient and family may fail to emphasize the preceding symptoms of dizziness, headache, and vomiting that had been interpreted as the flu. Other patients have laterally placed cerebellar hematomas that compress the cerebellopontine angle structures, and they develop dysfunction of the fifth, sixth, seventh, and eighth cranial nerves, in addition to ataxia. Rarer is hemorrhage into the vermis, with headache, vomiting, and sudden coma.[113]

Because the course of cerebellar hematomas is unpredictable and larger lesions frequently cause coma and death, it is probably wise to drain lesions that are 3 cm or greater, especially if there is any decrease in level of alertness.[125] Some patients have been successfully treated by medical decompression (steroids and osmotic diuretic agents) or ventricular drainage.[126] Ventricular shunts do not treat brainstem compression and have been followed by delayed deterioration.[127]

Diagnosis, Prognosis, and Treatment

Diagnosis

Accurate bedside diagnosis of ICH rests on the presence of an appropriate ecological background, such as hypertension or bleeding diathesis; the nonfluctuating, usually gradually progressive course over minutes or hours; accompanying symptoms such as headache and vomiting; and neurological signs compatible with a deep lesion. CT has proven to be an unparalleled instrument for the diagnosis of ICH. Blood provides dense contrast, even acutely. A reported patient with ICH had an abrupt increase in symptoms while in the CT scanner. The initial films had shown a small, round hyperdensity in the lentiform nucleus. A second film of the same area showed a very much larger, hyperdense, irregular zone, extending laterally from the putamen to the insula.[128] Other investigators have also described enlargement of hematomas on sequential CT scans.[14,15]

Findings on CT scan can help determine the age of the hematoma. Hematomas are at first regular and smooth. During the first 48 hours, large hematomas may show fluid-blood levels, indicating that the hematoma is partially liquid and has not solidified.[129] During the first 72 hours or more, edema produces a hypodense area around the lesion, and considerable mass effect is noted. From 3 to 20 days after bleeding, the dense area becomes smaller, beginning at the periphery, and the border develops an irregular contour, which is enhanced with the use of contrast.[130,131] Reduction of edema and mass effect also occurs during this period. Intraventricular blood has usually disappeared by the fifth week.[132] The absorption coefficient of the hematoma decreases gradually, and the lesion develops a lucent appearance, with absorption characteristics resembling edema fluid or CSF. By 9 weeks, mass effect and enhancement are usually gone, and a local circumscribed region of slight hypodensity remains.[132] On MRI or PET scans, the zone of altered attenuation or abnormal metabolism is usually much larger than the hypodensity seen on CT.

Acute hematomas are isointense or hypointense on T1-weighted scans, sometimes with a darker hypointense rim, and they are bright and hyperintense on T2-weighted images. Figure 13.8 shows a large acute hematoma in the thalamus, imaged by T2-weighted MRI. Later, the center of the hematoma appears dark on T2 and is surrounded by a bright rim. Chronic hematomas are bright on T2-weighted images.

Prognosis

The size and locale of the lesion on CT give useful prognostic information. In putaminal hemorrhages, lesions greater than 140 mm^2 in one slice had a poorer outcome.[22] In thalamic hemorrhage, lesions greater than 3.3 cm in maximal diameter had a poor prognosis,[23] as did cerebellar lesions greater than 3 cm.[133] In three other studies, large-volume hematomas were invari-

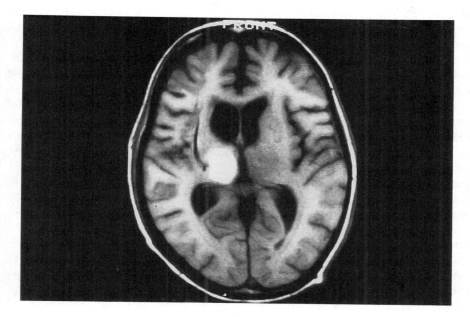

a

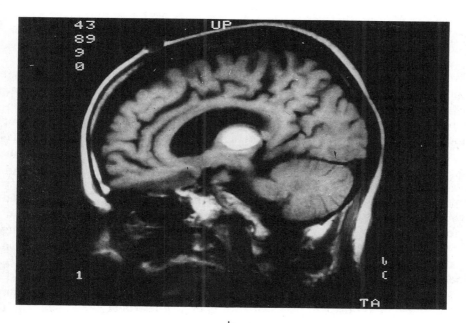

b

FIGURE 13.8 MRI T2-weighted axial (a) and sagittal (b) sections, showing a large thalamic hematoma.

ably associated with a poor outcome.[18,134,135] Pulse pressure and level of consciousness, as measured by the Glasgow coma scale, are also important prognostic variables.[18] Angiography is generally unnecessary unless the lesion is in an unusual locus or the patient has no risk factors for hemorrhage, such as hypertension or bleeding diathesis. Angiography is used to opacify AVMs or aneurysms that might have caused ICH.

During the acute phase of ICH, the mass effect of the developing hematoma presents a much larger risk of death than does a comparable-sized cerebral infarct. In the case of ICH, something extra (blood) has been added to the intracranial contents. In cerebral infarction, the already existing contents, brain tissue, are ischemic, but an acute mass has not been added. Later, both infarcts and hematomas become edematous, increasing ICP. In the chronic phase, if the patient with ICH has survived, the prognosis for recovery is actually much better than that for cerebral infarcts of similar size and location. Hematomas have dissected and separated the cerebral cortex and other brain parts, but usually the surrounding cortex is preserved. In contrast, infarcts leave dead, nonfunctioning cortex when they heal. Unlike SAH, recurrence of ICH during the acute illness is rare. These simple facts dictate the approach to ICH treatment—that is, aggressively try to limit the expanding hematoma, in order to prevent death and late morbidity. In patients with ICH, the concern is control of acute mass effect, whereas in SAH, the goal is to prevent rebleeding and arterial vasoconstriction.

Treatment

Careful medical management of patients with ICH may be lifesaving and is important even in those patients who will later have surgical drainage of their hematomas. Increased ICP causes decreased responsiveness and hypoventilation; in turn, hypoventilation causes a low arterial oxygen tension and high carbon dioxide tension, which lead to vasodilation and further increase in ICP. Maintenance of a good airway and mechanical hyperventilation can reverse this process and quickly lower ICP. Control of systemic blood pressure helps stop intracranial bleeding but must be done cautiously. In some patients with ICH, systemic blood pressure is further increased to ensure adequate perfusion of the brain. Increased ICP causes increased venous pressure, so elevated arterial pressure is needed to overcome the increased venous pressure in order to perfuse the tissues. Overzealous lowering of blood pressure can lead to underperfusion and clinical deterioration. Blood pressure should be lowered quickly but not to hypotensive levels, and patients must be watched carefully during the treatment.

So-called medical decompression with corticosteroids, mannitol, or glycerol is widely used in patients with ICH, but few data exist about their effectiveness. There is concern that hypertonic agents could diffuse into the ICH and cause a secondary increase in volume of the hematoma because of ingress of fluid. Langfitt noted that mannitol and forced hyperventilation were effective in reducing ICP in a group of patients with ICH.[136] When considering therapy, hematomas in practice can be divided into three main groups.

1. *Massive, rapidly developing lesions* that effectively have killed or devastated patients before they reach the hospital: For these lesions, little can or should be done.
2. *Small hematomas,* from which the patient will make an excellent spontaneous recovery: Treatment consists of controlling the etiological factors, such as hypertension, to prevent recurrences.
3. *Medium-sized hematomas*—between the two extremes—with developing mass effect after the patient reaches the hospital: Within this third group, medical measures and surgery can be most helpful.

Because hematomas represent the development of so-called benign masses, the logical treatment for life-threatening lesions is surgical drainage. The following factors should be considered in deciding on surgical therapy: size, location, mass effect and drainage patterns, etiology, timing, and clinical course.

Size.   Hematomas over 3 cm in their widest diameter have a higher mortality and a more delayed recovery rate than do smaller lesions. Thus, the larger the lesion is on CT, the more logical its drainage would be.

Location.   Some hematomas are more accessible surgically, such as those in the cerebellum or cerebral lobes. Though putaminal hemorrhages can be drained through the sylvian fissures and insular cortex, large left basal-ganglionic hemorrhages usually leave patients aphasic and dependent, so treatment should be less aggressive than for right-sided lesions. Cerebellar ICH can cause respiratory arrest without preceding gradual deterioration of neurological function or alertness, and surgical removal of a portion of the cerebellum often leaves no important residual handicap. For these reasons, the threshold for recommending surgery for cerebellar hematomas is lower than for other lesions of comparable size. Cerebellar, lobar, and right putaminal hemorrhages are most accessible to surgical drainage.

Mass Effect and Drainage Patterns.   The size of the hematoma does not, by itself, solely determine mass effect. Older patients may have sufficient preexisting atrophy to be able to accommodate a sizable hematoma without a critical rise in ICP or shift in intracranial compartments. Some lesions have a great deal of surrounding edema, while others have relatively little. Does the lesion compress the third or lateral ventricle? Is there a shift of the midline, or is there uncal herniation? In posterior fossa ICH, is there displacement of the fourth ventricle, and are the ambient, cerebellopontine, and other cisterns effaced? Does the lesion drain into the ventricles or superficially into the subarachnoid space? Entry into the CSF may spontaneously decompress the lesion. Surgical drainage would be indicated more strongly for lesions with greater mass effect and no spontaneous decompression.

Etiology.   Hematomas caused by CAA tend to bleed even after surgical drainage because of the fragility of the blood vessels.[125,137] Similarly, hemorrhages in patients with anticoagulant-related or other bleeding disorders will also continue to bleed unless the coagulopathy is reversed before surgery. When operating on hematomas caused by AVMs, ideally, surgeons would like to remove the AVM while also draining the hematoma. The threshold for surgical treatment should be most favorable for AVMs, moderately so for hypertensive accessible lesions, and least favorable for CAA or for ICH due to a bleeding diathesis.

Timing.   During the first 24 to 36 hours, hematomas are still at least partly liquid and can be more easily drained. Later, hematomas solidify and become technically more difficult to drain. After 7 to 10 days, blood begins to be absorbed, and again the lesion becomes softer. Thus, ideally, for technical reasons, drainage should occur either very early or after 7 to 10 days. In general, if the patient has survived the first week, improvement occurs as edema subsides, so there seems little argument for late drainage except for concurrent removal of an AVM. Some have wondered whether late surgery (1–2 weeks) would speed recovery, but this argument is unsupported by data.

Clinical Course.   Perhaps the most important factor to consider is whether the patient is improving, stable, or worsening. Patients who deteriorate and show a decrease in level of consciousness to severe lethargy or stupor have a poor outlook for recovery.[8,11] In patients with putaminal hemorrhage, other poor prognostic signs include the development of ipsilateral pupillary dilation, ipsilateral extensor plantar response, or an ipsilateral conjugate-gaze paresis; these signs are indicative of midline shift or early brainstem compression. In patients with cerebellar hemorrhage, the development of bilateral extensor plantar responses is a poor prognostic sign.[122] In deteriorating patients with accessible lesions, surgery should not be delayed if medical decompression is not quickly beneficial. Advances in neuroimaging capabilities since the mid-1980s have made it possible to drain hematomas percutaneously, using stereotaxic surgery:[138,139] A burr hole is made, and the drainage instrument is guided stereotactically, using CT or MRI, to the core of the hematoma, which is then evacuated. Fibrinolytic agents also can be instilled to soften and lyse the clot.[140] As yet, there is too little experience to allow comparison of open versus stereotactic drainage of hematomas.

A CT scan in JT showed a very large deep putaminal hemorrhage, with spread to the thalamus and lateral ventricles (Figure 13.6). At this time, he was comatose, had bilateral horizontal gaze palsies, dilated unreactive pupils, and bilateral extensor plantar reflexes. I judged that nothing could or should be done to reverse his mortal bleed.

There is still much to learn about therapy for patients with ICH. The remarkable technological revolution has made diagnosis easy. What are now needed are more well-designed studies of different modes of treatment.

References

1. Morgagni GB. De sedibus, et causis morborum per anatomen indagatis libri quinque. Vienna: Typographica Remondiana, 1761.
2. Cheyne J. Cases of apoplexy and lethargy with observations on comatose patients. London: Thomas Underwood, 1812.
3. Gowers W. A manual of diseases of the nervous system: vol 2, 2nd ed. London: J & A Churchill, 1892:384–421.
4. Osler W. The principles and practices of medicine. 5th ed. New York: Appleton, 1903:997–1008.
5. Aring C, Merritt H. Differential diagnosis between cerebral hemorrhage and cerebral thrombosis: clinical and pathological study of 245 cases. Arch Intern Med 1935;56:435–456.
6. Kunitz S, Gross C, Heyman A, et al. The Pilot Stroke Data Bank: definition, design, and data. Stroke 1984;15:740–746.
7. Caplan LR, Hier DB, D'Cruz I. Cerebral embolism in the Michael Reese Stroke Registry. Stroke 1983;14:530–540.
8. Mohr JP, Caplan LR, Melski J, et al. The Harvard Cooperative Stroke Registry: a prospective registry. Neurology 1978;28:754–762.
9. Whisnant J, Fitzgibbons J, Kurland L, et al. Natural history of stroke in Rochester, Minnesota, 1945–1954. Stroke 1971;2:11–22.
10. Matsumoto N, Whisnant J, Kurland L, et al. Natural history of stroke in Rochester, Minnesota, 1955–1969. Stroke 1973;4:20–29.
11. Caplan LR, Mohr JP. Intracerebral hemorrhage: an update. Geriatrics 1978;33:42–52.
12. Fisher CM. Pathological observations in hypertensive cerebral hemorrhages. J Neuropathol Exp Neurol 1971;30:536–550.
13. Herbstein D, Schaumburg H. Hypertensive intracerebral hematoma: an investigation of the initial hemorrhage and rebleeding using chromium Cr[51] labelled erythrocytes. Arch Neurol 1974;30:412–414.
14. Chen ST, Chen SD, Hsu CY, Hogan EL. Progression of hypertensive intracerebral hemorrhage. Neurology 1989;39:1509–1514.
15. Kelly R, Bryer JR, Scheinberg P, Stokes IV. Active bleeding in hypertensive intracerebral hemorrhage: computed tomography. Neurology 1982;32:852–856.
16. Kase C, Robinson K, Stein R, et al. Anticoagulant-related intracerebral hemorrhage. Neurology 1985;35:943–948.
17. Kornyey S. Rapidly fatal pontile hemorrhage: clinical and anatomic report. Arch Neurol Psychiatry 1939;41:793–799.
18. Tuhrim S, Dambrosia JM, Price TR, et al. Prediction of intracerebral hemorrhage survival. Ann Neurol 1988;24:258–263.
19. Borison H, Wang S. Physiology and pharmacology of vomiting. Pharmacol Rev 1953;5:193–230.
20. Faught E, Peties D, Bartolucci A, et al. Seizures after primary intracerebral hemorrhage. Neurology 1989;39:1089–1093.

21. Berger AR, Lipton RB, Lesser ML, et al. Early seizures following intracerebral hemorrhage. Neurology 1988;38:1363–1365.
22. Hier DB, Davis K, Richardson EP, et al. Hypertensive putaminal hemorrhage. Arch Neurol 1977;1:152–159.
23. Walshe T, Davis K, Fisher CM. Thalamic hemorrhage, a computed tomographic–clinical correlation. Neurology 1977;29:217–222.
24. Fisher CM. Some neuro-ophthalmological observations. J Neurol Neurosurg Psychiatry 1967;30:383–392.
25. Caplan LR. Intracerebral hemorrhage revisited. Neurology 1988;38:624–627.
26. Cole F, Yates P. Intracerebral microaneurysms and small cerebrovascular lesions. Brain 1967;90:759–768.
27. Rosenblum WI. Miliary aneurysms and "fibrinoid" degeneration of cerebral blood vessels. Hum Pathol 1977;8:133–139.
28. Santos-Buch CA, Goodhue W, Ewald B. Concurrence of iris aneurysms and cerebral hemorrhage in hypertensive rabbits. Arch Neurol 1976;33:96–103.
29. Takebayashi S, Kaneko M. Electron microscopic studies of ruptured arteries in hypertensive intracerebral hemorrhage. Stroke 1983;14:28–36.
30. Takebayashi S, Sakata N, Kawamura K. Re-evaluation of miliary aneurysms in hypertensive brain: recanalization of small hemorrhage. Stroke 1990;21(suppl I):59–60.
31. Caplan LR. Hypertensive ICH. In Caplan LR, Kase CS, eds. Intracerebral hemorrhage. Boston: Butterworth, 1993 (in press).
32. Bakemuka M. Primary intracerebral hemorrhage and heart weight: a clinicopathologic case-control review of 218 patients. Stroke 1987;18:531–536.
33. Brott T, Thalinger K, Hertzberg V. Hypertension as a risk factor for spontaneous intracerebral hemorrhage. Stroke 1986;17:1078–1083.
34. Caplan LR, Neely S, Gorelick PB. Cold-related intracerebral hemorrhage. Arch Neurol 1984;41:227.
35. Hines F, Brown G. A standard test for measuring the variability of blood pressure: its significance as an index of the prehypertensive state. Ann Int Med 1933;7:209–217.
36. Barbas N, Caplan LR, Baquis G, et al. Dental chair intracerebral hemorrhage. Neurology 1987;37:511–512.
37. Haines S, Maroon J, Janetta P. Supratentorial intracerebral hemorrhage following posterior fossa surgery. J Neurosurgery 1978;49:881–886.
38. Norregaard TV, Moskowitz MA. Substance P and sensory innervation of intracranial and extracranial feline cephalic arteries. Brain 1985;108:517–533.
39. Moskowitz MA. The neurobiology of vascular head pain. Ann Neurol 1984;16:157–168.
40. Caplan LR, Skillman J, Ojemann R, Fields W. Intracerebral hemorrhage following carotid endarterectomy: a hypertensive complication. Stroke 1978;9:457–460.
41. Bruetman MF, Fields WS, Crawford ES, DeBakey ME. Cerebral hemorrhage in carotid artery surgery. Arch Neurol 1963;9:458–467.
42. Wylie EJ, Hein MF, Adams JE. Intracerebral hemorrhage following surgical revascularization for treatment of acute strokes. J Neurosurg 1964;21:212–215.
43. Humphreys RP, Hoffman JH, Mustard WT, et al. Cerebral hemorrhage following heart surgery. J Neurosurg 1975;43:671–675.
44. Sila CA. Spectrum of neurologic events following cardiac transplantation. Stroke 1989;20:1586–1589.

45. Cole A, Aube M. Migraine with vasospasm and delayed intracerebral hemorrhage. Arch Neurol 1990;47:53–56.
46. Fisher CM, Adams RD. Observations on brain embolism with special reference to hemorrhagic infarction. In: Furlan A, ed. The heart and stroke. London: Springer-Verlag, 1987:17–36.
47. Wilson SAK, Bruce AN. Neurology. 2nd ed. London: Butterworth, 1955:1367–1383.
48. Askey JM. Hemorrhage during long-term anticoagulant drug therapy: intracranial hemorrhage. Calif Med 1966;104:6–10.
49. Babikian V, Kase CS, Pessin MS, et al. Intracerebral hemorrhage in stroke patients anticoagulated with heparin. Stroke 1989;20:1500–1503.
50. Kase CS, Pessin MS, Zivin JA, et al. Intracranial hemorrhage after coronary thrombolysis with tissue plasminogen activator. Am J Med 1992;92:384–390.
51. Caplan LR. Drugs. In: Caplan LR, Kase CS, eds. Intracerebral hemorrhage. Boston: Butterworth, 1993 (in press).
52. Caplan LR, Hier DB, Banks G. Stroke and drug abuse. Curr Concepts Cerebrovasc Dis (Stroke) 1982;17:9–14.
53. Harrington H, Heller HA, Dawson D, Caplan LR, Rumbaugh C. Intracerebral hemorrhage and oral amphetamine. Arch Neurol 1983;40:503–507.
54. Citron B, Halpern M, McCarron M, et al. Necrotizing angiitis associated with drug abuse. N Engl J Med 1970;283:1003–1011.
55. Rumbaugh C, Bergeron R, Fang H, et al. Cerebral angiographic changes in the drug abuse patient. Radiology 1971;101:335–344.
56. Rumbaugh C, Bergeron R, Scanlon R, et al. Cerebral vascular changes secondary to amphetamine abuse in the experimental animal. Radiology 1971;101:345–351.
57. Lukes SA. Intracerebral hemorrhage from an arteriovenous malformation after amphetamine injection. Arch Neurol 1983;40:60–61.
58. Cahill D, Knipp HJ, Mosser J. Intracranial hemorrhage with amphetamine usage. Neurology 1981;31:1058–1059.
59. Yu YJ, Cooper DR, Wellenstein DE, Block B. Cerebral and intracerebral hemorrhage associated with methamphetamine abuse: case report. J Neurosurg 1983;58:109–111.
60. Call G, Fleming MC, Sealfon S, et al. Reversible cerebral segmental vasoconstriction. Stroke 1988;19:1159–1170.
61. Levine SR, Welch KMA. Cocaine and stroke. Stroke 1988;19:779–783.
62. Levine SR, Brust JCM, Futrell N, et al. Cerebrovascular complications of alkaloid cocaine. N Engl J Med 1990;323:699–704.
63. Eastman J, Cohen S. Hypertensive crisis and death associated with phencyclidine poisoning. JAMA 1975;231:1270–1271.
64. Bessen H. Intracranial hemorrhage associated with phencyclidine abuse. JAMA 1982;248:585–586.
65. Stratton M, Witherspoon J, Kirtley T. Hypertensive crisis and phencyclidine abuse. Va Med 1978;105:569–572.
66. Lasagna L. Phenylpropanolamine: a review. New York: Wiley, 1988.
67. Kikta DG, Devereux MW, Chandar K. Intracranial hemorrhage due to phenylpropanolamine. Stroke 1985;16:510–512.
68. Kase CS, Foster TE, Reed JE, Spatz EL, Girgis GN. Intracerebral hemorrhage and phenylpropanolamine use. Neurology 1987;37:399–404.

69. McDowell JR, Leblanc H. Phenylpropanolamine and cerebral hemorrhage. West J Med 1985;142:688–691.
70. Glick R, Hoying J, Cerullo L, Perlman S. Phenylpropanolamine: an over-the-counter drug causing cerebral nervous system vasculitis and intracerebral hemorrhage. Neurosurgery 1987;20:969–974.
71. Mueller S, Muller J, Asdell S. Cerebral hemorrhage associated with phenyl-propanolamine in combination with caffeine. Stroke 1984;15:119–123.
72. Mueller S. Neurologic complications of phenylpropanolamine use. Neurology 1983;33:650–652.
73. Caplan LR, Thomas C, Banks G. Central nervous system complications of addiction to T's and blues. Neurology 1982;32:623–628.
74. Zenkevich GS. Role of congophilic angiopathy in the genesis of subarachnoid-parenchymatous hemorrhages in middle-aged and elderly persons. Zh Nevropatol Psikhiatr 1978;78:52–57.
75. Jellinger K. Cerebral hemorrhage in amyloid angiopathy. Ann Neurol 1977;1:604.
76. Jellinger K. Cerebrovascular amyloidosis with cerebral hemorrhage. J Neurol 1977;214:195–206.
77. Vinters H, Gilbert J. Cerebral amyloid angiopathy: incidence and complications in the aging brain: II. the distribution of amyloid vascular changes. Stroke 1983;14:923–928.
78. Lee S, Stemmerman G. Congophilic angiopathy and cerebral hemorrhage. Arch Pathol Lab Med 1978;102:317–321.
79. Gilbert J, Vinters H. Cerebral amyloid angiopathy: incidence and complications in the aging brain: I. cerebral hemorrhage. Stroke 1983;14:915–923.
80. Gilles C, Brucher J, Khoubesserian P, et al. Cerebral amyloid angiopathy as a cause of multiple intracerebral hemorrhages. Neurology 1984;34:730–735.
81. Finelli P, Kessimian N, Bernstein P. Cerebral amyloid angiopathy manifesting as recurrent intracerebral hemorrhage. Arch Neurol 1984;41:330–333.
82. Stein B, Wolpert S. Arteriovenous malformations of the brain: I. current concepts and treatment. Arch Neurol 1980;37:1–5.
83. Kelly J, Mellinger J, Sundt T. Intracranial arteriovenous malformations in childhood. Ann Neurol 1978;3:338–343.
84. Dobyns WB, Michels VV, Groover RV, Mokri B, et al. Familial cavernous malformations of the central nervous system and retina. Ann Neurol 1987;21:578–583.
85. Rigamonti D, Spetzler R, Johnson P, et al. Cerebral vascular malformations. B I Quarterly 1987;3:18–27.
86. Stein B, Wolpert S. Arteriovenous malformations of the brain: II. current concepts and treatment. Arch Neurol 1980;37:69–75.
87. Dawson RC III, Tarr RW, Hecht ST, et al. Treatment of arteriovenous malformation of the brain with combined embolization and stereotactic radiosurgery: results after 1 and 2 years. AJNR 1990;11:857–864.
88. Caplan LR. Traumatic ICH. In: Caplan LR, Kase CS, eds. Intracerebral hemorrhage. Boston: Butterworth, 1993 (in press).
89. Fisher CM. Clinical syndromes in cerebral hemorrhage in pathogenesis and treatment of cerebrovascular disease. In: Fields W, ed. Proceedings of the annual meeting of the Houston Neurological Society. Springfield, Ill.: Thomas, 1961:318–342.

90. Koba T, Yokoyama T, Kaneko M. Correlation between the location of hematoma and its clinical symptoms in the lateral type of hypertensive intracerebral hemorrhage. Stroke 1977;8:676–680.

91. Mizukami M, Nishijuma M, Kin H. Computed tomographic findings of good prognosis for hemiplegia in hypertensive putaminal hemorrhage. Stroke 1981;12:648–652.

92. Stein R, Caplan LR, Hier DB. Intracerebral hemorrhage: role of blood pressure, location, and size of lesions. Ann Neurol 1983;14:132–133.

93. Mizukami M, Kin H, Araki G, et al. Surgical treatment of primary intracerebral hemorrhage: I. new angiographical classification. Stroke 1976;7:30–36.

94. Metter EJ, Jackson C, Kempler D, et al. Left hemisphere intracerebral hemorrhages studied by (F-18)-fluorodeoxyglucose PET. Neurology 1986;36:1155–1162.

95. Stein R, Kase C, Hier DB, et al. Caudate hemorrhage. Neurology 1984;34:1549–1554.

96. Weisberg L. Caudate hemorrhage. Arch Neurol 1984;41:971–974.

97. Pedrazzi P, Bogousslavsky J, Regli F. Hematomes limites a la tete du Noyau Caude. Rev Neurol 1990;146:12:726–738.

98. Barraquer-Bordas L, Illa I , Escartin A, et al. Thalamic hemorrhage: a study of 23 patients with diagnosis by computed tomography. Stroke 1981;12:524–527.

99. Caplan LR. "Top of the basilar" syndrome: selected clinical aspects. Neurology 1980;30:72–79.

100. Mohr JP, Walters W, Duncan G. Thalamic hemorrhage and aphasia. Brain Lang 1975;2:3–17.

101. Ciemins V. Localized thalamic hemorrhage: a cause of aphasia. Neurology 1970;20:776–782.

102. Samarel A, Wright T, Sergay S, et al. Thalamic hemorrhage with speech disorder. Trans Am Neurol Assoc 1975;101:283–285.

103. Watson R, Heilman K. Thalamic neglect. Neurology 1979;29:690–694.

104. Kawahara N, Sato K, Muraki M, et al. CT classification of small thalamic hemorrhages and their clinical implications. Neurology 1986;35:165–172.

105. Ikeda K, Yamashima T, Uno E, et al. Clinical manifestations of small thalamic hemorrhages. Brain and Nerve 1985;37:171–179.

106. Caplan LR. Thalamic hemorrhages. In: Caplan LR, Kase CS, eds. Intracerebral hemorrhage. Boston: Butterworth, 1993 (in press).

107. Gilner L, Avin B. A reversible ocular manifestation of thalamic hemorrhage: a case report. Arch Neurol 1977;34:715–716.

108. Waga S, Okada M, Yamamoto Y. Reversibility of Parinaud syndrome in thalamic hemorrhage. Neurology 1979;29:407–409.

109. Kase C, Williams J, Wyatt D, et al. Lobar intracerebral hematomas: clinical and CT analysis of 22 cases. Neurology 1982;32:1146–1150.

110. Ropper A, Davis K. Lobar cerebral hemorrhages: acute clinical syndromes in 26 cases. Ann Neurol 1980;8:141–147.

111. Butler A, Partain R, Netsky M. Primary intraventricular hemorrhage in adults. Surg Neurol 1977;8:143–149.

112. Little JR, Blomquist G, Ethier R. Intraventricular hemorrhage in adults. Surg Neurol 1977;8:143–149.

113. Kase C, Caplan LR. Parenchymatous posterior fossa hemorrhage. In: Bar-

nett HJM, Mohr JP, Stein B, Yatsu F, eds. Stroke: pathophysiology, diagnosis and management. New York: Churchill Livingstone, 1985:621–641.

114. Caplan LR, Zervas N. Survival with permanent midbrain dysfunction after surgical treatment of traumatic subdural hematoma: the clinical picture of a Düret hemorrhage. Ann Neurol 1977;1:587–589.

115. Steegman T. Primary pontile hemorrhage. J Nerv Ment Dis 1951;114:35–65.

116. Silverstein A. Primary pontine hemorrhage. In: Vinken P, Bruyn G, eds. Handbook of clinical neurology: vol 12, pt 2. vascular diseases of the nervous system. Amsterdam: North Holland, 1972:37–53.

117. Caplan LR, Goodwin J. Lateral tegmental brainstem hemorrhage. Neurology 1982;32:252–260.

118. Kase C, Maulsby G, Mohr JP. Partial pontine hematomas. Neurology 1980;30:652–655.

119. Gobernado J, de Molina A, Gineno A. Pure motor hemiplegia due to hemorrhage in the lower pons. Arch Neurol 1980;37:393.

120. Schnapper R. Pontine hemorrhage presenting as ataxic hemiparesis. Stroke 1982;13:518–519.

121. Brennan R, Berglund R. Acute cerebellar hemorrhage: analysis of clinical findings and outcome in 12 cases. Neurology 1977;27:527–532.

122. Fisher CM, Picard E, Polak A, et al. Acute hypertensive cerebellar hemorrhage: diagnosis and surgical treatment. J Nerv Ment Dis 1965;140:38–57.

123. Ott K, Kase C, Ojemann R, et al. Cerebellar hemorrhage: diagnosis and treatment. Arch Neurol 1974;31:160–167.

124. Holmes G. The symptoms of acute cerebellar injuries due to gunshot wounds. Brain 1917;40:451–535.

125. Ojemann R, Heros R. Spontaneous brain hemorrhage. Stroke 1983;14:468–474.

126. Shenkin H, Zavala M. Cerebellar strokes: mortality, surgical indications and results of ventricular damage. Lancet 1982;2:429–432.

127. Richardson AE. Spontaneous cerebellar hemorrhage. In: Vinken P, Bruyn G, eds. Handbook of clinical neurology. Amsterdam: North Holland, 1972:54–67.

128. Longo M, Fiumara F, Pandolfo I, et al. CT observation of an ongoing intracerebral hemorrhage. J Comput Assist Tomogr 1983;7:362–363.

129. Zilkha A. Intraparenchymal fluid-blood level: a CT sign of recent intracerebral hemorrhage. J Comput Assist Tomogr 1983;7:301–305.

130. Pineda A. Computed tomography in intracerebral hemorrhage. Surg Neurol 1977;8:55–58.

131. Scott W, New P, Davis K, et al. Computerized axial tomography of intracerebral and intraventricular hemorrhage. Radiology 1974;112:73–80.

132. Herald S, Kummer R, Jaeger C. Follow-up of spontaneous intracerebral hemorrhage by computed tomography. J Neurology 1982;228:267–276.

133. Little J, Blomquist G, Ethier R. Cerebellar hemorrhage in adults: diagnosis by computerized tomography. J Neurosurg 1978;48:575–579.

134. Young WB, Lee KP, Pessin MS, et al. Prognostic significance of ventricular blood in supratentorial hemorrhage. Neurology 1990;40:616–619.

135. Radberg JA, Olsson JE, Radberg CT. Prognostic parameters in spontaneous intracerebral hematomas with special reference to anticoagulant treatment. Stroke 1991;22:571–576.

136. Langfitt T. Conservative care of intracranial hemorrhage. In: Thompson R, Green J, eds. Advances in neurology: vol 11. stroke. New York: Raven Press, 1977:169–180.

137. Tyler K, Poletti C, Heros R. Cerebral amyloid angiopathy with multiple intracerebral hemorrhages. Neurosurgery 1982;577:286–289.
138. Kandel EL, Peresadov VV. Stereotactic evacuation of spontaneous intracerebral hematomas. J Neurosurg 1985;62:206–213.
139. Matsumoto K, Honda H. CT guided stereotaxic evacuation of hypertensive intracerebral hematoma. J Neurosurg 1984;61:440–448.
140. Mohadjer M, Eggert R, May J, Mayfrank L. CT-guided stereotactic fibrinolysis of spontaneous and hypertensive cerebellar hemorrhage: long-term results. J Neurosurg 1990;73:217–222.

CHAPTER 14

Stroke in Children and Young Adults

Strokes are not especially common in the young, but when they do occur, clinical features and evaluation strategies are rather different from in the customary stroke age group (50–80 years). In this chapter, I briefly outline some of the key differences, and I review the differential diagnoses of strokes in the young. I do not repeat descriptions of stroke syndromes and vascular disorders covered in more depth elsewhere in this book.

General Features and Differences from Geriatric Age Strokes

Heterogeneity. The causes of stroke in the young are more heterogeneous. The differential-diagnosis list includes many genetic, congenital, metabolic, and systemic disorders that are rarely encountered in mature adult populations. Also, more often than in adults, the cause of childhood stroke remains obscure, even after evaluation.

Etiological Variations Associated with Age. The causes vary considerably with age. For example, the differential diagnosis of stroke in a young baby is quite different from that in a 40-year-old, yet both are often referred to as "stroke in the young." Three convenient groups can be distinguished: perinatal and neonatal, children (ages 1–15 years old), and adolescents and young adults (15–40 years). Each of these groups has different frequencies of various stroke etiologies. *Causes also vary considerably, depending on geographical–socioeconomic–environmental factors.* For example, tuberculosis meningitis is an important cause of stroke in India, while strokes due to oral contraceptive use are quite rare there.[1]

Prevalence of Hemorrhagic Stroke. Hemorrhagic strokes, including SAH and ICH are relatively more common in the young. In the geriatric years, the ischemic/hemorrhagic stroke ratio is about 4/1 (i.e., 80% of strokes are ischemic), while in the young, the ratio is close to 1/1.5 (i.e., 60% are hemorrhagic).[2,3] Because hemorrhagic strokes often are cared for on neurosurgical units and ischemic strokes are usually admitted to pediatric neurology services, accurate comparative statistics are hard to gather.

Prevalence of Particular Etiologies of Stroke. In my experience, *migraine, trauma (including dissection)*, and *cardiac disease* are especially important etiologies in children and young adults. *Systemic, genetic*, and *hematological* causes, and *drugs* are also very important. Occlusion of dural venous sinuses is a much more important cause of stroke in the young than in mature adults.

Locations of Lesions. The brain and vascular location of lesions is somewhat different in the young. *Cerebral infarcts tend to be more often limited to the deep regions of the hemisphere, especially the striatocapsular region.* Vascular-occlusive lesions are more often *intracranial*, affecting *especially the supraclinoid ICA*, the *proximal MCA*, and the *basilar artery.* Extracranial occlusive disease is much rarer. When the occlusive process affects the MCA before the lenticulostriate branches, the striatum and the internal capsule are involved. Because of the absence of extensive vascular disease, collateral circulation over the convexity is usually good, accounting for sparing of the cortical territory of the MCA.[4,5] Similarly, proximal PCA occlusion before the thalamogeniculate branches usually leads to thalamic infarcts, with sparing of the temporal and occipital lobes.[6] Vascular malformations are more often periventricular or intraventricular than in adults.

Clinical Presentations and Features. In youths, the clinical presentations and features of stroke are also different. In youths, *apoplectic sudden onset* is the rule, and TIAs are *unusual. Seizures* are very common and are often the presenting feature. *Brain edema* and *increased ICP* are common. Perhaps there is less reserve space in the cranium because of the absence of brain atrophy. Aphasias *in childhood are most often nonfluent*, regardless of *location of the brain lesion.*[7] In children, *agitation and general confusion are often described*, but specific disorders of higher cognitive function are harder to recognize and are less well characterized than in adults. *Abnormalities of posture and movement, such as dystonias, chorea, and athetosis are more frequent features and sequelae of stroke than in adults.*[8] These extrapyramidal disorders probably reflect the predominance of striatocapsular ischemia. In young children with ischemic damage to the basal ganglia and thalamus, these basal gray-matter tissues become hypermyelinated, giving them a marbled appearance, referred to as "status marmoratus."[9]

Prognosis. In youths, *the outlook for recovery is better than for adults with comparable lesions.* The absence of generalized vascular disease and the presence of good collateral circulation often minimize the eventual brain damage, making the ultimate infarct smaller than in adults. Also, the developing brain shows more plasticity. Undamaged areas can undoubtedly take over the functions of damaged regions. As a result, focal disorders of cognition and aphasia often improve, leaving no major speech deficit, although general intellectual function is less than that expected before the stroke.

Strokes in Neonates

Hypoxic–ischemic injury is relatively common in neonates. Hypoxia is most often caused by intrauterine asphyxia, respiratory insufficiency after birth due to aspirated meconium, recurrent apnea, and hyaline-membrane disease in premature infants, and to severe congenital heart disease with left-to-right shunts in both premature and full-term neonates.[10] The neonatal brain has very little autoregulatory capability, so it is much more vulnerable to falls or elevations in blood pressure. Neonatal ischemia is often due to cardiac disease, sepsis with vascular collapse, and hypertension. The most vulnerable areas for hypoxic–ischemic injury are the cortex, especially the hippocampus; the Purkinje cells of the cerebellar cortex; and the pontine nuclei in the brainstem.[10,11]

There are two particularly common distributions of hypoxic–ischemic lesions in neonates—the parasagittal regions, and the deep periventricular white matter. The *parasagittal cortex between the ACA and the MCA and PCA territories* is a *watershed zone, frequently selectively damaged by hypotension in the full-term newborn infant.*[10,12] The most frequent resulting clinical picture is weakness of the proximal limbs, especially the arms. Spastic quadriparesis, which is worse in the arms, is the most characteristic clinical picture.[10,13] CT, MRI, radionuclide studies, and PET scanning can show the parasagittal distribution of ischemic damage.[10,13,14]

In premature infants, hypoxic–ischemic injury often is reflected in damage to the white matter around the ventricles, a process usually termed *periventricular leukomalacia.*[15–17] Sometimes, there are small isolated foci of necrosis at the angles of the ventricles. Often, the lesions are extensive and spread out from the ventricles toward the cortex. The periventricular lesions can be hemorrhagic and are often associated with enlargement of the ventricular system. The predominant clinical sequela is spastic weakness of the legs (diplegia), with lesser involvement of the upper limbs. The white-matter lesions near the anterior horns intercept the fibers coming from the parasagittal motor cortex subserving the control of the thighs, legs, and feet. CT and ultrasound now allow diagnosis during the neonatal period and sequential evaluation of the lesions.

Focal arterial and venous infarcts are also often found in neonates with seizures or hemiparesis.[10,18,19] Most of these lesions are in the territories of the major cerebral arterial distribution, most often affecting the MCA. The lesions may be large and cystic and on occasion communicate with the ventricular system, forming porencephalic cysts. For reasons that are unclear, focal asymmetrical infarcts are sometimes found in asphyxiated infants with generalized hypoxia and ischemia. Focal infarcts are clearly more common than are presently diagnosed. In an autopsy study of 592 neonates, 32 (5.4%) had focal infarcts in a recognized arterial distribution.[18] Full-term neonates more often had focal infarcts than did premature infants. Arterial embolization with sepsis and DIC were common causes. Focal arterial territory infarcts in infants can also result from drug use, especially cocaine, by the mother.[20] Traumatic occlusions of the cervical, carotid, and vertebral arteries and intracranial vessels during delivery are another important cause of stroke in neonates.[21,22]

Brain hemorrhages are an even more frequent and important cause of stroke in the perinatal period. Premature infants are especially susceptible to developing hemorrhages in *the periventricular region, spreading into the ventricles*.[10,23,24] These hemorrhages originate in the *subependymal germinal matrix*, a structure located over the head and body of the caudate nuclei at the level of the intraventricular foramina. The matrix contains fragile capillaries and loose supporting tissue. By full term, the germinal matrix is no longer visible. In the absence of effective autoregulation, increase in blood pressure or blood volume can lead to breakage of these fragile vessels and to ICH. Also, an increase in venous pressure—as might be found in asphyxia or hyaline-membrane disease—might facilitate hematoma formation. Hemorrhages usually extend into the adjacent ventricle. Regions of necrosis often surround the hematomas. In full-term infants, periventricular and intraventricular hemorrhages arise from residual matrix tissue or directly from the choroid plexus vasculature.

Clinically, infants with germinal-matrix hemorrhages may appear desperately ill with coma, respiratory abnormalities, and poor muscle tone, or they may appear to be faring normally. At times, there is a gradual deterioration of function. Ultrasound and CT are effective ways to diagnose and follow children with hemorrhages. Intraventricular hemorrhages can cause temporary hydrocephalus, which resolves itself, or progressive hydrocephalus, requiring ventricular drainage or shunting. Lumbar puncture (LP), with removal of CSF, is another effective treatment. Ventricular size should be carefully followed by ultrasound or CT.

Since the mid-1970s, *cerebellar hemorrhage* has been recognized more often during the early neonatal period, especially in premature infants.[22,25,26] Cerebellar hemorrhage occurs in an estimated 15 to 25 percent of preterm infants.[22,27] In the late stages of gestation, a cerebellar germinal matrix is present, and this probably accounts for the high risk of bleeding in preterm babies. Asphyxia and hyaline-membrane disease are contributing factors. Trauma is the principal cause of parenchymatous cerebellar bleeding in full-term babies. Often, cerebellar hemorrhage causes catastrophic loss of function. Seizures, falling hematocrit, signs of brainstem compression such as ocular bobbing or skew deviation, and acute hydrocephalus may result. Ultrasound and CT allow diagnosis. Surgical decompression is often required and can be lifesaving.[22]

Subarachnoid bleeding is extremely common, and some RBCs are found in the CSF of nearly every baby delivered vaginally. Bleeding is most often trivial. More severe birth trauma or coagulation abnormalities can lead to more severe subarachnoid bleeding and diminished alertness in the neonate. Trauma can also cause significant *subdural* collections of blood.

Strokes in Children (1–15 Years of Age)

Infantile hemiplegia and childhood stroke have been recognized for centuries. Gowers commented in his 1888 textbook of neurology, "Hemiplegia of sudden onset is not uncommon in children, especially in young children."[28] Despite considerable interest, not until the work of Ford and Schaffer was there much information about etiology.[29] A study in Rochester, Minnesota, estimated the rate as 2.52 cases/100,000 children/year,[30] but in Japan and India, the rates are undoubtedly higher. In the Rochester study, 31 childhood strokes were hemorrhagic, while 38 were ischemic.[30]

Hemorrhagic Stroke in Children (1–15 Years Old)

In preadolescent children, AVMs are the most frequent cause of intracranial bleeding.[22,31,32] However, if all individuals under age 20 years are included, aneurysms are a more common cause of bleeding than are AVMs. Among 124 young patients with SAH in one series, 50 had aneurysms, and 33 had AVMs.[33] Among three series, 36 percent of young patients had aneurysmal bleeding while 27 percent bled from AVMs.[33]

Aneurysms generally become symptomatic either before the age of 2 years or after the age of 10.[22,34] Aneurysms are more common in individuals with coarctation of the aorta, polycystic renal disease, and Ehlers-Danlos syndrome.[22] In childhood, bacterial endocarditis with embolism to the vasavasorum of intracranial arteries, and mycotic aneurysm formation is an especially important cause of SAH. Aneurysms that rupture in childhood have a somewhat different distribution than those found in adults. Shucart and Wolpert analyzed the site of rupture of 100 congenital intracranial aneurysms in children under age 15 years.[35] Compared to adult series, the intracranial ICA was more often the site of anterior-circulation bleeding in children, while the posterior and anterior communicating arteries were less often implicated in children.[35] Posterior-circulation aneurysms were relatively more common in children (23% of the total) than in adults. They especially involved the VAs and basilar artery apex.[35] Evaluation and treatment of aneurysms is similar in children and adults.

Intracranial vascular malformations are undoubtedly present at birth but do not become symptomatic in most patients until adulthood. Although AVMs are the most frequent cause of intracranial bleeding in preadolescents, less than 10 percent of malformations are diagnosed before the age of 10 years.[22] Mackenzie noted in 1953 that 29 of his 50 patients (58%) with brain angiomas had developed initial symptoms before age 20 years.[36] In adolescents and older children, the most frequent symptoms relate to bleeding. Most often, bleeding is into the brain (ICH), but superficial lesions and those abutting on ependymal surfaces can cause SAH or primary intraventricular bleeding. About 20 percent or so of malformations in children are infratentorial, about equally divided between the cerebellum and brainstem.[37] Supratentorial malformations typically are superficial and cone-shaped, with the base located on the cortical surface and the apex nearer the ventricle.[38] Only about 10 percent are deep, involving the basal ganglia and thalamus.[38] Focal neurological signs often develop gradually and can be associated with signs of increased ICP. Epilepsy and headache are other less frequent presentations of vascular malformations.

Neonates and young children often harbor a type of malformation that is rarely if ever first discovered in adulthood—so-called *vein of Galen malformations*. In this condition, the vein of Galen is greatly enlarged, forming a large varix, and the straight sinus is also large and tortuous. The malformation is usually fed by posterior choroidal arteries. The typical CT appearance is that of a round hyperdense mass behind the third ventricle, connected to a prominent torcula by the dilated midline straight sinus. Hydrocephalus is also occasionally associated (in about one third of cases). The commonest presenting syndrome during the neonatal period and infancy is high-output congestive heart failure due to the large volume of shunted blood.[22] A loud cranial bruit is usually audible. Older infants and young children may present with SAH or intraventricular hemorrhage, seizures, or signs of hydrocephalus. If left untreated, these malformations usually prove fatal early in life.

Ischemic Strokes in Children

The differential diagnosis of brain infarcts in children is quite wide (Table 14.1), and many cases escape diagnosis even after rather full evaluation. In my experience and that of others, four risk factors are unusually common in children with stroke: cardiac disease, infection, trauma, and migraine. In addition, sickle-cell anemia may cause brain infarction, particularly among African-American youths.

Brain infarcts in patients with *cardiac disease* are most often due to embolism, but infection (bacterial endocarditis) and in situ arterial and

TABLE 14.1
Differential Diagnosis of Pediatric Brain Ischema (1–15 years)

1. Migraine.
2. Trauma: dissection and other vascular injuries; abuse including whiplash-shake injuries; oral foreign body trauma to the ICA.
3. Cardiac: congenital heart disease with right to left shunts; tetralogy of Fallot; transposition of great vessels; tricuspid atresia; atrial and ventricular septal defects; cardiomyopathies; endocarditis; pulmonary A-V fistula.
4. Drugs, especially cocaine and heroin.
5. Infections: bacterial meningitis, especially Hemophilus influenza, pneumono-cocci, and streptococci; facial, otitic, and sinus infections; AIDS; dural sinus occlusion and infection; tuberculous meningitis.
6. Genetic and metabolic: neurofibromatosis; hereditary disorders of connective tissue (Marfan's, Ehlers-Danlos); pseudoxanthoma elasticum; homocystinuria; Menke's kinky hair syndrome; hypoalphalipoproteinemia; familial hyperlip-idemias; methylmalonic aciduria; MELAS syndrome (mitochondrial myopathy, encephalopathy, lactic acidosis, strokes).
7. Hematologic and neoplastic: sickle-cell anemia; purpuras; leukemia; L-arginase and amicar treatment; radiation vasculopathy; hypercoagulable states, e.g., due to decrease in natural inhibitors such as antithromin III.
8. Arteritis: collagen vascular disease; local infections; Takayasu's; Behçet's.
9. Venous sinus thrombosis; head and neck infections; dehydration; coagulopathy; paroxysmal nocturnal hemoglobinuria; puerperal or pregnancy-related.
10. Systemic disease: rheumatic; gastrointestinal; renal; hepatic; pulmonary.
11. Moyamoya.

venous occlusion secondary to polycythemia also occur. Congenital heart disease, especially with shunting of blood (atrial and ventricular septal defects and patent ductus arteriosis), and complex congenital defects are especially frequent.[39] Patients with stroke and congenital heart disease often are cyanotic and have chronic hypoxia and polycythemia. Brain abscess is also common in this situation and must be distinguished from infarction. Rheumatic heart disease, endocarditis, cardiomyopathies, and myocarditis are important acquired heart diseases associated with brain embolism. Newer diagnostic techniques, especially transesophageal echocardiography (TEE) and transcranial Doppler (TCD) sonography after intravenous injection of air bubbles, have recently led to the detection of small atrial shunts (intra-atrial septal defects and patent foramen ovale) in children and young adults with otherwise unexplained brain infarcts.

Infection was cited as an important predisposing cause of hemiplegia in children in the 1927 report of Ford and Schaffer[29] and in other early writings.[22] Most often, the infections were respiratory or systemic and the mechanism of stroke was uncertain. In a 1991 study of childhood stroke in the Tohoku district of Japan, 10 of 54 patients (18.5%) had upper respiratory tract infections or fevers of unknown origin.[40] Tonsillitis can occasionally lead to occlusive changes in the adjacent pharyngeal portion of the ICA. Influenza and mycoplasma pneumoniae have been occasionally implicated as causes of brain infarction.[22,41,42] The mechanism is cerebral vasculitis. In herpes zoster in adults, the virus can be detected in the vascular endothelium, often without an inflammatory response. Endothelial viral infection could cause thrombosis by activating platelets and triggering the coagulation cascade. Systemic infection can lead to changes in circulating globulins, with activation of serine protein coagulation factors, such as Factor VIII.

Head and neck *traumas*, even trivial ones, are frequently mentioned as a predisposing factor by the parents of children with ischemic strokes. Ten of the 54 patients (18.5%) in the previously cited Japanese series of ischemic strokes in children had head trauma in the home 2 days before the stroke.[40] Oral trauma by penetrating objects such as pencils can lead to ICA occlusion.[43,44] Dissection of the extracranial carotid and vertebral arteries can also develop after either head or neck injuries, especially involving sudden twisting movements and blunt trauma to the neck. Neck, jaw, or throat pain or headache may be the earliest symptom. Brain infarction occurs when the blood within the arterial wall dissects into the arterial lumen and embolizes intracranially. At times, the intramural clot occludes the lumen sufficiently that a luminal thrombus forms in situ because of the sluggish flow and the activation of clotting factors.

I have seen several patients in whom seemingly trivial head trauma led to very severe intracranial dissections. A young girl developed a fatal intracranial ICA and MCA dissection after her head hit the top of a car when it hit a bump.[45] A young boy fell and hit his head while going trick-or-treating on Halloween. Although he appeared uninjured to his mother, the next day, he developed a hemiplegia and bilateral motor signs, later shown to be caused by an angiographically documented basilar artery dissection.

Migraine is also common in children with brain infarcts. The frequency of its recognition depends on how vigorously physicians have explored the past personal and family history of headache. In 1990, I reported a 6-year-old boy who had severe headache preceding a basilar-artery occlusion;[46] he also had a strong family history of migraine. In another young boy, a striatocapsular infarct, associated with narrowing of the MCA, was followed by the development of typical unilateral throbbing migraine headaches with photophobia, nausea, and vomiting. Migraine probably causes brain infarcts due to prolonged vasoconstriction, or the formation of local thrombi related to vascular narrowing and activation of the clotting system.[46]

Sickle-cell (S-C) anemia is an important cause of brain infarction, especially in black children and young adults. In the study of Wood, three quarters of the patients with cerebrovascular complications of S-C disease were less than 15 years of age.[47] Patients with stroke often have a more severe form of the disease, with frequent sickle crises and lower hematocrits than other patients with the disease. Strokes often occur during a clinical sickle crisis.[22,48] Strokes in S-C disease involve both large and penetrating small arteries.[49] Hemoglobin S-C disease is also occasionally complicated by ischemic strokes. Thrombocytosis, and congenital deficiency of antithrombin III, of protein C and protein S, and of the C_2 component of complement are also implicated among the causes of stroke in childhood.[22]

The true incidence of coagulopathies in childhood and the frequency with which they cause ischemic stroke are unknown because coagulation factors and functions have seldom been systematically investigated in large series of children, with or without strokes. Activation of clotting factors could underlie many brain infarcts in children with systemic diseases, infections, and injuries.

Strokes in Young Adults (15–40 Years)

The causes of brain hemorrhage and infarction change as individuals progress from childhood to become young adults. The differential diagnosis of ischemic stroke in this age group is listed in Table 14.2. The topic of stroke in young adults has received increasing attention in recent years, and many series report the relative frequencies of various conditions.[1,3,50–62] The series, however, are not comparable because of the wide variation in socio-economic–environmental factors, including age, sex, and race of patients; the time of accrual of the series data, with widely varying available technologies for investigation; and the investigations performed to arrive at the stroke etiology. Drug use, tuberculosis, and oral contraceptive use, for example, vary widely among the United States, India, and Japan, accounting for the variability of these specific etiologies. Cardiac disease was assiduously sought by some authors using modern echocardiography,[58,59] but in other series, this technology was not available. In some series, few patients had angiography, while in a series of 148 patients, all had angiography.[62]

In some diagnoses, the key data come from the history (e.g., history of the use of illicit drugs and oral contraceptive agents, historical features suggestive of migraine, and the presence of preceding head trauma). The frequency of detection of these causes varies, depending on the preliminary hypotheses and biases of the investigators and on whether the series was *prospective*, allowing the authors to collect the history, or *retrospective*, gleaned from the charts. Medical records are notoriously poor in historical detail, especially in terms of negative factors. The history in the medical record may not note that the patient did not have migraine, head or neck trauma, a recent infection, etc. In some series, various possible etiologies are not considered. In some series, factors such as oral contraceptive use, migraine, and trauma are only noted when they were considered etiologically related to the stroke, while others simply note the percentage of subjects in which the factors were present. Table 14.3 summarizes the data from those series that quantitated their data sufficiently to allow tabulation.

In nearly all series, premature atherosclerosis becomes an important cause of stroke in individuals over age 20 years. Louis and McDowell ana-

TABLE 14.2
Differential Diagnosis of Ischemia in Young Adults (15–40 years)

1. Migraine.
2. Arterial dissection.
3. Drugs, especially cocaine and heroin.
4. Premature atherosclerosis; hyperlipidemias, hypertension, diabetes, smoking, homocystinuria.
5. Female hormone-related (oral contraceptives, pregnancy, puerperium): eclampsia; dural sinus occlusion; arterial and venous infarcts; peripartum cardiomyopathy.
6. Hematologic: deficiency of antithrombin III, protein C, protein S; fibrinolytic system disorders; deficiency of plasminogen activator; antiphospholipid antibody syndrome; increased factor VIII; cancer; thrombocytosis; polycythemia; thrombotic thrombocytopenic purpura; disseminated intravascular coagulation.
7. Rheumatic and inflammatory: systemic lupus erythematosus; rheumatoid arthritis; sarcoidosis; Sjögren's syndrome; scleroderma; polyarteritis nodosa; cryoglobulinemia; Crohn's disease; ulcerative colitis.
8. Cardiac: intra-atrial septal defect; patent foramen ovale; mitral valve prolapse; mitral annulus calcification; myocardiopathies; arrhythmias; endocarditis.
9. Penetrating artery disease (lacunes): hypertension, diabetes.
10. Others: Moyamoya; Behçet's; neurosyphilis; Takayasu's; Sneddon's; fibromuscular dysplasia; Fabry's disease; Cogan's disease.

lyzed risk factors in their patients under age 50 years, with stroke due to atherosclerosis.[50] Among 50 patients, 21 were diabetic; 17 among 30 with available lipid measurement had hypercholesterolemia; and 31 (54%) of the patients had hypertension.[50] In the series of Adams et al., among 144 patients aged 15 to 45 years, with ischemic strokes, 38 (27%) were attributed to atherosclerosis.[56] Hypertension, smoking, and diabetes were the principal risk factors, while only 3 patients had hyperlipidemia.[56] Although in series of patients with severe familial hyperlipidemia, premature strokes and coronary artery disease are prevalent, among the series of young stroke patients reviewed, hyperlipidemia was not a very important risk factor.

Because angiography was not consistently performed in most series, the diagnosis of premature atherosclerosis was often based on the presence of risk factors. Among 148 patients studied by angiography in one series, atherosclerotic lesions were found in 22 percent of patients, and 19 percent had thrombotic occlusions (three fourths involving the carotid circulation and one fourth being vertebrobasilar).[62]

Cardiac-origin embolism is a very important cause of stroke in young adults. The cardiac disorders responsible are, however, somewhat different than those found in childhood series. Rheumatic heart disease, prosthetic valves, and various cardiomyopathies are frequently mentioned cardiac sources of emboli. Intra-atrial septal defects and patent foramen ovale are also detected commonly in some series, depending on the technology

TABLE 14.3
Strokes in the Young Series

	N	Age Sex %M	Premature Athero	Cardiac Embolism	OC Use	Peri-Partum	Trauma	Dissection	Dural Sinus Occ	Migraine	Hem	Uncertain
Hart, Miller (52)	100 ISCH	<40 Yrs NM	18%	23%	9%	5%	4% <-	->	NM	NM	—	27%
Snyder, Ramirez-Lassepas (51)	61 ISCH	16–49 yrs 62% M	47%	11%	11%	1%	NM	NM	NM	NM	—	20%
Bogousslavsky, Regli (58)	41 ISCH	<30 yrs 27% M	5%	29% MVP	41%	NM	NM	21%	5%	15%	—	10%
Gautier et al (59)	133	9–45 yrs 51% M	15%	12%	34%F	NM	13%	20.5%	8%	14%	9%	9%
Chopra (1)	>700	6-40 yrs 50% M	NM	10.5%	0	16.3%	NM	NM	NM	NM	27%	NM
Adams et al (56)	144 ISCH	15-45 yrs 56% M	27%	24%	4%	5%	NM	6%	NM	14%	—	7%
Hilton-Jones, Warlow (54)	75	<45 yrs 66% M	9%	7%	9%	NM	17%	NM	NM	13%	20%	
Berlit (60)	168 ISCH	<40 yrs 46% M	32%	9%	12%	4%	4%	2%	NM	10%	—	7%
Lisovoski Rousseaux (62)	148 ISCH	5-40 yrs 51% M	22%	13%	11%	NM	Nm	10%	NM	17%	—	20%

NM not mentioned; ISCH ischemic strokes; MVP mitral valve prolapse; Hem hemorrhage; OC oral contraceptive use.

available. Lechat and his French colleagues found that 40 percent of young patients with ischemic stroke had patent foramen ovale, compared to 10 percent of controls the same age without stroke.[59,63,64] Intracardiac shunts can now be detected readily by using bubbles introduced intravenously while studying patients with TEE or TCD ultrasound. None of the series cited used these new techniques. Mitral valve prolapse (MVP) was very common in the series of Bogousslavsky and Regli[58] (12/41, 29%) but was infrequent in other series (3/144,[56] 3/100,[52] 8/133[59]). In the series studied by Gautier et al., 5 of the 8 patients with MVP also had patent foramen ovale.[59]

Trauma was a surprisingly common risk factor for ischemia in young adults. In the series studied by Hilton-Jones and Warlow, 13 of 75 patients had head or neck trauma at varying intervals before stroke.[54] Few of these patients had other stroke risk factors. Dissection was also common; the incidence of its detection varied with the extent of angiography. Gautier et al. identified 23 cases of dissection among their 112 arterial infarcts (20%). One third of patients with dissection gave a history of recent trauma.[59] Lisovoski and Rousseaux, in their angiography series, found that 15 of 148 patients (10.1%) had arterial dissections.[62]

Many strokes in young women were related to *pregnancy, the puerperium,* or the *use of oral contraceptive agents.* In India especially, puerperal stroke—usually due to dural venous sinus occlusion—was especially important.[1,53] Srinivasan reviewed the experience in Madurai, India,[53] where puerperal stroke accounted for 15 to 20 percent of strokes in the young, and 145 cases had been seen during a decade. Usually, symptoms began during the first 3 weeks after normal childbirth in multiparous women. Seizures (80%), reduced alertness (50%), transient focal signs such as unilateral weakness (60%), and raised ICP (18%) were common early findings.[53] The vast majority of patients had dural-sinus occlusion. Fibrinogen levels were usually considerably raised in 104 out of 120 measured (86%). Mortality was high. Pulmonary embolism and puerperal cardiomyopathy were also problems in these patients.[53] Oral contraceptive use was very common among young women with strokes, although the relationship to etiology was usually uncertain. Although 34 percent of young women in the series of Gautier et al. used oral contraceptives, this was not significantly different from the estimated rate of use in the population of the same age (32%).[59]

In some series, oral contraceptive use and migraine were combined risk factors. Migraine was mentioned prominently in some series,[54,56,58,59,61] but the mechanism by which it related to stroke was most often not identified. Neurosyphilis is an important cause of stroke in young adults in India, as is tuberculous meningitis.[53]

Another key factor may have been overlooked: The use of illicit drugs, especially cocaine, has become a very important and frequent cause of both ischemia and hemorrhage in young adults' brains.[3] A history of drug use was seldom mentioned in the series reviewed and was seldom pursued vigorously as a possible etiology.

Few reports analyze the causes of *hemorrhagic stroke* in young adults. Because hemorrhagic stroke patients are often cared for on neurosurgical services, and ischemia is usually treated on neurologic units, the relative frequencies of the two types of stroke are difficult to determine. Clearly, hemorrhagic strokes make up a smaller proportion of strokes in the years 15 to 45 than in the years before age 15. Also, the ratio varies considerably with the race, sex, and location of stroke patients. In Osaka, Japan, for example, among 252 young stroke patients ages 16 to 40 years, there were 175 hemorrhagic strokes (70%),[61] while in a British series of patients under age 45 years, only 20 percent were hemorrhages,[54] and in a French series, only 9 percent of 133 patients had intracranial hemorrhages.[59]

In general, the etiology of ICH in patients under age 45 years is very similar to that over age 45, except for an overrepresentation of AVMs, drug abuse, and early life bleeding disorders such as hemophilia. Amyloid angiopathy is not encountered in very young adults, and warfarin-related hemorrhages are less frequent than in older patients. Hypertension remains a very frequent cause of intraparenchymatous bleeding in both age groups. Toffol and colleagues reviewed the Iowa experience with nontraumatic ICH in patients 15 to 45 years of age.[57] The commonest location was lobar (41/72, 57%); 11 were putaminal (15%); and 4 were intraventricular. Etiologies included AVMs (21/55, 39%), hypertension (11/72, 15%), aneurysm (7/72, 10%), and drug use with amphetamines and/or phenylpropanolamine (5/72, 7%).[57] Among the 15 cases of ICH included in the British series, 6 were due to AVMs and 2 to hypertension.[54] In a Japanese neurological series among 25 young patients with ICH, 7 had AVMs, and in 16, hemorrhages were attributed to hypertension.[61] Aneurysms (51%) accounted for more ICHs than did AVMs (19%) among Japanese patients treated on a neurosurgical service.[61] Aneurysms in young adults have the same locations and clinical findings as in older patients. SAHs before and after age 40 years are diagnosed and managed in the same fashion.

Differences in Evaluation

In young adults and children, clinicians face a dilemma about the extensiveness of the evaluation. The youth of the patient with nearly a lifetime left of potential risk of future stroke and other vascular disease and the vast number of diagnostic possibilities are factors that argue for extensive evaluation. On the other hand, the tendency for young patients to improve dramatically irrespective of treatment, the knowledge that a high proportion of cases go undiagnosed despite intensive testing, and the high cost of technology and testing argue for conservatism in ordering tests.

In my opinion, clinicians clearly should spend more time with the clinical encounter. The history should include questions about smoking, headache, trauma, cardiac symptoms, past bleeding, miscarriages, thrombophlebitis, and prior strokes or ischemic attacks. The use of medicines and drugs of any kind, especially cocaine and amphetamines and other illicit drugs and oral contraceptive agents, is particularly important. The history should include a thorough review of systems, searching for symptoms that might indicate systemic disease. Family history is very important. Information about premature atherosclerosis, hypertension, hyperlipidemia, migraine, and metabolic and hereditary diseases in family members should be sought.

The general physical examination should include careful inspection of the skin for rashes and other lesions. Palpation of pulses and cardiac, neck, and cranial auscultation are especially important. Blood tests, including coagulation studies, neuroimaging, and cardiac evaluation are probably needed in every young person with stroke. Ultrasound and angiography may be indicated, depending on the findings from the clinical encounter and the early investigations. The yield of angiography is high. In one series, two thirds of angiograms were abnormal, often allowing an etiological diagnosis.[62] Magnetic resonance angiography and extracranial and intracranial ultrasound may now allow clinicians to noninvasively acquire more data about the vasculature without risk to the patients.

References

1. Chopra JS, Prabhakar S. Clinical features and risk factors in stroke in young. Acta Neurol Scand 1979;60:289–300.
2. Nencini P, Inzitari D, Baruffi MC, et al. Incidence of stroke in young adults in Florence, Italy. Stroke 1988;19:977–981.
3. Stern B, Kittmer S, Sloan M, et al. Stroke in the young. Maryland Med J 1991;40:453–462,565–571.
4. Walsh LE, Garg B. Isolated acute subcortical infarctions in children: clinical description and radiographic correlation. Ann Neurol 1990;28:458–459.
5. Caplan LR, Babikian V, Helgason C, et al. Occlusive disease of the middle cerebral artery. Neurology 1985;35:975–982.
6. Caplan LR, DeWitt LD, Pessin MS, et al. Lateral thalamic infarcts. Arch Neurol 1988;45:959–964.
7. Ferro JM, Crespo M. Young adult stroke: neuropsychological dysfunction and recovery. Stroke 1988;19:982–986.
8. Dooling EC, Adams RD. The pathological anatomy of posthemiplegic athetosis. Brain 1975;98:29–48.
9. Malamud N. Status marmoratus: a form of cerebral palsy following either birth injury or inflammation of the central nervous system. J Pediatr 1950;37:610–619.
10. Hill A, Volpe JJ. Stroke and hemorrhage in the premature and term neonate. In: Edwards MB, Hoffman HJ, eds. Cerebral vascular diseases in children and adolescents. Baltimore: Williams & Wilkins, 1989:179–194.
11. Leech RW, Alvord EC Jr. Anoxic–ischemic encephalopathy in the human neonatal period: the significance of brain stem involvement. Arch Neurol 1977;34:109–113.

12. Volpe JJ. Value of MR in definition of the neuropathology of cerebral palsy in vivo. AJNR 1992;13:79–83.

13. Volpe JJ, Pasternak JF. Parasagittal cerebral injury in neonatal hypoxic–ischemic encephalopathy: clinical and neuroradiologic features. J Pediatr 1977;91:472–476.

14. Volpe JJ, Herscovitch P, Perlman JM, et al. Positron emission tomography in the asphyxiated term newborn: parasagittal impairment of cerebral blood flow. Ann Neurol 1985;17:287–296.

15. Banker BQ, Larroch JC. Periventricular leukomalacia of infancy: a form of neonatal anoxic encephalopathy. Arch Neurol 1962;7:386–410.

16. DeReuck J, Chattha AS, Richardson EP Jr. Pathogenesis and evolution of periventricular leukomalacia in infancy. Arch Neurol 1972;27:229–236.

17. Truwit CL, Barkovich AJ, Koch TK, Ferriero DM. Cerebral palsy: MR findings in 40 patients. AJNR 1992;13:67–78.

18. Barmada MA, Moossy J, Shuman RM. Cerebral infarcts with arterial occlusion in neonates. Ann Neurol 1979;6:495–502.

19. Mantovani JF, Gerber GJ. "Idiopathic" neonatal cerebral infarction. Am J Dis Child 1984;138:359–362.

20. Chasnoff IJ, Bussey ME, Savich R, et al. Perinatal cerebral infarction and maternal cocaine use. J Pediatr 1986;108:456–459.

21. Roessmann CC, Miller RT. Thrombus of the middle cerebral artery associated with birth trauma. Neurology 1980;30:889–892.

22. Roach ES, Riela AR. Pediatric cerebrovascular disorders. Mount Kisco, NY: Futura, 1988.

23. Ahmann PA, Lazzara A, Dykes FD, et al. Intraventricular hemorrhage in the high-risk preterm infant: incidence and outcome. Ann Neurol 1980;7:118–124.

24. Papile LA, Burstein J, Burstein R, et al. Incidence and evolution of subependymal and intraventricular hemorrhage: a study of infants with birth weights of less than 1500 gm. Pediatrics 1978;92:529–534.

25. Grunnet ML, Shields WD. Cerebellar hemorrhage in the premature infants. J Pediatr 1976;88:605–608.

26. Martin R, Roessmann U, Fanaroff A. Massive intracerebellar hemorrhage in low birth-weight infants. J Pediatr 1976;89:290–293.

27. Volpe JJ. Neonatal periventricular hemorrhage: past, present and future. J Pediatr 1978;92:693–696.

28. Gowers WR. A manual of diseases of the nervous system. Philadelphia: P Blakiston, 1888:839.

29. Ford FR, Schaffer AJ. The etiology of infantile acquired hemiplegia. AMA Arch Neurol Psychiatry 1927;18:323–347.

30. Schoenberg BS, Mellinger JF, Schoenberg DG. Cerebrovascular disease in infants and children: a study of incidence, clinical features, and survival. Neurology 1978;28:763–768.

31. So SC. Cerebral arteriovenous malformations in children. Childs Brain 1978; 4:242–250.

32. Ventureyra EC, Herder S. Arteriovenous malformations in children. Child Nerv Syst 1987;3:12–18.

33. Sedzimir CB, Robinson J. Intracranial hemorrhages in children and adolescents. J Neurosurg 1973;38:269–281.

34. Orozco M, Trigueros F, Quintana F, et al. Intracranial aneurysms in early childhood. Surg Neurol 1978;9:247–252.

35.   Shucart WA, Wolpert SM. Intracranial arterial aneurysms in childhood. Am J Dis Child 1974;127:288–293.

36.   Mackenzie I. The clinical presentation of the cerebral angioma. Brain 1953; 76:184–213.

37.   Humphreys RP. Infratentorial arteriovenous malformations. In: Edwards MS, Hoffman HJ, eds. Cerebral vascular disease in children and adolescents. Baltimore: Williams & Wilkins, 1989:309–320.

38.   Martin NA, Edwards MS. Supratentorial arteriovenous malformations. In: Edwards MS, Hoffman HJ, eds. Cerebral vascular diseases in children and adolescents. Baltimore: Williams & Wilkins, 1989:283–308.

39.   Terplan AK. Patterns of brain damage in infants and children with congenital heart disease. Am J Dis Child 1973;125:176–185.

40.   Satoh S, Shirane R, Yoshimoto T. Clinical survey of ischemic cerebrovascular disease in children in a district of Japan. Stroke 1991;22:586–589.

41.   Zilkha A, Mendelsohn F, Borofsky LG. Acute hemiplegia in children complicating upper respiratory infections. Clin Pediatr 1976;15:1137–1142.

42.   Parker P, Puck J, Fernandez F. Cerebral infarction associated with *Mycoplasma pneumoniae*. Pediatrics 1981;67:373–375.

43.   Pitner SE. Carotid thrombosis due to intraoral trauma—an unusual complication of a common childhood accident. N Engl J Med 1966;274:764–767.

44.   Pearl PL. Childhood stroke following intraoral trauma. J Pediatr 1987;110:574–575.

45.   Duncan A, Rumbaugh C, Caplan LR. Cerebral embolic disease: a complication of carotid aneurysms. Radiology 1979;133:379–384.

46.   Caplan LR. Migraine and vertebrobasilar ischemia. Neurology 1990;41:55–61.

47.   Wood DH. Cerebrovascular complications of sickle-cell anemia. Stroke 1978; 9:73–75.

48.   Grotta JC, Manner C, Pettigrew LC, et al. Red blood cell disorders and stroke. Stroke 1986;17:811–816.

49.   Adams RJ, Nichols FT, McKie V, et al. Cerebral infarction in sickle cell anemia: mechanism based on CT and MRI. Neurology 1988;38:1012–1017.

50.   Louis S, McDowell F. Stroke in young adults. Ann Int Med 1967;66:932–938.

51.   Snyder BD, Ramirez-Lassepas M. Cerebral infarction in young adults: long term prognosis. Stroke 1980;11:149–153.

52.   Hart RG, Miller VT. Cerebral infarction in young adults: a practical approach. Stroke 1983;14:110–114.

53.   Srinivasan K. Ischemic cerebrovascular disease in the young: two common causes in India. Stroke 1984;15:733–735.

54.   Hilton-Jones D, Warlow CP. The causes of stroke in the young. J Neurol 1985;232:137–143.

55.   Radhakrishnan K, Ashek PP, Sridharan R, Mousa ME. Stroke in the young: incidence and pattern in Benghazi, Libya. Acta Neurol Scand 1986;73:434–438.

56.   Adams HP, Butler MJ, Biller J, Toffol GJ. Nonhemorrhagic cerebral infarction in young adults. Arch Neurol 1986;43:713–796.

57.   Toffol GJ, Biller J, Adams HP. Nontraumatic intracerebral hemorrhage in young adults. Arch Neurol 1987;44:483–485.

58.   Bogousslavsky J, Regli F. Ischemic stroke in adults younger than 30 years of age. Arch Neurol 1987;44:479–482.

59. Gautier JC, Pradat-Diehl P, Loron PL, et al. Accidents vasculaires cérébraux des sujets jeunes. Une etude de 133 patients ages de 9 à 45 ans. Rev Neurol 1989;145:437–442.
60. Berlit P. Cerebral ischemia in young adults. Ann Neurol 1990;28:258.
61. Yamaguchi T, Yoshinaga M, Yonekawa Y. Stroke in the young—Japanese perspective. Abstracts International Conference on Stroke, Geneva, Switzerland, May 30–June 1, 1991.
62. Lisovoski F, Rousseaux P. Cerebral infarction in young people: a study of 148 patients with early angiography. J Neurol Neurosurg Psychiatry 1991;54:576–579.
63. Lechat P, Mas JL, Lescault G, et al. Prevalence of patent foramen ovale in patients with strokes. N Engl J Med 1988;318:1148–1152.
64. Lechat P, Lascault G, Thomas D, et al. Patent foramen ovale and cerebral embolism. Circulation 1985;72(Suppl 3):134.

CHAPTER 15

Spinal-Cord Strokes

Strokes do affect the human spinal cord, but spinal-cord strokes represent a minute fraction of all patients with CNS vascular disease. The rarity of spinal strokes and the relative lack of accessibility of the spinal-cord vascular system to study during life have been barriers to the understanding of spinal-cord vascular disease. To compound ignorance about this topic, the spinal cord and its vascular system are seldom examined in detail at necropsy. Nonetheless, when sought, spinal ischemic lesions can be found. In London, Ontario, Canada, a systematic search for examples of hypoxic myelopathy uncovered 52 cases among 1200 consecutive necropsies (4%).[1,2]

Unique Anatomy of the Spinal Cord

The unique anatomy of the spinal cord makes the clinicians' approach to spinal lesions quite different from the approach to brain lesions. Anatomic definition requires placing the lesion in two planes, in *longitude* (rostro-caudally) and in *depth*. Imaging the lesion with MRI or standard angiography requires localization to the craniospinal junction region, the cervical cord, the thoracic cord, the lumbar cord, or the cauda equina. Lesions at different rostrocaudal levels have different likely etiologies.

There are three depths of lesions with clinical importance: (1) within the epidural space, (2) inside the dura but outside of the spinal cord (intradural extramedullary), and (3) intramedullary. Most epidural lesions reflect disease of the bony fortress and its connective tissue elements that surround the spinal cord. Lesions inside the dura are most often benign tumors, hematomas, or abscesses. Intramedullary lesions have a very wide differential diagnosis that includes infarcts and hematomas.

Rostrocaudal localization depends on both the level of findings affecting the long motor (pyramidal) and sensory (spinothalamic and posterior column proprioceptive) tracts and the presence of local segmental signs.[3] Root or dermatomal distribution of sensory, reflex, or lower-motor-neuron loss accurately identifies the level of the process. Local bone tenderness and pain is also usually reliable in pointing to the segment involved.

Depth localization is more difficult. Epidural processes usually involve the vertebral column, and bone pain and root pain usually precede dysfunction of the cord. Intradural lesions cause root pain, but bony findings are absent clinically and by x-ray. Intramedullary lesions are most often, but not always, painless. Asymmetric signs, sparing of distal sensory fibers, and dissociated sensory loss are other clues to an intramedullary localization. This subject is discussed in more depth elsewhere.[3]

The Spinal-Cord Vascular System

I did not include diagnosis or discussion of the spinal vascular system in the general discussion of anatomy in Chapter 2. I find it easiest to understand and visualize the system by first focusing on a spinal-cord segment in axial section (Figure 15.1). A large single anterior spinal artery runs in the ventral midline rostrally from the spinomedullary junction at the foramen magnum, caudally to the tip of the spinal cord, the filum terminale. In contrast, on the dorsal surface are paired smaller posterior spinal arteries, which often form a plexus of small vessels. The anterior spinal artery gives off deep branches, which course along the ventral sulcus and then branch as they reach the central gray to supply left and right branches to the anterior horn regions on each side.[4,5] Lateral circumferential arteries and their penetrators course laterally from the midline anterior spinal artery to supply the ventral white matter, tips of the anterior horns, and the pyramidal tracts.[4,5] This pattern is very similar to that found in the brainstem, in which paramedian penetrators and short and long circumferential arteries branch from the vertebral and basilar arteries (see Figure 2.11). The posterior spinal artery plexus also gives off penetrating branches to the posterior columns and posterior gray horns.[1,4,5] The regions of supply of the anterior and posterior spinal arteries are shaded diagrammatically on Figure 15.1. The area between the two zones of supply in the central portion of the cord has often been called the "border zone" or "watershed region of supply."[6]

The anterior spinal supply comes from 5 to 10 usually single unpaired radicular arteries, which feed into the anterior spinal artery at various levels (Figure 15.2). The most rostral supply comes from the VAs intracranially. Each intracranial VA in its distal segment gives off a ramus, which joins with that of the contralateral VA, to form a midline anterior spinal artery, which feeds the medulla and descends in the midline through the foramen magnum to supply the cervical spinal cord. Branches from the thyrocervical and costocervical branches of the subclavian artery feed into the spinal cord at

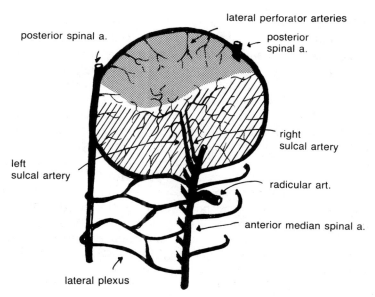

FIGURE 15.1 Cross-section of spinal cord, showing arterial patterns of supply: The anterior spinal artery is a single midline artery that courses in the anterior fissure. This artery divides into left and right sulcal arteries, which supply the anterior horns and white matter. There are usually two posterior spinal arteries, one on each side, which form an anastomotic rete from which branches emerge to supply the posterior gray horns and the posterior columns.

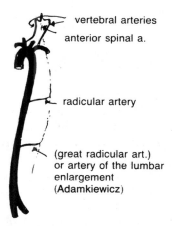

FIGURE 15.2 Aorta and its branches, showing important feeders at various levels: The cervical feeders come from the vertebral arteries. The others come from the aorta.

the cervical enlargement. The thoracic portion of the anterior spinal artery is fed by radicular branches of the deep cervical and intercostal arteries and by branches of the aorta. Blood supply is most marginal in the upper thoracic region (T_2–T_4), and this has been referred to as a longitudinal spinal cord watershed region. The largest artery usually arises in the lower thoracic or upper lumbar segments, most often between T_{12} and L_2. This artery is usually referred to as the artery of Adamkiewicz; it usually comes from the left and supplies the lumbar enlargement of the cord. The sacral cord and cauda equina are nourished anteriorly from the hypogastric or obturator arteries.

In contrast, there are many more posterior radicular arteries, which enter along nerve roots from each side at nearly every spinal level, to supply the plexus of vessels that lie on the posterior cord surface.[4] Some additional segmental arteries arise from the VAs and from the aorta and iliac arteries, to supply the paraspinous structures, and then end on the anterior and posterior nerve roots without supplying the spinal cord or penetrating the dura. These vessels are often the origin of spinal AVMs.[7]

The venous spinal cord anatomy has also been well worked out and studied.[8] Similar to the arterial supply, there are anterior and posterior venous drainage systems. Radicular veins are plentiful and drain into the paravertebral and intravertebral plexus into the pelvic veins. The posterior portions of the cord drain into a large midline posterior vein. The anterior and posterior venous system forms an extensive network, virtually encircling the spinal cord. Venous spinal-cord infarction is probably more common than venous brain infarcts and is most often due to mechanical compression, infection, and inflammation, which obliterate the veins, and to vascular malformations, which cause increased venous pressure.

Spinal Cord Ischemia and Infarction

In many ways, the history of the development of ideas about spinal-cord infarction parallels the evolution of knowledge about the mechanism of brain infarcts. Most of the details of the vascular anatomy of the spinal cord had been worked out by Düret and Adamkiewicz and others late in the nineteenth century.[1,6] Early in the twentieth century, clinicians recognized that most spinal infarcts involved the anterior cord, and these were attributed to anterior spinal-artery occlusion. The putative cause was intrinsic disease of this artery, especially due to syphilis, diabetes, or atherosclerosis. Recall that, during this same era, intracranial anterior circulation infarcts were invariably diagnosed as MCA occlusions. Later, it was shown that the intracranial arteries were less often the seat of disease than the extracranial arteries. Embolism was a more frequent explanation for intracranial arterial occlusion than in situ atherothrombosis. Similarly, in recent years, it has become clear that infarction in the distribution of the anterior spinal artery is most often due to disease of the parent artery (usually the aorta) or less often to embolism. Intrinsic disease of intraspinal arteries is much less common.

Disease of the aorta is undoubtedly the most commonly recognized cause of spinal cord infarction. Most often, paraplegia is recognized after repair of thoracic and abdominal aortic aneurysms.[5,6,9,10] During repair, flow through radicular supply arteries to the anterior spinal artery is compromised. When the thoracic cord is involved, usually a flaccid paraplegia is noted directly after surgery, with incontinence and a thoracic sensory level. Later, the lower limbs become spastic. When the lumbar cord is involved, a conus medullaris infarct develops with hypotonia, wasting and areflexia of the legs, loss of sphincter function, and variable loss of touch and pinprick sensation in the lower limbs, perineum, and lower abdomen.

Similar findings are noted in unruptured aneurysms, dissections of the aorta, and ulcerative aortic plaque disease. Thrombi and plaques can obstruct the orifices of radicular spinal arteries. Dissections can tear or interrupt the orifices of spinal-cord feeding arteries, sometimes over a long area. Cholesterol crystals and other plaque materials can embolize into spinal arteries and can block branches. In some patients, the spinal ischemia develops gradually and insidiously and can be misdiagnosed as motor-neuron disease or diabetic amyotrophy because of the selective ischemia in the anterior horns and sometimes the pyramidal tracts.[11] Usually, the posterior columns are spared, and vibration sense is retained. The regions of spinal-cord softening can now be imaged on newer-generation MRI scanners.[5]

Embolism can and does cause spinal-cord infarction. I have seen several patients with bacterial endocarditis with spinal and brain embolic infarcts, and such have been reported by others.[1] Atrial myxoma and nonbacterial thrombotic (marantic) endocarditis are other disorders in which small particles can embolize to the spinal cord.

Since the early 1980s, pathologists and clinicians have become aware that cartilaginous material from intervertebral discs can somehow invade the spinal arteries and veins and can cause devastating spinal-cord strokes.[3,12] Most reported cases are cervical and involve young women. Some patients have been pregnant, puerperal, or on oral contraceptives. Minor trauma, sudden neck motion, or lifting was commonly mentioned. The first symptom was usually pain in the neck or upper back or was radicular pain. Then a rapidly progressive, sometimes asymmetric, spinal-cord syndrome with quadriparesis developed. Syringomyelia-like dissociated sensory loss with loss of pain and temperature but preserved touch sensation may be found in the upper limbs or cape region. I have not seen or read of reversal of symptoms once paralysis developed. The same syndrome can affect the lumbar cord and can cause conus medullaris infarction. Myelography and other studies usually fail to show herniated discs with compression of the cord or nerve roots. Infarction is usually bland but can be hemorrhagic.[3] Undoubtedly, this syndrome occurs more often than is presently diagnosed.

Infarction and inflammation of the meningeal coverings of the cord can spread to the spinal arteries, causing acute spinal strokes. The phenomenon is similar to Heubner's arteritis found in the brain in the presence of tuberculosis and syphilis. These two disorders, as well as fungal infections and Lyme borreliosis, probably now account for the vast majority of infectious spinal arteritis. Almost invariably, the spinal fluid provides the clue to this problem.

Chronic adhesive arachnoiditis from any cause can also lead to scarring and obliteration of spinal penetrating arteries and ischemic necrosis of the central portion of the spinal cord.[13] The presenting picture is very similar to syringomyelia except that any level of the spinal cord can be involved. Arachnoidal scarring can be due to trauma, hemorrhage, or infection. The signs and symptoms develop gradually, sometimes years after the spinal injury, bleed, or meningitis.[13]

Spinal-cord ischemia may also develop during *shock* or *cardiac arrest*. Damage is most likely to affect the thoracic spinal cord near the T_4 segment, the most vulnerable region of the cord. Nearly always, the spinal-cord signs and symptoms are overshadowed by brain hypoxic–ischemic injury. The deeply comatose patient remains hypotonic and areflexic because of accompanying spinal ischemia. Very rarely, a pure spinal syndrome might complicate systemic hypoperfusion.

Venous infarction is an important cause of cord ischemia. The infarcts may remain bland[14] or become frankly hemorrhagic.[3,15] Venous infarcts are usually attributable to one of three different mechanisms: spinal dural AVMs,[3,7,16] coagulopathies with venous thrombosis, or mechanical compression of veins by epidural mass lesions.[14,15,17]

Spinal Vascular Malformations

Contrary to the situation within the cranium, spinal vascular malformations often present with ischemia rather than hemorrhage, and some malformations cause both bleeding and ischemia. Because of their distinctive characteristics and the fact that many neurologists and stroke experts are inexperienced with the usual findings and diagnosis in such cases, I thought it best to consider spinal vascular malformations separately rather than in relation to the topics of ischemia or hemorrhage.

Spinal malformations should be divided into two large groups, which have differing blood supplies, presentations, and clinical findings: the *dural* and the *intradural* groups.[18,19] So-called Type I malformations, often referred to as "dural," derive their blood supply from arteries located in the dural sleeves of spinal roots.[7,14] The small nidus of arteriovenous communication is fed by dural branches of a radicular artery. The arteriovenous fistulas drain intradurally by one or more arterialized, enlarged, usually tortuous veins, which course on the dorsal surface of the spinal cord, usually above but occasionally below the feeders. The dural feeding arteries *do not* participate in the blood supply of the spinal cord. These lesions occur predominantly in men (4/1 ratio) between 40 and 70 years of age, and they involve mostly the lower thoracic and lumbosacral segments. In one series, 26 of 27 Type I malformations were fed by arteries in the thoracic or lumbar regions, and the remaining 1 was sacral.[19] Most often, there is only one feeder, but at times two or at most three arterial feeders have been found.[7] Among a series of 27 such lesions, 24 had one feeder, and 3 had two.[19] Usually, this type of AVM is referred to as "low-flow" because angiography results only in very slow, low-volume filling of the lesions. These lesions are not associated with arterial or venous aneurysms.[7,19] Cutaneous angiomas are not seen, and bruits are not audible.

The most frequent presentation of dural malformations is that of progressive neurological worsening, often with acute deteriorations. *They do not cause subarachnoid bleeding.* Pain is present in about 40 percent of patients and can be radicular, sometimes mimicking sciatic pain. Symptoms often worsen after exercise. One of my patients had two episodes of leg paralysis and numbness that occurred while she was driving a car.[20] Her husband had to grab the wheel and foot controls to avert a crash. Soon, strength and feeling returned. Another patient had a Brown-Séquard distribution attack while in hospital that lasted several hours.[20] Activity worsened symptoms in 19 of 27 (27%) patients in the National Institutes of Health (NIH) series.[19] Signs usually progress if the lesion is untreated, and most patients become unable to walk within 5 years of the onset of weakness. These lesions probably cause symptoms because of venous hypertension and occasional thrombosis of the venous drainage system.

Type I dural lesions are often not well seen by MRI. Myelography is the key diagnostic test because usually, coiled enlarged veins are visible along the dorsal cord surface.[18] Often, the patients must be turned so that films are taken with the patients lying supine on their backs to show the abnormal veins. Selective spinal angiography in expert, experienced hands often shows the feeding arteries, but sometimes the feeding arteries cannot be opacified. In that case, I urge surgical exploration when the clinical findings are typical and abnormal veins are clearly present. Ligation of the arterial feeders usually prevents worsening, and the venous structures need not be removed.[7]

The remainder of spinal AVMs are intradural. The commonest type (referred to as Type II) are usually intramedullary but can be partially intramedullary and partially between the dura and the cord. Intradural malformations are divided into various types: *glomus*, referring to a tightly packed localized nidus of abnormal vessels within the cord; *juvenile*, in which abnormal vessels occupy the entire spinal cord and are fed by numerous arterial feeding vessels at different levels; direct *arteriovenous fistulas*, involving branches of arteries feeding the spinal cord; and *cavernous angiomas*, which have no major feeding arteries and resemble cavernous angiomas of the brain.

Usually, patients with intradural lesions are younger than those with dural lesions, but again, there is a strong male predominance. In one series, 65 percent of patients were less than 25 years old at first presentation.[19] These lesions have high flow, and hemorrhage is relatively common.[7,19] Intradural lesions are more widely distributed along the spinal axis and are often cervical. Spinal aneurysms, extraspinal aneurysms, other AVMs, and arterial bruits are common in patients with intradural AVMs. Most lesions are intramedullary (80% in the NIH series)[19] and symptoms and signs are progressive.

Intradural AVMs are usually well-imaged and diagnosed by MRI. Glomus and juvenile lesions and cavernous angiomas have a nidus in the cord parenchyma. The spinal cord is usually enlarged, and multiple serpiginous signal voids are seen.[21] Increased signal on T1-weighted images may represent methemoglobin from a prior hemorrhage, and low dark signals on T1- and T2-weighted images can represent hemosiderin.[21] Spinal angiography usually readily shows intradural AVMs. Surgical treatment is not as successful for intradural AVMs as for dural ones, but glomus lesions and cavernous angiomas can be removed.

Cavernous angiomas are now shown well by MRI, but little has been written about their usual presentations or course.[22] They may worsen with pregnancy or in the puerperium. They are angiographically occult. Appearance on MRI is similar to that of brain angiomas—heterogeneous, well-circumscribed discrete lesions.

Intradural AVMs can cause chronic arachnoiditis due to bleeding, with subsequent scarring of small cord-feeding arteries, and to cord ischemia. Veins can thrombose. The so-called Foix-Alajouanine syndrome,[23] a subacute necrotizing ascending myelopathy, probably in retrospect was due to such thrombosed vascular malformations, either of the dural or the intradural variety.[24]

Spinal Hemorrhages

Hematomyelia describes bleeding into the substance of the spinal cord parenchyma. The most common cause is trauma. Onset can be immediate or delayed. Usually, the area around the central canal and the central gray matter are involved, most often in the cervical region. Neck pain, weakness, and areflexia in the arms, associated with a capelike distribution of pain and temperature loss are the usual signs. Other causes include AVMs, anticoagulation, hemophilia and other bleeding disorders, and hemorrhage into spinal-cord tumors, as well as—rarely—syrinxes. The spinal fluid is bloody, and MRI and myelography reveal a swollen blood-filled cord.

Spinal SAH is unusual. Unlike intracranial SAH, the commonest causative lesions are AVMs. Rarely, aneurysms on spinal arteries can rupture.[25] Local back pain is often followed by a stiff neck and pain that radiates along a root distribution or down the back or legs. Often, headache ensues, due to spillage of blood intracranially. Bleeding diatheses and anti-coagulants may cause spinal SAH.

Spinal epidural and *subdural hematomas* are much rarer than intra-cranial hemorrhages in these compartments. Epidural hematomas are about four times more common than subdural hematomas. Each most often occurs in patients who are on anticoagulants.[26] Some patients have had liver disease and portal hypertension.[26] Lumbar punctures (LPs) have been known to precipitate these bleeds in patients on anticoagulants. At times, these hemorrhages begin after exertion or straining, and no cause is found even after full evaluation.[26] The earliest symptom is usually pain in the back usually in the neck. This is followed by radicular pain, usually in one or both arms. Within hours, or rarely days, sensory and motor signs develop in the legs, and bowel, bladder, and sexual dysfunction ensues. Usually, weakness and sensory loss are symmetric, but a Brown-Séquard distribution may be found.[26,27]

Diagnosis of spinal epidural or subdural hematoma has usually been made by myelography. Usually, a block is found. CT may show the blood. Few reported cases have had MRI. Signs are almost invariably progressive unless the lesions are decompressed. Anticoagulation should be reversed, using vitamin K or fresh frozen plasma. Decompression is urgent and should be pursued as soon as the PT reaches about 40 to 50 percent of the control values.[26] Outcome depends on the severity of the deficit before surgery, the duration of spinal-cord compression, and the rapidity of onset of the paraplegia. Rarely, chronic spinal subdural hematomas or hygromas can result, usually from prior trauma or small bleeds.[28]

References

1. Buchan AM, Barnett HJM. Infarction of the spinal cord. In: Barnett HJM, Mohr JP, Stern B, Yatsu F, eds. Stroke: pathophysiology, diagnosis and management. New York: Churchill-Livingstone, 1986:707–719.
2. Vinters HV, Gilbert JJ. Hypoxic myelopathy. Can J Neurol Sci 1979;6:380.
3. Caplan LR. Case records of the Massachusetts General Hospital: Case 5—1991. N Engl J Med 1991;324:322–332.
4. Gillilan L. The arterial blood supply of the human spinal cord. J Comp Neurol 1958;110:75–103.
5. Mawad ME, Rivera V, Crawford S, et al. Spinal cord ischemia after resection of thoracoabdominal aortic aneurysms: MR findings in 24 patients. AJNR 1990; 11:987–991.
6. Hogan EL, Romanul FCA. Spinal cord infarction occurring during insertion of aortic graft. Neurology 1966;16:67–74.
7. Heros R. Arteriovenous malformations of the spinal cord. In: Ojemann RG, Heros RC, Crowell RM, eds. Surgical management of cerebrovascular disease. 2nd ed. Baltimore: Williams & Wilkins, 1988:451–466.
8. Gillilan L. Veins of the spinal cord: anatomic details—suggested clinical applica-tions. Neurology 1970;20:860–868.

9. Dodson WE, Landau W. Motor neuron loss due to aortic clamping in repair of coarctation. Neurology 1973;23:539–542.
10. Ross RT. Spinal cord infarction in diseases and surgery of the aorta. Can J Neurol Sci 1985;12:289–295.
11. Herrick MK, Mills PE. Infarction of spinal cord: two cases of selective grey matter involvement secondary to asymptomatic aortic disease. Arch Neurol 1971; 24:228–241.
12. Srigley JR, Lambert CD, Bilbao JM, Pritzker KP. Spinal cord infarction secondary to intervertebral disc embolism. Ann Neurol 1981;9:296–301.
13. Caplan LR, Noronha A, Amico L. Syringomyelia and arachnoiditis. J Neurol Neurosurg Psychiatry 1990;53:106–113.
14. Kim RC, Smith HR, Henbest ML, Choi BH. Nonhemorrhagic venous infarction of the spinal cord. Ann Neurol 1984;15:379–385.
15. Hughes JT. Venous infarction of the spinal cord. Neurology 1971;21:794–800.
16. Larsson EM, Desai P, Hardin CW, et al. Venous infarction of the spinal cord resulting from dural arteriovenous fistula: MR imaging findings. AJNR 1991; 12:739–743.
17. Roa KR, Donnenfeld H, Chusid JG, Valdez S. Acute myelopathy secondary to spinal venous thrombosis. J Neurol Sci 1982;56:107–113.
18. DeChiro G, Doppman JL, Ommaya AK. Radiology of spinal cord arteriovenous malformations. Prog Neurol Surg 1971;4:329–354.
19. Rosenblum B, Oldfield EH, Doppman JL, DiChiro G. Spinal arteriovenous malformations: a comparison of dural arteriovenous fistulas and intradural AVMs in 81 patients. J Neurosurg 1987;67:795–802.
20. Teal PA, Wityk RJ, Rosengart A, Caplan LR. Spinal TIAs—a clue to the presence of spinal dural AVMs. Neurology 1992;42(Suppl 3):341.
21. Greenberg J. Neuroimaging of the spinal cord. Neurologic Clin 1991;9(3): 696–698.
22. Lopate G, Black JT, Grubb RL. Cavernous hemangioma of the spinal cord: report of two unusual cases. Neurology 1990;40:1791–1793.
23. Foix C, Alajouanime T. La myelite necrotique subaique. Rev Neurol 1926; 2:1–42.
24. Criscuolo GR, Oldfield EH, Doppman JL. Reversible acute and subacute myelopathy in patients with dural arteriovenous fistulas. J Neurosurg 1989; 70:354–359.
25. Garcia C, Dulcey S, Dulcey J. Ruptured aneurysm of the spinal artery of Adamkiewicz during pregnancy. Neurology 1979;29:394–398.
26. Mattle H, Sieb JP, Rohner M, Mumenthaler M. Nontraumatic spinal epidural and subdural hematomas. Neurology 1987;37:1351–1356.
27. Russman BS, Kazi K. Spinal epidural hematoma and the Brown-Séquard syndrome. Neurology 1971;21:1066–1068.
28. Black P, Zervas N, Caplan LR, Ramirez L. Subdural hygroma of the spinal meninges: a case report. Neurosurgery 1978;2:52–54.

CHAPTER 16

Strokes, Cerebrovascular Disease, and Surgery

Surgery is now performed in patients who are older and sicker than was the case in previous decades. Surgical considerations play an increasingly frequent role in the thoughts and activities of neurologists and other clinicians who care for individuals with cerebrovascular disease. Often, they or others are considering surgery on their own patients or in a patient seen in consultation. Clinicians are also often asked to see patients who have had surgery, in whom a stroke or other neurological complication has developed. Both surgeons and nonsurgeons must become fully knowledgeable about the indications, nature, and complications of surgical procedures. In this chapter, I selectively review the two most common surgical situations that confront clinicians: (1) coronary artery and other cardiac surgery, and (2) carotid endarterectomy (CEN) and other extracranial vascular surgery. I also touch briefly on some causes of stroke after general surgery.

Carotid Endarterectomy

Carotid-artery surgery is one of the most commonly performed procedures in the USA today. The frequency of CEN varies dramatically in various countries throughout the world. Chapter 5 (treatment) and Chapter 6 (anterior circulation disease) include discussions of CEN, so herein, I discuss only selected aspects.

Indications

The 1991 reports of North American[1] and European[2] CEN trials have shown that patients with symptoms (TIAs or small strokes) related to carotid stenosis that is severe (>70% luminal narrowing) clearly benefit from CEN when performed by selected surgeons with excellent past low

497

rates of complications. For the benefit/risk ratio to favor CEN, the operative morbidity and mortality should not exceed 2 percent mortality and 5–6 percent morbidity.[1-4] As yet, there are no data about CEN either in symptomatic patients with more severe deficits or in individuals with lesser degrees of carotid artery stenosis, with or without ulceration. The larger the brain infarct and the more severe the neurological deficit, the less is the residual at-risk ischemic tissue, and the less there is to gain by reperfusion. Also, complication rates are higher. The European trial showed that patients with minor degrees of carotid stenosis (<30% luminal narrowing) do not benefit from CEN.[2] There are now no definitive data about asymptomatic patients with carotid stenosis, but such are in progress.

I am not convinced that ulcers found on angiography should be an important factor favoring surgery. Recognition of ulcers is difficult, and the accuracy of the radiological diagnosis is low. As plaques grow and encroach further on the lumen, plaque complications, including ulceration and mural thrombi, become more frequent. Examination of CEN specimens from tightly stenotic arteries shows a very high incidence of these complications.[5] Ulcers do occur in nonstenotic arteries but not very often. The natural history of ulcers in nonstenosing plaques is unknown; they may very well heal. Agents that alter platelet function, such as aspirin, might be effective in preventing white platelet–fibrin clots from embolizing from these plaques. At present, I use the degree of luminal narrowing as the major vascular factor in deciding on CEN. A residual lumen of <2 mm favors surgery in symptomatic patients. I would only suggest CEN for ulceration in a nonstenotic artery if all medical therapy had failed, a circumstance I have not personally seen. At times, large thrombi are found within the ICA.[6,7] These can be attached to plaques or may be found without plaques and may be caused by a hypercoagulable state. Anticoagulants and surgery have been used to treat these thrombi, but I favor anticoagulants after evaluation of coagulation functions.

The patient's preferences should be considered. All of us live in different socioeconomic–psychological milieus. Given the same information, different folks would make different decisions. Some patients find the knowledge of a severe carotid lesion very difficult to live with. Told that they are at imminent, permanent risk of having a disabling stroke, they perceive the sword continually hovering over them. This leads to great stress and altered behavior. Some individuals will gamble some risk for removal of the sword. They choose the knife (CEN) over the sword (the stenotic artery). Others do not find the news untenable. They have heard before of risk to their health from lots of different things. They do not let the knowledge of their carotid artery disease interfere with their lives and are content to pursue medical therapy and clinical monitoring. These individuals usually would not gamble the risk of a surgical stroke complication if that risk is avoidable. I feel that the patient should be provided with the information and the pros and cons of each alternative. Doctors should convey their own advice and opinion, but ultimately, the patient has the right to choose.

When considering the decision about CEN, I follow the schema proposed by Sundt, with some modifications[8] (Table 16.1). Risks for CEN include neurological factors, vascular-specific factors, cardiac factors, and other comorbidity. The degree of neurological stroke deficit and the presence of neurological deficits (e.g., dementia) are clearly important considerations. Vascular risk factors include the length of the stenotic lesion, tandem intracranial disease in the ICA siphon and MCA, involvement of the CCA and the ECA, and location of the bifurcation (a very high bifurcation increases the technical difficulty of the vascular surgery). MI is the most important and severe nonneurological complication of CEN; the presence of coronary artery disease is also of great importance and is discussed in more depth subsequently. Other diseases, such as pulmonary disease and cancer, clearly affect surgical risk and other treatment decisions.

Also to be considered are indications and contraindications for alternative, nonsurgical treatment of carotid artery disease. Intolerance to aspirin and other antiplatelet aggregants, bleeding disorders, and active peptic ulcers might make aspirin and warfarin unattractive therapeutic alternatives.

The surgeon, hospital, and surgical team are also very important. Studies in Springfield, Illinois,[9] and in Cincinnati, Ohio,[10] showed very dramatic variability in the complication rates among hospitals and even among surgeons in the same hospital. In order to establish the benefit/risk ratio of CEN, the morbidity and mortality results of the individual surgeon

TABLE 16.1
Risks of Carotid Endarterectomies

Neurological risks
  Progressive course
  Recent stroke
Angiographic risks
  High bifurcation
  Very long lesion (>3 cm distally in ICA or 5 cm into CCA)
  Clot
  Contralateral ICA stenosis or occlusion
  Intracranial stenosis or occlusion
Medical risks
  Hypertension
  Coronary artery disease
  Diabetes
  Obesity
  Smoking
  Chronic obstructive pulmonary disease (COPD)
  Congestive heart failure

Data from Sundt TM, Sandok BA, Whisnant JP. Carotid endarterectomy complications and pre-operative assessment of risk. Mayo Clin Proc 1975;50:301–306.

are critical data to know. The patient deserves the very best surgical care, even if that care is in another hospital or locale.

Complications

The major complications of CEN are death, ischemic stroke, MI, and ICH. The most frequently fatal complications are medical, especially perioperative MI. Callow reviewed CEN complications at my hospital, the New England Medical Center, during two decades: 1958 to 1967 and 1968 to 1979.[11] During the first decade, the operative morbidity (3.4%) was nearly all accounted for by stroke, but during the second decade, all mortality was due to MI.[11] Patient selection and improved technique explain the difference. MI is especially common when there has been an MI within the preceding 3 months and when the operative procedure is performed under general anesthesia. In one series, there was a 27 percent rate of perioperative MI, all fatal, in such patients.[12] Cardiac evaluation is mandatory in any patient who will undergo CEN who has cardiac symptoms. Recent MI, unstable angina, gallop rhythm, and heart failure are high risk factors.[13] Noncardiac serious medical complications are unusual, except for pulmonary embolism. Most relate to preexisting disorders such as obstructive uropathy, chronic lung disease, and so forth.

Perioperative and postoperative strokes are a major cause of morbidity and a great worry for all concerned. Many episodes of ischemia are transient and may occur *after* the immediate postoperative period. Among a total of 358 CENs performed in a number of centers in Toronto, 18 patients had postoperative TIAs, 14 had brain infarcts, and there were 2 fatal brain hemorrhages.[14] Nine of the ischemic strokes and both hemorrhages occurred after the immediate postoperative period. Steed and colleagues timed the onset of neurological deficits in patients they operated on under local anesthesia.[15] Among 345 CENs, 3 TIAs occurred during ICA dissection, 1 stroke during carotid clamping, and 2 strokes on release of the clamp; 5 patients had TIAs immediately after surgery, and 10 had delayed onset of ischemia.[15] The mechanisms of perioperative ischemia include reocclusion of the ICA; embolization of plaque, clot, or fibrin during or after the surgery; and hemodynamic decrease in flow during surgery or during perioperative hypotension. Most ischemic events are due to artery-to-artery emboli. Reocclusion rates vary but are probably between 5 and 10 percent.[4,16]

Suddenly opening up the ICA into a chronically underperfused region can cause a so-called hyperperfusion syndrome,[17] characterized by headache and often severe, migrainelike neurological accompaniments,[18] and occasionally by seizures. More serious is brain hemorrhage after CEN. Careful monitoring of blood pressure after CEN shows that many patients become hypertensive, probably because of surgical injury to the baroreceptors in the carotid sinus.[19,20] This risk is higher in patients who have been hypertensive in the past. Severe hypertension can lead to brain hemorrhage either into an area of infarction or in sites common for hypertensive ICH (see

TABLE 16.2
Types of Carotid Endarterectomy Complications[4]

Serious	Death, usually cardiac
	MI
	Perioperative ischemic stroke
	Postoperative ICH
	Pulmonary embolism
Usually minor	Hypertension
	Wound hematoma
	Wound infection
	Numbness in local region of jaw or neck ipsilaterally
	Facial (VII), hypoglossal (XII), and superior laryngeal branch of vagus (X) nerve palsies

Chapter 13). If the patient has neurological signs and CT or MRI shows infarction, it is probably wise to delay CEN for 4 to 6 weeks. All patients must have careful monitoring of blood pressure in the days after CEN. I have seen an ICH develop as long as 3 days after CEN.[21]

Other complications are usually less serious and are reversible. They include wound hematomas and continued wound bleeding and wound infection. The local retraction on cranial and cervical nerves and their branches and the cutting of cranial nerve branches can lead to focal regions of numbness or weakness. Complications are listed in Table 16.2.

Overall morbidity and mortality figures are so variable that a standard rate is hard to choose. As I have noted, most important to the patient undergoing CEN are the results of the surgeon who will perform the procedure. The two largest and probably most representative series are those of the Toronto Cerebrovascular Surgeons[14] study previously cited, and a retrospective review audit undertaken by a neurosurgical society[22] (Table 16.3).

Combined Carotid and Cardiac Disease

Atherosclerosis is a systemic disease that hits hardest at the aorta, the coronary arteries, extracranial brain arteries, and the arteries to the limbs. *Severe coronary artery and cerebrovascular disease frequently coexist.* Asymptomatic neck bruits are found in about 10 percent of preoperative coronary bypass patients, and about half of the patients with bruits have significant carotid stenosis by ultrasound testing.[23] An arteriographic study of 100 coronary artery bypass graft (CABG) patients with neck bruits, of whom one third had some cerebrovascular symptoms, showed that one half had carotid stenosis.[24,25] Evaluation of patients with carotid artery disease shows a high incidence of concurrent symptomatic and asymptomatic coronary artery disease. Rokey and colleagues found significant coronary artery disease in 29 of 50 (58%) patients who presented with TIAs or stroke.[26,27] Hertzer et al. found, in a coronary angiography study, that 35 percent of all patients with symptomatic carotid artery disease or asymptomatic bruits had severe coronary artery disease.[28]

TABLE 16.3
Cardiac and Cerebrovascular Complications of Carotid Endarterectomy—
Two Large Series

	Fode et al.[22]	Toronto[14]
Cerebrovascular		
TIAs	82 (2.5%)	18 (5.4%)
Strokes	140 (4.2%)	16 (4.8%)
minor	44 (1.3%)	
major	96 (2.8%)	
Stroke deaths	40 (1.2%)	3 (0.8%)
Cardiac: MIs		8 (7 MI and 1 cardiac arrest)
Deaths		
Total	66 (2%)	5 (1.5%)
MI deaths	26 (0.8%)	1 (0.3%)
Stroke deaths	40 (1.2%)	3 (0.9%)

Fode et al.[22]—3328 patients/44 institutions
Toronto[14]—333 patients

I find that the data persuasively show that *patients undergoing CEN should be evaluated for coexistent coronary artery disease.* As has been discussed in relation to complications of CEN, both MI and cardiac death are frequent and important sequelae of CEN. Riles et al. studied the MI rate in 683 consecutive CEN procedures, among whom 203 patients had preexisting coronary artery disease.[29] Among the patients with coronary artery disease, 14 had MIs, 5 of which were fatal, while among the 288 patients without coronary artery disease, only 2 had MIs, and there were no deaths.[29] Similar results were found by Hertzer and Lees, who reported on 335 CEN patients treated at the Cleveland Clinic.[30] Five of 217 patients with coronary artery disease had an MI within 30 days of CEN, all of which were fatal, compared to only 1 fatal MI among those without historical or ECG evidence of coronary disease.[30]

Noninvasive testing for the presence of coronary artery disease is very effective. A careful history, looking especially for past MI and angina, is mandatory. ECG, echocardiography, and myocardial perfusion imaging, and exercise ECG are useful in predicting the presence and severity of coronary artery disease.[27,31] Particularly helpful is the thallium-201-dipyridamole test, which has a high sensitivity and specificity for the diagnosis of coronary artery disease.[31-33] Some patients with angina and positive findings from noninvasive testing will need coronary angiography to define the coronary disease. The presence of active coronary artery disease or unstable angina clearly presents a prohibitive risk if untreated. Patients with unstable angina who do not respond to medical therapy or who have evidence of silent ischemia have a reduced 1-year survival rate.

Physicians have long deliberated on the best way to manage patients with combined severe coronary artery and cerebrovascular disease. They worry that if CEN is performed first, the risk of MI and death from coronary disease will be high. If, on the other hand, CABG is performed first, they worry about the risk of stroke. I have already indicated that the risk of MI and death has been shown unequivocally to be high in patients with active coronary artery disease.[27,34,35] Studies show that the risk of stroke during CABG is high in those patients with past strokes and symptomatic carotid artery disease but is rather low in patients with asymptomatic carotid artery disease.[25,27]

Ropper and colleagues showed that bruits did not predict stroke complication risk after a variety of elective surgical operations.[36] Neck bruits were found in 104 of 735 (14%) patients preoperatively. One patient with a history of transient monocular blindness had a stroke within three days of CABG. Among 631 patients without bruits, 4 had strokes during the perioperative period. There was no difference in the incidence of stroke in patients with and without bruit.[36] Breslau et al. used duplex scanning in 102 patients undergoing CABG.[37] Eighteen had >50 percent carotid stenosis, and none of these had perioperative strokes, while 2 of 84 (2.4%) patients without stenosis had strokes.[27,37] Turnipseed and colleagues studied 330 CABG patients:[38] Severe carotid stenosis or occlusion was found in 103 patients, by Doppler, using spectral analysis of flow. The stroke rate after CABG in the patients with severe carotid disease and those without was an identical 5 percent.

The initial strategy in dealing with patients with combined coronary and carotid disease was to perform the two procedures, CEN and CABG, together, under the same anesthetic. Unfortunately, the perioperative stroke, MI, and mortality figures proved very high, much higher than with either procedure alone. Pettigrew tabulated 22 articles that described the results of staged or simultaneous cardiac and carotid surgery procedures among a total of 1076 patients.[27] Perioperative complications included 34 (3.2%) MIs, 57 (5.3%) TIAs or strokes, and 47 (4.4%) deaths.[27]

Considering the foregoing data, I advise a treatment paradigm similar to that of Hertzer and his Cleveland Clinic colleagues. The recommendations are summarized in Table 16.4.

What if the patient has severe coronary artery disease and asymptomatic carotid stenosis? CABG or coronary angioplasty, if indicated, are warranted. The patient could then be subsequently evaluated for possible CEN. Fisher said, "if the patient[s] can stand up, they can lie down." By this, he meant that if patients can perform daily living activities in an upright posture, they can safely lie down for surgery. The data bear this out.[26,36–39]

What if the patient has severe symptomatic carotid artery disease and the coronary disease is stable or inactive? I favor CEN in this circumstance, without concurrent CABG. The choice of medical therapy, coronary angioplasty, or a later CABG would be left to a cardiologist.

What if the patient has both active symptomatic coronary and carotid disease? These patients have unstable angina or silent myocardial ischemia

TABLE 16.4
Recommendations for Combined Carotid and Coronary Disease

Carotid Disease	Coronary Disease	Recommendation
Active, severe	Inactive	CEN
Inactive	Active, severe	CABG
Active, severe	Active, severe	CABG and CEN combined

Active carotid disease—ipsilateral hemispheral or retinal TIAs or recent stroke and severe ICA stenosis (<2 mm residual lumen or 75% stenosis). Active coronary disease—unstable angina, silent ischemia, or a recent MI with severe surgically operable disease by coronary angiography.

and TIAs or recent strokes in the territory of the narrowed carotid artery. In this circumstance, I advise combined CABG and CEN under the same anesthetic because the risk of either procedure alone or of the staged procedures is very high.

Vertebral Artery Surgery

The number of posterior-circulation surgical reconstructions is minimal, when compared with the number of anterior-circulation procedures. Yet surgery for posterior-circulation occlusive disease has been performed by selected surgeons with good results and low complication rates.[40–47] The commonest procedures involve the VA-origin region, including the parent subclavian artery.[40–42] Bypass intracranial procedures[43–45] and even endarterectomy of the ICVA[46,47] have been performed. Unfortunately, in sharp contrast to the situation in the anterior circulation, in which both CEN[1,2] and EC/IC bypass[48] have been and are being studied in formal trials, no trials or controlled data apply to the posterior circulation, and as far as I know, none are on the drawing board or planned.

Subclavian Artery Surgery for Subclavian Steal

Studies have shown that subclavian steal is generally a very benign syndrome, with a very low frequency of stroke.[49] There is a high incidence of concurrent carotid artery disease. Surgery on the subclavian artery is complex and often requires a thoracotomy for repair. The morbidity is higher than for neck surgery. In my opinion, only two circumstances warrant consideration for subclavian surgery: (1) when there is disabling arm ischemia (e.g., athletes—especially baseball pitchers and golfers—are susceptible to the development of subclavian artery disease, and arm ischemia may limit their performance);[50] and (2) when the occlusive disease involves the right side—the innominate or right subclavian artery. Subclavian clots may extend proximally and may embolize into the right carotid artery territory, causing right-hemisphere strokes.[51,52] As in the ICA, surgery should be considered in those circumstances only if the stenosis is severe.

Vertebral Artery Origin Disease

Although surgery on the VA-origin region can be done safely, the indications are unclear. Most surgeons do not do an endarterectomy but perform some type of shunting procedure into the carotid system. At times, the local VA bypass is accompanied by a CEN on the same side. After the stenotic ICA is repaired, the VA is divided, the proximal end is tied, and the distal end is anastomosed to the ICA.[41] Atherostenosis of the VA origin seldom causes persistent hemodynamic symptoms because even in the event of occlusion, excellent collateral circulation develops from the thyrocervical trunk and the ECA branches. Even bilateral VA-origin disease is usually well tolerated.[53] However, when one VA is stenosed or occluded intracranially, stenosis of the opposite VA can be problematic, especially if there also is some ipsilateral tandem intracranial disease. The VA can also serve as the nidus for embolism into the posterior circulation.[54] Possible indications for VA-origin surgery are embolism from the VA origin; persistent hemodynamic insufficiency, especially when there is contralateral intracranial VA disease; and at the time of CEN, when both the ICA and the VA on the same side are tightly stenotic.

Intracranial Posterior-Circulation Bypass Surgery

Shunts within the posterior circulation most often involve anastomoses between the occipital artery branch of the ECA and the PICA or one of its branches.[43–45] Less often, the occipital artery is grafted to the AICA. The superficial temporal artery can also be used as a donor, with the SCA or the PCA as recipients.[43,44] Nearly always, the indication for surgery has been persistent ischemic attacks despite medical therapy. In my own experience, bilateral ICVA disease, once symptoms develop, is a rather malignant disorder, with death or severe disability often due to bilateral motor and cerebellar signs. This is, in my opinion, the only indication for posterior-circulation bypass. When the basilar artery is occluded, usually collaterals from the ICA–posterior-communicating arteries provide natural collaterals to the distal basilar artery. The perforating arteries at the level of occlusion are not fed, but a bypass does not help this situation either.

Cardiac Surgery

In part, I have discussed the indications for CABG in patients with cerebrovascular disease earlier in this chapter. Neurologists are often called on to see patients after open-heart surgery, so they must be familiar with the common complications.

The reported incidence of neurological abnormalities during the postoperative period varies from 7 to 61 percent for transient and from 1.6 to 23 percent for permanent complications.[55-57] The complication rate is much higher in prospective series, in which patients are all routinely examined postoperatively, rather than in retrospective reviews of charts. In one study, among 312 patients, transient complications were noted in fully 61 percent of patients.[57] At the Cleveland Clinic, among a series of 421 CABG patients operated on, 16.8 percent had prolonged encephalopathy or stroke.[58] Complications can be readily divided into three groups: encephalopathy, stroke, and peripheral nervous system complications.

Encephalopathy

This term has been used to cover a wide spectrum of neuropsychiatric findings, including delirium, confusion, disorientation, drowsiness, and altered behavior, without focal neurological abnormalities. Imaging tests do not show new large focal brain infarcts. In the Cleveland Clinic series of CABG operations, 11.6 percent of patients were considered encephalopathic on the fourth postoperative day.[58] In another very large series, 57 of 1669 (3.4%) CABG patients had severe postoperative mental changes, including delirium and encephalopathy.[59] Undoubtedly, the causes are multiple. Some patients have a hypoxic–ischemic encephalopathy due to prolonged time on the pump, during which their brain was poorly perfused. An important number of cases are explained by medications. Sedatives, analgesics especially narcotics, and most important *haloperidol* are common offenders. Haloperidol very often produces depressed alertness, stiffness, inertia, and drowsiness, and the drug stays in the body a long time. Haloperidol has been shown to retard recovery in animals with brain lesions.[60,61] In my opinion, this drug should not be used in older surgical and medical patients, especially those with abnormal brains.

The initial recognition that the neurobehavioral changes were not psychiatric in origin was made by Gilman in 1965 when he prospectively followed a series of open-heart-surgery patients.[62] Early research led to the idea that embolization of particulate matter that was related to the pump and its filters had led to the encephalopathy.[63] The introduction of membrane rather than bubble oxygenators and in-line filtration led to a decrease in the risk of macroembolic particles (>25 μm).[63] A 1990 report of the necropsy findings in five patients and six dogs who all had cardiac surgery has aroused new interest in this subject.[64] Widely scattered in 10 of these 11 brains were focal small capillary and arteriolar dilations (SCADs). About one half of the SCADs contained birefringent crystalline material within the dilated capillary regions.[64] The vascular lesions affected medium-sized arterioles, terminal arterioles, and capillaries; they were often distributed in multiples in the same vessels or in clusters near each other. Two other patients had a small number of SCADs after arteriography. The authors thought that the findings were most consistent with iatrogenically induced release into the system of small particles of air or fat.[64] Microemboli are likely to be an important cause of encephalopathy.

Strokes

Focal neurological deficits are a most feared complication of cardiac surgery because they are often persistent and can be disabling. Among the Cleveland Clinic series were 22 of 421 (5.2%) patients who had postoperative strokes, but the deficits were severe in only 2 percent of the total series.[58] Twelve infarcts involved a cerebral hemisphere (7 right, 5 left), 5 involved the brainstem, 5 involved the retina, and 2 involved an optic nerve.[58]

In my opinion, the vast *majority of brain infarcts after cardiac surgery are due to embolism from the heart or aorta.* A major worry of cardiac surgeons, cardiologists, and neurologists has been that hemodynamic circulatory stress during heart surgery would lead to underperfusion of tenuous zones of preexisting extracranial vascular stenosis. This concern was the driving force behind early use of preoperative auscultation for bruits and behind later use of noninvasive and angiographic demonstration of the extracranial vascular systems prior to cardiac surgery. If carotid artery disease was found, CEN was performed before or during the same anesthetic as cardiac surgery. Unfortunately, the morbidity and mortality of this approach proved high.[39]

The data have also shown that true hemodynamic insufficiency in regions of prior vascular compromise is quite rare. Patients with carotid bruits have a very low rate of stroke after elective surgery.[36] I have already cited studies of patients with carotid stenosis documented by ultrasound who had a low rate of ipsilateral ischemic infarcts in the perioperative periods.[27,37,38] In a retrospective study of CABG patients with known carotid artery disease, 144 patients had severe atherostenosis (>50% luminal narrowing) affecting 155 arteries, as shown by preoperative angiography.[65] Strokes ipsilateral to the stenosis occurred in only 1.1 percent of arteries with 50 to 90 percent stenosis, in 6.2 percent of arteries with >90 percent stenosis, and in only 2 percent of arteries with carotid occlusion.[65] In 1988, von Reutern and colleagues monitored the MCA of patients, using TCD during cardiac surgery; even patients with severe carotid stenosis usually showed no important changes during surgery.[66]

Brain infarcts often develop in the period *after* cardiac surgery. Because hemodynamic stress is maximal intraoperatively, underperfusion should cause damage, noted on awakening after surgery. In one study, 5 of 30 postoperative strokes (17%) were noted immediately after cardiac surgery;[67] 14 others developed deficits within 24 hours, and 7 did so during the subsequent 24- to 48-hour period; in 2 patients, strokes occurred 5 and 11 days, respectively, after surgery. The distribution of the postoperative infarcts on CT scans and their multiplicity were most consistent with embolism.[67]

The authors concluded, "Our findings support the contention that in patients who suffer cerebral infarction associated with coronary artery bypass grafting, the main mechanism of injury is cerebral embolization rather than cerebral hypoperfusion."[67]

Some emboli are from cardiac lesions known to exist before heart surgery, such as valve lesions, ventricular aneurysms, and myocardial akinetic zones. Atrial fibrillation and other arrhythmias may have been present before surgery or may first appear during the postoperative period. Some patients had taken warfarin or aspirin before surgery, but this was discontinued before and during the operation and was not restarted until after the embolic stroke had occurred. Mounting evidence now also links postoperative embolism to ulcerative atherosclerotic lesions of the ascending aorta.[68-73] Aortotomy, or cross-clamping of the aorta in order to anastomose the vein graft, may liberate cholesterol crystals and calcific plaque debris. Yellow aortic plaques are often visible and can be palpated by the surgeon. When the aorta is clamped, an audible crunch is often heard.

The advent of TEE has now made it possible to detect ulcerative aortic plaques before surgery.[68-71] Tunick and colleagues identified 29 patients with protruding aortic plaques on TEE, one of whom had repeated peripheral emboli that led to surgical removal of the aortic plaque.[68] In another study, among 122 patients suspected of having brain embolism, 33 had protruding atheromas in the thoracic aorta. Mobile atheromas were seen only in patients with embolism.[69] Karalis et al. found that 38 patients among 556 TEE examinations (7%) had "intra-aortic atherosclerotic debris."[70] Nearly a third of those with debris had embolic events; the frequency of embolism was higher when the debris was pedunculated and mobile than when it was layered and immobile.[70] Among 15 patients in this study who had invasive aortic procedures (transfemoral angiography, intra-aortic balloon counterpulsation, and clamping during heart surgery), 27 percent had embolism.[70]

Marshall and colleagues used an intraoperative B-mode probe placed on the aorta in search of protruding plaques.[71] Ultrasonic imaging was more effective in showing plaques than was visual inspection and palpation. Furthermore, the amount and location of plaque often altered the procedure performed.[71]

In another study, cardiac surgeons retrospectively reviewed the cases of 3279 consecutive patients having CABG at Johns Hopkins, seeking risk factors for postoperative stroke.[72] Severe atherosclerosis of the ascending aorta was one of the most definitive risk factors found.[72] Manipulation (e.g., what occurs during aortography or clamping) can stir up recurrent bouts of embolization for days. Clearly, the aorta is a very important source of embolism, especially in patients having aortography or cardiac surgery. Occasionally, ICHs develop after cardiac surgery. Most often, this occurs after repair of congenital heart disease[73] and after cardiac transplantation.[74,75] Usually, cardiac output has been greatly increased by the surgery. The rather sudden change in brain blood flow usually caused the hemorrhages.[76]

Peripheral Nervous System Complications

Brachial plexus and peripheral nerve lesions often develop after heart surgery, and the symptoms can be confused with a stroke. In one large series, among 421 patients, 63 new peripheral nervous system deficits occurred among 55 patients (13% of patients).[77] The most common syndrome is characterized by shoulder pain and numbness and weakness of the hand. This results from a brachial plexus intraoperative injury related to positioning of the arm with traction on the plexus. Ulnar, peroneal, and saphenous nerve injuries are also common and also relate to positioning. Diaphragmatic and vocal-cord paralysis relate to local injury to the phrenic and recurrent laryngeal nerves during surgery.[77]

General Surgery

General anesthesia can augment brain edema and so should ordinarily not be given to patients recovering from a sizable brain infarct or hematoma. Stroke risk factors rarely, if ever, should postpone or delay general surgery unless the patient is having active brain ischemia (TIAs within 2 weeks or stroke within a month). Cardiac risk factors are more important because MI and cardiac death are larger surgical risks than is stroke. Goldman et al. have outlined the relative risk factors for cardiac morbidity and mortality in relation to general surgery.[13]

Strokes do occur after general surgery. Some relate to known medical disorders antedating surgery, such as polycythemia, thrombocytosis, arrhythmia, bleeding diathesis, etc. Puncture of the carotid artery[58] or VA[78] during attempted jugular-vein cannulation can lead to thrombosis of these arteries, with subsequent stroke.

As I and my colleagues reported in 1991, we studied a group of patients that developed posterior-circulation strokes after general, noncardiac, nonvascular surgery.[79] The surgical procedures were often minor (bunion removal, fracture repair, appendectomy). Most were orthopedic or gynecological. During the immediate postoperative period, or during the first 36 hours, the patients developed either vestibulocerebellar symptoms and signs or stupor with reduced levels of consciousness. CT showed cerebellar and rostral basilar-artery-territory infarcts. None of these patients had known atherosclerosis or a cardiac-source embolism. I think that the most likely mechanism of stroke was abnormal positioning in relation to surgery, which was performed using general anesthesia and intubation in all patients. Thrombus probably formed in one VA in the neck, during positioning in one neck posture. After the surgery was over and patients could move freely, clot then was discharged intracranially to block the ICVA (causing a cerebellar infarct) or the top of the basilar artery (causing thalamic, superior cerebellar, or posterior cerebral-hemisphere infarcts). These are the same areas affected by intra-arterial emboli in patients who have not had surgery.[54]

VA dissection can also complicate surgery, and it is possible that even carotid artery dissection might be precipitated by unusual head and neck positioning.[80] The incidence of stroke during general surgery is not known, but stroke occurrence is probably more common than is presently recognized. Careful preoperative screening for cardiac and hematological diseases and meticulous patient positioning are key factors in stroke prevention.

References

1. North American Symptomatic Carotid Endarterectomy Trial (NASCET) Collaborators. Beneficial effects of carotid endarterectomy in symptomatic patients with high-grade carotid stenosis. N Engl J Med 1991;325:445–453.
2. European Carotid Surgery Trialists' Collaborative Group. MRC European Carotid Surgery trial: interim results of symptomatic patients with severe (70–99%) or with mild (0–29%) carotid stenosis. Lancet 1991;1:1235–1243.
3. Caplan LR. Carotid artery disease [editorial]. N Engl J Med 1986;315:886–888.
4. Caplan LR, Pessin MS. Symptomatic carotid artery disease and carotid endarterectomy. Ann Rev Med 1988;39:273–299.
5. Fisher CM, Ojemann R. A clinico-pathological study of carotid endarterectomy plaques. Rev Neurol 1986;142:573–589.
6. Caplan LR, Stein R, Patel D, et al. Intraluminal clot of the carotid artery detected radiographically. Neurology 1984;34:1175–1181.
7. Pessin MS, Abbott BF, Prager R, et al. Clinical and angiographic features of carotid circulation thrombus. Neurology 1986;36:518–523.
8. Sundt TM, Sandok BA, Whisnant JP. Carotid endarterectomy complications and pre-operative assessment of risk. Mayo Clin Proc 1975;50:301–306.
9. Easton JD, Sherman DO. Stroke and mortality rate in carotid endarterectomy: 228 consecutive operations. Stroke 1977;8:565–568.
10. Brott TG, Thalinger K. The practice of carotid endarterectomy in a large metropolitan area. Stroke 1984;15:950–955.
11. Callow AD. An overview of the stroke problem in the carotid territory: the David M. Hume Memorial Lecture. Am J Surg 1980;140:181–191.
12. Tarhan S, Moffitt FR, Taylor W, Guiliani E. Myocardial infarction after general anesthesia. JAMA 1972;220:1451–1454.
13. Goldman L, Caldera DL, Nussbaum SR, et al. Multifactorial index of cardiac risk in non-cardiac surgical procedures. N Engl J Med 1977;297:845–850.
14. Toronto Cerebrovascular Study Group. Risks of carotid endarterectomy. Stroke 1986;17:848–852.
15. Steed DL, Pertzman AB, Grandy B, Webster M. Causes of stroke in carotid endarterectomy. Surgery 1982;92:634–641.
16. Diaz FG, Patel S, Bordas R, et al. Early angiographic changes after carotid endarterectomy. Neurosurg 1982;10:151–161.
17. Sundt TM. The ischemic tolerance of nerve tissue and the need for monitoring and selective shunting during carotid endarterectomy. Stroke 1983;14:93–98.

18. Leviton A, Caplan LR, Salzman EW. Severe headache following carotid endarterectomy. Headache 1975;13:201–210.

19. Lehv MS, Salzman EW, Silen W. Hypertension complicating carotid endarterectomy. Stroke 1970;1:307–313.

20. Caplan LR, Skillman J, Ojemann R, Fields WS. Intracerebral hemorrhage following carotid endarterectomy: a hypertensive complication. Stroke 1978; 9:157–160.

21. Pessin MS, Kwan ES, Scott RM, Hedges TR. Occipital infarction with hemianopia from carotid occlusive disease. Stroke 1989;20:409–411.

22. Fode NC, Sundt T, Robertson J, et al. Multicenter retrospective review of results and complications of carotid endarterectomy. Stroke 1986;17:370–376.

23. Hart RG, Easton JJ. Management of cervical bruits and carotid stenosis in preoperative patients. Stroke 1983;14:290–297.

24. Mehigan JT, Birch WS, Pipkin RD, Fogarty TJ. A planned approach to coexistent cerebrovascular disease in coronary artery bypass candidates. Arch Surg 1977;112:1403–1409.

25. Easton JD, Hart RG. Asymptomatic carotid artery disease in patients undergoing open heart surgery: a neurologic viewpoint. In: Furlan AJ, ed. The heart and stroke. London: Springer-Verlag, 1987:319–327.

26. Rokey R, Rolak LA, Harati Y, et al. Coronary artery disease in patients with cerebral vascular disease: a prospective study. Ann Neurol 1984;16:50–53.

27. Pettigrew LC. Surgical considerations. In: Rolak LA, Rokey R, eds. Coronary and cerebral vascular disease. Mount Kisco, NY: Futura, 1990:349–377.

28. Hertzer NR, Young JR, Beven EG, et al. Coronary angiography in 506 patients with extracranial cerebral vascular disease. Arch Intern Med 1985;145: 849–852.

29. Riles TS, Kopelman I, Imparato AM. Myocardial infarction following carotid endarterectomy: a review of 683 operations. Surgery 1979;85:249–252.

30. Hertzer NR, Lees CD. Fatal myocardial infarction following carotid endarterectomy. Ann Surg 1981;194:212–218.

31. Verani M, Rokey R. Coronary artery disease: diagnosis and clinical features. In: Rolak LA, Rokey R, eds. Coronary and cerebral vascular disease. Mount Kisco, NY: Futura, 1990:19–49.

32. Boucher CA, Brewster DC, Darling RC, et al. Determination of cardiac risk by dipyridamole–thallium imaging before peripheral vascular surgery. N Engl J Med 1985;312:389–394.

33. Gould KL, Sorenson SG, Albro P, et al. Thallium-201 myocardial imaging during coronary vasodilatation induced by oral dipyridamole. J Nucl Med 1986;27:31–36.

34. Gottlieb SO, Weisfeldt ML, Ouyang P, et al. Silent ischemia as a marker for early unfavorable outcome in patients with unstable angina. N Engl J Med 1986;314:1214–1219.

35. Gazes PC, Mobley EM Jr, Faris HM Jr, et al. Preinfarctional (unstable) angina—a prospective study: ten year follow-up. Circulation 1973;48:331–337.

36. Ropper AH, Wechsler LR, Wilson LS. Carotid bruit and the risk of stroke in elective surgery. N Engl J Med 1982;307:1388–1390.

37.   Breslau PJ, Fell G, Ivey TD, et al. Carotid arterial disease in patients undergoing coronary artery bypass operations. J Thorac Cardiovasc Surg 1981;82:765–767.
38.   Turnipseed WD, Berkhoff HA, Belzer FO. Postoperative stroke in cardiac and peripheral vascular disease. Ann Surg 1980;192:365–368.
39.   Hertzer NR, Loop FD, Beven EG. Management of coexistent carotid and coronary artery disease: a surgical viewpoint. In: Furlan AJ, ed. The heart and stroke. London: Springer-Verlag, 1987:305–318.
40.   Roon A, Ehrenfeld W, Cooke P, et al. Vertebral artery reconstruction. Am J Surg 1979;138:29–36.
41.   Lee RE. Reconstruction of the proximal vertebral artery. In: Berguer R, Caplan LR, ed. Vertebrobasilar arterial disease. St. Louis: Quality Medical, 1991:211–223.
42.   Spetzler RF, Hadley MN, Martin NA, et al. Vertebrobasilar insufficiency: pt I. microsurgical treatment of extracranial vertebrobasilar disease. J Neurosurg 1987;66:648–661.
43.   Hopkins LN, Martin NA, Hadley MN, et al. Vertebrobasilar insufficiency: pt II. microsurgical treatment of intracranial vertebrobasilar disease. J Neurosurg 1987;66:662–674.
44.   Sundt T, Whisnant J, Piepgras D, et al. Intracranial bypass grafts for vertebrobasilar ischemia. Mayo Clin Proc 1978;53:12–18.
45.   Roski R, Spetzler R, Hopkins L. Occipital artery to posterior inferior cerebellar artery bypass for vertebrobasilar ischemia. Neurosurgery 1982;10:44–49.
46.   Allen G, Cohen R, Preziosi T. Microsurgical endarterectomy of the intracranial vertebral artery for vertebrobasilar transient ischemic attacks. Neurosurgery 1981;81:56–59.
47.   Ausman JI, Diaz FG, Pearce JE, et al. Endarterectomy of the vertebral artery from C_2 to posterior inferior cerebellar artery intracranially. Surg Neurol 1982;18:400–404.
48.   The EC/IC Bypass Study Group. Failure of the extracranial–intracranial arterial bypass to reduce the risk of ischemic stroke. N Engl J Med 1985;313:1191–1200.
49.   Hennerici M, Aulich A, Sandmann W, Freund HJ. Incidence of asymptomatic extracranial arterial disease. Stroke 1981;12:750–758.
50.   Fields WS. Neurovascular syndromes of the neck and shoulders. Sem Neurol 1981;1:301–309.
51.   Symonds C. Two cases of thrombosis of subclavian artery with contralateral hemiplegia of sudden onset, probably embolic. Brain 1927;50:259–260.
52.   Fields WS, Lemak NA, Ben-Menachem Y. Thoracic outlet syndrome: review and reference to a stroke in a major league pitcher. AJNR 1986;7:73–78.
53.   Fisher CM. Occlusion of the vertebral arteries. Arch Neurol 1970;22:13–19.
54.   Caplan LR. The 1991 Graeme Robertson Lecture: vertebrobasilar embolism. Clin Exp Neurology 1991;28:1–23.
55.   Slogoff S, Girgis KZ, Keats AS. Etiologic factors in neuropsychiatric complications associated with cardiopulmonary bypass. Anesth Analg 1982;61:903–911.
56.   Gilman S. Neurological complications of open heart surgery. Ann Neurol 1990;28:475–476.
57.   Shaw PJ, Bates D, Cartledge NEF. Early neurological complications of coronary artery bypass surgery. Brit Med J 1985;391:1384–1387.

58. Breuer AC, Furlan AJ, Hanson MR, et al. Central nervous system complications of coronary artery bypass graft surgery: prospective analysis of 421 patients. Stroke 1983;14:682–687.

59. Coffey CE, Massey EW, Roberts KB, et al. Natural history of cerebral complication of coronary artery bypass graft surgery. Neurology 1983;33:1416–1421.

60. Feeney DM, Gonzalez A, Law WA. Amphetamine, haloperidol and experience interact to affect the rate of recovery after motor cortex injury. Science 1982; 217:855–857.

61. Houda DA, Feeney DM. Haloperidol blocks amphetamine induced recovery of binocular depth perception of the bilateral visual cortex abilities in the cat. Proc West Pharmacol Soc 1985;28:209–211.

62. Gilman S. Cerebral disorders after open heart operations. N Engl J Med 1965;272:489–498.

63. Sila C. Neuroimaging of cerebral infarction associated with coronary revascularization. AJNR 1991;12:817–818.

64. Moody DM, Bell MA, Challa VR, et al. Brain microemboli during cardiac surgery or aortography. Ann Neurol 1990;28:477–486.

65. Furlan AJ, Cracium AR. Risk of stroke during coronary artery bypass graft surgery in patients with internal carotid artery disease documented by angiography. Stroke 1985;16:797–799.

66. Von Reutern G, Hetzel A, Birnbaum D, et al. Transcranial Doppler ultrasound during cardiopulmonary bypass in patients with internal carotid artery disease documented by angiography. Stroke 1988;19:674–680.

67. Hise JH, Nipper MN, Schnitker JC. Stroke associated with coronary artery bypass surgery. AJNR 1991;12:811–814.

68. Tunick PA, Culliford AT, Lamparello PJ, et al. Atheromatosis of the aortic arch as an occult source of multiple systemic emboli. Ann Intern Med 1991; 114:391–392.

69. Tunick PA, Perez JL, Kronzon I. Protruding atheromas in the thoracic aorta and systemic embolization. Ann Int Med 1991;115:423–427.

70. Karalis DG, Chandrasekaran K, Victor MF, et al. Recognition and embolic potential of intra-aortic atherosclerotic debris. J Am Coll Cardiol 1991; 17:73–78.

71. Marshall WG, Barzilai B, Kouchoukos NT, et al. Intraoperative ultrasonic imaging of the ascending aorta. Ann Thorac Surg 1989;48:339–344.

72. Gardner TJ, Horneffer PJ, Manolio TA, et al. Stroke following coronary artery bypass grafting: a ten-year study. Ann Thorac Surg 1985;40:574–581.

73. Amarenco P, Duyckaerts C, Tzourio C, et al. The prevalence of ulcerated plaques in the aortic arch in patients with stroke. N Engl J Med 1992;326: 221–225.

74. Sila CA. Spectrum of neurologic events following cardiac transplantation. Stroke 1989;20:1586–1589.

75. Andrews BT, Hershon JJ, Calanchini P, et al. Neurologic complications of cardiac transplantations. West J Med 1990;153:146–148.

76. Caplan LR. Intracerebral hemorrhage revisited. Neurology 1988;38:624–627.

77. Lederman RJ, Breuer AC, Hanson MR, et al. Peripheral nervous system complications of coronary artery bypass graft surgery. Ann Neurol 1982;12: 297–301.

78.   Sloan MA, Mueller JD, Adelman LS, Caplan LR. Fatal brainstem stroke following internal jugular vein catheterization. Neurology 1991;41:1092–1095.
79.   Caplan LR, Tettenborn B, DeWitt LD. Brainstem and cerebellar infarcts after non-cardiac surgery. Neurology 1991;41(Suppl 1):346.
80.   Caplan LR, Zarins C, Hemmatii M. Spontaneous dissection of the extracranial vertebral artery. Stroke 1985;16:1030–1038.

PART **III**

Prevention, Complications, and Rehabilitation

CHAPTER 17

Stroke Prevention and Risk Factors

When meditating over a disease I never think of finding a remedy for it, but instead a means of preventing it.

Louis Pasteur[1]

Prevention of stroke is much more likely to have a major impact on the health and welfare of the population than even the most effective treatment after stroke has occurred. For this cogent reason, much effort is aimed at identifying risk factors for cerebrovascular disease. The declining incidence of stroke is tangible evidence that this strategy has had positive results.[2–4]

Despite these efforts, much of the population is woefully ignorant about stroke. The medical profession and the media have been relatively successful in educating the public about heart attacks, cancer, and AIDS. Unfortunately, stroke, although it is the third leading cause of death in the United States, has received much less public attention and remains only a poorly understood word to most Americans. The San Francisco Chapter of the American Heart Association sponsored a survey of 500 representative local residents to compare knowledge about stroke and heart disease.[5] Nearly half of those surveyed were unable to name any early warning signs of stroke; those who did answer often gave incorrect responses. On the other hand, 9 of 10 respondents could easily identify at least one major sign of heart attacks, and most could name two or more. On the positive side, nearly two thirds of those surveyed reported having changed a habit, activity, or way of life in order to reduce their perceived risk for heart attacks.

The American Heart Association's Stroke Subcommittee sponsored a national survey using a sample of 1253 respondents to study knowledge about stroke, compared with other common diseases.[6] The survey results included the following:

1. Most were aware that stroke is among the three major causes of death in the United States.

517

2. In answer to the question, "A stroke occurs when the blood supply is cut off to what part of the body?" 29 percent did not select the brain from the choices of "heart," "brain," "don't know," and "other."
3. Some (about 7%) thought that arthritis was a major cause of stroke.
4. Only 44 percent identified weakness or loss of feeling in one arm or leg as a symptom of stroke, as opposed to heart attack.
5. The respondents overestimated the proportion of stroke victims who are permanently disabled or require institutionalization after stroke.

Despite the lack of public knowledge about stroke, there has been a rather consistent decline in stroke incidence and mortality.[2-4] This fact probably is explained by a number of factors. First, the public is definitely more health conscious. Emphasis on preservation of health through good eating habits, regular exercise, and avoidance of cigarettes, alcohol, and dietary excesses has been an educational and media theme. Reduction in risk factors perceived in the public mind as related to heart attacks has, as its natural by-product, reduced cerebrovascular disease as well. An emphasis on check-ups and screening for high blood pressure, diabetes, and high cholesterol, and the availability of more health professionals also must have had an impact. Physicians' more aggressive treatment of hypertension and better technology for assessing vascular disease have also played a role. Clearly, more public and physician education is needed if we are to make further gains in stroke prevention.

Risk Factors

Extensive information has accumulated and been analyzed regarding risk factors for the general category of stroke[3,7,8] and particularly of brain ischemia.[9-11] With regard to some stroke mechanisms, such as SAH,[12] ICH, and cerebral embolism of cardiac origin, there are ample data. I discuss causes of hemorrhage in detail in Chapters 12 and 13. Obviously, the major risk factors for cardiac-origin embolism are those that predispose to the various cardiac conditions. These are described in Chapter 10. Relatively less information is available about other specific stroke mechanisms, especially within the broad group of patients with cerebral ischemia. Most analyses of risk factors do not differentiate among patients with stenotic lesions of the extracranial arteries, those with stenosis of the large intracranial vessels such as the MCAs, and those with disease of penetrating arteries such as the lenticulostriate arteries. There is evidence that various risk factors such as race and sex have a differential effect on various pathological lesions and on lesions at various loci within the vasculature.[13-15] Further data, especially in patients with specific stroke subtypes, studied prospectively, are needed.

Despite these limitations, the currently identified risk factors are of great significance. They help to identify individuals at risk for stroke, in whom modification of life-style might reduce the chance of stroke and other cardiovascular diseases. In this section, I briefly discuss only some of these risk factors because larger, more detailed reviews of the subject are available.[2,7,16] When risk factors are identified, the evidence is usually an epidemiological relationship between the factor and the occurrence of stroke; correlation does *not* mean causation. Being female is very strikingly associated with becoming pregnant but clearly does not cause the condition.

Age is probably the risk factor best correlated with stroke. The Framingham study showed that increasing age is associated with an increased risk of stroke, with incidence rates per 10,000 increasing from 22 to 32 to 83 in the age groups 45 to 55, 55 to 64, and 65 to 74 years, respectively.[16] The incidence of SAH also rises steadily with age.[12] Studies that have not found an increase in the oldest age group cite the lack of definitive evaluation of geriatric stroke patients.[17,18] Data on age in patients with ICH (Chapter 12) also document a high frequency in the elderly. Despite our best efforts, unless the alternative—death—prevents us, we will all continue to get older; also, stroke does occur in younger patients. Ischemic stroke in patients less than 45 years old is correlated with more frequent cardiac-origin embolism and less common occlusive lesions (Chapter 9), while in stroke patients over age 65, intrinsic large- and small-artery diseases are most common, followed by cardiac-origin embolism.

Following age, hypertension is the risk factor that most significantly correlates with stroke. The degree of elevation of both systolic and diastolic pressure is correlated with stroke risk. The risk curve is a continuum, without any clear point separating the stroke-prone from the non-stroke-prone individual.[16,19,20] Hypertension plays a role in multiple mechanisms of stroke. Without a prior history of diabetes or hypertension, lacunar disease is rarely found at necropsy. Also, the association between hypertension and cardiac disease is well known, making cardioembolic brain infarction more likely. Hypertension also plays a role in the atherodegenerative process in large blood vessels, resulting in both occlusive and artery-to-artery embolic strokes. Hypertension also plays a role in the rupture of cerebral aneurysms.[7,12] ICH in the basal ganglia, thalamus, pons, and cerebellum is more commonly found in the setting of acute and chronic hypertension.

For stroke in general and atherothrombotic brain infarction, there is no evidence that women tolerate hypertension better than men, nor does the effect of hypertension wane in the elderly.[7,16] The Framingham data strongly suggest that control of hypertension is as critical for stroke prevention in patients over age 80 years as it is in younger age groups.[19] Systolic blood pressure is as important as diastolic.[7,16,19] In the systolic hypertension in the elderly program (SHEP), studies show that treating isolated systolic hypertension in the geriatric years reduces the incidence of stroke and other cardiovascular events.[21] Antihypertensive treatment with low-dose chlorthalidone, lowering systolic pressure to 143 torr in the treatment group versus 155 torr in the placebo group, reduced the total stroke incidence by 36 percent—that is, by 30 strokes per 1000 patients during 5 years.[21] Other clinical studies have also shown a reduction in stroke incidence and mortality when hypertension is treated.[22–26] In the United States, between 1972 and 1977, age-adjusted death rates for hypertension-related cardiovascular diseases declined 20 percent, whereas unrelated cardiovascular disease declined only 9 percent.[7] It is generally agreed that aggressive and effective control of hypertension over many years has contributed to the decline in stroke incidence and mortality.

When caring for patients with acute stroke, the ravages of many years of hypertension on the blood vessel wall cannot be reversed in 1 or 2 days by precipitously lowering blood pressure. In fact, radical decrease in blood pressure may reduce cerebral perfusion, which can lead to profound worsening of neurological deficits. I aim for effective treatment of hypertension across many months. In some individuals with flow-dependent strokes, blood pressures that would usually be excessive must be tolerated during the weeks that collateral circulation is becoming firmly established.

Cardiac disease is also highly correlated with stroke. Cardioembolic stroke occurs in the setting of mitral- or aortic-valve disease, atrial fibrillation of any cause, prosthetic heart valves, endocarditis, myocardiopathies, akinetic myocardial segments, and ventricular aneurysms. Other indices of cardiac impairment—such as coronary artery disease, congestive heart failure, and left ventricular hypertrophy, as measured by electrocardiography, chest x-ray, or echocardiography—are associated with increased stroke risk. Particularly important is the fact that heart disease is the major cause of death in patients with stroke, TIA, or carotid bruits.[27,28] Stroke is a major risk factor for heart disease even if no overt cardiac disease is observed. We must diligently search for and treat heart disease in patients with stroke. The treatment of heart disease in association with stroke will play a major role in prolonging life and avoiding significant morbidity.

Diabetes is also associated with an increased risk of stroke.[29–31] Its relationship may be either direct or secondary to a strong correlation with hypertension.[29] The risk of stroke in diabetics does not diminish with advancing age in either sex.[7] Diabetes is a risk factor for both large extracranial disease and lacunar infarction. Unfortunately, no clear data exist to support the notion that strict control of diabetes alters the risk of stroke.

In the first edition of this book, the importance of cigarette smoking as a risk factor for stroke was still uncertain. Now, convincing epidemiological data strongly relate cigarettes with stroke and both extracranial and intracranial atherosclerosis.[32–34] The amount and duration of smoking are both important factors. In the Framingham study, smoking was a significant risk factor for atherothrombotic brain infarction only in men under 65 years of age.[35] Similarly, in a series of young adults (15–45 years old) in Iowa, a smoker was 1.6 times more likely to have a brain infarct than a non-smoker.[32] Paffenbarger and Williams found that smoking was one of the most important risk factors among college students who later had ischemic strokes.[36] In a series of patients with extracranial carotid artery disease studied at the Mayo Clinic, the total years of cigarette smoking was the single most significant independent predictor of the presence of severe occlusive disease.[33] Duration of cigarette smoking and hypertension were the most important predictors of intracranial ICA disease in another study.[34] In regard to SAH, cigarette smoking seems to be a risk factor only when combined with the use of high-dose estrogen and contraceptive-pill use in women.[12,37]

Asymptomatic carotid bruits are clear risk factors for stroke death and ischemic heart disease.[27] The location of the subsequent stroke does not reliably correlate with the side of the bruit. On the other hand, in patients who are about to undergo operative procedures, bruits have failed to identify a group who are at risk for perioperative stroke, which, when it occurs, is most commonly cardiac in origin.[38] Bruits in the neck can originate from the ECA, can radiate from the heart, or can result from hyperdynamic flow. Furthermore, significant stenosis can be present without a bruit.[39] Carotid artery and VA ultrasound and MRA, which can quantitate the degree of vascular narrowing, correlate much better with the risk of stroke than does the presence or absence of bruits. Pathologically elevated and high-normal hematocrits have been associated with increased stroke and TIA risk, even when hypertension and cigarette smoking are considered.[40,41] Higher hemoglobin levels are also correlated with larger brain infarcts.[42] This correlation might be partly due to the fact that chronic hypoxemia, pulmonary disease, and smoking may have caused the high hematocrits. The adverse effect of high hematocrits could also relate to increased viscosity.[42,43]

Abnormalities of blood lipids—especially cholesterol, triglycerides, and high- and low-density lipoproteins—are less closely correlated with stroke than with coronary heart disease. In the Framingham and other studies, the risk is primarily documented in those patients less than 55 years old.[44] A relationship between low cholesterol and SAH has been shown in several reports.[45,46] The risk of ICH is especially high in patients with very low cholesterol levels (< 160–190 mg/dl).[47,48] In one large series of more than 350,000 men, there was a significant relationship between morbidity from ischemic stroke and high serum cholesterol levels.[46] Elevated levels of low-density lipoproteins (LDL), *decrease* in concentrations of high-density lipoproteins (HDL), and the presence of lipoprotein (a) correlate better with coronary and extracranial atherosclerosis than do total cholesterol levels.[49,50] Serum lipids and lipoprotein levels are not as powerful predictors of extracranial ICA disease as are hypertension and cigarette smoking.[51]

No conclusive data link alcohol consumption with ischemic stroke.[7,12,52–55] There probably is, however, a relationship between alcohol consumption and brain hemorrhage. Finnish studies, not well controlled, clearly linked heavy alcohol consumption and recent alcohol use to the occurrence of SAH.[56,57] ICH can be caused by the hypoprothrombinemia accompanying cirrhosis of the liver. In the Honolulu Heart Study, alcohol consumption was associated with intracranial hemorrhage but not with ischemic stroke.[45,56]

Light to moderate regular consumption of alcohol seems to be inversely related to carotid artery and systemic atherosclerosis,[55] yet both acute and chronic heavy use of alcohol positively correlate with the incidence of ischemic stroke. The effect vanishes when the studies controlled for hypertension and cigarette smoking.[52,53]

Perhaps the most controversial of all the possible risk factors is the use of oral contraceptives. The American Heart Association Committee on Risk Factors in Stroke could not agree on whether the use of the pill was an independent risk factor and, if it was, to what degree.[7] Some retrospective case studies do suggest that oral contraceptive use conveys a 4- to 13-fold increase in the risk of cerebral infarction.[7,37,58–60] Hypertension, migraine, diabetes, hyperlipidemia, cigarette smoking, age over 35 years, and prolonged use of oral-contraceptive pills probably compound the risk of ischemic stroke in oral-contraceptive users.[7] Some evidence also indicates that the pill may also increase the risk for SAH.[12,61]

Most of the data on the relationship of stroke and oral contraceptives are in patients who used pills with a relatively high estrogen content. Now, lower-dose estrogen oral contraceptives are usually prescribed. These low-dose estrogen pills are posited to have much less tendency to predispose to venous and arterial thromboses, but few data now exist to confirm or refute this hypothesis.

TIAs are most often an indication that occlusive cerebrovascular disease has already become established. In fact, some patients with clinical TIAs have CT evidence of infarction in regions that correlate with the symptoms.[62–64] Nicolaides and Zukowski found that among 36 patients with clinical TIAs, 23 (64%) had CT-positive infarcts.[65] The incidence of infarcts in patients with clinical TIAs is even higher when MRI is performed.[63] Patients with TIAs are also, of course, at risk for subsequent TIAs, stroke, and MI.[3,66] Risk factors and prognosis are relatively similar for patients with TIAs and those with minor strokes because the underlying vascular diseases are identical.[10] Recognition and appropriate treatment of patients with TIAs will probably not influence the total stroke incidence as much as control of the factors that prevent the establishment of atherosclerotic disease.

Nevertheless, for the individual stroke patient, failure to recognize that a TIA has occurred, and failure to diagnose and treat potentially remediable abnormalities, can be a great personal and family tragedy. All too often, patients fail to understand the importance of temporary focal nervous system and ocular symptoms and so do not report them to their physicians. Even more lamentable, in my experience, all too often, doctors reassure patients that the spells are not important. This is most often the case with transient monocular blindness. When the nature of the spells is correctly identified, treatment often involves overzealous carotid artery surgery or automatic prescription of the latest panacea for ischemic stroke (warfarin, vasodilators, aspirin, etc.). Unfortunately, thoughtful evaluation of the cause in the individual patient is the exception, not the rule.

Prevention

When multiple risk factors are considered together, patients at particular risk for stroke can be identified. When systolic hypertension, elevated serum cholesterol, glucose intolerance, cigarette smoking, and ECG changes with left ventricular hypertrophy are combined, a population accounting for one third of the strokes can be identified.[35]

I actively encourage treatment of the remediable risk factors in such stroke-prone individuals, yet only treatment of hypertension has been shown to be correlated with lower stroke risk. Even when stroke has occurred, treatment of these factors has been shown in one study to decrease the expected mortality and stroke recurrence rate during the 5 years following the first stroke.[67]

The incidence of stroke is declining, but much more can and should be done. Advances will probably involve the following:

1. *Improved general health measures initiated by individuals concerned about their bodies*—A reduction in cardiopulmonary disease will clearly lower the incidence of stroke.
2. *Education of patients about the symptoms and significance of hypertension and TIAs*—They can and should become educated consumers who recognize and seek the most competent care.
3. *Education of general physicians*—They need to know about the warning signs of stroke, stroke risk factors, and how to manage cerebrovascular disease.
4. *Education of neurologists, vascular surgeons, neurosurgeons, and other stroke specialists*—These specialists need to know when and how to manage risk factors as well as to treat the present stroke problem.
5. *Research*—Advance the present capabilities for diagnosing and treating stroke patients and stroke-prone individuals.

References

1. Pasteur L. Address to the Fraternal Association of former students of the École Centrale des Arts et Manufactures, Paris, May 15, 1884.
2. Garraway WM, Whisnant JP, Furlan AJ, et al. The declining incidence of stroke. N Engl J Med 1979;300:449–452.

3. Wolf P. Risk factors for stroke. Stroke 1985;16:359–360.
4. Bonita R, Stewart A, Beaglehole R. International trends in stroke mortality: 1970–1985. Stroke 1990;21:989–992.
5. American Heart Association, San Francisco Chapter. San Francisco Public Awareness Survey: Study 62202. San Francisco: Opinion Research Corporation, 1984.
6. American Heart Association. Stroke Awareness Study. Dallas: SRI Research Center, 1985.
7. Wolf P, Dyken M, Barnett HJM, et al. Risk factors in stroke. Stroke 1984;15: 1105–1111.
8. Shaper AG, Phillips AN, Pocock SJ, et al. Risk factors for stroke in middle aged British men. Br Med J 1991;302:1111–1115.
9. Sobel E, Altu M, Davanipour Z, et al. Stroke in the Lehigh Valley: combined risk factors for recurrent ischemic stroke. Neurology 1989;39:669–672.
10. Dennis MS, Bamford JM, Sandercock PA, Warlow CD. A comparison of risk factors and prognosis for transient ischemic attacks and minor ischemic strokes. Stroke 1989;20:1494–1499.
11. Davis PH, Dambrosia JM, Schoenberg BS, et al. Risk factors for ischemic stroke: a prospective study in Rochester, Minnesota. Ann Neurol 1987;22: 319–327.
12. Longstreth WT, Koepsell T, Yerby M, et al. Risk factors for subarachnoid hemorrhage. Stroke 1985;16:377–385.
13. Gorelick PB, Caplan LR, Hier DB, et al. Racial differences in the distribution of anterior circulation occlusive cerebrovascular disease. Neurology 1984;34: 54–59.
14. Gorelick PB, Caplan LR, Hier DB, et al. Racial differences in the distribution of posterior circulation occlusive disease. Stroke 1985;16:785–790.
15. Caplan LR. Race, sex, and occlusive cerebrovascular disease: a review. Stroke 1986;17:648–655.
16. Kannel WB. Current status of the epidemiology of brain infarction associated with occlusive arterial disease. Stroke 1971;2:295–318.
17. Pakarinen S. Incidence, etiology and prognosis of primary subarachnoid hemorrhage: a study based on 589 cases diagnosed in a defined urban population during a defined period. Acta Neurol Scand 1967;43(Suppl 29):9–128.
18. Bonita R, Beaglehole R, North JD. Subarachnoid hemorrhage in New Zealand: an epidemiologic study. Stroke 1983;14:342–347.
19. Kannel WB, Wolf PA, Verter J, et al. Epidemiologic assessment of the role of blood pressure in stroke: the Framingham study. JAMA 1970;214:301–310.
20. Whisnant JP. Epidemiology of stroke: emphasis on transient cerebral ischemic attacks and hypertension. Stroke 1974;5:68–75.
21. SHEP Cooperative Research Group. Prevention of stroke by antihypertensive drug treatment in older persons with isolated systolic hypertension. JAMA 1991;265:3255–3264.
22. Management Committee. The Australian therapeutic trial in mild hypertension. Lancet 1980;1:1261–1267.
23. Taguchi J, Faris E. Partial reduction of blood pressure and prevention of complications in hypertension. N Engl J Med 1974;29:329–331.
24. Veterans Administration Cooperative Study Group on Antihypertensive Agents. Effect of treatment on morbidity in hypertension: I. results in patients

with diastolic blood pressures averaging 115 through 129 mm Hg. JAMA 1969;202:1028.

25. Veterans Administration Cooperative Study Group on Antihypertensive Agents. Effects of treatment on morbidity in hypertension: II. results in patients with diastolic blood pressures averaging 90 through 114 mm Hg. JAMA 1970;213:1143–1152.

26. Spence JD. Antihypertensive drugs and prevention of atherosclerotic stroke. Stroke 1986;17:808–810.

27. Heyman A, Wilkinson WE, Heyden S, et al. Risk of stroke in asymptomatic persons with cervical arterial bruits: a population study in Evans County, Georgia. N Engl J Med 1980;302:838–841.

28. Toole FJ, Janeway R, Choi K, et al. Transient ischemic attacks due to atherosclerosis: a prospective study of 160 patients. Arch Neurol 1975;32:5–12.

29. Schoenberg BS, Schoenberg DG, Pritchard DA, et al. Differential risk factors for completed stroke and transient ischemic attack (TIA): study of vascular disease (hypertension, cardiac disease, peripheral vascular disease) and diabetes mellitus. Trans Am Neurol Assoc 1980;105:165–167.

30. Olivares L, Castaneda E, Grife A, et al. Risk factors in stroke: a clinical study in Mexican patients. Stroke 1973;4:773–781.

31. Paffenbarger R Jr, Wing A. Chronic disease in former college students: XI. early precursors of nonfatal stroke. Am J Epidemiol 1971;94:524–530.

32. Love BB, Biller J, Jones MP, et al. Cigarette smoking: a risk factor for cerebral infarction in young adults. Arch Neurol 1990;47:693–698.

33. Whisnant JP, Homer D, Ingall TJ, et al. Duration of cigarette smoking is the strongest predictor of severe extracranial carotid artery atherosclerosis. Stroke 1990;21:707–714.

34. Ingall TJ, Homer D, Baker HL, et al. Predictors of intracranial carotid artery atherosclerosis: duration of cigarette smoking and hypertension are more powerful than serum lipid levels. Arch Neurol 1991;48:687–691.

35. Wolf P, Kannel WB, Verter J. Current status of risk factors for stroke. In: Barnett HJM, ed. Neurologic clinics: vol 1. cerebrovascular disease. Philadelphia: Saunders, 1983:317–343.

36. Paffenbarger R, Williams J. Chronic disease in former college students: V. early precursors of fatal stroke. Am J Public Health 1967;57:1290–1299.

37. Collaborative Group for the Study of Stroke in Young Women. Oral contraceptives and stroke in young women: associated risk factors. JAMA 1975;231:718–722.

38. Ropper AH, Wechsler LR, Wilson LS. Carotid bruit and the risk of stroke in elective surgery. N Engl J Med 1982;307:1388–1390.

39. Hennerici M, Aulich A, Sandman W, et al. Incidence of asymptomatic extracranial arterial disease. Stroke 1981;12:750–758.

40. Toghi H, Yamanouchi H, Murakami M, et al. Importance of the hematocrit as a risk factor in cerebral infarction. Stroke 1978;9:369–374.

41. Harrison MJG, Pollock S, Thomas D, et al. Hematocrit, hypertension, and smoking in patients with transient ischemic attack and in age and sex matched controls. J Neurol Neurosurg Psychiatry 1982;45:550–551.

42. Harrison MJG, Pollock S, Kendall B, et al. Effect of hematocrit on carotid stenosis and cerebral infarction. Lancet 1981;2:114–115.

43. Thomas DJ, Marshall J, Ross-Russel RW, et al. Effects of hematocrit on cerebral blood flow in man. Lancet 1977;2:940–943.
44. Kannel WB. Epidemiology of cerebrovascular disease. In: Ross-Russel RW, ed. Cerebral arterial disease. New York: Churchill Livingstone, 1976:1–23.
45. Kagan A, Popper J, Rhoads G. Factors related to stroke incidence in Hawaiian Japanese men: the Honolulu heart study. Stroke 1980;11:14–21.
46. Stemmerman G, Hayashi T, Resch J, et al. Risk factors related to ischemic and hemorrhagic cerebrovascular disease at autopsy: the Honolulu heart study. Stroke 1984;15:23–28.
47. Iso H, Jacobs DR, Wentworth D, et al. Serum cholesterol levels and six year mortality from stroke in 350,977 men screened for the multiple risk factor intervention trial. N Engl J Med 1989;320:904–910.
48. Yano K, Reed DM, Maclean CJ. Serum cholesterol and hemorrhagic stroke in the Honolulu Heart Program. Stroke 1989;20:1460–1465.
49. Steinberg D, Parthasarthy S, Carcio TE, et al. Beyond cholesterol: modification of low-density lipoprotein that increases its atherogenicity. N Engl J Med 1989;320:915.
50. Scance A, Lawin RM, Berg K. Lipoprotein (a) and atherosclerosis. Ann Intern Med 1991;115:209–218.
51. Homer D, Ingall TJ, Baber HL, et al. Serum lipids and lipoproteins are less powerful predictors of extracranial carotid artery atherosclerosis than are cigarette smoking and hypertension. Mayo Clin Proc 1991;66:259–267.
52. Gorelick PB, Rodin MB, Langenberg P, et al. Is acute alcohol ingestion a risk factor for ischemic stroke? Stroke 1987;18:359–364.
53. Gorelick PB, Rodin MB, Langengerg P, et al. Weekly alcohol consumption, cigarette smoking, and the risk of ischemic stroke. Neurology 1989;39:339–343.
54. Gorelick PB. Alcohol and stroke. Stroke 1987;18:268–271.
55. Bogousslausky J, Van Melle G, Despland PA, Regli F. Alcohol consumption and carotid atherosclerosis in the Lausanne stroke registry. Stroke 1990;21:715–720.
56. Hillborn M, Kaste M. Alcohol intoxication: a risk factor for primary subarachnoid hemorrhage. Neurology 1982;32:706–711.
57. Kagan A, Yano K, Rhoads G, et al. Alcohol and cardiovascular disease: the Hawaiian experience. Circulation 1981;64(Suppl 3):27–31.
58. Collaborative Group for the Study of Stroke in Young Women. Oral contraception and increased risk of cerebral ischemia or thrombosis. N Engl J Med 1973;288:871–878.
59. Handin R. Thromboembolic complications of pregnancy and oral contraceptives. Prog Cardiovasc Dis 1974;16:395–405.
60. Layde P, Beral V, Kay C. Further analyses of mortality in oral contraceptive users. Lancet 1981;1:541–546.
61. Longstreth W, Swanson P. Oral contraceptives and stroke. Curr Concepts Cerebrovasc Dis (Stroke) 1984;19:1–6.
62. Caplan LR. Are terms such as completed stroke or RIND of continued usefulness? Stroke 1983;14:431–433.
63. Caplan LR. TIAs: we need to return to the question, 'what is wrong with Mr. Jones?' Neurology 1988;38:791–793.

64. Waxman S, Toole J. Temporal profile resembling TIA in the setting of cerebral infarction. Stroke 1983;14:433–437.
65. Nicolaides A, Zukowski A. The place of computerized tomographic brain scanning in the classification of ischemic cerebral disease. In: Courbier R, ed. Basis for a classification of cerebral arterial disease. Amsterdam: Excerpta Medica, 1985:59–64.
66. Adams HP, Kassell N, Mazuz H. The patient with transient ischemic attacks: is this the time for a new therapeutic approach? Stroke 1984;15:371–375.
67. Leonberg SC, Elliot FA. Prevention of recurrent stroke. Stroke 1981;12: 731–735.

CHAPTER 18

Complications in Stroke Patients

Sometimes, the brain injury suffered during a stroke is not the only medical problem the patient, the family, and the doctor must battle. Strokes, like many other serious medical illnesses, can be followed by a host of other problems. As some families say, "Dad was okay when he got to the hospital, then complications set in." These complications can sometimes cause neurological deterioration; in other instances, the patient feels worse, and the deterioration is falsely attributed to worsening of the stroke.

The common causes of death in patients with stroke are shown in Table 18.1. Cerebral edema, cardiac abnormalities, and pulmonary embolism dominate during the first week.[1]

Pulmonary Embolism

The true frequency of pulmonary emboli is probably unknown because many are silent. In necropsy series of patients who died during the first week following stroke, pulmonary emboli, although not always the cause of death, are frequently noted by the pathologist. In one series, pulmonary emboli were responsible for death in 12 percent of the patients who died during the first week after stroke.

I consider all patients at risk for the development of deep venous thrombosis but pay particular attention to those who are immobile. Obesity, obtundation, congestive heart failure, paralysis of one or both legs, and abulia are risk factors for phlebothrombosis. I keep some patients with acute cerebral ischemia at bed rest, in order to maximize cerebral blood flow (CBF). I mobilize all other patients as soon as possible. Physical therapy is started at the bedside. I encourage patients to flex and extend the knees and ankles throughout the day. Support hose or special inflated stockings are often used. Patients who have not had a hemorrhagic stroke and are not otherwise on

TABLE 18.1
Causes of Death in Stroke Patients with Supratentorial Lesions

	Infarction		Hemorrhage	
Cause of Death	Week 1	Weeks 2–4	Week 1	Weeks 2–4
Transtentorial herniation	36	6	42	2
Pneumonia	0	28	1	2
Cardiac	7	17	0	2
Pulmonary embolism	0	4	0	0
Sudden death	2	8	0	0
Septicemia	1	4	0	0
Unknown	0	12	1	3
Brainstem extension (of hematoma)	—	—	1	1
Totals	46	79	45	10

Reprinted with permission from Silver F, Norris JW, Lewis A, Hachinski V. Early mortality following stroke: a prospective review. Stroke 1984;15:494.

anticoagulants are given low-dose subcutaneous heparin, 5000 units ("mini" heparin) twice per day.

Patients who have sudden shortness of breath, chest pain, hypotension, hemoptysis, change in respiratory pattern, agitation, confusion, or other worsening are suspected of having a pulmonary embolism. Depending on the index of suspicion, evaluation should include arterial blood gases, chest x-ray, ECG, noninvasive studies of the venous circulation in the legs, venography, nuclear lung ventilation and perfusion scans, and pulmonary angiography.

A very recent brain hemorrhage contraindicates anticoagulation. Antifibrinolytic therapy with urokinase or streptokinase therapy is also contraindicated in the presence of a recent stroke. If the pulmonary emboli were multiple and life-threatening, the patient might require placement of a venous umbrella or other procedure to occlude the venous circulation. Unfortunately, pulmonary embolism remains a vexing problem throughout the rehabilitation process in patients who remain paretic.

Cardiac Abnormalities

Cardiac dysfunction is another frequent accompaniment of stroke. The dysfunctioning heart may be the source of stroke, may coexist with stroke, or may be caused by the stroke. Patients with both ischemic and hemorrhagic stroke have been demonstrated at necropsy to have subendocardial hemorrhages and focal regions of necrosis of cardiac muscle cells.[2,3] ECG changes consistent with ischemia, elevated creatine-phosphokinase–myoglobin (CPK–MB) levels, and various cardiac arrhythmias are found in stroke patients, even without previous heart disease.[4] In some series, one third to one half of the patients with stroke have serious rhythm disturbances, including ventricular tachycardia, salvos or couplets of premature ventricular beats, greater than 10 premature beats per minute, second- or third-degree heart block, or asystole.[5,6] In a control population matched for age and history of cardiac disease, such arrhythmias were seen in only 15 percent. Mortality, fortunately, has rarely been related to these arrhythmias.[6]

The CPK elevations, when they occur, tend to be longer lasting than those associated with primary cardiac disease, peaking at the fifth day, then persisting until the twelfth. When levels of norepinephrine, epinephrine, and dopamine are measured in patients with stroke, TIAs, and nonstroke controls, a spectrum of values is found. The highest levels are seen in stroke, the next levels in transient disorders, and normal values occur in the control population.[7] Those patients with stroke and the highest CPK values have the highest values of norepinephrine. These data suggest that stroke causes an increase in sympathetic tone, elevating levels of catecholamines, which in turn cause focal myocardial damage and subsequent arrhythmias.

Older patients with hemispheric infarction seem to be at greater risk for cardiac arrhythmias.[6] All patients need careful attention to the cardiovascular system, both clinically and by the laboratory. In addition to surveillance for symptoms, the clinician should carefully monitor vital signs, regular cardiovascular examinations, echocardiography, and routine (and, if needed, follow-up) ECGs. In some patients, continuous monitoring may be needed. Although its efficacy is unproved, propranolol or other beta-blockers are theoretically useful in patients with neurogenic cardiac arrhythmias, treating both the arrhythmia and its cause.[6] Propranolol could, however, worsen sinus bradycardia, heart block, and episodes of asystole. In experimental animals, the cardiac rhythm disturbances secondary to cerebral ischemia can be effectively treated with propranolol and atropine.[8] If rhythm disturbances occur, I treat with standard antiarrhythmics, according to the cardiology consultant's suggestions.

Cerebral Edema

The most lethal complication of stroke is cerebral edema following large ischemic and hemorrhagic strokes. In stroke units, where the first two complications (pulmonary embolism and cardiac abnormalities) can be avoided, cerebral edema represents the major cause of early death.[9] An infarct is a rapidly evolving process, whereas cerebral edema will not only vary with time but also in its nature and severity in different parts of the lesion.[10] The two main components of the edema are (1) *intracellular cytotoxic edema*, which results from damage to the sodium–potassium pump, with failure of the cell to maintain the normal osmotic gradient across its membrane; and

(2) *extracellular vasogenic edema,* with fluid occupying the interstitial spaces, especially at the edge of infarcts and hemorrhages.

Cerebral edema may begin within hours but usually does not become clinically obvious until 1 to 4 days after the stroke. Ropper and Shafran analyzed the fluctuating clinical course of patients with stroke and brain edema.[11] With the ictus, patients may be drowsy. There is subsequent improvement in the level of consciousness, and by the second or third day, patients are usually more alert. However, as brain edema increases, patients again become drowsy. In the series of Ropper and Shafran, drowsiness was not the only sign but was accompanied by one or more of the following:

1. pupillary asymmetry or lack of pupillary response to light—the larger pupil was, in most patients, on the side ipsilateral to the brain infarct; pupillary asymmetry varied from 0.5 to 2 mm
2. periodic breathing patterns
3. sixth nerve paresis
4. extensor plantar responses on the previously spared side
5. papilledema
6. headache or vomiting
7. bilateral spontaneous extensor posturing

The clinical findings clearly need not follow the typical "central" or "uncal" herniation syndrome described by Plum and Posner.[12]

CT and MRI show mass effect from the edema with compression of the lateral ventricles and shift of the midline structures. As expected, except in posterior fossa strokes, patients with the largest infarcts and most mass effect have the poorest prognosis. When intracranial pressure monitoring is performed, pressures consistently greater than 15 torr as determined by subarachnoid screw devices are usually fatal.[11] In strokes involving the cerebellum, small amounts of swelling can compress the brainstem, injure its vital structures, and cause a rapidly progressive obstructive hydrocephalus. CT may show crowding of the perimesencephalic, ambient, and cerebellopontine-angle cisterns and lack of visibility or displacement of the fourth ventricle. The typical syndrome includes headache, vertigo, nausea, vomiting, and ataxia. Drowsiness may start almost immediately but usually develops during the next 12 hours to 4 days. It is not unusual for patients with cerebellar infarction to be sent home from the emergency ward with the diagnosis of labyrinthitis, only to return in 24 to 48 hours in coma. This serious mistake can be avoided if the patient's gait is tested at the time of the initial evaluation. In the presence of increased posterior fossa pressure, suboccipital decompressive surgery or venting of CSF by a shunt can be lifesaving.[9,13–15] Some neurosurgeons are wary of ventricular drainage in posterior fossa lesions because of the risk of upward herniation of cerebellar tissue through the tentorium. For this reason, if the patient is medically able to survive the more major procedure, I favor decompressive operation with removal of necrotic cerebellar tissue.

In supratentorial lesions, the therapy for increased pressure is twofold. The first is avoidance of factors that exacerbate increased ICP and fluid retention. These include unusual head and neck positions, fever, increased central venous pressure, overhydration, hypoxia, hypercapnia, increased mean airway pressure, and agitation. Second, specific measures can be attempted to decrease pressure. Hyperventilation with reduction of the arterial carbon-dioxide tension to between 20 and 34 torr will reduce ICP during the short term, but the pressure will usually soon return to pretreatment levels. Infusion of mannitol and glycerol to maintain blood osmolality between 300 and 310 mOsm/l will also decrease pressure. This osmotic therapy is effective only when the cell endothelium and membranes are intact. Thus, it will not be effective in the area of the infarction or for cytotoxic edema but rather will help reduce the extracellular edema that surrounds infarcts.[10]

Steroids may also be tried. The effectiveness and mechanism of action of steroids in decreasing ICP is obscure. They may ameliorate the extracellular edema that surrounds the infarct (as they do in brain tumors), or in areas where the cell membrane is not severely damaged, they may protect against free-radical generation. The efficacy of steroids is in doubt, and increased risk of gastrointestinal bleeding, infections, and exacerbation of diabetes are reported when steroids are used in stroke patients.[16,17] Therefore, I rarely use steroids after ischemic infarction. In occasional patients, especially young individuals, there is very impressive edema despite a relatively small zone of infarction. In this rare situation, steroids can be very helpful. Also, in patients with brain hematomas, I use steroids and osmotic agents to reduce pressure. In patients with very large infarcts, although steroids occasionally allow survival for the short term, patients remain in very disabled states and succumb later from pneumonia or other complications; thus, I rarely use steroids in patients with massive infarcts.

Seizures

Seizures may also follow strokes. As early as 1864, Jackson recognized seizures as a complication of the recovery phase of stroke.[18] While they might not be a cause of mortality, seizures complicate the care of the patient. Preliminary unpublished data from the Stroke Data Bank indicate that seizures during the first 6 months after an ischemic stroke occur in 7 percent of patients. Other series have estimated that seizures will occur in 7.7 percent to 20 percent of patients with stroke.[19–21] In one series, 60 percent of poststroke seizures occurred during the first month after stroke. Gupta and colleagues analyzed in more detail the timing of postinfarction seizures.[22]

In their series of 70 patients with seizures after ischemic strokes, a third occurred within the first 2 weeks, and 90 percent of the 30 early seizures occurred within the first 24 hours.[22] Nearly three fourths of seizures were within the first year, and only 2 percent developed more than 2 years after stroke.

The EEG may have prognostic value.[20] Patients with periodic lateralizing epileptiform discharges are particularly likely to develop seizures. Patients who have focal spikes are also at increased risk, with 78 percent developing seizures. In patients with focal slowing, diffuse slowing, or normal EEG records, only 20 percent, 10 percent, and 5 percent, respectively, had seizures.[20] Early seizures are usually focal spells with secondary generalization. Late-onset seizures are more often generalized.[22] Patients with cortical infarcts, especially large ones, with persistent hemiplegia are most susceptible to postinfarction epilepsy.[21,22] Patients with subcortical slit hemorrhages are also prone to early seizures. Usually, poststroke seizures are readily controlled with one anticonvulsant.[22]

Metabolic and Nutritional Disorders

Fluid, electrolyte, and nutritional abnormalities may also occur during the recovery period. Joynt et al. suggested that poststroke hyponatremia is usually related to inappropriate secretion of antidiuretic hormone (ADH).[23] They demonstrated excess ADH even in the presence of normal serum sodium levels. Though the exact etiology of the inappropriate ADH secretion is unknown, Joynt et al. reviewed some of the possible mechanisms:[23] damage to the anterior hypothalamus, effects on ADH secretion related to recumbency, resetting of osmoreceptors, damage to a more widespread vasopressin neuronal system, and increased release of ADH, secondary to stroke-related elevations in serum catecholamines and cortisol. Since their report, changes in the levels of atrial natriuretic factor have also been hypothesized as a cause of abnormalities of serum sodium concentrations.

In hyponatremic patients, both volume depletion and volume overload must be excluded as contributing factors. In the assessment of this problem, it must be remembered that fluid may accumulate in the sacral regions during prolonged bed rest. If volume status is normal, the syndrome of inappropriate ADH secretion can be diagnosed if there is, in addition to hyponatremia, decreased serum osmolality, continued urinary excretion of sodium, urine that is less than maximally dilute, normal renal function, and normal thyroid function. In the acute stroke period, I carefully follow the patient's volume status by clinical examination; uniform charting of input, output, and daily weights; and monitoring of electrolytes.

Prolonged undernutrition is an important but seldom recognized complication of stroke, especially in elderly patients whose nutritional intake was poor or marginal before their stroke. To help maintain an adequate nutritional state, I give multivitamins and especially thiamine, either by mouth, if the patient is able, or parenterally. If the patient is unable to eat by the fourth or fifth day, I insert a small nasogastric feeding tube through which nutritional supplements can be given. Prolonged inability to swallow may require the more permanent placement of gastric feeding tubes.

Aspiration and Pneumonia

Dysphagia and aspiration are very common after stroke. Dysphagia is noted in 25 to 32 percent of stroke patients[24,25] and is common after both brainstem and hemispheral strokes.[24] So-called silent aspiration is also very common when the clinician looks for it. Now, videofluoroscopic studies can detect abnormalities of swallowing in nearly 50 percent of stroke patients.[26] Patients with brainstem strokes, combined cerebral and brainstem strokes, and bilateral cerebral lesions are most susceptible to aspiration. Physical therapy with guidance in positioning, choice of foods, thermal stimulation, and instructions to the patient can be very helpful in preventing aspiration. Most patients are able to resume oral feeding within months, although feeding tubes may be needed temporarily.

Pneumonia is common after stroke, in both the immediate and the late period. The true incidence of this complication is unknown. In one retrospective postmortem study of patients dying with cerebrovascular disease, pneumonia was recorded as a complication in 33 percent.[27] The cause of the pneumonia in patients with stroke, like urinary-tract infections, is probably multifactorial. In a recumbent position, there is often atelectasis and poor mobilization of secretions. Difficulty in swallowing also may lead to aspiration. Coughing and deep breathing may not be done or may be only poorly performed. Chest movements are also decreased on the hemiplegic side.[28,29] Kaldor and Berlin suggested that pneumonia is more likely on the affected side because of the decreased thoracic movements and impaired pulmonary circulation.[30] Both respiratory drive and the function of interstitial muscles are often abnormal on the hemiplegic side.[29]

It is not clear whether physiotherapy or nursing techniques help to prevent pneumonia after stroke. I encourage deep breathing, coughing, frequent turning, and early mobilization of patients. If signs of infection develop despite these measures, the lung is aggressively evaluated as the potential source. Swallowing function should be tested before putting the patient on oral feedings.

Infections, Bedsores, and Nerve Compression

Infections and bedsores are common complications in both the early and late phases of recovery from stroke. Late deaths not caused by cardiac or renal disease are usually related to infections. The urinary tract and lungs are probably the most common sites for infection.

Urinary-Tract Infections

The high frequency of urinary-tract infections is probably caused by two factors. First, an indwelling catheter is often placed to empty the urinary bladder. This foreign body allows for the introduction and growth of bacteria. Whenever possible, continuous catheter drainage should be avoided. Intermittent catheterization, using strict sterile techniques is preferable. In some male patients, condom catheters will suffice. A Foley catheter should never be used as a convenience for the staff.

Second, the functioning of the urinary bladder and the external sphincter can be altered by the stroke. Urinary symptoms are common, even in patients with uninfected bladders, and they include urinary urgency, frequency, and retention. Tsuchida et al. documented these symptoms and attempted to establish their relationship to brain lesions.[31] Patients with frontal and internal-capsular lesions showed either a hyperactive bladder or uninhibited sphincter relaxation, with subsequent urinary frequency or incontinence. Patients with putaminal lesions had hyperactive bladders, with usually normal sphincter function. Patients who had urinary retention showed an inactive or hypoactive bladder, with an uncoordinated or normal sphincter; localization of the offending lesion could not be accomplished in these patients. Male patients in the stroke age group are often geriatric and also have large prostates, which can contribute to the obstructive uropathy.

When confronted with patients with these genitourinary symptoms, I survey for and treat bacterial urinary-tract infections when present. In addition, I attempt to define other mechanisms that may be operative in causing symptoms, such as inability to reach the commode or urinal because of gait or limb abnormalities, communication difficulty that may make it hard to signal the nurse, and unavailable nursing personnel. Measurement of post-voided residual urine may be all that is needed, but at times, cystometrics and IV pyelography are required to define the problem. I encourage frequent voiding during both the day and the night, in an effort to train the bladder. If these maneuvers fail to help alleviate the problem, urinary pharmacotherapy is used.

Decubitus Ulcers

The development of bedsores is an iatrogenic and preventable complication of stroke that significantly hinders the rehabilitation process. The skin should be kept clean and dry; the patient should be turned frequently. Adequate nutrition should be given. Pressure on anesthetic or immobilized limbs must be avoided. The use of padded heel boots can spare the heels from ulcers. Egg-crate mattresses, waterbeds, or soft cotton padding may help retard the development of sacral pressure sores. Physicians and nursing personnel should periodically examine the entire skin surface, looking for any area of early breakdown. Particular attention should be paid to susceptible areas such as the sacrum, buttock, heels, elbows, wrists, between the toes, and occiput. If an ulcer develops, pressure on that area should be totally avoided, special mattresses should be used, and the wound should be dressed and—if necessary—debrided and the skin grafted.

Peripheral-Nerve Injuries

Peripheral-nerve compression is also a hazard in limbs with weakness and reduced sensation. The peroneal nerve is probably the nerve most commonly involved; its compression causes a foot drop. Ulnar palsy due to compression of the nerve at the elbow is also common, especially in wheelchair-bound patients. Subluxation of the shoulders is another complication of hemiparesis. The weak arm should not be left to hang without support.

Depression and Other "Psychological" Effects

One of the most important and yet most frequently overlooked complications of stroke is depression. Family members will often say that Mom or Dad is no longer significantly weak and is able to get around well but is not her or his usual self. New personality traits can emerge or old ones become accentuated. The patient may become inflexible, rigid, impulsive, insensitive to others; may adopt a poor perception of self; or may become guilt-ridden, paranoid, or suicidal. The family must deal with these new personality traits. If the patient is very dependent on family members for care, the main caregiver can develop feelings of entrapment, isolation, anger, and depression. In some families, it seems as if a new dependent child has been thrust upon them. Depression is reported to occur in 26 to 60 percent of stroke patients.[32-34] I do not know the frequency of emotional disorders in family members but would suspect the number is substantial. Diagnosis may often be difficult, as functional psychogenic reactions are hard to separate from organic behavioral changes related to the stroke, such as abulia, aprosodia, impersistence, and anosognosia.

Aprosodia is the inability to express or understand the meaning of phrases, which is conveyed by the aprosodic speaker's changes in the accent on syllables within words or words within sentences. For example, patients with right parasylvian strokes may be unable to communicate emotion in spoken language, and thus, an observer might erroneously believe that they are depressed. Binder has noted additional factors complicating the recognition of depression.[35] An accurate history may not be available because of aphasia or slowed responses. Vegetative signs also may be difficult to interpret. Stroke may suppress appetite, change sleep patterns, or create a pseudobulbar state, with rapid shifts from laughing to crying.

Often, sexual function in patients with stroke is ignored. For some patients, stroke may make sexual relations cumbersome and may decrease their frequency. The patient and family need to be reassured that for most mechanisms of stroke, sex is very unlikely to cause a recurrent stroke. Sexual activity should be encouraged, although it may require some creativity on the part of the participants.

Ross and Rush proposed guidelines for the diagnosis of depression.[36] Depression should be considered in patients who are not making expected recovery, are uncooperative in rehabilitation, or lose previously achieved milestones. There may be emotional outbursts, inflexibility, irritability, insensitivity to others, and suicidal ideations. A flat affect must be distinguished from a depressed affect. Collateral history from friends and caregivers is also needed.

Depression is more common after left- than after right-hemisphere strokes.[33,37–39] In the left hemisphere, the more anteriorly placed infarctions are correlated with a higher frequency of depression.[38,39] When cortical and basal-ganglia lesions, infarcts, and hemorrhages affect the left hemisphere, especially anteriorly, they are more likely to be associated with depression than similarly placed right-cerebral lesions. Six months after stroke, there is an increased prevalence of symptoms of both major and minor depressive symptoms, increasing from 23 and 20 percent, respectively, immediately following the stroke, to 35 and 26 percent at 6 months.[40,41]

Finkelstein et al. used the dexamethasone suppression test to assess patients with mood and vegetative disturbances after stroke.[34] An abnormal test is defined as failure to suppress cortisol secretion in response to exogenously administered dexamethasone. This test is reported to be abnormal in 60 to 80 percent of psychiatric patients with endogenous depression. Abnormal dexamethasone suppression tests in patients with stroke were associated with occurrence of moderate to severe mood, sleep, and appetite disturbances.[34]

The etiology of the late depressive reaction is unknown. Whether it is a reaction to the loss the patient feels or a result of brain injury is unclear. Injury may result in depletion of noradrenergic neurotransmitters, resulting in depression. Nortriptyline has been reported to ameliorate significantly the symptoms of depression in patients with stroke.[42] I have had anecdotal experience with the use of antidepressants in this population and have enjoyed some success.

Beyond pharmacological therapy, the clinician should try to adopt a hopeful and fighting attitude. I encourage activity and independence for both the family and the patient. Attempt to promote continued affection, understanding, and respect between the family and the patient. Reassure all involved that efforts are intended to maximize rehabilitation and prevent recurrent stroke. Promote the patient's self-confidence and emphasize the old adage, "When the going gets tough, the tough get going!"

References

1. Ng L, Nimmannitya J. Massive cerebral infarction with severe brain swelling. Stroke 1970;1:158–162.
2. Norris JW, Kolin A, Hachinski VC. Focal myocardial lesions in stroke. Stroke 1980;11:130.
3. Connor RC. Focal myocytolysis and fuchsinophilic degeneration of the myocardium of patients dying with various brain lesions. Ann NY Acad Sci 1969; 156:261–270.
4. Dimant J, Grob D. Electrocardiographic changes in patients with acute cerebrovascular accidents. Stroke 1977;8:448–455.
5. Myers MG, Norris JW, Hachinski VC, et al. Cardiac sequelae of acute stroke. Stroke 1982;13:838–842.
6. Mikolich JR, Jacobs WC, Fletcher GF. Cardiac arrhythmias in patients with acute cerebrovascular accidents. JAMA 1981;246:1314–1317.
7. Myers MS, Norris JW, Hachinski VC, et al. Plasma norepinephrine in stroke. Stroke 1981;12:200–204.
8. Weidler DJ, Das SK, Sodeman TM. Cardiac arrhythmias secondary to acute cerebral ischemia: prevention by autonomic blockade. Circulation 1976; 53(Suppl 2):102.
9. White DB, Norris JW, Hachinski VC, et al. Death in early stroke: causes and mechanisms. Stroke 1979;10:743.
10. O'Brien MD. Ischemic cerebral edema: a review. Stroke 1979;10:623–628.
11. Ropper AH, Shafran B. Brain edema after stroke. Arch Neurol 1984;41:26–29.
12. Plum F, Posner JB. Diagnosis of stupor and coma. 3rd ed. Philadelphia: Davis, 1980.
13. Taneda M, Ozaki K, Wakayama A, et al. Cerebellar infarction with obstructive hydrocephalus. J Neurosurg 1982;57:83–91.
14. Wood MW, Murphy F. Obstructive hydrocephalus due to infarction of a cerebellar hemisphere. Neurosurg 1969;30:260–263.
15. Greenberg J, Skubick D, Shenkin H. Acute hydrocephalus in cerebellar infarct and hemorrhage. Neurology 1979;29:409–413.
16. Norris JW. Steroid therapy in acute cerebral infarction. Arch Neurol 1976; 33:69–71.
17. Ottonello GA, Primavera A. Gastrointestinal complications of high dose corticosteroid therapy in acute cerebrovascular patients. Stroke 1979;10:208–210.
18. Taylor J. Selected writings of John Hughlings Jackson on epilepsy and epileptiform convulsions: vol. 1. London: Hodder & Stoughton, 1931:230–235.
19. Louis S, McDowell F. Epileptic seizures in nonembolic cerebral infarction. Arch Neurol 1967;17:414–418.
20. Holmes GL. The electroencephalogram as a predictor of seizures following cerebral infarction. Clin Electroencephalogr 1980;11:83–86.
21. Olsen TS, Hogenhaven H, Thage O. Epilepsy after stroke. Neurology 1987;37:1209–1211.
22. Gupta SR, Naheedey MH, Elias D, Rubino F. Postinfarction seizures: a clinical study. Stroke 1988;19:1477–1481.
23. Joynt RJ, Feibel JH, Sladek CM. Antidiuretic hormone levels in stroke patients. Ann Neurol 1981;9:182–184.

24. Horner J, Massey EW. Silent aspiration following stroke. Neurology 1988; 38:317–319.

25. Groher ME, Bukatman R. The prevalence of swallowing disorders in two teaching hospitals. Dysphagia 1986;1:3–6.

26. Horner J, Massey EW, Risler JE, et al. Aspiration following stroke: clinical correlates and outcome. Neurology 1988;38:1359–1362.

27. Mulley GP. Pneumonia, stroke, and laterality. Lancet 1981;1:1051.

28. Fluck DC. Chest movements in hemiplegia. Clin Sci 1966;31:383–388.

29. Przedborski S, Brunko E, Hubert M, et al. The effect of acute hemiplegia on intercostal muscle activity. Neurology 1988;38:1882–1884.

30. Kaldor A, Berlin I. Pneumonia, stroke, and laterality. Lancet 1981;1:843.

31. Tsuchida S, Noto H, Yamaguchi D, et al. Urodynamic studies on hemiplegia patients after cerebrovascular accident. Urology 1983;21:315–318.

32. Feibel JH, Springer CJ. Depression and failure to resume social activities after stroke. Arch Phys Med 1982;63:276–277.

33. Robinson RG, Szetela B. Mood change following left hemisphere brain injury. Ann Neurol 1981;9:447–453.

34. Finkelstein S, Benowitz LI, Baldessarini RJ, et al. Mood, vegetative disturbances, and dexamethasone suppression test after stroke. Ann Neurol 1982; 12:463–468.

35. Binder LM. Emotional problems after stroke. Stroke 1984;15:174–177.

36. Ross ED, Rush AJ. Diagnosis and neuroanatomical correlates of depression in brain-damaged patients. Arch Gen Psychiatry 1981;38:1344–1354.

37. Robinson RG, Starr LB, Kubos K, et al. A two-year longitudinal study of poststroke mood disorders: findings during the initial evaluation. Stroke 1983; 14:736–741.

38. Robinson RG, Kubos KL, Starr LB, et al. Mood disorders in stroke patients: importance of location of lesion. Brian 1984;107:81–93.

39. Robinson RG, Kubos KL, Starr LB, et al. Mood changes in stroke patients: relationship to lesion location. Compr Psychiatry 1983;24:555–566.

40. Robinson RG, Price TR. Poststroke depressive disorders: a follow-up study of 103 patients. Stroke 1982;13:635–641.

41. Robinson RG, Starr LB, Price TR. A two-year longitudinal study of mood disorders following stroke. Br J Psychiatry 1984;144:256–262.

42. Lipsey JR, Robinson RG, Pearlson GD, et al. Nortriptyline treatment of poststroke depression: a double-blind study. Lancet 1984;1:297–300.

CHAPTER 19

Rehabilitation

Rehabilitation services are quite different from most traditional medical and surgical units, and therefore, rehabilitation is an unfamiliar process to many physicians. Rehabilitation has a different goal and emphasis than that of traditional medicine: adaptation to a functional handicap. In contrast, the usual goal of traditional medical care is to prevent and treat disease, a pathological and pathophysiological emphasis. Rehabilitation is usually performed in buildings or units separated from acute-care hospital facilities. Personnel include a much higher ratio of nonphysician-to-physician staff members. Although the physician usually captains the team, the role of other paramedical personnel is more important than in most acute-care units. Rehabilitation units have a slower pace, longer patient stays, and at times, different reimbursement rules for third-party payers.

Rehabilitation encourages and relies very heavily on family involvement and on the education of patient and family. It employs a lot of gadgetry—braces, walking aids, parallel bars—foreign to most medical units. Parts of rehabilitation units look more like gyms, exercise areas, workshops, or schools than like standard medical facilities.

Because of this perceived strangeness, many physicians are reluctant to refer their patients to rehabilitation facilities, and many patients who should have rehabilitation do not receive it. I feel strongly that rehabilitation is very important and is underutilized. In some patients, it can make the difference between a vegetative, bedridden existence at home or in an institution and active reentry into a productive life. Immobile patients discharged directly home or to nursing homes and not mobilized during the first months are very unlikely to become more active later. A bed or bed-and-chair existence is physically and psychologically destructive. If the same immobile patients are trained in rehabilitation units and if they can be trained to sit and walk, the probability is very high that they can remain self-reliant and can improve. Time is of the essence; training must occur in the weeks after the stroke, or it probably will never occur. The major recovery from stroke takes place during the first 3 to 6 months, and only small numbers improve during the next 18 months.[1,2]

Patient Selection

Although rehabilitation is very important, not all stroke patients will benefit. If every stroke patient were referred, rehabilitation facilities would be swamped, and the cost to taxpayers would greatly increase, while effective retraining for those who could benefit most would suffer from dilution. Selection of appropriate patients is important. Patients who are already ambulatory and who have only slight or temporary deficits do not need a stay in a rehabilitation unit; they will do well on their own or with outpatient care. At the other end of the spectrum, the patient who is stuporous, completely immobile, or has severe right-hemisphere dysfunction also will not be helped by rehabilitation. Most observers agree that the middle group between these two extremes is the appropriate target for rehabilitative care. How should this group be identified? What factors should be considered in making the triage decision?

Patients of all ages can be offered rehabilitation. By decade, no difference in outcome has been shown; substantial recovery is noted in all age groups.[3,4] Those patients who have serious cognitive impairment or severe underlying medical illness may be unable to participate in effective rehabilitation programs; these patients will be either unable to learn compensatory techniques or unable to tolerate the physical activity required. Aphasia, however, does not preclude stroke rehabilitation; when outcome is measured by performance of activities of daily living, ability to walk, and discharge disposition, no difference is found between aphasic and nonaphasic patients referred for rehabilitation.[4-6] Higher cortical function abnormalities other than aphasia—such as anosognosia, neglect, impersistence, reduplicative paramnesia, prosopagnosia, and extinction—may make rehabilitation more difficult but not impossible. These cognitive abnormalities tend to improve with time, allowing the stroke rehabilitation process to proceed.[7]

Neurological findings such as limb paralysis are prognostically important,[8] but neurological disability and accompanying medical illness are not the only factors that predict outcome. A host of nonmedical social, psychological, and environmental factors are of equal or even greater importance. Two of the most accurate prognostic predictors in patients with head trauma are (1) the presence of a "significant other" person to help the patient, and (2) whether the patient had a job prior to the injury.

Similarly, in stroke patients, a number of seemingly mundane factors apply: What was the patient's prestroke level of capability? Does the patient have financial support to help with special equipment, transportation, and so forth? Does the patient have a car or ready access to other transportation? Is there someone at home who is motivated, capable, and available to help the patient and to encourage him or her to regain former activity?[9] How is the home set up? With stairs? With a bathroom on each floor? Is "Meals on Wheels" or a store that delivers and takes phone orders accessible to the patient? What community services are available? All these prognostic factors and many others must be considered in order to offer rehabilitation to those who will benefit most. I feel that when the prognosis is very uncertain, the patient should be given the benefit of the doubt, and a trial period of rehabilitation should be offered.

Coordination of Acute and Long-Term Care

Rehabilitation, to be optimally successful, should be fully integrated with traditional medical care. Therapy should begin as early as possible, while the patient is still on the acute medical or neurological unit. Physicians, nurses, and other ward personnel must be involved. Therapy should not be completely delegated to the 30 minutes or so each day spent with therapists. Passive and active range-of-motion exercises and other physical therapy should be encouraged by the ward personnel. If the patient goes to a rehabilitation unit, whenever possible, the acute-care team should continue to follow the patient while there and afterward. Acute medical problems do not suddenly disappear when the patient is transferred. Subsequent strokes and medical complications are common among recuperating patients.

Also, the patient receives mixed signals if treatment and advice begun on the acute service are not followed. The patient may have been impressed by a doctor about the need for a low-salt, low-cholesterol diet, only to be served butter, cream, and eggs on the rehabilitation unit. Medical treatment and surveillance should be continued during rehabilitation and afterward. Similarly, when the patient leaves the rehabilitation unit, the physician must continue to emphasize the need to use and follow through with various rehabilitation techniques. Rehabilitation and traditional medical care need to be intertwined and overlapped, not seen by the patient as unrelated phases, one succeeding the other.

The Rehabilitation Team

The general theme of stroke rehabilitation is a disability-oriented, multidisciplinary team approach. Team members include the patient, the patient's family, the primary physician, neurologist, physical therapist, occupational therapist, speech therapist, social worker, and rehabilitation nurse. Members of the team should meet regularly to identify specific rehabilitation goals, strategies for their attainment, and methods of implementation. These team members educate and train patients and family members in their areas of expertise. Start the team rehabilitation process early in the course of treating the illness, so that the routine of working for improvement in quality of life can be established.

The formal multidisciplinary approach has clearly been shown to improve outcome.[10,11] When a formal rehabilitation program is followed, 82 percent of the patients can be cared for at home, 69 percent will be capable of self-care, and 54 percent will retain a vocation. Without a formal rehabilitation program, only 56 percent will return home, 47 percent will be independent in self-care, and 42 percent will be gainfully employed.[10,11]

Each team member plays an important role. The *physical therapist's* main function is training for ambulation. Balancing, weight-shifting techniques, parallel bars, braces, and quad canes are all employed. Severe weakness in a lower extremity does not preclude ambulation. Often, patients will be unable to lift the leg from the bed yet will become ambulatory. Increased extensor tone, combined with minimal bracing, will permit walking. Even before ambulation training begins, physical therapists perform range-of-motion, strengthening, and endurance exercises. In addition, physical therapists can help provide appropriate supporting apparatus, such as lap boards, chair arm supports, and swings. Range-of-motion exercises are both passive and active and should be performed at least four times daily. Patients can use the normal arm to passively move the paralyzed extremity through a full range of motion. These exercises help prevent deconditioning, excessive spasticity, joint contractures, and peripheral edema. Range-of-motion exercises combined with upper extremity support are the keys to preventing a painful shoulder, caused by subluxation or spasticity. Both the family and the nursing staff should take active roles, using the recommendations of the physical therapist, for remobilization throughout the day.

Occupational therapists perform upper-extremity retraining, with particular attention on teaching practical activities of daily living. Patient and therapists work on improving fine-motor skills, so that activities such as feeding, dressing, personal hygiene, and cooking can be accomplished. These skills allow the development of independent function. Often, special devices such as a reacher, utensil holder, specially placed rails or handles, commodes, tub benches, or hand-held showers are used. If possible, a home visit by the occupational therapist will allow customization of these techniques and physical changes in the home, which adapt to the patient's deficits.

Speech therapists work to improve communication skills. Early in the patient's rehabilitation, the goal is to facilitate communication. The methods may be verbal or nonverbal, using spoken or written words, gestures, or word boards. The boards may contain letters that the patients point to in order to spell words, or may contain words or pictures that the patients use to designate their needs or wishes. Often, for a severely aphasic patient, therapists can develop techniques of nonverbal communication among patients, family, and staff, so that patients' needs can be met and the feeling of isolation eliminated. During the first 3 months after a stroke, much spontaneous language recovery occurs. Beyond 3 months, the therapist's role is to enhance further recovery of language function. Do not accept a nihilistic attitude toward speech therapy. Start all aphasic patients early on a comprehensive program of speech therapy. Continue to pursue a vigorous course of treatment in most patients, withholding it only in those who are demented or severely globally aphasic. Speech therapists also provide help in the evaluation and treatment of dysarthria and dysphagia, breath control, and articulation, and they can often suggest types of foods and liquids and eating techniques that might be best tolerated by patients.

The two members of the team who must coordinate all rehabilitation efforts are the family and the *rehabilitation nurse*. This nurse must adopt an attitude unusual in the nursing profession. A nurse is usually the provider of direct care, but on a rehabilitation unit, the nurse must sit back and let the patient accomplish tasks at hand, providing teaching, encouragement, and help, as needed. Extreme patience is required. Nurses must synthesize all the recommendations of the other team members and must directly apply these ideas in the everyday care of patients.

Next to the patient, the *family* has the most difficult task. Usually medically unsophisticated, they must learn new skills from all the team members and must directly supervise the care of the impaired family member. The family's questions and concerns should be carefully addressed by each team member. It is often useful for the family member who will be most directly involved in home care to spend a few days at the hospital, directly caring for the patient, so that necessary skills can be acquired effectively. Once patients return home, continued contact with the team is crucial so that progress can be monitored, new problems identified, and solutions implemented. This contact may be in the form of visits to the home or appointments at the medical center with individual team members.

Perhaps most important is the spirit and milieu of the unit. An optimistic, forward look must be accompanied by empathy and acknowledgment of how difficult the task may be for the patient. Planning should be practical and goals realistic.

The Pitfall of Exaggerated Emphasis on Physical Therapy

I have been impressed with the frequency after discharge of a phenomenon that I have referred to as the "hyper-PT [physical therapy] syndrome," in which patients strive to improve hand, arm, or limb function, to exercise actively, and to return to normal. Instead of expending energy on readapting to their former life-style, which probably does not require absolutely normal function, they continue to exercise and focus attention on their limb dysfunction. These patients exchange a practical, reachable goal—that is, a return to all their prior activities—for an impractical, unreachable, and unimportant goal—a return to premorbid strength. Many patients also attribute their recovery to the PT and are fearful of stopping or decreasing it. Much of their energies and time are taken up in going to and from therapy, doing therapy at home, and resting after therapy is over. They have little time and energy left during which to live. Patients should be gradually weaned from PT at the appropriate time and should be encouraged to adapt to their deficit and to turn their attention away from their limb impairment and toward their enjoyment of life.

Loss of self-image and oversensitivity to minor disabilities are other common problems. Sometimes, exposure to others who have regained full prestroke activities despite unresolved neurological deficits is of great help to patients.

References

1. Andrew K, Brocklehurst JC, Richard B, et al. The rate of recovery from stroke and its measurement. Rehab Med 1981;3:155–161.
2. Katz S, Ford AB, Chinn AB, et al. Prognosis after stroke: II. long-term course of 159 patients. Medicine 1966;45:236–246.
3. Feigenson JS. Neurological rehabilitation. In: Baker AB, ed. Clinical neurology. New York: Harper & Row, 1983:1–66.
4. Feigenson JS, McDowell FH, Meese P, et al. Factors influencing outcome and length of stay in a stroke rehabilitation unit: I. analysis of 248 unscreened patients—medical and function prognostic indication. Stroke 1977;8:651–656.
5. Feigenson JS, McCarthy ML, Greenberg SD, et al. Factors influencing outcome and length of stay in a stroke rehabilitation unit: II. comparison of 318 screened and 248 unscreened patients. Stroke 1977;8:657–662.
6. Feigenson JS, McCarthy ML, Meese P, et al. Stroke rehabilitation: factors predicting outcome and length of stay—an overview. NY State J Med 1977;77:1426–1430.
7. Hier DB, Mondlock J, Caplan LR. Recovery of behavioral abnormalities after right hemisphere stroke. Neurology 1983;33:345–350.
8. Prescott RJ, Garraway WM, Akhtar AJ. Predicting functional outcome following acute stroke using a standard clinical examination. Stroke 1982;13:641–647.
9. DeJong G, Branch LG. Predicting the stroke patient's ability to live independently. Stroke 1982;13:648–655.
10. Anderson TP, McClure G, Athelstan G, et al. Stroke rehabilitation: evaluation of its quality by assessing patient outcomes. Arch Phys Med Rehabil 1978;59:170–175.
11. Anderson TP, Baldridge M, Ettinger MG. Quality of care for completed stroke without rehabilitation: evaluation by assessing patient outcome. Arch Phys Med Rehabil 1979;60:103–107.

Index